Treatment of Primary Glomerulonephritis

SECOND EDITION

Edited by

Claudio Ponticelli

Senior Consultant
Division of Nephrology
Scientific Institute Humanitas
Milano, Italy

and

Richard J. Glassock

Emeritus Professor
The David Geffen School of Medicine
UCLA
Los Angeles, CA, USA

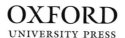

OXFORD
UNIVERSITY PRESS

OXFORD

UNIVERSITY PRESS

Great Clarendon Street, Oxford OX2 6DP

Oxford University Press is a department of the University of Oxford.
It furthers the University's objective of excellence in research, scholarship,
and education by publishing worldwide in

Oxford New York

Auckland Cape Town Dar es Salaam Hong Kong Karachi
Kuala Lumpur Madrid Melbourne Mexico City Nairobi
New Delhi Shanghai Taipei Toronto

With offices in

Argentina Austria Brazil Chile Czech Republic France Greece
Guatemala Hungary Italy Japan Poland Portugal Singapore
South Korea Switzerland Thailand Turkey Ukraine Vietnam

Oxford is a registered trade mark of Oxford University Press
in the UK and in certain other countries

Published in the United States
by Oxford University Press Inc., New York

British Library Cataloguing in Publication Data
Data available

Library of Congress Cataloging-in-Publication Data
Data available

Typeset by Cepha Imaging Private Ltd., Bangalore, India
Printed in Great Britain
on acid-free paper by
CPI Antony Rowe, Chippenham, Wiltshire

ISBN 978–0–19–955288–7

10 9 8 7 6 5 4 3 2 1

Preface

It has been a dozen years since the first edition of *Treatment of Primary Glomerulonephritis* was published. In this period progress in this field has been noteworthy. However, the treatment of glomerulonephritis remains a difficult and demanding task. A number of agents are currently available that are designed to optimize the benefits of both symptomatic and specific therapy. Use of these drugs in individual patients requires expertise in diagnosis, knowledge of actions and adverse consequences of each of the agents, and careful monitoring of the response of the patient to treatment. Paradoxically, the treatment of glomerulonephritis has become even more complicated in recent years, largely due to the introduction of a number of newer immunosuppressive drugs.

This book reviews the state-of-the-art in the treatment of primary glomerular diseases. It is comprehensive yet concise and contains not only an evidence-based review of the topic but also practical recommendations from experts in the field. The co-editors of the book have each made a contribution to all chapters in the book, thus encouraging a degree of uniformity of approach to the topic. Information to guide the day-to-day management of individual patients with primary glomerular disease can be easily accessed in this compact volume. A number of tables summarize the most important clinical aspects of any single disease in the various chapters. An Atlas of the pathology of primary glomerular disease is also supplied in the book.

The monograph is divided into eleven chapters the first three chapters are devoted respectively to symptomatic therapy, pharmacology of glucocorticoids and immuno-modulating agents, and evaluation of observational and controlled clinical trials. Each of the other chapters deals with a single primary glomerulonephritis with the exception of the last chapter which covers the less common types of primary glomerular disease.The chapters dealing with the single diseases follow a similar format that includes: an overview of the disease (definition, pathology, pathogenesis, aetiology, clinical presentation, epidemiology): the natural history and factors that may influence the outcome; specific treatment (with emphasis to the studies supported by randomized clinical trials); and practical recommendations. A final sub-chapter is devoted to the management of de-novo and recurrent glomerular diseases after kidney transplantation.

It is always a very difficult task to choose among the many important contributions to the literature when prefacing a monograph on such a broad topic. The authors and editors have tried to select an appropriate mix of citations to guide the reader in additional investigations of specific subjects but it has not been possible to cite all the relevant articles. Apologies are due to those authors whose work we have overlooked or failed to cite.

Our goal was to provide practical information organized in an easy to read manner. We hope that we have succeeded.

Special thanks to our co-authors for their excellent and enthusiastic collaboration and to doctors Banfi and Cohen for the beautiful illustrations that complement the text.

CP, Milan

RJG, Laguna Niguel

2008

Dedications

To my beloved wife, Titti.
– Claudio Ponticelli, M.D.

To my son Mark, for being a constant source of inspiration.
– Richard J. Glassock, M.D., M.A.C.P.

Contents

Contributors

Giovanni Banfi
Divisione Nefrologia Ospedale
Maggiore Policlinico Mangiagalli e
Regina Elena
Milano, Italy

Daniel Cattran
Toronto General Hospital
ON, Canada

Arthur H. Cohen
Department of Pathology
Cedars-Sinai Medical Center and
UCLA School of Medicine
Los Angeles, CA, USA

Rosanna Coppo
Director of Nephrology
Dialysis and Transplantation Unit
Regina Margherita Children's
Hospital
Torino, Italy

Richard J. Glassock
Emeritus Professor
The David Geffen School of
Medicine, UCLA
Los Angeles, CA, USA

Grace Lee
Grace Lee Renal and Medical Clinic
Singapore

Gabriella Moroni
Divisione Nefrologia Ospedale
Maggiore Policlinico Mangiagalli e
Regina Elena
Milano, Italy

Patrick Nachman
University of North Carolina
Chapel Hill, USA

Patrzia Passerini
Divisione Nefrologia Ospedale
Maggiore Policlinico Mangiagalli e
Regina Elena
Milano, Italy

Claudio Ponticelli
Senior Consultant
Division of Nephrology
Scientific Institute Humanitas
Milano, Italy

Francesco Scolari
Divisione di Nefrologia Ospedale di
Montichiari
Brescia, Italy

Chapter 1

Symptomatic therapy

Richard J. Glassock

Introduction and overview

Patients with glomerular diseases develop a wide variety of biochemical disturbances and pathophysiologic alterations leading to overt clinical manifestations (Remuzzi, 1993; Glassock et al., 1995, Remuzzi and Bertani, 1998; Schrier and Fassett, 1998; Vaziri, 2003; Floege and Feehally, 2007; Kim et al., 2007; Haraldsson et al., 2008). These occur as a direct result of injury to the capillary wall and disturbances in normal glomerular function, including loss of filtration capacity and excessive transfer of erythrocytes and/or plasma proteins from blood to tubular lumina eventuating in hematuria and/or proteinuria. Proteinuria—which is believed to be the consequence of disturbed glomerular capillary wall permselectivity (Haraldsson et al., 2008)—when substantial, can lead to hypoproteinemia and thereby to a reduction in plasma oncotic pressure. Changes in the synthesis, turnover, and plasma concentration of various proteins and lipids develop and can lead to an imbalance of pro-thrombotic and anti-thrombotic factors promoting a 'thrombophilic' state (Vaziri, 2003; Crew et al., 2004; Glassock, 2007) Disturbances in the renal handling of sodium chloride (NaCl) and water are often associated with edema formation and/ or hypertension (Perico and Remuzzi, 1993; Schrier and Fassett, 1998). Finally, the rapid or slow loss of the glomerular filtration capacity (glomerular filtration rate, GFR) due to damage of single nephrons (perhaps mediated by filtered proteins and their reabsorption) as well as by the 'drop out' of functioning nephrons from the overall population of nephrons in the two kidneys is responsible for ultimate progression to end-stage renal disease (ESRD) in many, but not all, of the primary glomerular disorders (Drummond et al., 1994; Remuzzi and Bertani, 1998; Squarer, et al., 1998; Floege and Feehally, 2007).

Collectively these abnormalities give rise to 'syndromes' of glomerular disease. These 'syndromes' can be arbitrarily, but usefully, grouped into five categories which may overlap to some degree; namely, the *acute nephritic syndrome*, *rapidly progressive glomerulonephritis, the nephrotic syndrome, 'symptomless'*

Table 1.1 Symptomatic therapy of nephrotic syndrome

Edema
Hypertension
Hyperlipidemia
'Hypercoagulable state'
Hypoproteinemia/proteinuria
Progressive renal failure
Trace metal deficiencies
Endocrine disturbances
Infectious/immunodeficiency states

Reproduced with permission from Ponticelli C and Glassock RJ (eds) (1997). *Treatment of Primary Glomerulonephritis.* Oxford University Press, Oxford.

haematuria and/or proteinuria, and slowly progressive 'chronic' nephritis (Glassock et al., 1995). The cardinal features of these syndromes and the diseases to which they are most closely associated are discussed in this monograph. This monograph will deal largely with those glomerular diseases which *primarily* affect the kidneys and in which the extra-renal manifestations are the consequence of the impairment or disturbance of kidney function itself (the so-called *primary glomerular diseases*).

The clinical abnormalities resulting from these disturbances in pathophysiology require management in order to minimize or avoid disabling symptoms, often referred to as *symptomatic therapy*, in order to distinguish the measures employed from those which are used in an attempt to ameliorate the specific underlying disease detailed in the chapters which follow, under the heading of 'Specific therapy.' Several aspects of *symptomatic therapy* will be discussed here (see also Table 1.1), namely:

- ◆ Management of edema arising from altered NaCl and fluid handling by the diseased kidney and the associated disturbances in the Starling forces operating within the peripheral capillaries.

- ◆ Treatment of hypertension developing because of extracellular and intravascular fluid volume expansion and vasoconstriction, possibly related incomplete suppression of the renin–angiotensin system, and other factors (such as reduced vasodilatory capacity and/or reduced vascular compliance).

- ◆ Therapy of hyperlipidemia and the tendency for accelerated atherogenesis;

- ◆ Management of the 'hypercoagulable' or 'thrombophilic' state accompanying hypoproteinemic forms of glomerulonephritis.

◆ Non-disease-specific treatment of hypoproteinemia and proteinuria, including protein-deficiency states.

◆ Non-disease-specific strategies designed to retard the progression of renal disease (loss of GFR) and prevention of the inexorable development of ESRD.

◆ Management of other disturbances, including trace metal deficiencies, endocrine perturbations, immunodeficiency states, and enhanced risk of infection (usually bacterial in origin) occurring in the absence of the use of immunosuppressant agents for 'specific therapy.'

The extent to which each of these 'symptomatic' management principles can be successfully applied to specific glomerular diseases and to individual patients will vary depending upon the extent and magnitude of the underlying biochemical or pathophysiologic disturbances and their interactions with each other.

Edema

Clinical features, pathogenesis, and pathophysiology

Edema is common in glomerular disease, especially in those accompanied by marked proteinuria (nephrotic syndrome) (Glassock, 1980, 1997; Schrier and Fassett, 1998; Vande Walle and Donckerwolcke, 2001; Kim et al., 2007). The acute nephritic syndrome may also be associated with edema, even when hypoproteinemia is absent or mild, but it is usually less severe than that seen in nephrotic states. Edema in glomerular disease usually first accumulates about the peri-orbital areas (where the interstitial pressure is low) and in dependent sites (ankle, feet, and pre-sacral areas). Pericardial effusions are very rare but pleural effusions and ascites may develop if the disease is severe and prolonged.

In glomerular disease (acute nephritis and the nephrotic syndrome), the occurrence of edema is usually related to hypoproteinemia and/or augmented primary NaCl resorption at distal nephron (collecting duct) sites, conditioned by abnormalities of the Starling forces in the peripheral capillaries governing interstitial fluid formation and its re-uptake. Complicating congestive heart failure, advanced liver disease, pericardial effusions, or obstructions to venous/lymphatic disease may be a concomitant cause of edema in some patients. Except in oliguric patients or those with markedly impaired renal function, reduced NaCl excretion is not usually the consequence of reduced delivery to tubular reabsorptive sites because of impaired GFR per se.

The pathogenesis of edema in glomerular disease in the absence of ESRD or severe acute renal failure is not fully understood (see Fig. 1.1), but considerable progress has been made in unraveling the complex processes underlying edema formation in both the nephrotic syndrome and in acute nephritis (Perico and Remuzzi 1993; Lee and Humphreys, 1996; Schrier and Fassett, 1998; Deschenes et al., 2001; Donckerwolcke et al., 2003; Kim et al., 2006; de Seigneux et al., 2006; Doucet et al., 2007).

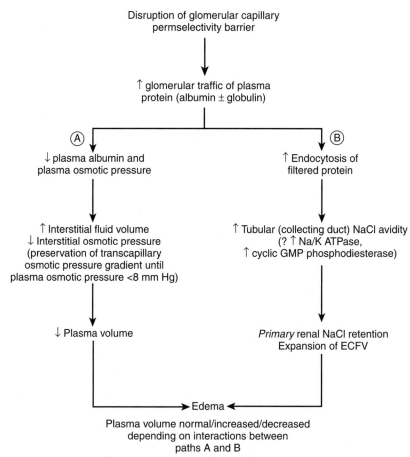

Fig. 1.1 Pathophysiology of oedema formation in nephrotic syndrome. Reproduced with permission from Ponticelli C and Glassock RJ (eds) (1997). *Treatment of Primary Glomerulonephritis.* Oxford University Press, Oxford.

Two quite distinct pathophysiologic processes appear to be involved:

- Disruption of the Starling equilibrium at the peripheral capillary level, particularly alterations in the factors governing the permeability of peripheral capillaries participating in the transfer of fluid from the vascular to the interstitial compartment (Joles et al., 1993; Joles and Koomans, 2001). In the nephrotic syndrome these abnormalities contribute to the redistribution of retained NaCl and water from the vascular to the interstitial compartments. If such transfers did not occur the degree of primary NaCl retention seen in nephrotic syndrome would quickly lead to marked intravascular volume expansion and severe hypertension. Primary renal NaCl retention *without* an accompanying marked transfer of the retained fluid to the interstitial space appears to be involved in the development of volume-dependent hypertension observed in the acute nephritic syndrome

- Marked primary renal NaCl retention occurring at distal (collecting duct) sites (Perico and Remuzzi 1993; Schrier and Fassett, 1998; Doucet et al., 2007) is the proximate cause of the retention of fluid in both nephritic and nephrotic states. Circulating hormones (e.g., aldosterone) play little role in the initiation of the salt-retaining state in these disorders.

While a decrease in plasma osmotic pressure (π) due to hypoalbuminemia should result in a major displacement of intravascular fluid into the interstitial compartment, this generally does not occur unless the plasma π value falls well below 8 mmHg or 1 kPa (normal about 25 mmHg or 3.3 kPa) because of a corresponding fall in interstitial osmotic pressure, thus maintaining the transcapillary osmotic gradient (Joles et al., 1993; Joles and Koomans, 2001). However, a very *acute* decline in plasma π value, such as might occur in rapidly developing nephrotic syndrome, may not be accompanied by a corresponding rapid decline in the interstitial π value, so a major displacement of fluid from the vascular compartment into the interstitial compartment may occur, leading to profound hypovolemia. In more slowly developing conditions, edema with expansion of the total extracellular volume occurs even when plasma π is only modestly reduced, thus factors in addition to the transcapillary osmotic gradient must be involved in edema formation (Joles et al., 1993; Dorhout Mees and Koomans, 1990; Joles and Koomans, 2001). In the nephrotic syndrome the peripheral capillaries increase the transfer of fluid from the intercapillary space to the interstitial space, irrespective of the fundamental disease casing the abnormal glomerular permeability. Thus, the accumulation of retained fluid in the interstitial space (edema) is the consequence of disturbed Starling forces in the peripheral capillary, but not usually due to the decrease in serum proteins (chiefly albumin) and thereby the plasma oncotic pressure (Joles and Koomans, 2001). This accounts for the variability in the severity of edema in patients with the nephrotic syndrome, independent of the plasma albumin concentration and the π of the circulating fluids.

As a result, it is very clear that edematous patients with hypoproteinemia (hypoalbuminemia) due to glomerular disease may have normal, expanded, or decreased intravascular volume (Joles et al., 1993; Joles and Koomans, 2001). The 'underfilling' theory of renal NaCl retention in the nephrotic syndrome has been largely discarded, except in unusual circumstances. Those patients with clearly and unequivocally reduced intravascular volume constitute the minority of patients with nephrotic syndrome. Such patients typically have relatively *rapid* development of edema and minimal glomerular structural abnormalities of glomeruli. Expansion of extracellular volume combined with normal or even increased intravascular volume in many patients with nephrotic syndrome points to an important contribution of primary renal processes in NaCl and fluid retention in the edema of nephrotic syndrome (Joles, 1993; Perico and Remuzzi, 1993; Doucet et al., 2007). On the other hand, the hypothesis that the great majority of subjects with the nephrotic syndrome have an 'overfilled' vascular volume (due to primary renal NaCl retention) can be criticized (Schrier and Fassett, 1998). These critiques have clinical implications as to how aggressively edema is treated with diuretics. Subjects with 'underfilling' of the intravascular volume in nephrotic syndrome may be very susceptible to decrements in arterial blood pressure or GFR with overly aggressive diuretic treatment of edema.

Strong experimental evidence suggests that primary renal retention of NaCl is caused by intrarenal disturbances rather than by circulating hormonal factors or neural effects (Ichikawa et al., 1983; Doucet et al., 2007). Excess plasma renin activity or elevated circulating aldosterone levels, deficient atrial natriuretic factor production, or activation of the sympathetic nervous system do not fully account for the disturbances in NaCl handling by the kidney observed in nephrotic syndrome (Perico and Remuzzi, 1993; Doucet et al., 2007). Furthermore, renal NaCl retention is related more to the onset and magnitude of proteinuria than the status of intravascular volume or the degree of hypoalbuminemia. Indeed, NaCl retention appears before any reduction in serum protein concentration and a diuresis ensues in the absence of any significant change in serum protein concentration in nephrotic subjects. Infusions of hyperoncotic albumin, in the absence of diuretics, do not increase NaCl excretion, despite a rise in plasma oncotic pressure. Plasma renin activity, although sometimes modestly elevated, may show little clear relationship to intravascular volume thus it is possible that renin–angiotensin system may be stimulated by intrarenal events rather than necessarily by a depletion of intravascular volume depletion.

The abnormal NaCl reabsorption within the nephron appears to be localized to the distal nephron and collecting ducts (Ichikawa et al., 1983). Post-receptor resistance to the action of atrial natriuretic factor due to enhanced activity of cyclic GMP phosphodiesterase may be involved (Perico and Remuzzi, 1993; Lee and Humphrey, 1996), but the dominant process appears to be an increased activity of Na^+/K^+ activated ATPase, perhaps abetted by alteration in the density of epithelial sodium channels (ENaC) in the cortical collecting ducts (Deschenes et al., 2001, Kim et al., 2006, 2007; de Seigneux et al., 2006; Doucet et al., 2007). Increased abundance and apical targeting of the subunits of ENaC have been demonstrated in the cortical collecting ducts in experimental nephrotic syndrome (Doucet et al., 2007). ENaC activation is secondary to hyperaldosteronism (by recruitment of an intracellular pool of channels), but sodium retention and induction of Na^+-K^+ ATPase in the cortical collecting ducts are independent of hyperaldosteronism and increased ENaC may not be the rate limited step in renal NaCl retention in experimental models of nephrotic syndrome (PAN nephrosis) (Lourdel et al., 2005). Primary renal NaCl retention can occur in the absence of aldosterone in experimental nephrotic syndrome (Doucet et al., 2007), Due to the *unilateral* retention of NaCl demonstrated in experimental models of nephrotic syndrome (Ichikawa et al., 1983) it is unlikely that any circulating factor is directly involved in primary renal NaCl retention observed in nephrotic states (Doucet et al., 2007).

A distinct linkage exists between abnormal glomerular permeability, increased exposure of tubules to, and subsequent reabsorption of, protein and primary renal NaCl retention. This indicates that enhanced glomerular permeability to protein may govern primary renal NaCl retention at the *individual* nephon level in nephrotic edema. Functional changes in tubular cellular function consequent to expression of factors governing NaCl reabsorption in the collecting ducts (such as Na/K ATPase, ENaC) resulting from abnormally high concentrations of protein (including albumin) in tubular lumina appear to be involved, although this remains controversial (Zandi-Nejad et al., 2004; Yu et al., 2005; Doucet et al., 2007) (see also 'Proteinuria and hypoalbuminemia,' below). Specific filtered proteins (albumin, high-molecular weight proteins) may have differing effects on tubular reabsorptive phenomena. Intrinsic proteins may also have direct effects on NaCl reabsorption. For example, parvalbumin has recently been shown to have effects on the thiazide-sensitive Na^+-Cl^- co-transporter and thus may be involved in both Na^+ and Ca^{++} handling in the distal convoluted tubule (Belge et al., 2007; Zacchia and Capasso, 2008).

It is important to re-emphasize that the proteinuria-driven changes (luminal protein concentration) in cortical collecting tubule sodium avidity operates at the *individual nephron level*. Tubules which are not exposed to abnormal luminal protein concentration (i.e., tubules which are not affected in a focal glomerular disease process involving some but not all nephrons) are capable of excreting NaCl in a normal manner and these '*normal*' nephrons would be expected to excrete the NaCl retained by the *abnormal* nephrons in the mixed diseased/non-diseased nephron population. This phenomenon may explain why edema is quite uncommon in subjects with very focal and segmental permselectivity defects (e.g., obesity-related glomerulopathy and other 'secondary' forms of focal segmental glomerulosclerosis). Tubular reabsorption of NaCl at more proximal sites (proximal tubule and ascending limb of the loop of Henle is normal in nephrotic states, at least in the absence of acute hypovolemia, diuretics, or advanced decline in GFR. Reabsorption of NaCl at distal convoluted tubule sites where Na^+ and K^+ exchange occurs is also initially normal. Thus, potassium retention or potassium loss is not seen in nephrotic states in the absence of diuretics or aldosterone deficiency. However, potassium retention may be severe in the acute nephritic syndrome, usually because of the attendant secondary hypo-reninemic, hypo-aldosteronism and reduced capacity for K^+ excretion (Don and Schambelan, 1990).

Therapy

Mild edema

If edema is mild and well tolerated, the best approach is to reduce dietary NaCl intake to levels below 3g per day (42mM Na^+ or about 0.5–0.6mM/kg/d) (Table 1.2). Bed rest should be avoided because of the tendency of these patients to develop thromboembolic complications (see below). Support stockings and nocturnal leg elevation may be of value in some patients with mild edema. Many patients will not require any more than these simple measures. However, if they are unsuccessful, a diuretic may be added to the regimen (Glassock et al., 1996). An oral thiazide diuretic (e.g., hydrochlorothiazide 12.5–50mg per day or chlorthalidone 12.5–25mg per day) is a reasonable first choice, providing the GFR is normal or near normal since the effectiveness of this class of agents is blunted when GFR is <30mL/min (Ellison and Wilcox, 2008). If the serum creatinine is elevated (above 1.4mg/dL; 120μmol/L), thiazide-type diuretics are not likely to be very effective. Loop-acting diuretics (furosemide, ethacrynic acid, bumetanide, piretanide, or torsemide) are more effective choices when the GFR is reduced and when edema is troublesome (Brater, 1986; Ellison and Wilcox, 2008). Because of the duration of action, furosemide should be given on a twice-daily regimen. Once-daily administration of loop-acting diuretics is not recommended. Because severe hypoproteinemia may impair the rate of refilling of the plasma volume, overly vigorous diuresis is to be avoided. Excessive diuresis may also activate the renin–angiotensin system and thereby promote thrombosis (see below). Oral furosemide 40–80mg per day or oral bumetamide 1–2mg per day given in two or three divided doses, along with modest dietary NaCl (3g/d) should suffice in most instances of mild edema.

Moderate edema

More severe edema may require more intensive regimens, such as high-dose oral furosemide (160–480mg) given in two or three divided doses daily or by continuous intravenous infusion (see below) (Glassock et al., 1995) (Table 1.2). Synergistic combinations of oral furosemide 160–320mg daily or bumetanide 4–8mg daily and the distally acting diuretic, metolazone 2.5–10mg daily, are particularly effective, but may lead to pronounced kaliuresis requiring intensive potassium replacement (Suki and Eknoyan 1992). Very high

Table 1.2 Management of edema in nephrotic syndrome

Mild

Dietary NaCl restriction (to 3–4 g NaCl per day)
Support stockings
Hydrochlorothiazide 12.5–50 mg per day (if GFR >50 mL/min)
Furosemide 40–80 mg per day (if GFR <70 mL/min)

Moderate

Continue NaCl restriction, add
Furosemide 160–480 mg per day or bumetamide 1–2 mg per day or torsemide
   40–160 mg per day

Severe

Continue NaCl restriction, add
Oral or IV furosemide 160–480 mg per day (or bumetamide or torsemide) plus metalozone
   2.5–10 mg per day

Refractory

Continuous IV infusion of furosemide (20 mg/h) or bumetanide (1 mg/h) after a loading
   dose
or
Hyperoncotic salt-poor albumin (25–50 g) mixed with 120 mg of furosemide

or
Slow continuous veno-venous ultrafiltration using a highly permeable (polysulfone)
   membrane

Reproduced with permission from Ponticelli C and Glassock RJ (eds) (1997). *Treatment of Primary Glomerulonephritis.* Oxford University Press, Oxford doses of loop-acting diuretics, oral or intravenous, should be used with caution in patients with markedly impaired renal function because of the risks of transient or permanent deafness (Ellison and Wilcox, 2008). Mild diarrhea may also be seen with very high doses of loop diuretics. The natriuretic effects of loop-acting diuretics are related to the urinary concentration of the diuretic (Brater, 1993). The relationship between diuretic excretion rate (in µg/min) and sodium excretion rate (in µEq/min) is described by a steep sigmoid curve. Different loop-acting diuretics differ only in potency, not in the shape of the curve (Brater, 1993).

Potassium-spring diuretics, such as spironolactone, eplerenone, triamterene, or amiloride, given alone, are also of limited value but they may blunt the kaliuresis seen with thiazides or loop-acting diuretic and augment the resulting natriuresis when used in combination with other diuretics acting at different sites within the nephron. Thus, they are not usually very effective when used as monotherapy, but they augment the effectiveness of both loop-acting diuretics and thiazide-type diuretics. These potassium-sparing diuretics should be used with great caution or not at all in patients with impaired GFR (<25mL/min) or when hyperkelemia is present. More rigorous dietary NaCl restriction (1g/d) may also be required for short periods of time, but this will usually not be tolerated (or adhered to) over a period of longer than a few weeks.

Severe or refractory edema

A severe edematous state (anasarca) in which increasing doses of loop-acting diuretics combined with potassium-sparing diuretics and/or metolazone become increasingly less effective in inducing a natriuresis is relatively common, especially in patients with severe and massive proteinuria (>10.2 g per day), marked hypoalbuminemia (<2.5 g/dL) and/or impaired renal function (serum creatinine >2.0mg/dL) (Glassock, 1997) (Table 1.2).

At one time the poor response to loop-acting diuretics (e.g., furosemide) was thought to be caused by binding of the drug to tubule fluid albumin, thereby preventing the action of the diuretic on the luminal side of the ascending limb of the loop of Henle to inhibit the $Na^+/K^+/2Cl^-$ reabsorptive pathway (Brater, 1993; Kirchner, 1993). This is no longer thought to be the case. An intravenous loading dose of furosemide or bumetanide followed by a slow intravenous infusion of the diuretic over 12–24h (20mg/h for furosemide and 1mg/h for bumetanide) (Brater, 1993) may sometimes be effective, when oral administration is not accompanied by a diuresis.

Excess compensatory 'upstream' distal-NaCl reabsorption (sites prior to the cortical collecting duct) may also be overcome by concomitant administration of a thiazide-type diuretic (Paton and Kane, 1977). Hyperoncotic (25%) or iso-oncotic (5%) human albumin infusions alone are seldom indicated to expand plasma volume, except when a rapid diuresis has resulted in clinical features of a plasma volume deficit, such as hypotension or a low central venous pressure. Such infusions should be used cautiously, if at all, in patients with impaired renal function and intrinsic cardiac disease because of the risk of precipitating congestive heart failure. Because of continued abnormal permselectivity, the infused albumin will be rapidly excreted in the urine (usually within 24–48 h). Thus, the beneficial effects are short lived. The increased filtration of albumin can also result in further injury to the glomerular epithelial cells and or tubule. Indeed, some studies have suggested that use of intravenous albumin may inhibit therapeutic responses to glucocorticoids in minimal change disease (Yoshimura et al., 1992). On the other hand, some investigators believe that intravenous albumin may be regarded as a useful vehicle for augmenting the delivery of loop-acting diuretics to tubular sites of action as mentioned above. A natriuresis can be potentiated by the concomitant administration of a loop-acting diuretic and hyper-oncotic albumin (frosemide mixed with 25% human serum albumin) in equimolar concentrations (Brater 1993; Kirchner 1993), but the effect is usually limited and of short-duration. In addition, some clinicial investigators have challenged the usefulness of intravenous albumin in the treatment of nephrotic edema, either alone or combined with diuretics, based on an exhaustive survey of the literature (Dorhout Mees, 1996). Loop-acting diuretics circulate bound to albumin and are delivered to their site of action in the ascending limb of the loop of Henle via the organic anion secretory pathway in the proximal tubule. When hypoalbuminemia is present, both the volume of distribution and the extrarenal catabolism of loop diuretics are increased. Less drug is therefore delivered to secretory sites in the proximal tubule and the urinary excretion is diminished, leading to a blunted effect even at high doses of the drug.

Intrinsic unresponsiveness of the renal tubule and impaired gastrointestinal (GI) absorption of frosemide have also been suggested as potential causes of diuretic refractoriness (Kirchner et al., 1992) but this does not appear to be of major importance, at least in the usual case of nephrotic syndrome. Non-steroidal anti-inflammatory drugs (including aspirin) *antagonize* and angiotensin-converting enzyme inhibitors *potentiate* the action of loop-acting diuretics (Brater, 1990).

In exceptional patients who are truly refractory to all oral or parenterally-based treatments (including high-dose loop-acting diuretics, metolazone and/or amiloride), a course of slow, continuous ultrafiltration using a highly permeable (polysulfone) dialysis membrane and a veno-venous circuit with systemic heparin anticoagulation can be used for temporary relief of anasarca

(Fauchald et al., 1985). Because the edema in the interstitial compartment can be partially mobilized when serum albumin concentration is increased by ultrafiltration, rapid rates of ultrafiltration (3–5 L/h) are usually well tolerated.

Hypertension

Clinical features, pathogenesis, and pathophysiology

Elevation of systolic and/or diastolic blood pressure (BP) commonly occurs in patients with glomerular disease (Glassock et al., 1995). The degree of hypertension is usually worse and the frequency more common in the acute nephritic syndrome and much less prominent in the nephrotic syndrome, unless a severe decrease in the GFR is present. Indeed, severe hypertension (and volume overload) can lead to congestive heart failure and encephalopathy in patients with the acute nephritic syndrome but this seldom occurs in those with the nephrotic syndrome, due to primary glomerular disease. Patients with hypertension due to primary glomerular disease tend not to have the normal decline in BP during sleep ('non-dipper') when studied by 24-h ambulatory BP monitoring (Tamura et al., 2008). The underlying pathophysiology of hypertension in primary glomerular disease remains a subject of intense investigation but several factors appear to be involved, namely:

- Primary renal NaCl retention leading to expansion of intravascular and extracellular fluid volumes (see above); this is especially important in the acute nephritic syndrome.

- Intrarenal activation of the renin–angiotensin system despite relative vascular volume expansion; plasma renin activity and plasma aldosterone levels are markedly suppressed in the acute nephritic syndrome, but they may be inappropriately elevated in the presence of extracellular volume overload.

- Activation of the sympathetic nervous system, perhaps a consequence of the central actions of angiotensin II.

- The release, at the level of the vascular endothelial cell, of vasoconstrictor substances (e.g., thromboxane or endothelin) or deficiencies in the generation of vasorelaxant factors (e.g., nitric oxide, prostaglandins) may also participate (Campese, 1995; Galla and Luke, 1995).

A more pronounced effect on systolic pressure with widening of the pulse pressure suggests a prominent volume-mediated component and/or an effect of the disease on vascular compliance. Acute post-streptococcal glomerulonephritis is a classic example of volume-mediated hypertension in which the renin–angiotensin–aldosterone system is markedly suppressed (Don and Schambelan, 1990). Chronic forms of glomerulonephritis nearly always show an admixture of volume-mediated and vasoconstrictor pathophysiology (Galla and Luke, 1995). The concomitant presence of hypertension and nephrotic syndrome may alter the distribution of fluid between the intravascular and interstitial spaces and thus blunt the expected hypertensionogenic effect of fluid retention (Geers et al., 1984). In some exceptional patients with nephrotic syndrome 'secondary' hyperreninemia and hyperaldosteronemia are present without hypertension, indicative of a reduced plasma volume. These patients usually have minimal change nephropathy and the rapid development of nephrotic syndrome (Meltzer et al., 1979).

Therapy

The management of hypertension accompanying glomerular disease is very important not only to reduce the risks of cardiovascular disease (stroke, myocardial infarction, peripheral vascular disease, congestive heart failure) but also potentially to blunt progressive renal insufficiency (see below). The management of hypertension in glomerular disease is based on two fundamental precepts:

1) Dietary NaCl restriction and/or diuretics in order to affect the volume-mediated influence on blood pressure, and

2) To reduce the vasoconstrictor effect of an inappropriately activated renin–angiotensin or sympathetic nervous system.

Thiazide or loop-acting diuretics may suffice in many patients but if not accompanied by NaCl restriction will often be ineffective, particularly when short-acting agents such as bumetamide or furosemide are used. When GFR is normal, the natriuretic effect of the furosemide lasts approximately six hours and thus, if this agent is administered on a once-daily basis, *in the absence of sodium restriction*, once the diuretic effect has dissipated, the sodium-avid kidney will reabsorb sodium to an extent that the 24-h balance will be neutral (Ellison and Wilcox, 2008). Diuretics with more prolonged action such as thiazides or chlorthalidone will not have this disadvantage. However, the natriuretic potency of these agents is considerably attenuated when the GFR is <30 mL/min.

If NaCl restriction and/or diuretics do not 'adequately' control blood pressure (see below for a discussion of what constitutes 'adequate' BP control), then additional antihypertensive agents can be added. For a variety of reasons, listed below, angiotensin-converting enzyme inhibitors (ACEi) or angiotensin II receptor blockers (ARB) or both combined appear to be the agents of choice. A new class of agents, the direct renin inhibitors (e.g. aliskerin), has also been recently introduced and may have a role in the management of hypertension.

The use of drugs interfering with the action of the renin–angiotensin system is preferred because:

- They tend also to reduce protein excretion, presumably because of their intra-renal hemodynamic and other BP independent effects (Cravedi et al., 2007).

- They may have renoprotective properties *independent* of lowering BP and even their anti-proteinuric effects, thus reducing the likelihood of future progression to ESRD (see below) (Cravedi et al., 2007; Ruggenenti et al., 2008).

- They are well tolerated and are associated with minimal side effects (except cough [see below] and occasionally anaphylaxis with ACEi) and a good quality of life.

- They are quite effective, particularly when combined with thiazide and/or loop diuretics and/or NaCl restriction. Hyperkalemia, allergic reactions (including angio-edema), and agranulocytosis are relatively uncommon.

A common troublesome side effect is a dry, non-productive cough associated with the use of ACEi but not with ARB, and is perhaps related to change in bradykinin activity. Cough is seen more commonly in individuals of Asian ancestry but may also be seen in Caucasians. Combinations of ACEi and ARB may produce more side effects, including acute reductions of GFR, when used in patients with underlying cardiac disease (Cravedi et al., 2007). Theoretically, ACEi may also reduce thrombotic tendency because they lower plasminogen activation inhibitor-1 levels (see below) (Kerins et al., 1995). Other antihypertensive agents such as β-adrenergic blockers (propanolol, atenolol), combined alpha/beta blockers (labetolol), central or peripherally acting adrenergic inhibitors (clonidine), α-1 receptor blockers (doxazosin), dihydropyridine or non-dihydropyridine calcium channel blockers (CCB), and direct-acting vasodilators (e.g., hydralazine, minoxidil, nitroprusside) may also be quite effective in lowering BP (Campese, 1995), but are not preferred as front-line agen`ts in glomerular disease with proteinuria. Non-dihydropyridine CCB (e.g., diltiazem, verapamil) may also reduce proteinuria, but to a lesser extent than ACEi (Gansevoort et al., 1995). Dihydropyridine CCB have little effect on proteinuria or may actually increase protein excretion rates. Dihydropyridine CCB should not be given in the absence of concomitant ACEi or ARB. Combinations of loop-acting diuretics, ACEi and/or ARB, and non-dihydropyridine calcium antagonists may be useful in difficult-to-manage cases. Refractory hypertension requires a multi-drug approach, but control of volume expansion with diuretics and NaCl restriction is a critical component of therapy. Dihydropyridine CCB (nifedipine, nisoldipine, amlodipine) are quite useful adjunctive antihypertensive agents but they tend not to be associated with a reduction in protein excretion and may aggravate edema (Gansevoort et al., 1995). Furthermore, these latter agents do not appear to have reno-protective actions, independent of BP lowering. Small doses of spironolactone or eplerenone may be very helpful for the control of BP in those subjects (mainly diabetics) who do not respond favorably to thiazides or loop-acting diuretics agents or ACEi/ARB, but caution about hyperkalemia is warranted (Schjoedt et al., 2006).

Agents which can be administered on a once-a-day basis are preferred for chronic therapy. Administration of doses at bedtime may be helpful for subjects with 'non-dipping' BP elevations. Newer anti-hypertensive agents, such as direct renin inhibitors (aliskiren) can also be used (alone or in combination with other angiotensin-II inhibing agents), but there is only limited short-term little experience in their use in primary glomerular disease with nephrotic syndrome or acute nephritis (Parving et al., 2008). This class of agents would not be expected to be beneficial if plasma renin activity is depressed (see also Table 1.3 for a description of recommendations for treatment of hypertension).

Table 1.3 Therapy of hypertension in primary glomerular disease

Goals:	Maintain systolic blood pressure of 120–130 mmHg and diastolic BP of 70–80 mmHg. Do not allow diastolic BP to fall below 70 mmHg if symptomatic coronary artery disease is present
Agents:	Angiotensin converting enzyme inhibitors (ACEi) or angiotensin receptor blockers (ARB) preferred
	Use NaCl restriction and/or diuretics (thiazides, loop acting, spironolactone oreplerenone) to augment effectiveness
	Combinations of ACEi and ARB may be used, with careful attention to serum potassium levels
	Direct renin inhibitors may also be used selectively
	Adjuctive therapy with calcium channel blockers (CCB) may be used for optimal BP control
	Change in serum creatinine and potassium levels should be monitored at frequent intervals during the first month of initiating therapy. If serum creatinine levels rise >25% from baseline, therapy may have to be interrupted.
Dosage:	For monotherapy with ACEi or ARB, the maximum tolerated dosage should be used, preferably to assure both daytime and night-time control of BP to desired goals. Ambulatory monitoring of 24-h BP may be needed
	For combination ACEi and ARB therapy the maximum recommended dosage of each agent should be used, with monitoring of serum potassium levels.

The extent to which BP should be lowered for optimal or 'adequate' control remains a subject of ongoing investigation. For the time being, a goal of 120–130 mm Hg for the systolic BP and 70–80 mmHg for the diastolic BP (mean arterial pressure of around 92 mmHg) appears prudent. Acute lowering of BP to these levels in subjects with encephalopathy (or carotid arterial stenoses) may be hazardous due to reduction in cerebral perfusion. Intravenous, short-acting antihypertensive agents (such as labetolol, enalaprilat, or nitroprusside) may be useful for severe hypertension and associated acute left ventricular dysfunction with congestive heart failure. In more chronic states, it is not known whether lower levels of BP (<120 mmHg systolic or <70 mmHg diastolic) will be associated with any better protection from progressive renal failure and a low diastolic pressure (<70 mmHg) should be avoided in older patients with established coronary artery disease because of the risk of impairing coronary perfusion which is highly dependent on diastolic pressure gradients (Messerli, et al., 2006). Too low BP should also be avoided in those with carotid artery stenoses. 24-h ambulatory BP recordings may be useful to detect 'non-dipping' status, which is associated with a greater degree of left-ventricular hypertrophy and a higher mortality rate from CVD (Hermida, 2007).

Hyperlipidemia

Clinical features, pathogenesis, and pathophysiology

Elevation of plasma total cholesterol and triglycerides is commonly found to accompany glomerular disease, especially in those situations associated with heavy proteinuria and hypoalbuminemia (nephrotic syndrome) (Table 1.4) (Vaziri, 2003). The lowering of plasma albumin concentration and the increased protein excretion contribute separately to changes in lipoprotein metabolism in the nephrotic syndrome (Shearer et al., 2001; Vaziri, 2003). The underlying pathophysiology of hyperlipidemia is only partially understood but appears to involve both enhanced synthesis and decreased metabolism of lipoproteins (Joles and Kaysen 1991; Vaziri, 2003). The characteristic perturbation seen in nephrotic syndrome is an increase in low density lipoproteins (LDL), very low density lipoproteins (VLDL), and/or intermediate density lipoproteins (IDL), but no change or a decrease in high density lipoproteins (HDL). Apolipoprotein B and apolipoprotein CIII are increased but apolipoprotein AI, AII, and CII are unchanged. The ratio of apolipoprotein CIII/CII is increased and contributes to a prevailing state of inhibition of lipoprotein lipase. HDL_3 is increased whereas HDL_2 is decreased. The combination

Table 1.4 Plasma lipid concentrations in nephrotic syndrome

Increased

Very low density lipoproteins
Intermediate density lipoproteins
Low density lipoproteins
Apolipoprotein B
Apolipoprotein CIII
High density lipoprotein$_3$
Lipoprotein (a)
Total cholesterol
Triglycerides (when serum albumin <2 g/dl)

Unchanged

Apolipoprotein AI
Apolipoprotein AII
Apolipoprotein CII

Decreased

High density lipoprotein$_2$

See Wheeler and Bernard (1994) and Kaysen *et al.* (1991) for details.

of reduced HDL$_2$ and increased LDL/IDL increases greatly the *potential* risk for atherosclerotic cardiovascular disease, especially with the concomitant presence of smoking, obesity, diabetes, hyperuricemia, and hypertension. Circulating levels of lipoprotein (a) [Lp(a)] and fibrinogen are also increased in nephrotic syndrome and may have an additive effect on atherogenesis and on the predisposition to thrombotic events (Stenvinkel et al., 1993). The synthesis and cellular expression of LDL receptors is diminished in experimental nephrotic syndrome (Vaziri and Liang, 1996; Vaziri, 2003).

The hepatic synthesis of apolipoproteins A, B, E, and VLDL is often, but not invariably, increased perhaps as a result of decreased serum albumin concentration and plasma osmotic pressure, but other processes are probably also involved (Vaziri, 2003). The catabolism of VLDL and LDL is also greatly reduced in nephrotic syndrome and this does not appear to be the direct consequence of reduced albumin concentration (Vega et al., 1995). Reduced catabolism of apolipoprotein B LDL is also present when increased plasma cholesterol is not accompanied by hypertriglyceridemia, but hepatic production of apolipoprotein B LDL is increased in combined hypercholesterolemia and hypertriglyceridemia (Vega et al., 1995).

It has been suggested that proteinuria per se results in a disturbance of lipoprotein metabolism, perhaps because of the renal generation or urinary loss of a lipoprotein regulatory substance (Garber et al., 1984; Vaziri, 2003). It has long been known that elevated serum lipoproteins can occur even in glomerular proteinuria unaccompanied by nephrotic syndrome or hypoalbuminemia.

These lipid abnormalities (increased LDL, reduced HDL_2, and increased Lp(a)) have important long-term consequences which deserve careful attention and appropriate management (Radhakrishnan et al., 1993; Appel, 2001), but here is little evidence-based data (such as randomized clinical trials) to guide rational management. Observational and controlled trials have proven atherogenesis to be accelerated in hypercholesterolemic states (high LDL and low HDL cholesterol) and this leads to an increased risk for cardiovascular disease, including angina, myocardial infarction, strokes, and peripheral vascular disease. Concomitant hypertension, heavy smoking, obesity, diabetes (insulin resistance), physical inactivity, and/or a positive family history of coronary artery disease (Radhakrishnan et al., 1993). By inference, it is believed that the abnormal lipid patterns seen in glomerular disease also predispose to accelerated atherogenesis, but this is much less proven than in subjects without glomerular disease. It is also postulated that abnormal plasma lipid concentrations also contribute to progressive glomerular injury (see below) (Keane, 1994). However, the benefits and risks of 'statin' therapy to slow progression of renal disease (independent of its benefits for dyslipidemia) remains unproven and controversial (Rahman et al., 2008; Strippoli et al., 2008; Tonelli, 2008). Further randomized trails in progress will likely resolve this controversy. Statins may have lowering effects on established albuminuria but whether this will translate into better outcomes is unknown (Douglas et al., 2006).

Therapy

Unfortunately, the management of hyperlipidemia accompanying nephrotic syndrome is only fully successful in restoring the elevated levels to normal values when the underlying cause is remedied and long-term complete remissions of proteinuria are induced (see Table 1.5). Dietary therapy consisting of reduced cholesterol and saturated fat intake is generally relatively ineffective and can make the HDL_2 reductions worse. Restriction of total fat intake has never been proven to alter the natural history of atherogenesis in subjects with the nephrotic syndrome. Even with strict dietary prescription and full compliance, LDL levels will usually fall a maximum of 15–20% from baseline values. The long-term use of agents which interfere with the GI absorption of dietary cholesterol (such as ezetimide [Zetia®]) or exchange resins (e.g. cholestyramine, colestipol, psyllium colloids, oat bran) is incompletely evaluated in nephrotic

Table 1.5 Therapy of lipid disturbances in nephrotic syndrome

Prudent diet, low in total cholesterol and saturated fat (relatively ineffective); vegetarian/soy diet

Stop smoking

Modest exercise

Avoid excessive alcohol

HMG co-reductase inhibitors (lovastatin, simvastatin, pravastatin, atorvastatin, rosuvastatin, fluvastatin)

Probucol (may lower HDL_2)

Bile acid sequestering agents (cholestyramine, colestipol, psyllium colloid)

Reproduced with permission from Ponticelli C and Glassock RJ (eds) (1997). *Treatment of Primary Glomerulonephritis.* Oxford University Press, Oxford.

syndrome, and they cannot be recommended at the present time. A vegetarian–soy diet supplemented with amino acids may achieve the best results but long-term compliance and overall efficacy of this dietary approach is not well known (D'Amico et al., 1992). Oral administration of bile-acid sequestering agents, such as cholestyramine, colestipol, or psyllium colloid, are able to reduce modestly the total cholesterol but are relatively poorly tolerated and may aggravate underlying vitamin D deficiency.

Fibric acid derivatives (gemfibrozil) and nicotinic acid are more effective for hypertriglyceridemia but are not very useful for the hypercholesterolemia which accompanies nephrotic syndrome (Grundy, 1990). They may also be associated with muscle injury (Bridgman et al., 1972). Nicotinic acid (niacin) will lower both LDL cholesterol and triglycerides and also increase HDL cholesterol but is not well tolerated at the high dosage required. Extended-release preparations of niacin may be better tolerated. Probucol may be a useful agent since it lowers LDL cholesterol concentration by approximately 20–35% and it may have other beneficial effects as an antioxidant (Neale et al., 1994). Unfortunately, it may also modestly reduce HDL_2 levels further.

Hydroxymethylglutaryl co-enzyme A reductase (HMG co-A reductase) inhibitors ('statins') are the current treatments of choice for hypercholesterolemia of nephrotic syndrome (Appel, 2001). All currently available preparations (lovastatin, simvastatin, pravastatin, fluvastatin, atorvastatin, rosuvastatin,) will lower LDL and total cholesterol by approximately 25–45% (atorvastatin and rosuvastatin are the most potent) despite continued proteinuria. (See Table 1.6 for a listing of preparations and recommended dosage).

Table 1.6 Hydroxy methyl glutaryl co-enzyme A reductase ('statin') therapy for hypercholesterolemia in the nephrotic syndrome (adults)

◆ *Lovastatin:*	10–20mg once daily in the evening (80mg/d maximum dosage)
◆ *Simvastatin:*	20–40mg once daily in the evening (80mg/d maximum dosage)
◆ *Pravastain:*	10–40mg once daily (maximum dose 80mg/d)
◆ *Fluvastatin:*	20–40mg once daily (maximum dose 80mg/d)
◆ *Atorvastatin:*	10–40mg once daily (maximum dose 80mg/d)
◆ *Rosuvastatin:*	5–20mg once daily (maximum dose 40mg/d)

These agents cause no changes or only a mild-modest elevation in HDL_2 and are generally well tolerated but rarely they may produce rhabdomyolysis and even acute renal failure, particularly at high dosage or combined with fibric acid derivatives (or possibly cyclosporin). Asian patients might be more susceptible to these effects. Unfortunately, statins have no or very limited effects on Lp(a) or fibrinogen levels (Wanner et al., 1994).

Although lowering serum cholesterol levels with a statin has the *potential* for significantly reducing the risk of coronary heart disease events in patients with and without preexisting coronary heart disease in the absence of nephrotic syndrome or renal disease, their effects on prevention or regression of atherogenesis complicating human glomerular disease or on the progression of renal have not been unequivocally proven in a large prospectively designed randomized clinical trial in nephrotic subjects (Strippoli et al., 2008; Tonelli, 2008; thus, treatment is largely 'on faith' that modest lowering of an atherogenic lipid (but not to normal ranges) will be accompanied by a lowered risk of subsequent cardiovascular events. (Scandinavian Simvastatin Survival Study, 1994; Tonelli et al., 2004). Meta-analyses of existing trials have suggested that statins may reduce cardiovascular event rate in patients with chronic kidney disease (CKD) (Tonelli, et al., 2006; Tonelli and Pfeffer, 2007), and may also very modestly slow the rate of progression of CKD *not* accompanied by diabetes, hypertension or glomerulonephritis (Sandhu et al., 2006), but as stated above this is quite controversial. Large prospective randomized trials are in progress to test this hypothesis (SHARP, AURORA) and their results are eagerly anticipated.

The overall cost of this therapy is relatively high and the long-term benefits and risks uncertain, but most patients are so concerned about elevated total cholesterol and/or LDL levels that treatment can be justified as a means of reducing apprehension. Some evidence has been generated suggesting that statins given alone modestly reduce the level of proteinuria (Douglas et al., 2006), although at high doses in normal subjects they paradoxically increase albuminuria by interfering with tubular re-absorption of normally filtered protein by a direct action on tubules. Thus, for the present time at least, the indications for the use of statins in CKD, even accompanied by the nephrotic syndrome are the same as for their use in the general population (Clase, 2008).

Regular moderate exercise, a prudent anti-atherogenic diet (low in total cholesterol, low in saturated and transfat, low in fructose and sucrose, high in anti-oxidant content 'Mediterranean' style diet), complete avoidance of smoking, rigorous control of BP (with ACEi and/or an ARB) and obesity may offer as much or more than drug management of serum cholesterol levels (see below) with respect to prevention of cardiovascular disease and slowing the rate of progression of renal disease.

Hypercoagulability

Clinical features, pathogenesis, and pathophysiology

It has been known for many decades that patients with glomerular disease and marked (nephrotic range) proteinuria are at increased risk for thromboembolic events ('*thrombophilia*'), such as deep venous thrombosis (DVT), renal vein thrombosis, pulmonary embolism, and arterial thrombi (Vaziri, 1983; Glassock, 2007). This '*thrombophilic*' phenomenon has been attributed to an ill-defined 'hypercoagulable' state in which an imbalance between naturally occurring pro-coagulant/pro-thrombotic factors and anti-coagulant/anti-thrombotic factors promote *in situ* thrombosis in deep veins or arteries (Table 1.7) (Vaziri, 1983; Cameron, 1984; Glassock 2007).

Table 1.7 Coagulation abnormalities in nephrotic syndrome

Increased (prothrombotic)

Fibrinogen

Platelets (and platelet adhesiveness)

Plasma viscosity (cholesterol, lipid)

Lipoprotein (a)

Plasminogen activator inhibitor

Decreased (antithrombotic)

Active protein C

Active protein S

Antithrombin III

Reproduced with permission from Ponticelli C and Glassock RJ (eds) (1997). *Treatment of Primary Glomerulonephritis.* Oxford University Press, Oxford

The biochemical nature of this *thrombophilic* state is probably multifactorial. The plasma concentration of fibrinogen is markedly increased in nephrotic syndrome. When this is combined with a low albumin level it leads to an almost universal increase in the erythrocyte sedimentation rate irrespective of underlying inflammation. A mild thrombocytosis is frequently present. Hypercholesterolemia leads to an increase in plasma viscosity. Urinary losses of proteins C, S, and antithrombin III may predispose to a low plasma concentration of these factors (Vaziri, 1983; Kauffman et al., 1978; Cameron, 1984). A genetically determined background of impaired resistance to activation of factor V (Leiden trait) may also predispose to thrombosis in the presence of these disturbances (Ridker et al., 1995). Elevated Lp (a) levels may also contribute to impaired fibrinolysis (Kronenberg et al., 1996).

Evidence has accumulated linking local activation of the renin–angiotensin system with impaired endogenous fibrinolysis and a pro-thrombotic tendency. Angiotensin IV (AT-IV), a hexapeptide produced by the action of aminopeptidase on angiotensin II (AT-II), promotes endothelial cell synthesis of plasminogen activation inhibitor-1 (PAI-1) via interaction with an AT-IV specific receptor, not via the well recognized AT-I and AT-II receptors (Kerins et al., 1995). Fibrinolysis may thus be inhibited leading to a prothrombotic state. It is possible that TGFβ (transforming growth factor β) is also involved in this interaction since angiotensin II is a strong promoter of TGFβ synthesis in tissue and TGFβ stimulates PAI-1 synthesis (Border and Noble 1994). Angiotensin-converting enzyme inhibitors may reduce PAI-1 synthesis and because of concomitant elevated bradykinin levels, endothelial cell synthesis of tissue plasminogen activator (tPA) is enhanced (Kerins et al., 1995). The net effect of ACEi is to tilt the tPA/PAI-2 ratio in favor of a pro-fibrinolytic rather than a pro-thrombotic state. Angiotensin II receptor antagonists (ARB) would not be expected to have as favorable an effect on this ratio, and could even theoretically promote increased PAI-1 levels, because of high AT-II (and thereby AT-IV) levels (Johnston 1995). Similarly, diuretics which promote activation of the renin–angiotensin system and thereby the AT-II and AT-IV levels could also promote a pro-thrombotic state by altering PAI-1 levels. High PAI-1 levels are known to be associated with increased risk of recurrent myocardial infarction in survivors of acute coronary thrombosis (Ridker et al., 1993).

Excess mortality from cardiovascular events in nephrotic syndrome could theoretically be explained, at least in part, by both hyperlipidemia-related increased atherogenesis and a pro-thrombotic state induced by elevated PAI-1 levels driven by an activated renin–angiotensin system. Other concomitant processes such anti-phospholipid auto-antibodies (usually seen in connection with systemic lupus erythematosus) and anti-plasminogen auto-antibodies seen in systemic vasculitis (Wegener's granulomatosis) may greatly affect the tendency to thrombosis in these diseases (Merkel, et al., 2005; Bu et al., 2008). Anti-enolase auto-antibodies, strongly associated with membranous nephropathy and exerting an anti-fibrinolytic effects, could also be involved in the marked tendency of this disorder for thrombosis (Wakui et al, 1999).

Many of the disturbances associated with the thrombophilic state in nephrotic syndrome are correlated with the magnitude of depression of serum albumin levels (Kauffman et al., 1978; Glassock, 2007). The concentration of albumin may therefore be used as 'surrogate' to approximate the magnitude of the 'hypercoagulable' state and thereby the potential risk of thromboembolic events. Serum albumin concentrations <2.0–2.5g/dL appear to be associated with an increased risk of thromboembolism. High levels of fibrinogen, low plasminogen activity, low antithrombin III, and high levels of PAI-1 may also predict the tendency for thrombosis (Glassock, 2007). A preceding thrombotic event (such as a DVT), recent abdominal, gynecologic or orthopedic surgery, recent trauma, the presence of a lupus anticoagulant (anti-phospholipid antibody), an anti-plasminogen antibody, systemic vasculitis (Wegener's granulomatosis), prolonged inactivity, obesity, and a family history of 'thrombophilia' (such as might be present with a factor V Leiden trait) are all predisposing factors for thrombotic events. The presence of *one or more* of these predisposing factors should influence the decision regarding use of measures to prevent thrombosis (oral anti-coagulation with warfarin or use of heparin or enoxaparin) in individual patients (Glassock, 2007).

It also must be appreciated that the tendency for thrombosis is not uniform among the primary glomerular diseases leading to the nephrotic syndrome. The disorders most prominently associated with thrombophilia are membranous nephropathy (MN), membrano-proliferative glomerulonephritis (MPGN) and minimal change nephropathy (MCN) (see Chapters 5, 7, and 9) (Glassock, 2007). The reasons underlying these disparities are incompletely understood. Membranous nephropathy has been best studied (Glassock, 2007). DVT and renal vein thrombosis (RVT) may develop. The combined burden of both DVT and RVT in MN has been estimated to be about 45% in MN. The development of RVT in MN is highly variable with reported prevalences ranging from 1.6% to 60%. The development of DVT is highly dependent on serum albumin concentration. A DVT prevalence of <3% has been reported in those with a serum albumin >2.5g/dL and 40% in those with a serum albumin level of <2.5g/dL (Bellomo and Atkins, 1993). In many cases the DVT or RVT are asymptomatic. Ventilation-perfusion lung abnormalities can be found in about 10% of asymptomatic patients without any overt RVT or DVT and in about 20% of those with RVT alone accompanying the neph-rotic syndrome. Higher values have been reported when pulmonary angiogra-phy is used for diagnosis. Thus, all patients with nephrotic syndrome should be considered at increased risk for thrombotic events, but those with MN, MPGN, and MCN appear to be at the highest risk. DVT is the most common, but spontaneous arterial thrombosis (pulmonary artery, axillary artery) may also occur when the nephrotic syndrome is very severe (Glassock, 2007).

Therapy

Management of the thromboembolic complications of the '*thrombophilic*' state accompanying nephrotic syndrome in glomerular diseases may be divid-ed into *prophylactic* and *therapeutic* strategies. As stated above, certain catego-ries of renal diseases appear to be at higher risk for thromboembolic events, not entirely explained by the magnitude of proteinuria or hypoalbuminemia. Such patients may be candidates for *prophylactic* anticoagulation with long-term oral warfarin or short-term anticoagulation with parenteral high molecu-lar weight heparin or low molecular weight heparin derivatives, or even oral or parenteral direct anti-thrombin (hirudin-like) agents in order to prevent thromboembolic phenomena (DVT, RVT, pulmonary embolism, arterial thrombosis). The latter agents (direct thrombin inhibitors) have not yet received an evaluation for safety and efficacy in nephrotic subjects. Decision analyses as well as systematic reviews have shown that an approach using oral warfarin theoretically will reduce the overall risk for serious thromboembolic events (e.g., pulmonary embolism) in excess of the induction of serious bleed-ing manifestations (Sarasin and Schifferli 1994; Glassock, 2007) in subjects with nephrotic syndrome due to MN. However, no prospective, randomized controlled studies have ever examined the overall efficacy and safety of a pro-phylactic approach to anticoagulation for patients with the nephrotic syn-drome judged clinically to be at 'high-risk' for thromboembolic phenomenon, including those with MN. It is noteworthy that thromboembolism is rare in the 'placebo' arm of reports of controlled trials of therapy in MN (Glassock, 2007). Whether prophylactic oral warfarin anticoagulation is indicated in other glomerular diseases associated with hypoalbuminemia is unknown. Short-term prophylactic, low-dose, subcutaneous heparin or enoxaparin may be indicated in patients with severe nephrotic syndrome who are massively edematous and who are placed at bed rest or hospitalized for diuresis, trauma, surgery, or congestive heart failure.. Low molecular weight heparin should be used with caution in subjects with reduced renal function and only with appro-priate dosage adjustment. Low-dose oral aspirin could also theoretically be of benefit but this has not been proven in a randomized clinical trial. A profound reduction in antithrombin III levels may be associated with resistance to the heparin anticoagulant effect. Patients with the Leiden trait (see above) may be at special risk and therefore may be candidates for a prophylactic approach (Glassock, 2007). A family history of venous thrombosis should always be sought and if positive, serious consideration should be given to prophylactic anticoagulation. The risk of anticoagulation cannot be overlooked, especially in the elderly and those with CNS or GI lesions (Glassock, 2007).

In summary, the decision to employ *prophylactic* anticoagulation in subjects with the nephrotic syndrome is dependent upon:

- The nature of the underlying disease (e.g. membranous nephropathy
- The severity of the nephrotic state (especially the level of serum albumin).
- The presence or absence of other predisposing factors (e.g., immobility, CHF, obesity, a family history of thrombophilia).
- A prior history of thrombosis.
- The risks of anticoagulation (e.g., a central nervous system lesion, a prior history of GI bleeding, advanced age).

The final decision can only be made on a case-by-case basis (Glassock, 2007).

Patients who have already experienced a thromboembolic event, such as DVT or pulmonary emboli, should probably be treated with long-term oral warfarin, after an initial course of intravenous standard high or low molecular weight heparin, unless some serous contraindication exists. Warfarin should never be administered alone, without initial heparin anticoagulation, because deficiency in active protein C and/or S may increase the risk of warfarin-induced skin necrosis. The warfarin should be continued for as long as the patients have hypo-albuminemia and heavy proteinuria. The precise 'cut-off-point' for continuing or discontinuing warfarin is unknown, but I believe that it would be prudent to consider withdrawal of warfarin after at least six months of therapy if serum albumin is above 3.0g/dL and urine protein is <3.5g per day. The international normalized ratio (INR) for prothrombin time should be followed with the goal of maintaining the INR at about 1.8–2.0. Values over 3.0 are be associated with a marked increase in the risk of bleeding, particularly in the elderly. Values for INR between 2.0 and 2.9 are associated with a low risk of bleeding (about 5/100 patient years of treatment, but this risk may be higher in elderly subjects).

Initially, a search for an origination site of the thrombosis (DVT and/or RVT) in patients with an *overt* pulmonary embolus may not be very useful, since long-term anticoagulants will be used irrespective of the source of emboli. Patients with repeated episodes of pulmonary emboli despite anticoagulation should probably receive percutaneously placed inferior vena cava filters positioned above the renal veins.

The investigation of patients having *no* clinical, laboratory, or radiologic evidence of a thromboembolic event for the existence of a *covert* thrombosis, such as a RVT or asymptomatic DVT, is probably not routinely warranted especially if prophylactic warfarin is to be administered in any case, based on the individualized assessment of risks and benefits. Non-invasive screening studies, such as duplex Doppler ultrasonography, computed tomography, or magnetic resonance imaging are relatively sensitive and specific for RVT but contrast venography is the standard used for these comparisons (Rostoker et al., 1992). In most situations a non-invasive test would be considered adequate and renal venous angiography is seldom required. At present, despite the demonstrated utility of these non-invasive studies, there is little reason to investigate asymptomatic patients for occult renal-vein or DVT since a *negative* non-invasive screening study at a particular point in time does not mean that a thrombosis cannot develop later. A *positive* non-invasive screening study, even in the absence of an *overt* pulmonary embolus, would likely be an indication for consideration of anticoagulation, but there are no studies to evaluate the safety or efficacy of such an approach to investigation and treatment in asymptomatic patients (Glassock, 2007).

Proteinuria and hypoalbuminemia

Clinical features, pathogenesis, and pathophysiology

The mechanisms underlying proteinuria and hypoalbuminemia in glomerular disease have been the subject of many recent reviews (Haraldsson et al., 2008). Proteinuria in glomerular disease is believed to be a consequence of a breakdown in the permselectivity barrier of the glomerular capillary wall (comprised of the endothelial cell, glomerular basement membrane, and the slit-pore diaphragm of the podocyte), although this time-honored concept has been recently challenged by some experimental observations suggesting a role for impaired, proximal tubular reclamation of normally filtered proteins (Russo et al., 2007). Plasma proteins, principally albumin but including other plasma proteins as well, are allowed to pass through the glomerular capillary wall and into Bowman's space in variable amounts. The reabsorption of the filtered proteins is governed by the activity of cubulin and megalin in the brush border of the proximal tubular epithelial cell. The maximum tubular protein reabsorptive capacity is quickly exceeded resulting in overt proteinuria, which can range from barely above normal (200mg per day) to massive (>20g per day). Values >3.5g per day in the adult signify nephrotic-range proteinuria (Glassock et al., 1995). The overall quantity of protein excreted above 3.5g/d has little diagnostic significance per se although 'massive' proteinuria (>20g/d) is most commonly seen in amyloidosis, focal and segmental glomerulosclerosis (FSGS, collapsing variant), MN, and MCN. The excretion of higher molecular weight proteins in the urine (IgG, IgM- 'non-selective' proteinuria) is thought to represent a more severe permselectivity defect and a greater degree of glomerular pathologic alterations (such as is seen in FSGS). The depression in serum albumin concentration and total-body albumin mass is the result of both increased renal catabolism and urinary excretion of albumin accompanied by an augmentation of hepatic albumin synthesis which is insufficient to offset catabolic and excretory losses (Kaysen et al., 1986; Kaysen 1993b). Alteration in the plasma and interstitial distribution of albumin may also contribute to altered plasma concentration. Hypoalbuminemia is not the inevitable consequence of nephrotic-range proteinuria. Modest levels of nephrotic-range proteinuria (4–8g per day) can be well tolerated by well-nourished, robust individuals and serum albumin concentrations may remain normal presumably because of augmented hepatic synthesis (or alternatively to slower rates of transfer of albumin into the interstitial space). Urinary protein excretion rates are influenced by dietary protein intake, transglomerular hydraulic pressure gradients, by serum protein concentrations and GFR (Kaysen, 1993a). Increased dietary protein intake will augment urinary protein excretion and vice versa (Hutchinson et al., 1995). Lowered glomerular capillary pressure, as a result of ACEi or ARB induced efferent glomerular arteriolar dilatation, will lower urinary protein excretion (Heeg et al., 1987; Gansevoort et al., 1995; Hutchinson et al., 1995; Hemmelder et al., 1996). Abnormal traffic of filtered protein along and through tubular epithelial cells can induce a phenotypic transformation in these cells which then promote local inflammation and fibrosis, contributing to the progressive nature of renal disease (Abbate et al., 2006).

The degree of proteinuria seen in glomerular disease is generally classified according to quantity. Non-nephrotic or '*sub-nephrotic*' proteinuria is defined as protein excretion between 1 and 3.5 g/d while '*nephrotic*' proteinuria is judged to be present when >3.5g of protein are excreted per day in an adult (or 40mg/h/m^2 in a child). Protein excretion above the normal level (about 150–200mg/d) but <1 g is generally regarded as 'asymptomatic' proteinuria. Measurement of protein excretion based on 24-h (timed) collections of urine has largely been abandoned, because of the inaccuracies in urine collection. Estimation of urinary total protein (or albumin) excretion can be satisfactorily obtained by collection of a first-voided morning specimen and by analyzing it for protein (or albumin) concentration (by chemical or immunochemical means) and also for creatinine concentration. The protein to creatinine (or albumin to creatinine) ratio in g/g, mg/g, or mM/μM can then be calculated. The values for the first morning specimen (obtained after overnight recumbency) will generally be less than that obtained during the day with normal upright activity—so one should always collect serial specimens at the same time of the day and under similar condition of hydration. However, even with meticulous care, the protein excretion rate in patients with glomerular disease can spontaneously vary over time, perhaps due to differences in physical activity, salt intake, or dietary protein intake. This sample-to-sample biologic variation is usually <20–25%. A total protein to creatinine ratio of >3.0g/g generally indicates a 'nephrotic range' proteinuria while values of <0.2g/g would be regarded as normal. One must be sure to exclude 'tubular' proteinuria or 'overflow' proteinuria associated with primarily tubular disease or the presence of lower-molecular weight monoclonal proteins (light chains) respectively before concluding that the proteinuria is of 'glomerular' origin. Tubular and glomerular proteinuria can co-exist. Elevated β_2 macroglobulin excretion relative to albumin excretion is a feature of tubular proteinuria. The 'quality' of the proteinuria, believed by some to have diagnostic, prognostic, or therapeutic significance, can be determined by measuring the rate of IgM, α, or β_2 microglobulin excretion, by assessing the fractional excretion of IgG (FE IgG) or by comparing the IgG to transferrin clearance in 'spot' urine samples (Bazzi et al., 2003; D'Amico and Bazzi, 2003; Deegens and Wetzels, 2007; Hofstra et al., 2008). The significance of these estimates of the 'selectivity' of proteinuria will be discussed further in the individual chapters which follow. I should also point out that the magnitude of proteinuria has different associations with the likelihood of progression of disease according to the individual diseases and is also influence by gender (Cattran et al., 2008). The same amount on 24-h proteinuria has much different associations with the rate of decline in GFR in membranous nephropathy, focal glomerular sclerosis and IgA nephropathy.

Therapy

It is obvious that the best approach to the management of proteinuria and hypoalbuminemia in patients with glomerulonephropathies is to identify and correct the underlying disease. However, as pointed out in later chapters dealing with specific glomerular diseases (Chapters 4–11), this is not always possible. Exogenous infusion of hyperoncotic (salt-poor) human serum albumin will transiently increase the serum albumin concentration but in the absence of any change in glomerular permselectivity, the infused albumin will be rapidly excreted in the urine, perhaps with adverse effects on glomerular and tubular structure and function.

Therefore, except in unusually difficult circumstances, such as profound edema (anasarca) unresponsive to loop-thiazide-potasssium sparing diuretic combinations (see 'Edema,' above) this approach is not routinely recommended. Dietary measures which supplement oral protein intake are also often quite unsuccessful since urinary protein excretion almost invariably increases and total body albumin pools do not increase (Kaysen 1993b; Kaysen et al., 1998). Concomitant administration of ACEi and/or ARB will frequently reduce protein excretion rate by 30–60%, depending upon the dose and prevailing NaCl intake (Gansevoort et al., 1995; Talal and Brenner, 2001; Pisoni et al., 2002). As noted above, these effects are probably mediated by intra-renal hemodynamic alterations independent of systemic arterial BP levels, but other specific effects of angiotensin II inhibition on glomerular permeability can also participate. The antiproteinuric effects of ACEi, but not ARB may be partially dependent on elevated bradykinin levels (Hutchinson et al., 1995). In addition, a fall in systemic arterial BP appears to initiate the antiproteinuric effects of ACEi/ARB but the magnitude of the persistent antiproteinuric effect of ACEi/ARB are independent of the extent of BP reduction (Gansevoort et al., 1995). Modest protein restriction, combined with sufficient dosage of ACEi/ARB in the presence of restricted NaCl intake and/or diuretics, can not only reduce protein excretion rates but can also increase the total body albumin pool and serum albumin concentration (Kaysen 1993b). In addition, as noted previously, diuretic responsiveness may be restored in edematous patients with the use of these agents along with NaCl restriction. The addition of an inhibitor of the action of aldosterone (spironolactone or eplerenone, but not other potassium sparing diuretics, such as amiloride), even in rather low doses not associated with a prominent risk of hyperkalemia, can also lead to an additive anti-proteinuric effect, it is not yet clear whether this effect is independent of the systemic arterial BP lowering effects of such agents.

Combinations of ACEi and ARB given in maximum recommended dosages appear to have a greater anti-proteinuric effect compared to monotherapy with individual agents also given in maximum recommended dosage (Kunz, et al., 2008). However, this effect may be 'disease-dependent' and is not seen in all primary glomerular diseases. 'Supra-maximal' doses of some angiotensin inhibiting agents may also have augmented anti-proteinuric effects compared to 'conventional' doses even though blood pressure is not further reduced (Pisoni et al., 2001, 2002). The anti-proteinuric response to ACEi and ARB, alone or combination, varies among the categories of primary glomerular diseases (for example, the anti-proteinuric response to ACEi/ARB is poor in MN), and it is difficult to predict in individual patients what the response to this therapy will be in advance of a 'trial' of treatment, in adequate dosage. However, if urine protein excretion falls to 'sub-nephrotic' levels or below (partial remission) on such treatment and remains at or below this level, it is *likely* that the prognosis, in terms of progression to ESRD, is improved (Troyanov et al., 2004, 2005; Reich et al., 2007).

The effects of ACEi/ARB on protein excretion rates may not be observed for several weeks and usually continue for several weeks when the drug is discontinued. The antiproteinuric effects of ACEi may also be related to polymorphisms in the ACE gene (Yoshida et al., 1995). Patients with the DD polymorphism tend to have higher levels of plasma renin activity and plasma angiotensin II concentrations and may respond better to an ARB than to an ACEi (Hadjadj et al., 2007) but this has not been as well established for the primary glomerular diseases as in diabetic neprhopahty. Chronic administration of an ACEi may be associated with 'escape'—defined as a loss of the effect of ACEi on angiotensin II levels and aldosterone secretion rates (Werner et al., 2008). This phenomenon may have consequences for long-term use of agents in this class as monotherapy of proteinuria in glomerular disease.

Non-steroidal anti-inflammatory drugs (NSAID, e.g., indomethacin, meclofenamate, ibuprofen, celecoxib) also exert a dose-dependent, antiproteinuric effect which is potentiated by NaCl depletion and which is independent of a change in GFR (Pisoni et al., 2001). The effects may be additive to the effects of ACEi in some circumstances but are more rapid in onset and quickly dissipate when the drug is discontinued. NSAID will also interfere with the action of loop-acting diuretics and may, at times, cause acute renal failure, due to an interstitial nephritis or acute tubular necrosis. The combination of ACEi and NSAID may also produce serious hyperkalemia. For reasons of undesired side effects, NSAID are seldom used for their anti-proteinuric effects.

Omega$_3$ polyunsaturated fatty acids (O3FA; e.g., eicosapentaenoic and docosohexanoic acid) may have a renoprotective actions in certain diseases (see also Chapter 8 on IgA nephropathy), but these appear to be independent of any effect on protein excretion.

In very unusual and fortunately rare circumstances, ablation of renal function by administration of nephrotoxic agents (medical nephrectomy) may become necessary if continued massive proteinuria results in severe life-threatening malnutrition (Glassock et al., 1995). Surgical bilateral nephrectomy or intentional arterial embolic infarction of the kidneys is almost never performed for massive proteinuria in current times.

Reduction in GFR and progressive renal failure

Clinical features, pathogenesis, and pathophysiology

Many glomerular diseases are associated with an acute or even progressive, albeit variable, degree of depression of GFR. In the acute nephritic syndrome the loss of GFR may be quite abrupt and spontaneously reversible, even in the absence of 'specific' therapy. In the syndrome of rapidly progressive nephritis the loss of GFR may be abrupt or more insidious and, in the absence of specific therapy, the development of ESRD may be inexorable. In the nephrotic syndrome the loss of GFR is highly variable and some cases progress to a picture of the 'chronic' nephritic syndrome. Patients with 'symptomless' hematuria and/or proteinuria, by definition, have a normal GFR at the onset or presentation of disease, but in some instances, slow progression to ESRD may subsequently be observed.

The pace of development and progression of abnormal GFR varies widely among patients and between diseases and is determined by a multitude of factors (Jaber and Madias, 2005). These include:

♦ The severity of the initial insult to glomerular architecture (proliferation, necrosis, obliteration of capillary network, obstruction or misdirection of the flow of the glomerular ultrafiltrate, and reduction of the trans-capillary hydraulic conductivity [Lp or Kf].

♦ The pathophysiologic response to injury (including maladaptive glomerular capillary hypertension/hypertrophy).

♦ The continued activity of the underlying disease process.

♦ Concomitant systemic biochemical and circulatory abnormalities (such as hyperlipidemia and hypertension).

♦ The noxious effect of proteinuria and/or hematuria on tubulointerstitial structure.

♦ The activity and dysregulation of the balance of mediator systems (such as complement, TGFβ, platelet-derived growth factor, and PAI-1).

♦ The loss of angiogenic factors contributing to capillary 'drop-out.'

♦ The underlying genetic milieu.

Each of these interact to determine the rate and manner of changes in individual nephron filtration rate as well as the extent and pace of nephron loss and thereby the concomitant decline in GFR and its potential for reversibility (Meyer et al., 1995). *The level of renal function at the time of discovery of disease and during follow-up, the magnitude, quality, and duration of proteinuria, the severity of systemic and glomerular capillary hypertension and their control, and the extent of capillary loss, podocyte deficiency, tubular atrophy, and interstitial fibrosis stand out as major predictors of the long-term outcome of disease with respect to the eventual occurrence of ESRD.* Once a proportion of the functioning nephron mass is lost, a vicious cycle of events, unrelated to the initiating processes, is brought into play. Intra-glomerular hypertension, glomerular hypertrophy, visceral epithelial cell (podocyte) injury, and tubulo-interstitial damage are principal components of these processes. Until we have a full and complete understanding of how the various pathophysiologic, cellular, and molecular events participate in progressive disease, our approach to ameliorating progression will remain relatively empiric, but as knowledge of these mechanisms improve so does the prospects for a rational and specific therapeutic approach to reduction, arrest, or even reversal of the progressive disease process (generically called 'reno-protection') (Pisoni et al., 2001). Indeed, systematic clinical efforts to this end (called 'renal remission clinics') are growing (Ruggenenti et al., 2008).

Increased filtration of protein and its eventual partial rebsorption by the proximal tubule is thought to play a major role in progression of renal injury (see Remuzzi and Bertani, 1998, for a reviw). Such events can lead to marked phenotypic changes in the tubule and the development of interstitial inflammation and fibrosis. The precise nature of proteins involved in stimulating this sequence of events and how injury to the glomerular filtration barrier produces their undesired effects is a subject of intense research interest (Remuzzi and Bertain, 1998; Kriz and LeHir, 2005; Zandi-Nejad et al., 2004). *Nevertheless, a reduction in urinary protein excretion (by whatever method) can slow the rate of progressive loss of GFR in many renal diseases (Ruggenenti et al., 2008).*

Assessment of GFR is the *sine qua non* for evaluating the degree of renal functional depression and its progression. Classically, serial measurements of serum creatinine concentrations have been used for this purpose. In recent years, formulae have been devised to use serum creatinine concentration to 'estimate' true GFR, since measurement of the 'true' value may not always be practical, e.g., estimated GFR (eGFR), corrected for body surface area (e.g., to standard body surface area of $1.73m^2$) using the modification of diet in renal disease (MDRD) abbreviated equation (see Table 1.8 and http://www.kidney.org/professionals/KDOQI/gfr_calculator.cfm for an online Internet based calculation method) (Stevens et al., 2006). This formula, derived from subjects with CKD, takes into account variables of age, gender, and race. These factors are added as 'surrogates' for the estimation of endogenous creatinine generation, a requirement for translation of serum creatinine levels into estimated clearance or GFR values. The MDRD abbreviated formula is widely used but not well verified in diverse populations (according to diet, body habitus, ancestry, or geography) and the derived eGFR tends to have a negative bias (underestimate true GFR) at values above $60mL/min/1.73m^2$ and in the presence of obesity. The estimates of eGFR by the MDRD formula are not very accurate relative to true GFR, particularly at GFR levels $>60mL/min/1.73m^2$ (Froissart et al., 2005; Issa et al., 2008). For accurate results the MDRD eGFR also requires that the serum creatinine be 'calibrated' to the standards used in the derivation

Table 1.8 Estimation of the glomerular filtration rate (eGFR) by the modification of diet in renal disease (MDRD) abbreviated equation and the estimation of the endogenous creatinine clearance (C-G –Ccr) by the Cockcroft–Gault formula

MDRD eGFR (mL/min/1.73m^2 = 186.3 × (serum creatinine in mg/dL)$^{-1.154}$× (age in years)$^{-0.203}$ × (1.212 if black) × (0.742 if female)
C-G Ccr (mL/min) = (140 – age in years) × (weight in kg)/72 × serum creatinine in mg/dL (× 0.85 if female)

of the equation. Serum creatinine values are reproducible within laboratories but vary considerably between laboratories. This state of affairs will continue until a universal 'gold-standard' approach to quantifying serum creatinine concentration is adopted on a world-wide basis. This appears to be a likely outcome of intense efforts over the next few years (Levey et al., 2007).

Another formula, to estimate the creatinine clearance is the Cockcroft–Gault equation (which takes into account age and body weight and estimates creatinine clearance not adjusted for standard body surface rather than GFR) (Cockcroft and Gault, 1976). Creatinine clearance may be significantly altered in the present of proteinuria, due to augmented tubular creatinine secretion (Branten et al., 2005). Creatinine clearance or its estimation by the Cockcroft–Gault formula tends to provide values which are higher than true GFR, especially when marked proteinuria is present, at least when values are >60mL/min. Current recommendations are to use the MDRD equation for estimating eGFR in monitoring patients with primary glomerular disease, but due to biases caution should be exerted in interpreting the results of serial measurements of eGFR using the MDRD formula (Xie et al., 2008). The determination of whether the values obtained are normal or abnormal should also take into account the expected decline in GFR with aging and the fact that GFR is lower in females than in males, even after correcting for differences in body surface area (Wetzels et al., 2007). Non-creatinine based methods for estimating GFR, such as the serum cystatin C concentration, are also gaining favor as they eliminate the variability of endogenous creatinine production and extra-renal elimination that complicate the MDRD and Cockcroft–Gault equations (Hoja et al., 2008). Application of cystatin C measurement for eGFR is not yet widespread or well-tested in primary glomerular disease of various etiologies.

Therapy

Obviously, eradication or control of the *underlying* disease process itself represents the best chance for improving GFR and preventing progression providing it can be accomplished prior to the induction of irreversible or self-perpetuating injury. Falling short of this, consideration should be given to the employment of non-specific strategies designed to ameliorate the pathophysiologic processes contributing to progressive renal damage, such as glomerular capillary (maladaptive) hypertension, proteinuria, glomerular and interstitial fibrosis, and capillary 'drop-out.' *Renoprotective agents* are a class of therapeutic compounds which affect these processes by slowing further nephron loss and delaying the development of the ESRD, quite independent of control of the basic disease process itself (Pisoni et al., 2002; Ruilope, 2008). Control of systemic and/or intracapillary hypertension, reduction of plasma lipid concentrations, inhibition of thrombosis, retardation of fibrogenesis, promotion of angiogenesis to counteract capillary loss, alteration of the regulation of cell cycle/cell growth could all be properly classed as potentially *renoprotective* strategies. ACEi and ARB both have renoprotective properties, independent of their BP lowering effects, as do certain non-dihydropyridine calcium channel-blocking agents (e.g., diltiazem, verapamil). Additional agents, including dihydropyridine calcium antagonists, do not have renoprotective actions, even though they reduce systemic arterial BP. Theoretically, HMG co-reductase inhibitors (statins) and NSAID may also be renoprotective, but randomized controlled trials are lacking (Tonelli, 2008). NSAID should be used with great caution and in the lowest effective dose in patients with primary glomerular disease as they have a propensity to induce acute interstitial nephritis and may also produce a sudden fall in GFR because of hemodynamic effects.

Systematic reviews, meta-analyses, and observational studies have suggested a rather modest but variable renoprotective action for statins (Strippoli, 2008). Randomized controlled trials are in progress (SHARP, AURORA). Modest protein restriction (0.6–0.8 g/kg/d) combined with an ACEi/ARB *may* slow the rate of progression of renal disease in patients with heavy proteinuria and reduced GFR (25–50 mL/min) (see below) (Klahr et al., 1994; Levey et al., 2006; Mandayam and Mitch, 2006; Menon et al., 2008), but protein malnutrition is a potential hazard of such an approach in patients with nephrotic syndrome. The benefit appears to be magnified by the concomitant use of ACEi/ARB.

As a class, renoprotective agents such as ACEi/ARB should be considered in the management of *all* forms of glomerular disease accompanied by persisting proteinuria which have a demonstrated potential to progress to ESRD, providing contraindications to their use do not exist (e.g., hypersensitivity, hyperkalemia, bilateral renal arterial stenosis). Patients with heavy and persistent proteinuria, those with impaired GFR, and those whose renal biopsies demonstrate tubular atrophy and/or interstitial fibrosis should be considered as potential candidates for such treatment. Systemic arterial hypertension requires vigorous therapy, preferably with ACEi, ARB, and/or non-dihydropyridine CCB (see 'Hypertension,' above). The goal should be to reduce BP to the lowest level possible, usually 120–130/70–80 mmHg, around a mean arterial pressure of 90–92 mmHg, without impairing quality of life or inducing disabling symptoms. At times, three or even four drugs may be needed.

It must be recognized that the degree to which ACEi and/or ARB reduce proteinuria or delay the progression of declining GFR vary considerably between and among the individual diseases to be discussed in this monograph. Thus, for example, a dosing regimen of an ACEi or ARB alone (or perhaps in combination) may be much more effective in IgA nephropathy than in MN. Unfortunately, very few large, long-term studies have been conducted in homogeneous groups of patients to provide us with information regarding the likely 'responsiveness' of the individual diseases to such therapy. In addition, the precise 'optimal' goals for proteinuria reduction have not been well defined for each entity. We do suspect that they will not be the same, since the relationship of the magnitude of persistent proteinuria to prognosis varies among the primary glomerular diseases (see Table 1.9) (Cattran et al., 2008). In other

Table 1.9 The relationship of time averaged proteinuria (in g/d) to the progression of renal disease (in decline of eGFR in mL/min/year) in three primary glomerular diseases (adapted from Cattran et al., 2008)

	Decline in eGFR (mL/min/year)					
	Time averaged proteinuria					
	<1g/d	1–2gs/d	2–3g/d	3–5gs/d	5–7g/d	>7g/d
IgA nephropathy:						
Males	<1	3.8	6.1	7.0	10.7	na
Females	<1	3.0	6.0	9.1	9.8	na
Focal segmental glomerulosclerosis:						
Males	2.1	2.5	3.1	4.0	10.9	18
Females	2.7	2.8	5.0	5.6	9.8	12
Membranous nephropathy:						
Males	1.3	1.5	1.6	1.4	4.0	12.0
Females	0.9	1.6	1.4	1.5	4.8	7.3

Adapted from Cattran, et al., (2008). The impact of sex on primary glomerulonephritis. *Nephrol Dial Transplant* 23:2247–2253.

words, reduction of proteinuria from 4 g a day to 2 g per day (a 50% reduction) may have differing effects on the rate of subsequent progression of renal disease in each primary glomerular disease entity. It does appear that reduction of proteinuria is more dose-dependent when an ACEi or an ARB is used than hypertension and that 'supra-maximal' doses (above those recommended by regulatory agencies and manufacturers) of these agents might have further beneficial effects on proteinuria without further lowering of blood pressure (Pisoni, 2002; Weinberg et al., 2003). Combinations of an ACEi and an ARB are possibly more effective than either given alone in maximal recommended doses (such as in IgA nephropathy, less well understood in other lesions), but side effects (such as hyperkalemia) need to be monitored more closely. If combinations of an ACEi and an ARB are to be used at all it would be appropriate to limit their use to patients with proteinuria >1.0g/day (Epstein, 2009). One should also be cognizant of the potential risks (hyperkalemia and sudden declines in GFR). The addition of spironolactone or eplerenone, in low dosage, appears to have an additive effect on BP control and proteinuria reduction in patients who fail to achieve goal BP or proteinuria with ACEi and/or ARB, but again caution must be exercised regarding the risk of hyperkalemia in these combinations (Schjoedt et al., 2006; Chrysostomou et al., 2006; Epstein 2006). When using ACEi and/or ARB for their anti-proteinuric effects, one must pay careful attention to the need for concomitant NaCl restriction and the addition of diuretic appears to potentiate the anti-proteinuric (and anti-hypertensive) action of these agents. Not uncommonly, the serum creatinine may rise following initiation of therapy with an ACEi and/or ARB. This rise is largely due to blunting of the intra-glomerular maladaptive capillary hypertension and a reduction in the transcapillary hydraulic pressure gradients favoring filtration (due to efferent glomerular arteriolar dilatation). When the rise in serum creatinine is <25% (e.g., a serum creatinine increases from 2.0mg/dL to 2.3mg/dL) one need not stop or modify therapy. However, progressive increase in serum creatinine above this threshold (e.g., a serum creatinine increases from 2.0mg/dL to 2.6mg/dL), then the regimen should be interrupted. Such patients may have an underlying bilateral renal arterial stenosis or a unilateral stenosis in a solitary functioning kidney. ACEi and/or ARB can be used to retard progression even when the GFR is substantially reduced, but the risks of hyperkalemia may require more intense monitoring (Hou et al., 2006).

General management principles

Patients with glomerular disease should be encouraged to consume a prudent diet, low in saturated fats, trans-fatty acids, cholesterol, and in NaCl content (6g per day in the absence of edema or 3g per day in the presence of edema). Caloric intake should be sufficient to maintain ideal body weight, around

35 kcal/kg. Caloric restriction is indicated in obese subjects with BMI >30kg/m^2. Protein intake should be 0.8–1.0g/kg per day plus any urinary protein losses if the GFR is >70 mL/min. Modest protein restriction to the level of 0.6–0.8g/kg per day plus urinary losses could be used for patients with reduced GFR so long as malnutrition is not present. Protein should be of high biologic value and red meat should be discouraged. Fish, white meat, fruits, and colored vegetables should be encouraged. A vegetarian/ Mediterranean diet is best if the GFR is reduced. Increased protein intake (above 1.0–1.2g/kg per day) is usually accompanied by increasing urinary protein excretion and has little or no effect on albumin stores (see above). Total fat should be limited to <30% of total calories. Saturated fat should represent no more than 10% of total calories. Cholesterol intake should be limited to 200mg per day. Modest alcohol consumption (<60mL of 30–40% ethanol daily) is permitted. Supplementation of the diet with O3FA is permissible, but the benefits are uncertain.

Supplementation of the diet with antioxidant vitamins (e.g., vitamin C, ascorbic acid) is reasonable, but in the absence of malnutrition, supplementation with soluble vitamins B1, B2, B6, B12, or folate is not necessary, but no harm would be done if such vitamins were given in doses equivalent to minimum daily requirements (especially to older patients) A normal intake of the fat soluble vitamin E and K is suggested and supplementation is not needed. Vitamin D supplements (ergocalciferol, cholecalciferol) are useful in patients with heavy proteinuria since they are often deficient in 25-hydroxy vitamin D2 or D3 and may have a mild form of secondary hyperparathyroidism due to urinary losses of vitamin D combined with its receptor protein (Goldstein et al., 1977). Estrogen, androgen, and glucocorticoid-binding proteins are all excreted in the urine in excess in heavily proteinuric subjects (Harris and Ismail 1994). Mild hypogonadism and altered glucocorticoid metabolism may ensue but usually these abnormalities do not require active intervention. Copper, zinc, and iron are all excreted in the urine in patients with heavy proteinuria and deficiencies of these metals may occur (Harris and Ismail 1994). Copper supplementation can be helpful for leg cramps. Zinc supplementation may be useful for dysgeusia, impotence, or poor wound healing. Iron supplementation is only indicated if iron deficiency is documented. Oral or IV iron preparations may not be efficacious if serum transferrin levels are very low due to excessive urinary losses not offset by enhanced hepatic transferrin synthesis (Prinsen, et al., 2001). Oral calcium intake should be at least 1500mg/day and supplementation of dietary calcium may be necessary. Phosphate intake need not be restricted unless GFR is <25mL/min. Phosphate-binding compounds (calcium carbonate, calcium acetate, sevalamer hydrochloride or carbonate, lanthanum carbonate) can be prescribed if serum phosphorus is elevated. Aluminum-containing compounds should be avoided.

While less frequently observed now than prior to the steroid-treatment era (circa 1960), infections remain a troublesome problem particularly among children and in developing countries (Glassock et al., 1995). Not infrequently, spontaneous bacterial peritonitis may complicate severe edema/ascites in children (Rubin et al., 1975). Encapsulated *Streptococcus* and *Hemophilus* species (e.g., *S. pneumoniae*) are frequently implicated, and in pediatric patients with severe edema and ascites a prophylactic approach with oral penicillin or IM benzanthine penicillin (Bicillin®) is be indicated. Pneumoccocal immunization programs may also reduce the incidence of this dreaded but now rare complication of nephrosis in children. The occurrence of fever, abdominal pain, and ascites is an indication for emergent paracentesis with culture and leukocyte counts. Cellulitis may become severe in profoundly edematous patients and demands vigorous therapy with advanced generation cephalosporins and/or anti-staphylococcal agents (e.g., nafcillin, methicillin, vancomycin, linezolid. daptomycin). Other localized and systemic infections, such as bacterial pneumonia, urinary tract infection, infectious diarrhea, or meningitis, can be treated in a standard fashion, taking into account the potential effects of hypoalbuminemia and/or reduced GFR on pharmacokinetics and pharmacodynamics of individual agents. In patients who have or are receiving therapy with immunosuppressive agents, special care must be given to evaluation for opportunistic infections such as candidiasis, tuberculosis, toxoplasmosis, cryptococcosis, cytomegalovirus, herpesvirus, BK virus, or JC virus. Patients at high risk for human immunodeficiency viral (HIV) infection should always be studied with an appropriate serologic test for HIV antibody or by polymerase chain reaction (PCR) for virions.

IgG deficiency can arise, either from excessive urinary losses, extrarenal catabolism, or perhaps impaired synthesis (Giangiacomo et al., 1975). Sometimes this can be severe enough to impair the defense against bacterial infection (usually with encapsulated organisms). Exogenous polyvalent intravenous or intramuscular Ig replacement could be considered if bacterial infections are severe and recurrent. Vaccination with live, attenuated viruses are ordinarily well tolerated (but should be used with great caution in heavily immunosuppressed patients), however, protective humoral immune responses may be impaired, particularly when renal failure is present (Garin et al., 1983). Some vaccines (e.g Variclla) are well tolerated and highly effective even in the face of nephrotic syndrome (Furth et al., 2003) Although cell-mediated immunity may be impaired in patients with heavy proteinuria and/or mild renal insufficiency, there is no tendency for opportunistic infections unless severe renal failure is present or unless patients are receiving concomitant immunosuppressive therapy (Glassock et al., 1995).

Regular aerobic or anaerobic exercise, and even engagement in competitive sport activities requiring short-time exposure to vigorous exercise, are not contraindicated. Indeed, such activity may promote fibrinolysis and prevent thrombotic events in those with the nephrotic syndrome. On the other hand, short-periods of bed rest may be advised for those with acute glomerulonephritis during periods of active NaCl retention and serious hypertension and edema. Prolonged bed rest does not improve the chances for recovery from acute nephritis. Forced and extended periods of inactivity in overtly nephrotic subjects may have disastrous consequences by augmenting DVT or even pulmonary embolization. It is well appreciated that vigorous prolonged exercise (such as in marathon running) can result in an increase of proteinuria and/or hematuria. This effect is quite transient. While theoretically this can be harmful, no prospective studies have yet demonstrated that modest, regular exercise has any deleterious (or beneficial) effects on the progression of primary glomerular disease. Regular swimming may be the best advice, since it may be good for maintaining conditioning and does not apparently have any adverse effects (other than the potential for drowning or hypothermia).

References

Abbote M, Zoja C, Remuzzi G (2006). How does proteinuria cause progressive renal damage? *J Am Soc Nephrol* **17**: 2974–84.

Appel G (2001). Lipid abnormalities in renal disease. *Kidney Int* **39**:169–83.

Bazzi C, et al. (2003). Fractional excretion of IgG predicts renal outcome and response to therapy in primary focal segmental Glomerulosclerosis: a pilot study. *Am J Kidney Dis* **41**:328–35.

Belge H, et al. (2007). Renal expression of parvalbumin is critical for NaCl handling and response to diuretics. *Proc Nat Acad Sci USA* **104**: 14849–54.

Bellomo R, Atkins RC (1993). Membranous nephropathy and thromboembolism: is prophylactic anticoagulation warranted. *Nephron* **63**: 249–54.

Border W, Noble N (1994). Transforming growth factor-β in tissue fibrosis. *New Engl J Med* **331**:1286–92.

Branten AJ, Vervoot G, Wetzels JF. (2005). Serum creatinine is a poor marker od GFR in nephrotic syndrome. *Nephrol Dial Transplant* **20**:707–11.

Brater D (1986). Disposition and response to bumetanide and frusemide. **57**:20–5A.

Brater DC (1993). Diuretic resistance in patients with chronic renal insufficiency. In J Puschett, A Greenberg (eds), *Diuretics IV: chemistry pharmacology and clinical application*, pp.417–25. Elsevier, Amsterdam.

Bridgman J, Rosen S, Thorp J (1972). Complications during clofibrate therapy of nephrotic syndrome hyperlipoproteinaemia. *Lancet* **ii**:506–9.

Bu C, et al. (2008) IgG antibodies to plasminogen and their relationship to IgG anti-beta(2) glycoprotein 1 antibodies and thrombosis. *Clin Rheumatol* **27**:171–8.

Cameron JS (1984). Coagulation thromboembolic complications in the nephrotic syndrome. *Adv Nephrol* **13**:75–97.

Campese V (1995). Pathophysiology of essential hypertension. In S Massry and R Glassock (eds), *Textbook of Nephrology*, (eds), pp.1169–85. Lippincott, Williams and Wilkins. Philadelphia, PA.

Cattran DC, et al. (2008). The impact of sex on primary gloemrulonephritis. *Nephrol Dial Transplant* **23**:2247–53.

Chrysostomou A, et al. (2006). Double-blind placebo-controlled study on the effect of the aldosterone receptor antagonist spironolactone in patients who have persistent proteinuria and are on long-term angiotensin-converting enzyme inhibitor therapy, with or without an angiotensin II receptor blocker. *Clin J Am Soc Nephrol* **1**:256–62.

Clase CM (2008). Statins for people with kidney disease. *BMJ* **336**:624–5.

Cockcroft DW, Gault MH (1976). Prediction of creatinine clearance from serum creatinine. *Nephron* **16**:31–41.

Cravedi P, et al. (2007) Intensifiedd inhibition of renin-antiotensin system- a way to improve renal protection? *Curr Hypertens Rep* **9**:430–6.

Crew RJ, et al. (2004). Complications of the nephrotic syndrome and their treatment. *Clin Nephrol* **62**:245–59.

D'Amico C, Gentile M, Manna G, et al. (1992). Effect of vegetarian soy diet on hyperlipidaemia in nephrotic syndrome. *Lancet* **339**:1131–4.

D'Amico G, Bazzi C. (2003). Pathophysiology of proteinuria. *Kidney Int* **63**:809–25.

Deegens JK, Wetzels JF. (2007). Fractional excretion of high and low molecular weight proteins and outcome in primary focal and segmental Glomerulosclerosis. *Clin Nephrol* **68**:201–8.

de Seigneux S, Kim SW, Hemmingsen SC, et al. (2006). Increased expression but not targeting of ENaC in adrenalectomized rats wtih PAN-induced nephrotic syndrome. *Am J Physiol Renal Physiol* **29**:F208–17.

Deschenes G, et al. (2001). Increased synthesis and AVP responsiveness of Na-K-ATPase in collecting duct from nephrotic rats. *J Am Soc Nephrol* **12**:2241–52.

Don B, Schambelan M (1990). Hyperkalemia in acute glomerulonephritis due to transient hypoproteinemic hypoaldosteronism. *Kidney Int* **38**:1159–63.

Donckerwolcke RA, et al. (2003) Distal nephron sodium-potassium exchange in children with nephrotic syndrome. *Clin Nephrol* **59**:259–66.

Dorhout Mees E J (1996). Does it make sense to administer albumin to the patient with nephrotic oedema. *Nephrol Dial Transplant* **11**:1224–6.

Doucet A, Favre G, Deschenes G (2007). Molecular mechanisms of edema formation in nephrotic syndrome: therapeutic implications. *Pediatr Nephrol* **22**:1983–90.

Douglas K, O'Malley PG and Jackson JL (2006). Meta-analysis of the effect of statins on albuminuria. *Ann Intern Med* **145**:117–24.

Drummond MC, et al. (1994). Structural basis for reduced glomerular filtration capacity in nephrotic humans. *J Clin Ivest* **94**: 1187–95.

Ellison DH, Wilcox C (2008). Diuretics. In B Brenner (ed), *The Kidney*, 8th edn, pp. 1646–78. Saunders Elsevier, Philadelphia, PA.

Epstein M (2006). Aldosterone blockade: an emerging strategy for abrogating progressive renal disease. *Am J Medicine* **119**: 912–9.

Epstein M (2009). Re-examining RAS blocking treatment regimens for abrogating progression of chronic kidney disease. *Nat Clin Pract Nephrol* **5**: 12–3.

Fauchald P, Noddeland H, and Norseth J (1985). An evaluation of ultrafiltration as treatment of diuretic resistant edema in nephrotic syndrome. *Acta Med Scand* **17**:127–31.

Floege J, Feehally J (2007). Introduction to glomerular disease: Clinical Presentations. In J Feehally, J Floege, R Johnson (eds), *Comprehensive Clinical Nephrology*, 2nd edn, pp.193–207. Mosby, Elseveir, Edinburgh.

Froissart M, et al. (2005). Predictive performance of the modification of diet in renal disease and Cockcroft–Gault equations for estimating renal function. *J Am Soc Nephrol* **16**:763–73.

Furth SL, et al. (2003). Varicella vaccination in children with the nephrotic syndrome: a report of the Southwest Pediatric Nephrology Study Group. *J Pediatr* **142**:145–6.

Galla J,Luke R (1995). Hypertension in renal parenchymal disease. In B Brenner (ed), *The Kidney*, 6th edn, pp.2215–47. W B Saunders, Philadelphia, PA.

Gansevoort R, Slinter W, Aemmelder M, et al. (1995). Antiproteinuric effect of blood pressure lowering agents: a meta analysis of comparative trials. *Nephrol Dial Transplant* **10**:1963–74.

Garber D, Gottlieb B, Marsh J, et al. (1984). Catabolism of very low density lipoproteins in experimental nephrosis. *J. Clin Invest* **79**:1375–83.

Garin E, Sansville P, Richard G (1983). Impaired primary antibody response and experimental nephrotic syndrome. *Clin Exp Immunol* **52**:595–603.

Geers A, Koomans H, Boer P, et al. (1984). Plasma and blood volumes in patients with the nephrotic syndrome. *Nephron* **38**:170–3.

Giangiacomo J, Cleary T, Cole B, et al. (1975). Serum immunoglobulins in the nephrotic syndrome. *New Engl J Med* **293**:8–13.

Glassock RJ (1980). Sodium homeostasis in acute glomerulonephritis and the nephrotic syndrome. *Contrib Nephrol* **23**:181–203.

Glassock RJ (1997). Management of intractable edema in the nephrotic syndrome. *Kidney Int* (Supplement) **58**:s75–9.

Glassock R (2007). Prophylactic anticoagulation in nephrotic syndrome: a clinical conundrum. *J Am Soc Nephrol* **18**:2221–5.

Glassock R, Cohen A, Adler S. (1995). Primary glomerular disease In B Brenner (ed), *The Kidney*, 6th edn, pp.1423–4. W B Saunders, Philadelphia, PA.

Goldstein D, Oda Y, Kurokawa K, et al. (1977). Blood levels of 25-hydroxy vitamin D in nephrotic patients. *Ann Int Med* **87**:664–73.

Grundy SM (1990). Management of hyperlipidemia of kidney disease. *Kidney Int* **37**:847–55.

Hadjadj S, et al. (2007). Association between angiotensin-converting enzyme gene polymorphisms and diabetic nephropathy: case–control, haplotype and family-based study in three European populations. *J Am Soc Nephrol* **18**:1284–91.

Haraldsson B, et al. (2008). Properties of the glomerular barrier and mechanisms of proteinuria. *Physiol Rev* **88**:451–87.

Harris R, Ismail N (1994). Extrarenal complications of the nephrotic syndrome. *Am J Kidney Dis* **23**:477–97.

Heeg JE, de Jong P, van de Hern G, et al. (1987). Reduction of proteinuria by angiotensin converting enzyme inhibitor. *Kidney Int* **32**:78–86.

Hemmelder M, de Zeeuw D, Gansevoort R, et al. (1996). Blood pressure reduction initiates the antiproteinuric effect of ACE inhibitors. *Kidney Int* **49**:174–80.

Hermida RC (2007). Ambulatory blood pressure monitoring and the prediction of cardiovascular events and effects of chronotherapy: rationale and design of the MAPEC study. *Chronobiol Int* **24**:749–75.

Hofstra JM, et al. (2008) Beta-2-microglobulin is superior to N-acetyl-beta-glucosamine in predicting prognosis in idiopathic membranous nephropapthy. *Nephrol Dial Transplant* **23**:2546–51.

Hoja R, et al. (2008). Serum Cystatin C-based equations compared to serum creatinine based equations for estimation of glomerular filtration rate in patients with chronic kidney disease. *Clin Nephrol* **70**:10–17.

Hou FF, et al. (2006). Efficacy and safety of benazepril for advanced chronic renal insufficiency. *N Engl J Med* **12**:131–40.

Hutchinson F, Cui X, Webster, S (1995). The antiproteinuric effects of angiotensin-converting enzyme is dependent on kinin. *J Am Soc Nephrol* **6**:1216–22.

Ichikawa, I, Rennke, H, Hoijer, J, et al. (1983). Role in intrarenal mechanisms in the impaired salt secretion of experimental nephrotic syndrome, *J Clin. Invest* **71**:91–103.

Issa N, et al. (2008). Evaluation of creatinine-based estimates of glomerular filtration rate in a large cohort of living donors. *Transplantation* **86**:223–30.

Jaber BL, Madias NE (2005). Progression of chronic kidney disease: can it be prevented or arrested? *Am J Med* **118**:1323–30.

Johnston C (1995). Angiotensin receptor antagonists: focus on losartan. *Lancet* **346**:1403–7.

Joles JA, Koomans HA (2001). Transcapiullary fluid exchange in normal and pathologic states. In S Massry, R Glassock (eds), *Textbook of Nephrology*, 4th edn, pp.235–8. Lippincott, Williams and Wilkins. Philadelphia, PA.

Joles JA, Rabelink T, Braam B, et al. (1993). Plasma volume regulation: defenses against edema formation (with special reference on hypoproteinemia). *Am J Nephrol* **13**: 399–412.

Kauffman R, Veltkamp J, van Tilburg N, et al. (1978). Acquired anti-thrombin-III deficiency and thrombosis in the nephrotic syndrome. *Am J Med* **65**:607–14.

Kaysen GA (ed.) (1993a). The nephrotic syndrome: pathogenesis and consequences. *Am J Med* **13**:309–428.

Kaysen G (1993b). Plasma composition in the nephrotic syndrome. *Am J Nephrol* **13**:347–59.

Kaysen G, Myers B, Couser W, et al. (1986). Biology of disease: mechanisms and consequences of proteinuria. *Lab Invest* **54**:479–89.

Kaysen GA, et al. (1998). High-protein diets augment albuminuria in rats with Heymannn nephritis by angiotensin II-dependent and –independent mechanisms. *Miner Electrolyte Metab* **24**:238–45

Keane WF (1994). Lipids and the kidney. *Kidney Int* **46**:910–20.

Kerins D, Hao Q, Vaughan D (1995). Angiotensin induction of PAI-1 expression is mediated by the hexapeptide angiotensin IV. *J Clin Invest* **96**:2515–20.

Kim SW, et al. (2006) Increased apical targeting of renal ENaC subunits and decreased expression of 11betaHSD2 in HgCl2-induced nephrotic syndrome in rats. *Am J Physiol Renal Physiol* **290**:F674–87.

Kim SW, et al. (2007).Pathogenesis of oedema in nephrotic syndrome: role of epithelial sodium channel. *Nephrology* (Carlton) **3**(Suppl.):s8–s10.

Kirchner K (1993). Mechanisms of diuretic resistance in nephrotic syndrome. In J Puschett, A Greenberg (eds), *Diuretics. IV: Chemistry, pharmacology and clinical applications,* pp. 435–44. Elsevier, Amsterdam.

Kirchner K, Voelker J, Brater D (1992). Tubular resistance to frusemide contributes to the attenuated diuretic response in nephrotic rats. *J Am Soc Nephrol* **2**:1201–7.

Klahr S, Levey A, Beck G, et al. (1994). The effects of dietary protein restriction and blood pressure control on the progression of renal disease. *New Engl J Med* **330**:877–84.

Kriz W, LeHir M (2005). Pathways to nephron loss from glomerular diseases-insights from animal models. *Kidney Int* **67**:404–19.

Kronenberg F, Utermann G, Dieplinger H (1996). Lipoprotein (a) in renal disease. *Am J Kidney Dis* **27**:1–25.

Kunz R, et al. (2008). Meta-analysis: effect of monotherapy and combination therapy with inhibition of the renin–angiotensin system on proteinuria in renal disease. *Ann Intern Med* **148**:30–48.

Lee EY, Humphries MH (1996). Phosphodiesterase activity as a mediator of renal resistance to ANP in pathological salt retention. *Am J Physiol* **271**:F3–F6.

Levey AS, et al. (2006). Effect of dietary protein restriction on the progression of kidney disease: long term follow-up of the Modification of Diet in Renal Disease (MDRD) Study. *Am J Kidney Dis* **48**:879–88.

Levey AS, et al. (2007). Expressing the Modification of Diet in Renal Disease Study equations for estimating glomerular filtration rate with standardized serum creatinine values. *Clin Chem* **53**:766–72.

Lourdel S, et al. (2005) Hyperaldosteronism and activation of the Epithelail Sodium Channel are not reqruired for sodium retention in Puromycin induced nephrotic syndrome. *J Am Soc Nephrol* **16**:3642–50.

Mandayam S, Mitch WE (2006). Dietary protein restriction benefits patients with chronic kidney disease. *Nephrology* (Carlton) **11**:53–7.

Meltzer JI, et al.(1979) Nephrotic syndrome: vasoconstriction and hypervolemic types indicated by renin-sodium profiling. *Ann Intern Med* **91**:688–96.

Menon K, et al. (2008). Long-term outcome in non-diabetic chronic kidney disease. *Kidney Int* **73**:1310–15.

Merkel PA, et al. (2005). Brief communication: high incidence of venous thrombotic events among patients with Wegener's granulomatosis: The Wegener's Clinical Outcome Occurrence of Thrombosis (WeCLOT) Study. *Ann Intern Med* **19**:620–6.

Messerli FH, et al. (2006). Dogma disputed: Can aggressive lowering of blood pressure in hypertensive patients with coronary artery disease be dangerous? *Ann Intern Med* **144**:884–93.

Neale T, Ojha P, Exner M, et al. (1994). Proteinuria in passive Heymann nephritis is associated with lipid peroxidation and formation of adducts on type IV collagen. *J Clin Invest* **94**:1577–84.

Parving HH, et al. (2008). Aliskiren combined with losartan in Type 2 diabetes and nephropathy. *N Engl J Med* **358**:2433–46

Paton R, Kane R (1977). Long-term diuretic therapy with metolazone of renal failure and the nephrotic syndrome. *J Clin Pharmacol* **17**:243–51.

Perico N, Remuzzi G (1993). Renal handling of sodium in the nephrotic syndrome. *Am J Nephrol* **13**:415–21.

Pisoni R, Ruggenenti P, Remuzzi G (2001). Renoprotective therapy in patients with non-diabetic nephropathies. *Drugs* **61**:733–45.

Pisoni R, et al. (2002). Effect of high dose ramipril with or without indomethacin on glomerular selectivity. *Kidney Int* **62**:1010–19.

Prinsen BH, et al. (2001). Transferrin synthesis is increased in nephrotic patients insufficiently to replace urinary losses. *J Am Soc Nephrol* **12**:1017–25.

Radhakrishnan J, Appel A, Valeri A, et al. (1993). The nephrotic syndrome, lipids and risk factors for cardiovascular disease. *Am J Kidney Dis* **22**:135–42.

Rahman M, et al. (2008) Progression of kidney disease in moderately hypercholesterolemic hypertensive patients randomized to pravastatin vs usual care: A report from the Antihypertensive and Lipid Lowering Treatment to Prevent Heart Attack Trial (ALLHAT). *Am J Kidney Dis* **52**:412–24.

Reich HM, et al. (2007). Remission of proteinuria improves prognosis in IgA nephropathy. *J Am Soc Nephrol* **31**:3177–83.

Remuzzi G (1993). Renal Pathophysiology. *Current Opin Nephrol Hypertens* **2**:597–601.

Remuzzi G, Bertani T (1998). Pathophysiology of progressive nephropathies. *N Engl J Med* **339**:1448–556.

Ridker P, Hennekens C, Lindpainter K, et al. (1995). Mutations in the gene coding for coagulation factor V and the risk of myocardial infarction, stroke and venous thrombosis in apparently healthy men. *New Engl J Med* **332**: 912–17.

Rostoker G, Texier J, Jeandel B. (1992). Asymptomatic renal vein thrombosis in adult nephrotic patients: ultrasonography and urinary fibrin–fibrinogen products — a prospective study. *Eur J Med* **1**:19–22.

Rubin H, Blau E, Michaels A (1975). Hemophilus and pneumonococcal peritonitis in children with the nephrotic syndrome. *Pediatrics* **56**:598–603.

Ruggenenti P, et al. (2008) Role of remission clinics in the longitudinal treatment of CKD. *J Am Soc Nephrol* **19**:1213–24.

Ruilope LM (2008). Angiotensin receptor blockers: RAAS blockade and renoprotection. *Curr Med Res Opin* **24**:1285–93.

Russo LM, et al. (2007). The normal kidney filters nephritic levels of albumin retrieved by proximal tubule cells: retrieval is disrupted in nephrotic states. *Kidney Int* **71**:504–13.

Sarasin, F, Schifferli J (1994). Prophylactic oral anticoagulation in nephrotic patients with idiopathic membranous glomerulonephritis. *Kidney Int* **45**:578–85.

Sandhu S, Wiebe N, Fried LF, Tonelli F. (2006). Statins for improving renal outcomes: a meta-analysis. *J Am Soc Nephrol* **17**: 2006–16.

Scandinavian Simvastatin Survival Study (1994). A randomized trial of cholesterol lowering in 4444 patients with coronary heart disease. *Lancet* **344**:1383–9.

Schrier R, Fassett RG (1998) A critique of the overfill hypothesis of sodium and water retention in the nephrotic syndrome. *Kidney Int* **53**:1111–17.

Shearer GC, et al. (2001). Hypoalbuminemia and proteinuria contribute separately to reduced lipoprotein metabolism in the nephrotic syndrome. *Kidney Int* **59**:179–89.

Squarer A, et al.(1998) Mechanisms of progressive glomerular injury in membranous nephropathy. *J Am Soc Nephrol* **9**:1389–98.

Schjoedt KJ, et al. (2006). Beneficial impact of spironolactone on nephrotic range albuminruria in diabetic neprhopathjy. *Kidney Int* **70**:536–42.

Stenvinkel P, Berglund L, Heimburger D. (1993). Lipoprotein (a) in nephrotic syndrome. *Kidney Int* **44**:1116–23.

Stevens LA, et al. (2006). Assessing kidney function—measured and estimated glomerular filtration rate. *N Engl J Med* **354**:2473–83.

Strippoli GF, et al. (2008). Effects of statins in patients with chronic kidney disease: meta-analysis and meta-regression of randomized controlled trials. *BMJ* **336**:645–51.

Talal MW, Brenner BM (2001). Evolving strategies for renoprotection: non-diabetic renal disease. *Curr Opin Nephrol Hypertens* **10**:523–31.

Tamura K, et al. (2008). Ambulatory blood pressure and heart rate in hypertension with renal failure: Comparison between diabetic nephropathy and non-diabetic glomerulopathy. *Clin Exp Hypertens* **30**:33–43.

Tonelli M, Isles C, Curhan GC, et al. (2004). Effect of pravastatin on cardiovascular events in people with chronic kidney disease. *Circulation* **110**: 1557–67.

Tonelli M, Wiebe N, Culleton B, et al. (2006). Chronic kidney disease and mortality risk: a systematic review. *J Am Soc Nephrol* **17**: 2034–47.

Tonelli M, Pfeffer M (2007). Kidney disease and cardiovascular risk. *Annual Review of Medicine* **58**: 123–39.

Tonelli M (2008). Statins for slowing kidney disease progression: an as yet unproven indication. *Am J Kidney Dis* **52**:391–4.

Troyanov S, et al. (2004). Idiopathic membranous nephropathy: definition and relevance of a partial remision. *Kidney Int* **66**:1199–1205.

Troyanov S, et al. (2005). Focal and segmental glomerulosclerosis: definition and relevance of a partial remission. *J Am Soc Nephrol* **18**:1061–8.

Vande Walle JG, Donckerwolcke RA (2001). Pathogenesis of edema formation in the nephrotic syndrome. *Pediatr Nephrol* **16**:283–93.

Vaziri N (1983) Nephrotic syndrome and coagulation and fibrinolytic abnormalities. *Am J Nephrol* **3**:1–6.

Vaziri N (2003). Molecular mechanisms of lipid disorders in nephrotic syndrome. *Kidney Int* **63**:1964–76.

Vaziri N, Liang KH (1996). Down regulation of hepatic LDL- receptor expression in experimental nephrosis. *Kidney Int* **50**:887–93.

Vega G, Toto R, Grundy S (1995). Metabolism of low-density lipoproteins in nephrotic dyslipidemia: comparison of hypercholesterolemia alone and combined hyperlipidemia. *Kidney Int* **47**:579–86.

Wakui H, et al. (1999). Circulating antibodies against alpha-enolase in patients with primary membranous nephropathy (MN). *Clin Exp Immunol* **118**:445–50.

Wanner C, Bohler J, Eckhardt H (1994). Effects of simvastatin on lipoprotein (a) and lipoprotein composition in patients with nephrotic syndrome. *Clin Nephrol* **41**:138–43.

Weinberg MS, Kaperonis N, Bakris GL (2003). How high should an ACE inhibitor or angiotensin receptor blocker be dosed in patients with diabetic nephropathy. *Curr Hyperten Rep* **5**:418–425.

Werner C, et al. (2008). RAS blockade with ARB and ACE inhibitors: current perspectives on rationale and patient outcome. *Clin Res Cardiol* **97**:418–31.

Wetzels JF, et al. (2007). Age- and gender- specific reference values of estimated GFR in Caucasians: The Nijmegen Biomedical Study. *Kidney Int* **72**:632–7.

Xie D, et al. (2008). A comparison of change in measured and estimated glomerular filtration rate in patients with nondiabetic kidney disease. *Clin J Am Soc Nephrol.* **3**:1332–1338.

Yoshida H, Mitarai T, Kawamura T, et al. (1995). Role of deletion polymorphisms of the angiotensin converting enzyme gene in the progression and therapeutic responsiveness of IgA nephropathy. *J Clin Invest* **96**:2162–9.

Yoshimura H, Idenra T, Iwasaki S, et al. (1992). Aggravation of minimal change nephrotic syndrome by administration of serum albumin. *Clin Nephrol* **37**:109–14.

Yu Z, et al. (2005). Regulation of epithelial sodium channel in puromycin aminonucleoside-induced unilateral experimental nephrotic syndrome in normal and analbuminemic Nagase rats. *Nephron Physiol* **101**:51–62.

Zacchia M, Capasso G (2008). Parvalbumin: a key protein in early distal tubule NaCl reabsorption. *Nephrol Dial Transplant* **23**:1109–11.

Zandi-Nejad K, et al. (2004). Why is albuminuria an ominous biomarker of progressive kidney disease. *Kidney Int* **92**(Suppl):s576–s89.

Chapter 2

Glucocorticoids and immunomodulating agents

Claudio Ponticelli

Although the rationale for an etiological treatment of primary glomerulonephritis is still lacking, a number of clinical studies have shown that some subtypes of these diseases may benefit from empirical treatment based upon the use of glucocorticoids or immunomodulating agents. In this chapter the clinical pharmacology, the mechanisms of action, and the toxic effects of these drugs will be reviewed.

Glucocorticoids

Glucocorticoids are synthesized from cholesterol and secreted by adrenal glands in response to adrenocorticotropic hormone (ACTH). The adrenal cortex synthesizes two classes of steroids: corticosteroids (21 carbons) and androgenic steroids (19 carbons). Corticosteroids may be divided according to their metabolic activity into glucocorticoids (which interfere with intermediate metabolism, immunity, and inflammation) and mineralocorticoids (which regulate water and electrolyte metabolism).

Clinical pharmacology

The three natural glucocorticoids are cortisol (or hydrocortisone), cortisone, and corticosterone. They contain groups that are essential for anti-inflammatory activity, namely a carbonyl group (CO) in position 17, a hydroxyl group (OH) in 11, an oxygen (O) in 3, and a double bond in 4–5. Substitutions adjacent to critical sites increase anti-inflammatory activity and reduce mineralocorticoid activity.

Cortisol represents about 90% of corticosteroid output in humans. The secretion of cortisol increases in the morning around 3 to 4 a.m., peaks around 8 a.m., and then begins to decline. The release decreases through the afternoon and evening and reaches its lowest levels at midnight. The release of cortisol and ACTH occurs in pulses with intervals between them of 40min to 8h.

A variety of physical or psychological events can interrupt this circadian rhythm of secretion. Endogenous glucocorticoids may be suppressed by adipocyte-derived leptin and elevated by dietary acidity.

In blood, 90–93% of cortisol is bound to plasma proteins. About 80% is bound to transcortin (also called corticosteroid-binding globulin), an α-2 globulin synthesized in the liver; another 10% is bound to albumin; and a negligible amount is bound to other proteins. When the binding capacity of transcortin (about 25mg/dL) is exceeded, binding to albumin increases. In normal conditions only 10% of cortisol circulates free in the blood; this fraction represents the active hormone. The hydrophobic glucocorticoids are filtered by the glomeruli but almost 99% are reabsorbed by the tubuli. To render them capable of renal elimination, glucocorticoids are first converted in the liver to inactive compounds through a series of reduction reactions and are then conjugated with glucuronide or sulfate. These water-soluble compounds are finally excreted by the kidney.

Synthetic glucocorticoids bind less efficiently to transcortin and therefore diffuse more rapidly into tissues where they are metabolized, particularly in the liver, to active 11β-hydroxyl compounds by 11β-hydroxysteroid dehydrogenase enzymes. The conversion of inactive 11-ketoglucocorticoids (cortisone and 11-dehydrocorticosterone) into active 11β-hydroxyglucocorticoids (cortisol and corticosterone) is catalyzed by 11β-hydroxysteroid dehydrogenase, which is expressed in many tissues (Atanasov and Ondermatt, 2007).

Cortisol is cleared from the plasma with a half-life of 70–120min but its tissue half-life ranges between 8–12h. The half-lives of synthetic analogs are longer since their hepatic metabolism is lower. According to their duration of action, glucocorticoids may be divided into those that are *short acting* (prednisone, prednisolone, methylprednisolone, deflazacort), with a plasma half-life of 60–200min and a tissue half-life between 12–36h; *intermediate acting* (paramethasone, triamcinolone), with a plasma half-life of about 300min and a tissue half-life of about 48h; and *long acting* (dexamethasone, betamethasone), which suppress ACTH for more than 48h.

Mechanisms of action

After dissociation from its plasma carrier protein, the active moiety of cortisol and its fat-soluble synthetic analogs enter tissue cells. Their actions in the cells are mediated by a specific receptor protein, the glucocorticoid receptor (GR), a member of a superfamily of ligand-inducible transcription factors which is predominantly localized within cytoplasm but rapidly and efficiently translocates to the nucleus following hormone binding (Heitzer et al., 2007).

Cytosolic receptors are single polypeptides of 90–95kDa with three functional domains: the ligand-binding domain (or domain A) which is located in the carboxyl terminal region and interacts with the specific steroid; the DNA-binding domain (or domain B) which is located in the center of the molecule and recognizes specific sequences of the DNA called hormone-responsive elements; and an immunogenic domain (or domain C) in the amino terminal region. The three domains are separated by less defined regions. The non-activated GR complex resides in the cytosol in the form of a hetero-oligomer with other highly conserved proteins such as heat-shock proteins (a family of proteins produced by cells in response to various insults, including heat), and cyclophilin (a family of proteins that plays a role in the folding of proteins). When the ligand binds, the receptor dissociates from the rest of the complex and translocates into the nucleus, through an allosteric change in conformation (Fig. 2.1). This conformational change is probably centered around a hinge region at the border between domain A and domain B. Once having traversed the nuclear membrane, probably through nucleopores, the activated receptors bind to their acceptor sites alongside the genes. This enables specific transcriptional factors to gain access to the genome and triggers the transcription of DNA to RNA transcripts in order to synthesize new proteins, usually enzymes, which activate or inhibit several metabolic processes. In other instances, however, glucocorticoids decrease the expression of some genes at the transcriptional level and inhibit the synthesis of some proteins. Glucocorticoids may also exert their effects post-transcriptionally by either

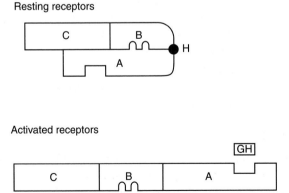

Fig. 2.1 Activation of the glucocorticoid receptor complex. The binding of glucocorticoid hormone (GH) to the ligand-binding domain causes a conformational change of the complex which rotates around a hinge region (H). A = ligand-binding domain; B = DNA-binding domain; C = immunogenic domain. Reproduced with permission from Ponticelli C and Glassock RJ (eds) (1997). *Treatment of Primary Glomerulonephritis.* Oxford University Press, Oxford.

increasing the degradation of messenger RNA or by inhibiting the synthesis or secretion of the protein (Fig. 2.2). Glucocorticoids can elicit both rapid and delayed effects. Rapid glucocorticoid actions are mediated by the activation of one or more membrane-associate receptors, while delayed effects are mediated by classical steroid mechanisms involving transcriptional regulation.

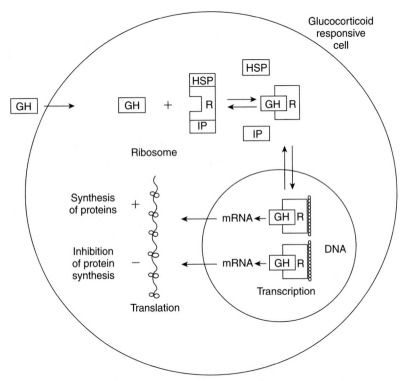

Fig. 2.2 Mechanisms of glucocorticoid action. Glucocorticoid hormone (GH) enters the cell and binds to receptors (R) that reside in the cytosol complexed to heat-shock protein (HSP) and immunophilin (IP) (also called cyclophilin). Binding of ligand to the receptor complex causes dissociation of HSP and IP from the receptors. The receptor–glucocorticoid ligand translocates into the nucleus where it binds certain DNA sequences, thus modifying their expression. In the case of increased expression (+) glucocorticoids favour the synthesis of certain proteins by increasing the transcription of messenger RNA. In the case of decreased expression (−) glucocorticoids inhibit the secretion of proteins by reducing the transcription of certain genes. The final result is an altered function of the target cell. Reproduced with permission from Ponticelli C and Glassock RJ (eds) (1997). *Treatment of Primary Glomerulonephritis*. Oxford University Press, Oxford.

In proteinuric renal diseases, glucocorticoids might exert their beneficial action by restoring the integrity of the podocyte and on the maintenance of the permselectivity barrier. Experimental studies showed that dexamethasone upregulated expression of nephrin and tubulin-alpha and downregulated vascular endothelial growth factor. Effects on cell cycle were complex with downregulation of cyclin kinase inhibitor p21 and augmentation of podocyte survival, without any effect on apoptosis. Cytokine production by human podocytes, especially interleukin (IL)-6 and -8; IL-6 expression was suppressed by dexamethasone (Xing et al., 2006).

The biological mechanisms of glucocorticoids largely depend on the number and availability of receptors, the affinity for the receptors which varies from analog to analog, transcriptional factors, and the receptor isoforms. Increasing numbers of human GR isoforms, generated from one single gene via mutations or polymorphism, have been reported. It has been speculated that composition and relative proportions of the unique receptor within a cell can determine the specific responses to glucocorticoids (Lu and Cidlowski, 2004). In this regard it is of interest to remind that the composition of GR in the podocytes may change the expression of proteins that may protect cells from injury (Ransom et al., 2005).

When given intravenously at very high doses, glucocorticoids can rapidly and completely saturate the cytosolic receptors of the target cells and can also stabilize the cell membrane. Cell membranes consist of a bilayer of fluid lipids in which inactive enzymatic proteins and activator proteins flow together to perform enzymatic reactions. At normal concentrations glucocorticoids would intercalate into lipids without affecting the fluidity, but at very high doses they can harden the membrane lipids, diminish protein interaction, and block enzymatic activities (Lamche et al., 1990).

Anti-inflammatory and immunosuppressive effects

Glucocorticoids are the most effective anti-inflammatory agents and also interfere with the immune response, cellular immunity being more susceptible than humoral immunity. These and other actions which involve most cells of the body, occur simultaneously.

Effects on inflammation

Inflammation is characterized by the increased expression of multiple inflammatory genes that are regulated by proinflammatory transcription factors, such as nuclear factor-κB(NF-kB) and activator protein-1(AP-1). These transcription factors bind to and activate coactivator molecules, which acetylate core histones and switch on gene transcription. Glucocorticoids suppress multiple inflammatory genes (cytokines, enzymes, receptors, and adhesion molecules) mainly by reversing histone acetylation of activated inflammatory genes through binding of glucocorticoid receptors to coactivators and recruitment of histone deacetylase-2 to the activated inflammatory gene transcription complex (Barnes 2006). Besides distinct genomic targets, there are non-genomic effects of glucocorticoids on the basis of the interference with membrane-associated receptors as well as with membrane lipids.

Glucocorticoids interfere also with the traffic of inflammatory cells. They cause neutrophilia both by increasing the release of polymorphonuclear cells by bone marrow and by decreasing their margination. Marginated neutrophils first stick to the endothelium and then rapidly leave the vascular bed to enter the inflamed area by diapedesis. Glucocorticoids decrease margination and therefore many neutrophils move from the endothelium to the circulating blood and fewer leukocytes pass through the capillary walls in the case of inflammation. Glucocorticoids induce a reduction of circulating lymphocytes and monocytes, because of their redistribution into bone marrow. Eosinopenia may be caused both by decreased delivery from the bone marrow and by increased margination. The causes of basopenia are still far from clear. Glucocorticoids cause vasoconstriction and block the increase in capillary permeability induced by acute inflammation. These effects oppose the leakage of proteins and fluids into the site of inflammation and therefore combat edema formation. Moreover, since less plasma protein leaks, less vasoactive kinin is released. Finally, glucocorticoids also interfere with macrophage recruitment and function, and inhibit the production by macrophages of some enzymes that promote tissue destruction, such as collagenase, elastase, and plasminogen activator.

When given intravenously at high doses, glucocorticoids can also reduce the generation of superoxide anion radicals; can inhibit the production of the platelet-activating factor, a lipid mediator of glomerular inflammation; can modify the chemical composition of the glomerular basement membrane, with consequent reduced proteinuria; and can inhibit complement-induced granulocyte aggregation without producing long-lasting abnormalities of polymorphonuclear functions.

Effects on the immune response

Glucocorticoids can exert both negative and positive effects on immune response with a dynamic and bi-directional spectrum of activities on various limbs and components of the immune response. Their impact on the immune response is mainly mediated by the nuclear factor-kB, which promotes and regulates the cytokine gene transcription.

As already mentioned, glucocorticoids produce a transient lymphopenia. Rather they have profound effects on cytokines. In particular, glucocorticoids reduce IL-2 production as well as the action of IL-2 on activated T cells, inhibit IL-1, IL-3, IL-4, IL-6, interferon-γ (IFNγ), and tumor necrosis factor-α (TNFα). Through the inhibition of cytokines, glucocorticoids reduce generation, proliferation, and function of helper and suppressor T cells and inhibit cytotoxic T-cell response. Glucocorticoids interfere with macrophage functions that are associated with antigen presentation to T cells. They can also induce tolerance to specific antigens by inhibiting dendritic cell maturation and function and promoting the development of regulatory IL-10-producing T cells. Through these mechanisms glucocorticoids may systemically cause a selective suppression of the Th1-cellular immunity axis, and a shift toward Th2-mediated humoral immunity. On the other hand, in clinical situations characterized by overactivation of Th2 inflammatory response glucocorticoids may suppress Th 2 released cytokines. The peripheral counts of CD4 lymphocytes rapidly decrease after administration of glucocorticoids.

In contrast to T cells, B cells are relatively resistant to glucocorticoids. These agents inhibit the proliferation of B cells if they are given before or immediately after stimulation. However, once B cells are already activated, glucocorticoids exert only minimal, if any, effects. The interference of glucocorticoids with antibody production is dose-related. Low doses do not affect the synthesis of antibodies but high doses may decrease serum immunoglobulin levels. This suppression is the result of an increased catabolism of immunoglobulin coupled with the decreased activity of helper T cells.

When given intravenously at very high doses, glucocorticoids can inhibit the alternative and amplification pathways of complement, can inhibit some cytokines that may alter glomerular permeability, and can inhibit immune-complex-induced changes in vascular permeability.

A key role in regulating the immunosuppressive actions of glucocorticoids is exerted by the macrophage migration inhibitory factor (MIF), which can counter-regulate the inhibitory effects of glucocorticoids. MIF is released from macrophages and T lymphocytes stimulated by glucocorticoids. Once released, MIF overcomes the inhibitory effects of glucocorticoids on TNFα, IL-1, IL-6, and IL-8 production by monocytes. MIF also antagonizes glucocorticoid inhibition of T-cell proliferation in vitro by restoring IL-2 and IFNγ production.

Toxic effects

Glucocorticoids can elicit a variety of symptoms and signs which are usually dose- and time-dependent.

Gastrointestinal complications

It is generally thought that high-dose glucocorticoids may contribute, along with stress, to increase the risk of peptic ulcer. However, this view has been challenged by some investigators. In recent experimental studies (Filaretova et al., 2007) it has been shown that an increase in glucocorticoid production following ulcerogenic stimuli may exert a protective effect on gastric mucosa, by both maintaining local defensive factors (mucosal blood flow and mucus production) and inhibiting pathogenic elements (gastric motility and microvascular permeability).

Cardiovascular disease

Glucocorticoid excess elicits *arterial hypertension* and *atherosclerosis.* Hemodynamic changes, salt and water retention, increased arterial contractile sensitivity, diabetes, hyperlipidemia, and obesity may concur in triggering or aggravating arterial hypertension and to accelerate atherosclerosis. The sodium and fluid retention caused by glucocorticoids may also aggravate a pre-existing congestive heart failure. Glucocorticoids may also cause overproduction of reactive oxygen species and thereby perturb nitric oxide availability in the vascular endothelium, leading to vascular complications (Iuchi et al., 2003).

Diabetes mellitus

Glucocorticoids increase the synthesis of glucose, decrease β-cell insulin production and reduce the effectiveness of insulin to suppress hepatic glucose production and to increase glucose uptake in muscle and fatty tissue (Fardet et al., 2007). The risk of diabetes is increased in patients with familial diabetes, in pregnant women, and in elderly patients. Usually diabetes develops after some weeks or months of oral glucocorticoid therapy. However, immediately after the administration of intravenous high-dose methylprednisolone, severe hyperglycemia can occur. It usually reverses spontaneously but in a few patients this hyperglycemia heralds the development of an often severe diabetes requiring the chronic administration of insulin or hypoglycemic agents.

Hyperlipidemia

Glucocorticoids may enhance the activity of acetyl-coenzyme A carboxylase and free fatty acid synthetase, may increase hepatic synthesis of VLDL, may downregulate LDL receptor activity of 3-hydroxy-3methylglutaryl coenzyme A (HMG-CoA) reductase, and may inhibit lipoprotein lipase. These effects can result in increased levels of VLDL, total cholesterol, and triglycerides, and decreased levels of HDL depending on the doses and duration of treatment.

Obesity and metabolic syndrome

Body weight gain is common in patients given glucocorticoids and some patients may develop a true obesity. High leptin stores in adipose tissue of obese humans are maintained by glucocorticoids acting at pre- and posttranslational levels (Lee et al., 2007). Steroid-induced obesity can aggravate other risk factors triggered by glucocorticoids and eventually lead to a true metabolic syndrome, characterized by obesity, insulin resistance, type 2 diabetes, and cardiovascular complications. Chronically elevated local glucocorticoid action as a result of increased 11β-HSD1 activity rather than elevated systemic glucocorticoid levels has been associated with metabolic syndrome. Compounds inhibiting 11β-HSD1 activity can ameliorate the adverse effects of excessive glucocorticoid concentrations on metabolic processes, providing promising opportunities for the development of therapeutic interventions (Atanasov and Ondermatt 2007). A low-calorie diet should be prescribed to patients for whom a prolonged administration of glucocorticoids is foreseen. Some suggestions have been made that glucocorticoids increase the risk for deep venous thrombosis. This increased risk could be due to immobility (due to weakness), to obesity, or to direct effects of glucocorticoids on the coagulation system.

Dermatologic effects

The most typical esthetic complication is represented by *Cushingoid appearance*, with facial and neck fullness, 'buffalo hump,' increased supraclavicular and suprasternal fat, and truncal obesity. These features are usually dose-dependent and are caused by abnormal adipose tissue redistribution. They may be reversible after interruption of steroids.

Acne is extremely frequent. Its severity is usually dose-related. Facial erythrosis and rosacea can also occur. Acne occurs early on the cheeks, forehead, chin, and chest. Rarely, the lesions may progress to nodulocystic transformation (acne conglobata). Doxycycline, 100mg daily, may be effective in reducing acne. Severe cases can be successfully treated with isotretinoin or acitretin, a second-generation retinoid. A complication seen almost constantly in patients given prolonged glucocorticoid administration is the so-called *Bateman's purpura*. It consists of irregular purpuric areas that develop spontaneously or after minor trauma, mainly on the extensor surfaces of the hands, forearms, and legs, often with spontaneous star-shaped pseudo-scars. *Striae rubrae* are wide and violaceous stripes, mainly located over the abdomen, thighs, and buttocks. They are usually irreversible, although they tend to become pale after interruption of glucocorticoids. Some patients have increased *hair growth* mainly on the face and back. Finally, the skin of patients under prolonged glucocorticoid treatment can become thin, *atrophic*, and *friable*. Topical retinoic acid at concentrations ranging from 0.01–0.05%, may improve this complication. Some patients, however, complain of irritation. Ammonium lactate 6–12% creams are usually better tolerated.

Adrenal insufficiency

Synthetic glucocorticoids suppress the release of ACTH and cortisol. To prevent suppression of the hypothalamic–pituitary–adrenal axis, *steroids should be administered in a single morning administration, between 7–9 a.m.* It should be taken into account that some synthetic glucocorticoids (such as betamethasone) induce more profound adrenal suppression than others (e.g., prednisolone). Whenever possible the administration of a dose every other day may reduce the inhibitory effect of synthetic glucocorticoids. As severe suppression of ACTH release and cortisol secretion can occur after long-term steroid administration, the dosage of glucocorticoids should be gradually reduced and discontinued only after reaching minimal doses (i.e., prednisone 2.5mg every other day). In case of serious infection, operation, or injury, patients should receive supplementary steroid administration. The degree of the hypothalamic–pituitary–adrenal axis suppression cannot be reliably estimated from the dose of glucocorticoid, the duration of therapy, or the basal plasma concentration. More reliable tests to assess the pituitary–adrenal response are considered to be the corticotrophin-releasing hormone test and the insulin–hypoglycemia test.

Infection

The risk of infection increases as the dose of glucocorticoid increases but may vary according to the age, the clinical conditions of the patient, the concomitant administration of other drugs interfering with the immune response, and the type of underlying disease. Any kind of infection—bacterial, viral, fungal, parasitic—can occur. Attention should be given to the possibility of a preexisting infection before starting glucocorticoid therapy. Reactivation of tuberculosis can occur but may be masked by the steroid-induced inhibition of tuberculin reaction.

Neuropsychiatric complications

Psychiatric reactions may occur in up to 1/3 of patients. Patients with psychological difficulties experience more frequent and more severe reactions. Decreasing the doses of steroids may improve the symptoms. Lithium carbonate is effective, while tricyclic antidepressants may worsen the steroid-induced depression.

Sleeplessness is frequent. It may be reduced by administering short-acting glucocorticoids in a single morning administration.

Pseudotumour cerebri, characterized by intracranial hypertension and papilledema, may occur in children when glucocorticoid doses are rapidly decreased. Pseudotumor cerebri can be managed with lumbar taps or increased doses of glucocorticoids.

Muscular complications

Steroid-induced *myopathy* symmetrically involves proximal muscles especially of the lower extremities. The first complaint is an inability to climb stairs. Muscle enzymes are normal. Myopathy is not related to the patient's age or to the dosage of therapy. Improvement occurs after steroids are discontinued.

Spontaneous *tendon rupture* is a rare complication which occurs mainly with prolonged therapy. This should be taken into account for patients engaged in active sports (e.g., tennis, basketball).

Bone complications

Glucocorticoids may cause an imbalance in bone remodeling which can lead to osteopenia and even to severe *osteoporosis*, through different mechanisms. Glucocorticoids decrease the net intestinal calcium absorption, increase urinary calcium excretion, inhibit the secretion of growth hormone, and decrease the production and/or the bioactivity of some skeletal growth factors, such as insulin-like growth factor 1 and transforming growth factor-β1 (TGFβ1). However, the main deleterious effect of glucocorticoids is a direct inhibition of bone formation, as they inhibit osteoblast differentiation, induce apoptosis in mature osteoblasts as well as osteocytes, and stimulate the proliferation and differentiation of human osteoclast precursors (Hirayama and Athanasou 2002). While trabecular bone is particularly vulnerable, cortical bone is relatively spared even in the long-term therapy. Calcium, vitamin D, hormone-replacement therapy, calcitonin, and biphosphonates can be used to prevent and/or treat osteoporosis. Bisphosphonates, which are potent inhibitors of bone resorption, are considered the most effective and first-line agents for increasing bone mineral density and decreasing the risk of fracture. Human parathyroid hormone has emerged as a promising agent for the treatment of severe osteoporosis when used alone or in combination with a bisphosphonate.

Aseptic necrosis of hips and more rarely knees or shoulders usually occurs after long-term therapy but may also develop in the first weeks of treatment. Unilateral hip or knee pain is the most common initial symptom. Although the cause of aseptic necrosis is still unknown, there are few doubts that glucocorticoids are important contributors in its development.

Ocular complications

Bilateral, posterior subcapsular *cataract* is a common complication. It is usually dose- and time-related but can occur even after short-term steroid therapy. *Increased intraocular* pressure, caused by decreased aqueous outflow, is a dose-related complication which can reverse after prompt cessation of therapy. Patients with diabetes myopia or a familial history of glaucoma have an increased risk.

Growth retardation

Glucocorticoids impair statural growth in children and adolescents. This effect is due to an abnormal spontaneous secretion as well as to a reduced response to the stimulation of growth hormone. Glucocorticoids also interfere with growth hormone receptors and reduce the local production of insulin-like growth factor. Since the major growth spurts occur in infancy before the age of two years and at puberty, steroid therapy may cause severe loss of height at these times. Recombinant human growth hormone may be effective and safe for pediatric patients with growth retardation (Harris et al., 2004).

Pregnancy

Glucocorticoids easily traverse the placenta, but 90% of the maternal dose is metabolized within the placenta before reaching the fetus, so that the fetus is protected from adverse effects. However, sporadic cases of fetal adrenal suppression have been reported. Prednisone is associated with scattered reports of birth defects, particularly at doses exceeding 20mg per day (McKay and Josephson 2006). There is an increased risk of cleft lip or cleft palate for newborns of mothers receiving glucocorticoids. It has been estimated to be about one case every 1000 newborns (Chambers et al., 2006).

Clinical use in glomerulonephritis

Glucocorticoids have been used with variable success in all the subtypes of primary glomerulonephritis. One of the main problems with the use of glucocorticoids is represented by their low therapeutic index. Prednisone, prednisolone, and methylprednisolone are the short-acting glucocorticoids most frequently used in clinical practice. These agents have a similar anti-inflammatory activity, but methylprednisolone has a considerably higher antilymphocyte potency than prednisolone. Deflazacort is a synthetic glucocorticoid which is an oxazoline derivative of prednisolone. Deflazacort has reduced lipid solubility compared to prednisolone. Deflazacort has few adverse effects on glucose and calcium metabolism but it is less potent. At least in rheumatic patients, the correct equivalence ratio of deflazacort to methylprednisolone is 1.875:1, and to prednisolone 1.5:1 (Saviola et al., 2007).

Table 2.1 Recommendations to avoid toxicity when long-term administration of glucocorticoids is required)

- Prefer short-term acting agents (prednisone, prednisolone, methylprednisolone, deflazacort).
- Give the entire daily dose in a single-morning administration between 7 and 9 a.m.
- Whenever possible use alternate-day administration (see text).
- Use intravenous high-dose methylprednisolone as burst therapy (see text).
- Administer the glucocorticoid during or after the breakfast.
- Recommend low-calorie intake to prevent obesity, diabetes, hyperlipidemia.
- Recommend low-salt intake to prevent hypertension, edemas.
- Recommend physical activity to prevent myopathy, osteopenia, obesity.
- Avoid sudden cessation after prolonged therapy; rather taper off the daily or the alternate-day dosage gradually.
- Consider the use of prophylactic biphosphonates for osteopenia (except if renal function is abnormal).

Waiting for new classes of glucocorticoids with reduced toxicity, some measures can be adopted to minimize the toxicity of glucocorticoids without diminishing efficacy (Table 2.1).

Methylprednisolone pulse (MPP) therapy

High-dose (500mg to 1000mg per dose) 'pulses' of intravenous methylprednisolone are mainly used to initiate therapy in patients with rapidly progressive renal disease. Theoretically, intravenous megadoses of methylprednisolone should show prompter and greater interference with the inflammatory and immune processes than oral glucocorticoids. Unfortunately, no formal studies have compared conventional high-dose and pulse steroid therapy in these instances. Pulse therapy, followed by moderate doses of oral prednisone, has also been used in patients with minimal change nephropathy or with membranous nephropathy in order to reduce the steroid-related side effects, as there is evidence from an older study that in patients with idiopathic nephrotic syndrome a short course of MPP followed by moderate doses of oral prednisone is as effective as, but less toxic than, standard high doses of prednisone (Imbasciati et al., 1985).

MPP administration is generally safe, but, exceptionally, severe complications—including seizures, sudden death, and anaphylaxis—have been reported, particularly when the steroid was injected rapidly and/or was given through a central venous line. These complications occurred generally in severely ill patients and the relationship with methylprednisolone has not always been established.

Some patients may suffer from complex ventricular arrhythmias, others complain of flushing, tremor, nausea, and altered taste. These symptoms, which may be exacerbated by the use of high-dose furosemide, spontaneously disappear within a few hours. Steroid pulses can produce severe hyperglycemia and a transient hypercoagulable state through the activation of the tissue factor factor VII. Intravenous MPP may also induce a transient reduction of glomerular filtration rate (GFR). Renal dysfunction is more likely to occur in patients with renal insufficiency or severe nephrotic syndrome, suggesting that sodium and water retention may be responsible for interstitial edema. Renal dysfunction spontaneously reverses within few days. To minimize the possible side effects of intravenous high-dose methylprednisolone, some precautions should be taken (Table 2.2).

Single morning-dose therapy

Endogenous cortisol has peak values at about 8 a.m. and a nadir at about 12 p.m. As a consequence, a synthetic short-acting agent given in a single morning dose will produce only a slight adrenal suppression, while the same dose given at midnight will bring about a nearly complete suppression of the adrenal secretion for at least 24h. Furthermore, while 10mg of prednisone given at 8 a.m. does not cause adrenal suppression, four administrations of 2.5mg each given to the same subjects at spaced-out intervals produce a considerable adrenal suppression. Therefore, for long-term therapy, one should prefer a short-acting agent and try to give the entire amount in a single dose, between 7 and 9 a.m., so allowing normal hypothalamic stimulation.

Alternate-day therapy

Even more innocuous is alternate-day therapy based on the administration of a short-acting agent in a single double dose between 7 and 9 a.m. every 48h.

Table 2.2 Precautions with the use of intravenous high-dose MPP

- ◆ Serum potassium should be checked and abnormal levels should be corrected before infusion.
- ◆ Methylprednisolone should be infused in a peripheral vein over 30–60min.
- ◆ Patients with cardiac problems should have an electrocardiographic monitoring during infusion.
- ◆ Outpatients should stay at hospital for at least 2h after MPP to verify the absence of side effects.
- ◆ Nephrotic patients should be given prophylactic subcutaneous heparin for at least 3d.
- ◆ In case of hyperglycemia persisting for 24h after MPP, further administration of MPP should be delayed until basal glycemia returns to normal values.

This regimen minimizes the interference with the pituitary-adrenal axis and reduces the deleterious side effects of a divided-dose regimen. It can also be used to help restoration of the pituitary–adrenal axis following prolonged daily administration. Alternate-day therapy is particularly indicated for maintenance therapy when the activity of a renal disease has been quenched by previous treatment. A sudden switching from daily to alternate-day therapy can be complicated by fever, arthralgias, and asthenia on the 'off' day. In the case of previous prolonged daily steroid therapy, it is advisable to switch to alternate-day administration by modifying the doses gradually.

New glucocorticoids

As both the anti-inflammatory and the adverse events of glucocorticoids are related to the ligand-binding domain of GR, efforts have been done to find selective GR ligands, with preserved beneficial anti-inflammatory activity, but reduced side-effect profile. Novel 21-*NO-prednisolone* which releases low levels of nitric oxide is much more potent than prednisolone in models of acute and chronic inflammation while reducing the bone side effects. *Long-circulating liposomal glucocorticoids* accumulate at sites of inflammation and have low levels in plasma. This characteristic should enhance their anti-inflammatory activity while reducing side effects. *Selective GR agonists* might optimize genomic GC effects as they, by modulating NF-kB and AP-1, induce transrepression with little or no transactivating activity. However, further studies are needed to confirm the better therapeutic index of these new glucocorticoids in clinical practice (Löwenberg et al., 2008).

Synthetic adrenocorticotropic hormone (ACTH)

Tetracosactide acetate is a synthetic peptide which contains the same sequence of the first 24 amino acids of ACTH. This preparation is known as Cortrosyn® (Amphastar, Rancho Cucamonga) in the US and as Synacthen® (Novartis, Basel) in Europe. Synthetic ACTH is mainly used for diagnostic purposes. There are sporadic reports suggesting a potential therapeutic role for synthetic ACTH in membranous nephropathy (see Chapter 7). Synthetic ACTH is available in single-dose vials and may be administered by intravenous, intramuscular, or subcutaneous injection.

Clinical pharmacology

Natural ACTH is a polypeptide containing 39 amino acids. The biologic activity of ACTH resides in the N- terminal portion of the molecule and the 1–20 amino acid residue is the minimal sequence retaining full activity. Thus, the sequence of 24 amino acids allows the synthetic ACTH to exert the same activities of natural ACTH. The pharmacologic profile of synthetic ACTH is also similar to that of purified natural ACTH. At a dose of 0.25mg, tetracosactide stimulates the adrenal cortex maximally and to the same extent as 25 units of natural ACTH. Following intravenous administration of 0.25mg in patients with normal adrenocortical function, plasma cortisol concentrations begin to increase within 5min and are approximately doubled within 15–30min. After intramuscular administration of 0.25mg in patients with normal adrenocortical function, peak plasma cortisol concentrations are usually achieved within 1 h and begin to decrease after 2–4h. The drug is rapidly removed from the plasma by many tissues, so that the duration of action of tetracosactide is short. A long-acting synthetic b1–24-corticotropin has been developed. This depot formulation, which allows less frequent administration, exhibits the same activity as natural ACTH with regard to all its biological activities.

Mechanism of action

In the early 1960s tetracosactide was used for treating idiopathic nephrotic syndrome but was rapidly replaced by the more active glucocorticoids. More recently tetracosactide has been used successfully in a few patients with membranous nephropathy (see Chapter 7). The main function of ACTH is to stimulate the production of cortisol from adrenal glands. However, it is unlikely that this mechanism may explain the response of membranous nephroapthy to tetracosactide. Berg et al. (2006) showed that, differently from glucocorticoids, ACTH may reduce the concentration of apo B-containing lipoproteins and increase the serum apo E concentrations. On this basis we speculated that ACTH could also restore normal levels of apolipoprotein J (clusterin) in podocytes, which are reduced in membranous nephropathy. As clusterin compete with the terminal component of complement C5b-C9 for the podocyte receptor megalin, a return to normal levels of clusterin might protect the podocyte from the attack of C5b-C9 (Ponticelli et al., 2006). Another possible hypothesis is that ACTH may act peripherally by inhibiting inflammation through the activation of the melanocortin type 3 receptor, as it may occur in acute gout (Schlesinger 2008).

Toxic effects

Hypercorticism

A prolonged administration of tetracosactide may result in symptoms and signs of hypercorticism (see above), although the risk is lower than that observed with glucocorticoids. As ACTH has a chemical structure similar to that of melanocyte-stimulating hormone, the administration of tetracosactide may cause a bronze coloration of the skin.

Allergic and anaphylactic reactions

Some patients may suffer from rash, itching, hives, or flushing. In exceptional cases patients may develop an anaphylactic reaction with difficult breathing, swelling of the face, lips, tongue, or other parts of the body. The risk is higher in patients with a history of allergy or in asthmatic patients. Patients under treatment with tetracosactide should carry a vial of adrenaline for a first aid in case of anaphylactic reaction.

Injection site

Some patients may suffer of redness or pain at the injection site.

Clinical use in glomerulonephritis

In Europe tetracosactide was approved decades ago for treating patients with idiopathic nephrotic syndrome, but no preparation is approved for this use in the USA. Tetracosactide, given intramuscularly or subcutaneously at a dose of 1mg twice a week for 9–12 months, proved to be able to induce remission in patients with membranous nephropathy (see Chapter 7). Further studies are needed to confirm the preliminary data based on a small number of patients with short-term follow-up.

Nucleotide synthesis inhibitors (Table 2.3)

Azathioprine

Azathioprine is an N-methylnitroimidazole thiopurine which was developed in the early 1950s. It is a prodrug, being a modification of 6-mercaptopurine, which in turn is an analog of the purine base hypoxanthine. Azathioprine has been mainly used in clinical transplantation and in autoimmune diseases. The possible indications for azathioprine in primary glomerulonephritis are still a matter of controversy. The drug is available for oral use, in the form of tablets, and as a sodium salt for intravenous injection.

Clinical pharmacology

The bioavailability of azathioprine is poor, with large interindividual variability and a less pronounced intraindividual variability. After oral administration, about 40–44% of azathioprine is absorbed and rapidly transformed into 6-mercaptopurine by hepatic and erythrocytic glutathione. The peak plasma concentration of 6-mercaptopurine ranges between 1 and 2h after oral administration. The mean half-life of 6-mercaptopurine is about 74min but there is wide day-to-day variability. The compound is rapidly biotransformed into mercaptopurine-containing nucleotides (thioinosinic acid and 6-thioguanine

Table 2.3 Main characteristics of nucleotide synthesis inhibitors

	Mechanism of action	**Side effects**	**Dosage**
Azathioprine	Releases 6-mercaptop-urine which inhibits both the *de novo* and salvage pathways of nucleotide synthesis	Bone marrow toxicity, liver toxicity (rare), infection, increased risk of tumor when given long term	Given orally at doses of 1.5–3.0mg/kg/d **Warning:** do not associate azathioprine and allopurinol (risk of bone marrow aplasia)! If the association is needed, reduce the dose of aza-thioprine to one-third
Mycophenolic acid salts	Mycophenolic acid inhibits guanine synthesis necessary for the *de novo* pathway of nucleotide synthesis	Bone marrow toxicity (mild), gastrointestinal troubles, viral infec-tion	1–2 g/d orally for mofetil mycophenolate and 720–1440mg/d for sodium mycophenolate
Mizoribine	Inhibits the guanine synthesis necessary for the *de novo* pathway of nucleotide synthesis	Bone marrow toxicity (mild), gastrointestinal troubles	100–200mg/d orally or intermittent pulses of 10mg/kg
Fludarabine	Purine analog which inhibits DNA synthesis of dividing and resting cells	Severe bone marrow toxicity, opportunistic infections, hemolytic anemia, neurological complications, liver toxicity, acute renal failure, graft-versus-host disease after blood transfusions	In oncology fludarabine is administered intrave-nously at a dose of 25mg/m^2 over a period of approximately 30min daily for five consecu-tive days. Each 5-d course of treatment should commence every 28d
Brequinar sodium	Inhibits the *de novo* pyrimidine synthesis and therefore blocks the synthesis of DNA and RNA	Bone marrow toxicity, mucositis, gastrointestinal troubles	Administered intrave-nously at weekly doses of 1200mg/m^2 or at a dose of 250mg/m^2 daily for 5d at week
Leflunomide	Inhibits the *de novo* synthesis of pyrimidine and/or tyrosine kinase.	Gastrointestinal trou-bles, infection (rare), liver toxicity (rare)	Given orally at a dose of 100mg/d for 3d followed by a dosage of 10–20mg/d

nucleotides) that exert effects on the synthesis and utilization of precursors of RNA and DNA. These compounds are integrated into the DNA and RNA. These nucleotides are eliminated slowly. The two main pathways of degrada-tion are direct oxidation by the enzyme xanthine oxidase and *S*-methylation, via the enzyme S-methyltransferase, with subsequent oxidation of the methylated derivatives. Both these degradation processes lead to formation of 6-thiouric acid, a final product devoid of immunosuppressive effects which is eventually eliminated by the kidney. There are racial differences in S-methylation. About 65% of Japanese people, 59% of black people, and only 42% of Caucasian people are 'fast methylators' and may therefore be considered as 'poor responders' to azathioprine (Chocair et al. 1993).

Mechanisms of action

The pharmacological activity of azathioprine rests on the formation of the active intracellular nucleotides thioinosinic acid and 6-thioguanine. Thioinosinic acid inhibits enzymes that mediate the first step of *de novo* pathways of purine synthesis from smaller molecular weight precursors, while 6-thioguanine interferes with the salvage pathway, by inhibiting enzymes required for the interconversion of purine bases. By depleting cellular purine stores, these nucleotides inhibit the synthesis of DNA, RNA, and various proteins and coenzymes, so halting the proliferation of lymphocytes which require purines during their proliferative phase. The immunosuppressive effects of azathioprine are more potent on T than on B cells. The drug may also block antigen recognition by alkylating thiol groups on T-cell surface membranes.

Toxic effects

Bone marrow inhibition This complication is usually dose-dependent but, in rare cases, myelotoxicity is caused by a genetic defect of thiopurine methyltransferase which mediates S-methylation of 6-mercaptopurine. 'Slow methylators' are particularly susceptible to myelotoxicity from the drug. Some have suggested that subjects who are prescribed azathioprine should have the S-methyltranferase activity measured beforehand so as to avoid unexpected toxicity (particularly profound myelosuppression with 'normal' dosage. Leukopenia is the most common manifestation of bone marrow toxicity, although thrombocytopenia and megaloblastic anemia may also occur. As only inactive metabolites are excreted by the kidney, renal insufficiency does not lead to accumulation of metabolites with immunosuppressive effects. However, due to the increased sensitivity of uremic bone marrow to the products of azathioprine metabolism, a reduction of the dose is advisable in patients with renal failure.

Concomitant administration of azathioprine and allopurinol, which blocks xanthine oxidase, engenders the hazard of severe bone marrow suppression because the oxidation of 6-mercaptopurine to inactive metabolites is blocked by allopurinol. *Whenever allopurinol is introduced azathioprine should be reduced to one-third of the previous dosage and blood cell count should be checked every week for the first 4 weeks.*

Hepatic toxicity Azathioprine may cause *cholestasis* which presents with a reversible increase in serum transaminases and bilirubin. At liver biopsy, lobular necrosis and biliary stasis may be seen.

A rare but severe complication, described in renal transplant recipients, is represented by *veno-occlusive hepatic disease*, characterized histologically by a fibrous obliteration of terminal hepatic venules. This condition causes mild liver enzymatic increases and eventually leads to portal hypertension and death. Early discontinuation of azathioprine may improve the outcome. Another exceptional complication, again described in renal transplant recipients, is *nodular regenerative hyperplasia* of the liver characterized by a diffuse nodular involvement of the liver and by absence of fibrosis. This condition may lead to intrahepatic portal hypertension and/or chronic anicteric cholestasis. Exceptionally, idiosyncratic reactions with acute leukopenia, fever, rash, and hepatitis may develop a few days after the first administration of azathioprine.

Gastrointestinal complications About 10% of patients may complain of gastric discomfort, which only exceptionally leads to drug discontinuation.

Dermatological complications Azathioprine may cause thinning of the hair and scalp hair loss. Azathioprine may also be responsible for changes of color or texture of the hair. Actinic keratoses may occur in azathioprine-treated patients particularly after extensive sunlight exposure. Rarely, azathioprine may favor the development of dermatitis or alopecia.

Neoplasia As with other immunosuppressive drugs azathioprine can lead to an increased risk of malignancy. The risk mainly depends on the duration and cumulative dosage of azathioprine treatment as well as by the association with other drugs or infections that may impair the immunological surveillance. It is also possible that the DNA substitution by 6-thioguanine increases chemical reactivity of DNA 6-thioguanine and contributes to the increased risk of acute myeloid leukemia and skin cancer.

A high incidence of cancer has been reported in organ transplant recipients treated with azathioprine and steroids. Malignancies commonly seen in the general population do not increase, while squamous cell carcinoma, '*in situ*' carcinoma of the cervix, non-Hodgkin's lymphomas, lip cancers, carcinomas of the vulva and perineum, and sarcoma have a high incidence in azathioprine-treated transplant patients (Penn 1991). The incidence of squamous cell carcinomas are strikingly elevated in countries with high ambient UV light exposure (such as Australia), and UV absorbing skin creams should be routinely prescribed when azathioprine is used in these circumstances. Immunosuppression can increase the risk for Kaposi's sarcoma, which is particularly frequent in Mediterranean countries, in Sub-Saharan areas, and in Jewish descent.

The oncogenic risk of azathioprine in autoimmune diseases is more difficult to assess. A systematic review aimed to determine the trade off between the benefits and risks of azathioprine in multiple sclerosis, hypothesized that a long-term risk of cancer from azathioprine may be related to a treatment duration above 10 years and cumulative doses above 600 g (Casetta et al., 2007). There is little information about the risk of malignancy in primary glomerulonephritis but sporadic cases of cancer in azathioprine-treated patients have been reported. The problem is complicated by the fact that in some cases glomerulonephritis is secondary to cancer.

Infections The interference of azathioprine with cellular immunity may theoretically account for a high rate of infections, particularly in leukopenic patients. Usually, however, azathioprine is well tolerated and its use does not account for an increased risk of infections, except for patients with bone marrow suppression.

Hypersensitivity reactions While hypersensitivity reactions are uncommon, an acute hypersensitivity interstitial nephritis has been observed. Such patients may have fever, rash, and renal failure. The hypersensitivity can be due to the parent 6-mercaptopurine compound or to the imidazole ring only.

Pregnancy Only inactive metabolites pass into the fetal circulation. The FDA classified azathioprine as a drug at risk of teratogenic effects on the basis of animal studies. Sporadic congenital malformations were reported in babies of women who were receiving azathioprine,and dose-related fetal myelosuppression and transient neonatal immunosuppression were also reported. However, the transplantation community has not recommended that transplant recipients should avoid taking azathioprine during pregnancy. The long-term consequences of *in-utero* exposure to azathioprine are unknown (McKay and Josephson 2006).

Clinical use in glomerulonephritis

Azathioprine has been used in several types of primary glomerulonephritis. The results have not been very impressive and after initial enthusiasm azathioprine has almost been abandoned, although some studies reported a possible benefit.

The drug is administered at doses ranging between 1.5 and 3mg/kg per day. During treatment, circulating leukocytes should be checked regularly, every 7–10d initially and at longer intervals when leukocytes maintain stable levels with a fixed dose of azathioprine. We suggest not to attempt to induce leukopenia deliberately with this drug, since there is no evidence that leukopenia improves the response to treatment while it certainly does increase the risk of infections. Therefore, the dose should be halved whenever the leukocyte count falls below 5000 per mm³, and azathioprine should be stopped if the leukocyte level falls below 3000 per mm³. The concomitant use of allopurinol and azathioprine should be avoided, since bone marrow toxicity is dangerously increased by this association. Should the use of allopurinol be necessary, the dose of azathioprine must be reduced to one-third. Liver transaminases should be checked regularly in the case of prolonged therapy with azathioprine.

Mycophenolic acid (MPA)

MPA inhibits the enzyme inosin monophosphate dehydrogenase, by which guanine is synthesized from inosine. As a consequence the *de novo* pathway of purine synthesis is inhibited. Unlike azathioprine it is not incorporated into DNA. Since activated lymphocytes rely more than other cells on *de novo* pathway, T and B cells are preferentially affected by MPA, which causes an accumulation of lymphocytes at the G1–S phase of the cell cycle. There are two salts of mycophenolic acid, *mycophenolate mofetil (MMF)* and an enteric coated formulation of *sodium mycophenolate*. These drugs are largely used in organ allotransplantation and in lupus nephritis. Non-randomized studies also reported promising results in primary glomerulonephritis, but randomized trials in some primary glomerular disease are less encouraging i.e IgA nephropathy. The two drugs are available for oral use, in the form of tablets. A tablet of the enteric coated formulation of 360mg is equivalent to a tablet of 500mg of MMF.

Clinical pharmacology

MMF and enteric coated sodium mycophenolate are prodrugs of mycophenolic acid. After oral administration MMF is rapidly reabsorbed and hydrolyzed by esterases to the active moiety MPA. There is a peak in plasma concentration of MPA between 0.5–1.0h after oral administration of MMF and a second peak between 6–12 h post-dose, caused by enterohepatic cycle. Differently from MMF the enteric coated formulation does not release MPA under acidic conditions (pH <5) as in the stomach but is highly soluble in neutral pH conditions as in the intestine. Therefore it reaches a peak concentration in plasma later than MMF. Following oral administration the median time to maximum concentration of MPA ranges between 1.5–2.75h.

In the liver, MPA is mainly metabolized by glucuronyl transferase to acid glucuronide MPA (MPAG) which does not manifest pharmacological activity. A minor metabolite is acyl glucoronide which has a pharmacologic activity comparable to MPA. A dynamic equilibrium occurs between MPAG and free MPA in the blood. MPA is highly protein-bound to albumin, >98%. Thus the free MPA concentration may increase in the presence of hypoalbuminemia. The protein binding of MPAG is 82%.

The majority of MPA dose administered is eliminated in the urine primarily as MPAG (>60%) and approximately 3% as unchanged MPA. The mean renal clearance of MPAG is approximately 15mL/min. MPAG is also secreted in the bile and available for deconjugation by gut flora. MPA resulting from the deconjugation may then be reabsorbed and produce a second peak approximately 6–8 h after drug administration. The mean elimination half-life of MPA and MPAG ranges between 8–16h, and 13–17h, respectively. MPA exposure is not appreciably influenced by impaired renal function.

Mechanisms of action

MPA is an uncompetitive and reversible inhibitor of inosine monophosphate dehydrogenase (IMPDH) and induces a striking conformational change in IMPDH protein in intact cells, resulting in the formation of annular aggregates of protein with concomitant inhibition of IMPDH activity. As a result MPA produces a marked reduction of guanosine triphosphate necessary for DNA synthesis and inhibits the *de novo* pathway of guanosine nucleotide synthesis without incorporation to DNA. MPA is not a nucleotide and therefore does not require incorporation into DNA, as does azathioprine. Because T- and B-lymphocytes are critically dependent for their proliferation on *de novo* synthesis of purines, whereas other cell types can utilize salvage pathways, MPA has potent cytostatic effect on lymphocytes. Experimental studies have also found that MMF diminished the fibroblasts contractily and motility. This may result in beneficial therapeutic effects of MMF against fibrotic lesions.

Toxic effects

Bone marrow toxicity The risk of leukopenia with *mycophenolate salts* is increased in patients with high circulating levels of free MPA, which may occur in case of hypoalbuminemia. Interaction between MPA and valacyclovir may also lead to neutropenia. In renal transplant recipients it has been reported that anemia is more frequent with MMF than with azathioprine (Vanrenterghem et al., 2003). Thrombocytopenia is uncommon.

Gastrointestinal toxicity Nausea, vomiting, and in particular diarrhea are relatively frequent in patients treated with mycophenolate salts. These complications are related to the doses of the drug and to the peak concentration of MPA in the blood (Behrend and Braun 2005). The gastric adverse effects are irritative in nature and are often reversible. However, in a number of patients they may require a dose change or even the discontinuation of the drug. As gastric symptoms are related to the peak blood concentration, it is advisable to subdivide the daily dose of MMF in two or even three administrations. The enteric coated formulation of mycophenolate sodium has a later and lower peak concentration in the blood and might mitigate the incidence and the impact of gastrointestinal disturbs.

Hepatic toxicity Rare cases of increased liver enzymes, which returned to normal levels after reducing the dosage of MMF, have been reported.

Pulmonary toxicity In rare cases MMF may cause dry cough and dyspnea. In most patients symptoms develop within the third month and may raise problems of differential diagnosis with pnemonitis. Exceptionally, MMF may lead to pulmonary fibrosis and acute respiratory failure. The clinical symptoms reverse only after MMF discontinuation.

Acute inflammatory syndrome A paradoxical pro-inflammatory reaction of polymorphonuclear cells, characterized by fever, arthralgias, oligoarthritis, and increased levels of reactive C protein may exceptionally occur. The syndrome is completely reversible with the discontinuation of the drug.

Neoplasia Although MPA may theoretically favor an increased risk of tumor through an impairment in the immune surveillance, it has been shown to have an antiproliferative activity against leukemia and lymphoma and an anti-tumor effect against colon and prostate cancer. In renal transplant recipients the use of mycophenolate is associated with a reduced incidence of lymphoproliferative disorder (Vasudev and Hariharan 2007).

Infections As all other immunosuppressive agents mycophenolate may render the patients more susceptible to infections. In organ transplant recipients given mycophenolate the risk of cytomegalovirus infection is increased. The risk is dose dependent and is highly influenced by the concomitant use of glucocorticoids or other immunosuppressive agents. An increased risk of polyoma BK virus interstitial nephritis has been reported in patients given the association tacrolimus with mycophenolate (Hirsch et al., 2002).

Pregnancy Use of mycophenolate salts during pregnancy is associated with an increased risk of first trimester pregnancy loss and increased risk of congenital malformation, especially external ear and other facial abnormalities including cleft lip and palate and anomalies of the distal limbs, heart, esophagus, and kidney (McKay and Josephson 2006) (FDA Category D). Female patients being considered for treatment with either of the mycophenolate salts should always have a negative pregnancy test and should employ at least two methods of contraception during its use. If pregnancy occurs, the drug should be stopped. Azathioprine can be substituted for mycophenolate under these circumstances.

Clinical use in glomerulonephritis

Both MMF and mycophenolate sodium might be indicated for prolonged treatments in view of their relative safety. However, the indications, the dosage, the duration of treatment, and the possible associations in primary glomerulonephritis are still unclear. Good results have been reported in minimal change nephropathy. In focal glomerular sclerosis and in membranous nephropathy some uncontrolled studies reported the effectiveness of MMF in reducing proteinuria in patients who failed to respond to conventional treatments, but complete remission was rare, relapses were common, and kidney function deterioration was not affected in a number of patients. Controlled trials of MMF in membranous nephropathy have been less encouraging, at least when MMF was given without steroids. The results with IgA nephropathy are very inconsistent. Although these drugs may well find a place in the management of proteinuric renal diseases, well designed randomized trials are needed to better evaluate their proper evidence-based role in patients with primary glomerulonephritis.

Mizoribine

Mizoribine, also called bredinin, is an imidazole nucleoside which demonstrated immunosuppressive activity in various animal models, in renal transplant recipients and in Japanese patients with steroid-resistant nephrotic syndrome. Clinical advantages with this imidazole have also been reported in patients with rheumatoid arthritis, lupus nephritis, and other rheumatic diseases. It is administered orally in the form of tablets. It is not approved for use in USA or in Europe, only in Asia.

Clinical pharmacology

Pharmacokinetic studies of mizoribine showed that the peak serum level appeared 2-4h after oral administration of 50–200mg, with a linear relationship between the dose and the peak serum mizoribine level. The elimination rate from serum depends on kidney function, and the elimination rate constant is well correlated with the endogenous creatinine clearance. No circadian rhythm is apparent in the elimination rate constant. The absorption rate of bredinin from the gastrointestinal tract may be affected by gastrointestinal diseases. Dosage adjustment based on the renal function is suggested

Mechanisms of action

Mizoribine and its metabolites exert activity through selective inhibition of inosine monophosphate synthetase and guanosine monophosphate synthetase, resulting in the complete inhibition of guanine nucleotide synthesis without incorporation into nucleotides. Thus, mizoribine blocks the *de novo* synthesis of the purine guanosine. The proliferation of T and B cells is especially sensitive to inhibition by mizoribine. On the other hand, most non-immune cells are resistant to the drug because they can meet their requirements for guanosine by using enzymes in the salvage pathway. Mizoribine has immunosuppressive effects comparable to those of azathioprine but exerts less toxicity on bone marrow and liver. A major problem is enterotoxicity, which can be prevented by once-daily administration, keeping the serum levels below 0.5mcg/mL.

Clinical use in glomerulonephritis

The mechanisms of action and the indications of mizoribine are similar to those of mycophenolic acid. Most reports on this drug come from Japan, where mizoribine is produced. In the field of renal diseases mizoribine has been mostly used in lupus nephritis. The drug has also been successfully administered in patients with focal segmental glomerular sclerosis, membranous nephropathy, and IgA nephritis without serious adverse effects. Unfortunately there are no controlled randomized trials. It is also unclear which is the best regimen. Usually mizoribine was administered daily at a dose of 100–200mg either given in a single dose or three times in a day. Other investigators used intermittent pulse therapy (10mg/kg) to obtain higher peak serum levels and higher efficacy in severe cases of lupus nephritis. As for MPA it is difficult to assess the role of mizoribine in primary glomerulonephritis until well designed, prospective, randomized trials will be available.

Fludarabine

Fludarabine is a purine analogue which is used in the treatment of chronic lymphocytic leukemia, indolent non-Hodgkin's lymphomas, and acute myeloid leukemia. Because of its immunosuppressive effects, fludarabine has been used in cryobulinemic nephritis and lupus nephritis. It can be administered orally or by intravenous infusion in a central vein.

Clinical pharmacology

Fludarabine is the phosphate salt of a fluorinated nucleotide antimetabolite analog of the antiviral agent vidarabine. After intravenous administration, Fludarabine phosphate is rapidly dephosphorylated to 2-fluoro-ara-A (F-ara-A) and then phosphorylated intracellularly by deoxycytidine kinase to the active triphosphate, 2-fluoro-ara-ATP. After oral administration the bioavailability ranges between 50–55% with large interindividual but minimal intraindividual variability. There are wide variations in the half-life (7–33h) and in the area under the curve. F-ara-A is eliminated by the urine (50–60%). Therefore the doses of fludarabine should be adjusted to the levels of creatinine clearance and the use of the drug should be avoided in patients with a creatinine clearance < 30mL/min.

Mechanisms of action

F-ara-A is the major intracellular metabolite of fludarabine and the only metabolite with known cytotoxic activity. This metabolite inhibits DNA synthesis by interfering with ribonucleotide reductase and DNA polymerase. It is active against both dividing and resting cells. The immunosuppressive effect is related to the inhibition of a key component of signal transduction of lymphocyte activation.

Toxic effects

Myelosuppression Fludarabine causes profound and long-lasting lymphopenia. Moreover anemia, thrombocytopenia, and neutropenia are frequent and severe, with a nadir ranging between 13–16d after fludarabine administration. Regular blood count monitoring is mandatory. Some patients require blood or platelet transfusion, and injections of granulocyte-colony stimulating factor to boost neutrophil counts.

Opportunistic infections The profound lymphopenia increases the risk of opportunistic infections significantly. Patients who have been treated with fludarabine should take co-trimoxazole or use monthly nebulized pentamidine to prevent *Pneumocystis jiroveci* pneumonia.

Transfusions The profound lymphopenia caused by fludarabine renders patients susceptible to transfusion-associated graft-versus-host disease, a fatal complication of blood transfusion. For this reason, all patients who have ever received fludarabine *should only be given irradiated blood components.*

Autoimmune hemolytic anemia Fludarabine is associated with the development of severe autoimmune hemolytic anemia in a proportion of patients. Hemolysis may occur after infusion or in the intervals.

Neurological complications An irreversible neurotoxic syndrome with cortical blindness, optic neuritis, enecephalopathy, seizures, and coma may occur after administration of high doses of fludarabine. A milder reversible neurotoxicity is relatively frequent even at normal doses in the elderly patients.

Hepatotoxicity An increase in transaminase may occur in a number of patients treated with fludarabine for hematological malignancies.

Renal toxicity Cases of acute renal failure or even crescentic glomerulonephritis have been reported.

Pregnancy Fludarabine phosphate is teratogenic in rats and in rabbits causing an increased incidence of various skeletal malformations. There are no adequate and well-controlled studies in pregnant women but the drug has been classified by the FDA among the drugs that can cause human malformation. If a woman becomes pregnant while taking fludarabine, she should be appraised of the potential hazard to the fetus. Women of childbearing potential or fertile males must take contraceptive measures during and at least for 6 months after cessation of therapy.

Clinical use in glomerulonephritis

In spite of some good results with fludarabine in lupus and cryoglobulinemic glomerulonephritis, fludarabine has not found a role in treatment of primary glomerulonephritis mainly because of its elevated toxicity. Some good results have been observed in patients with membranous nephropathy (Boumpas et al., 1999).

Brequinar sodium

Brequinar is a synthetic quinolinecarboxylic acid analog with antineoplastic properties. Brequinar inhibits the *de novo* biosynthesis of pyrimidines and can interfere with the production of T and B cells. The drug has been used in organ transplantation.

Clinical pharmacology

The pharmacokinetics of brequinar in patients with cancer are characterized by an oral clearance of approximately 30mL/min and a long terminal half life (13–18 h). In organ transplant recipients the clearance is lower either because of a drug interaction with cyclosporine or because of altered clearance or metabolic processes.

Mechanisms of action

Brequinar inhibits the human mitochondrial enzyme dihydroorotate dehydrogenase which catalyses the conversion of dihydroorotate to orotate concurrent with the reduction of ubiquinone. Human dihydroorotate dehydrogenase has two domains: an α/β-barrel domain containing the active site and an α-helical domain that forms the opening of a tunnel leading to the active site.

Brequinar has a binding site in this tunnel. By inhibiting dihydroorotate dehydrogenase, brequinar causes a blockage in the pyrimidine *de novo* biosynthesis and therefore reduces the synthesis of proliferating T and B cells without interfering with the production of cytokines.

Toxic effects

In humans, brequinar can be responsible for bone marrow toxicity, mucositis, nausea, and vomiting. There is little information about its potential teratogenic effects.

Clinical use in glomerulonephritis

Brequinar is particularly active on proliferating T cells and may therefore find a role in autoimmune diseases. Brequinar might be synergistic with cyclosporine and tacrolimus. It could also be synergistic with mycophenolic acid, since the two drugs interfere with two different steps of the *de novo* synthesis. However there are no studies with this compound in primary glomerulonephritis.

Leflunomide

Leflunomide is an isoxazole derivative, a prodrug that releases the active compound A771726. Leflunomide has been shown to be active in some models of lupus nephritis and Heymann nephritis. It has proved to be effective and well tolerated in patients with rheumatoid arthritis and is currently approved for this use by the FDA and EMEA. Leflunomide produces neither myelotoxicity nor nephrotoxicity and does not require dose adjustment in case of renal insufficiency. It is available in the form of tablets. The initial dosage in patients with rheumatoid arthritis is 100mg/24h for 3d followed by a dose of 10–20mg/d.

Clinical pharmacology

After absorption leflunomide is converted to its active metabolite A771726, a malononitrilamide, possibly in the gut wall, in plasma, and in the liver. Peak plasma concentrations of A771726 are reached 6–12 h after leflunomide administration and appear to be linear across the dosage range of 5–25mg daily. The drug undergoes enterohepatic circulation and biliary recycling may contribute to its long elimination half-life (15–18d). The active metabolite is extensively protein bound (>99%) and is cleared by biliary and renal excretion. Plasma levels of A771726 remain above 0.02mg/L (the level above which teratogenic effects could still occur) for up to 2 years after stopping leflunomide.

Mechanisms of action

The exact mode of action of leflunomide is still poorly defined. The active metabolite A771726 binds to mitochondrial enzyme dihydroorotate dehydrogenase, which is involved in the synthesis of pyrimidines. This leads to a reduction in uridine triphosphate levels and pyrimidine synthesis by lymphocytes. The action of the enzyme tyrosine kinase is also reduced. These effects result in changes in DNA and RNA synthesis and T- and B-cell proliferation in addition to suppression of immunoglobulin production and interference with cell adhesion. Leflunomide inhibits the T-cell receptor signal and CD28 signal, which are resistant to CsA. Moreover, leflunomide inhibits the T–B cell interaction and T-independent antibody formation. Leflunomide may also exert anti-viral effects against polyoma BK virus and herpes virus 1 while its efficacy against cytomegalovirus infection is controversial.

Toxic effects

Gastrointestinal effects Diarrhea, nausea, and dyspepsia may occur in 10–20% of patients when leflunomide is administered at a dose of 20mg/d.

Bone marrow toxicity Transient cases of thrombocytopenia, leukopenia, and eosinophilia may occur.

Infections The risk of infections in patients with rheumatoid arthritis given leflunomide at a dose of 20mg/day is similar to that observed with standard methotrexate therapy.

Hepatotoxicity Increase in liver enzymes may occur in 2–4% of patients treated with leflunomide. There was a public statement on leflunomide from the EMEA regarding severe and serious hepatic reactions, but an extensive review made by FDA concluded that there was no consistent signal of serious level injury in rheumatic patients treated with leflunomide.

Pregnancy Animal studies indicate that the exposure to leflunomide during pregnancy has teratogenic and fetotoxic effects. The drug should not be used in women who are pregnant or who are contemplating pregnancy.

Malignancy To date, leflunomide has not been associated with an increased risk of malignancy.

Clinical use in glomerulonephritis

Apart from its use in rheumatoid arthritis, leflunomide has been used in association with glucocorticoids in lupus nephritis and in Wegener's granulomatosis. Studies in rats suggested a possible role for leflunomide in glomerulonephritis induced by antibasement membrane antibody. A small controlled trial in patients with IgA glomerulonephritis reported that in patients treated with leflunomide the mean proteinuria decreased from 1.6g /d to 0.6g/ d, a result non-significantly different from that observed in the arm assigned to the ACE-inhibitor fosinopril (Lou et al., 2006). It is not approved for use in glomerular disease by the FDA or by the EMEA.

Alkylating agents

These agents derive from nitrogen mustards, which are compounds with marked cytotoxic action on proliferating cells. This property has been exploited for cancer chemotherapy and many variants of nitrogen mustards have been prepared in order to improve their effectiveness and to reduce their side effects. Alkylating agents have in common the capacity to contribute alkyl groups to biologically vital macromolecules such as DNA. They are therefore called alkylating agents.

These drugs have been used by many clinicians in most subtypes of primary glomerulonephritis, unfortunately with variable results. No alkylating agent is approved for use in glomerular disease in the USA or in Europe. The two alkylating agents most frequently used in clinical nephrology are cyclophosphamide and chlorambucil.

Cyclophosphamide

Cyclophosphamide is an oxazaphosphorine with two chloroethyl groups on the exocyclic nitrogen atom. The drug is supplied as tablets and as a powder for injection.

Clinical pharmacology

Cyclophosphamide is a prodrug that is activated primarily in the liver. The hepatic cytochrome P-450 monooxygenase enzyme converts cyclophosphamide to 4-hydroxycyclophosphamide. Tautomerization of this metabolite yields the ring-opened aldophosphamide from which the active metabolites derive. Aldophosphamide and 4-hydroxycyclophosphamide are in a steady state; the two compounds can be further oxidized to inactive metabolites such as carboxycyclophosphamide (detoxification). Aldophosphamide is transported by the circulatory system to the target cells, where it is cleaved to phosphoramide mustard which alkylates target sites in susceptible cells, and to acrolein. The cytotoxic effects of cyclophosphamide are related to the total amount rather than to the velocity of generation of activated metabolites. Thus the biological activity of the drug is more affected by detoxification and by elimination than by changes in the rate of generation of the activated metabolites Some individuals, termed 'low carboxylators,' have been reported to excrete minimal amounts of inactive metabolites. This could have considerable clinical importance since variations in detoxification may lead to an accumulation of aldophosphamide with increased toxicity and efficacy of cyclophosphamide.

There is a large interpatient variability in the pharmacokinetics and metabolism of cyclophosphamide. Its protein binding capacity is low, 13–20%; maximal concentrations in plasma are usually achieved 1h after oral administration, and the drug is nearly completely cleared from plasma by 24h after its administration. The half-life of cyclophosphamide ranges between 5–8h in adults and between 3–6h in children. Phosphoramide mustard, carboxycyclophosphamide, and acrolein are the principal metabolites found in urine.

Mechanisms of action

Alkylating agents form covalent linkages by alkylating various nucleophilic moieties such as phosphate, amino, sulphydryl, hydroxyl, carboxyl, and imidazole groups. Thus the most important pharmacological actions are those that disturb the fundamental mechanisms concerned with cell growth, mitotic activity, differentiation, and function. The alkylating agents exert a marked action against cells in the dividing phase and may also alkylate quiescent cells, but in non-proliferating cells the process of alkylation is not a lethal event since the DNA repair systems correct lesions in the DNA prior to the next cellular division.

The biologic activity is based upon the presence of a bis-(2-chloroethyl) grouping. In the case of cyclophosphamide, bis-(2-chloroethyl) groups are linked to a cyclic phosphamide ester, which replaces the N-methyl of mechlorethamine. This makes cyclophosphamide relatively inert, compared with mechlorethamine, because the bis-(2-chloroethyl) groups do not ionize until the cyclic phosphamide is cleaved. However, after the drug undergoes metabolic activation it shows marked chemotherapeutic effects.

Both T and B lymphocytes, which are relatively resistant to some nitrogen mustards, are sensitive to the effects of cyclophosphamide. The drug is particularly effective at reducing antibody production by B cells. These actions can explain its important immunosuppressive effects.

Toxic effects

Bladder toxicity The excretion in the urine of acrolein, an inactive metabolite of aldophosphamide, can exert toxic effects on the bladder epithelium. As a consequence a sterile hemorrhagic cystitis characterized by gross or microscopic hematuria (typically isomorphic/normomorphic) and voiding symptoms (dysuria, frequency, urgency) can develop. More rarely, prolonged treatments with cyclophosphamide may be complicated by bladder fibrosis and, exceptionally, by bladder cancer (transitional cell carcinoma). There is no doubt that hemorrhagic cystitis is an inflammatory process. Many cytokines such as tumor necrosis factor and the interleukin family and transcription factors such as NF-kB and AP-1 also play a role in its pathogenesis. When these molecular factors are taken into account, pathogenesis of cyclophosphamide-induced bladder toxicity can be summarized in three steps:

♦ Acrolein rapidly enters into the uroepithelial cells.

♦ It activates intracellular reactive oxygen species and nitric oxide production (directly or through NF-kB and AP-1) leading to peroxynitrite production.

♦ The increased peroxynitrite level damages lipids (lipid peroxidation), proteins (protein oxidation), and DNA (strand breaks) leading to overactivation of poly(adenosine diphosphate-ribose) polymerase, a DNA repair enzyme, resulting in the depletion of oxidized nicotinamide-adenine dinucleotide and adenosine triphosphate, and consequently in necrotic cell death (Korkmaz et al., 2007).

Usually hemorrhagic cystitis develops after prolonged therapy but there is a large individual variability. To prevent bladder toxicity, frequent voiding, generous fluid intake, or diuretic therapy in the case of nephrotic syndrome, are recommended. For these reasons it is more convenient to give the drug in the morning. Some drugs can bind acrolein and reduce urotoxicity. The two most used agents are acetylcysteine, which can be administered orally or parenterally, and sodium 2-mercaptoethanesulphonate (MESNA) which binds acrolein and prevent its direct contact with uroepithelium. MESNA can be given orally or intravenously. In patients with prolonged exposure to the drug, urine cytology should be performed every 6–12 months. Treatment with MESNA appears effective and safe and can be considered early in severe hemorrhagic cystitis to reduce the risk of morbidity and mortality.

If, in spite of these measures, any voiding symptom occurs, the drug should be discontinued. A number of treatments have been used with a variable degree of success, e.g., intravesical formalin, conjugated estrogens, hyperbaric oxygen therapy, and recombinant factor VII.

Bone marrow toxicity The hematopoietic system is particularly susceptible to the toxic effects of cyclophosphamide. Leukocytes are the most vulnerable cells while significant thrombocytopenia is less common. Agranulocytosis is more frequent in patients with serum cholinesterase activity lower than 200 U/L. If cyclophosphamide is given orally, leukocytes should be checked regularly, every 7–10d. With intravenous administration the nadir for leukocytes is generally reached 8–14d later, with recovery after 1–2 weeks. While some clinicians think that the immunosuppressive effect is related to the degree of leukopenia, we do not seek to produce leukopenia in patients with renal diseases. On the contrary, we reduce the dose if the white blood cell count decreases below 5000 per mm^3, and we stop the drug if leukocytes fall below 3000 per mm^3 in order to reduce the risk of infection. Since the bone marrow of elderly patients is particularly susceptible to the toxic effects of alkylating agents, it is advisable to halve the standard doses in patients over 65 years.

Both cyclophosphamide and its metabolites are cleared from the kidney, moreover renal insufficiency seems to reduce the resistance of the bone marrow to cytotoxic agents. Thus in patients with creatinine clearance values lower than 40mL/min it is more prudent to halve the standard doses of cyclophosphamide and to reduce it to one-third or less for those on dialysis treatment. Either granulocyte colony-stimulating factor or granulocyte-macrophage colony-stimulating factor can obtain a rapid leukocyte mobilization in cases of agranulocytosis following an intensive treatment with cyclophosphamide.

Water retention Cyclophosphamide can cause a syndrome of inappropriate secretion of antidiuretic hormone with water retention. This complication, however, usually develops at doses higher than 50mg/kg which are not used in clinical nephrology.

Gonadal toxicity In males, cyclophosphamide can induce aplasia of the germinal epithelium of the testis, with consequent oligospermia or even permanent azoospermia. This complication is dose-, time-, and age-dependent. Although it is not easy to find out the threshold dosage, it is generally accepted that oligospermia does not develop for cumulative doses lower than 200mg/kg and that doses greater than 300mg/kg are required to induce azoospermia. In a study of meta-analysis in children with idiopathic nephrotic syndrome (Latta et al., 2001) no safe threshold for a cumulative amount of cyclophosphamide was found in males, but there was a marked increase in the risk of oligo- or azoospermia with higher cumulative doses. The authors recommended not to exceed 2–3mg/kg body weight for 8–12 weeks (maximum cumulative dosage of 250mg/kg) as the standard scheme. In some cases recovery from azoospermia can be observed 3 or more years after drug discontinuation, but permanent azoospermia is the rule. Males who will receive prolonged cyclophosphamide therapy and who wish to retain 'fertility' should have semen stored before starting the drug.

In females, the ovary is more resistant than the testis to the toxic effects of cyclophosphamide, but amenorrhea and ovarian failure may develop when prolonged treatment are used, particularly in women over the age of 30 years. Studies in women with lupus nephritis have reported amenorrhea in 50–70% of patients receiving regimens of daily oral cyclophosphamide or intermittent intravenous cyclophosphamide for 6–48 months. In a multivariate analysis the most important risk factors for menstrual abnormalities were duration of treatment and cumulative dose of cyclophosphamide. Lower dose reduced the number of premature ovarian failures significantly (Appenzeller et al., 2008). A logistic regression analysis showed that in women with lupus older age, high damage index at the initiation of intravenous pulse therapy, and high cumulative dosage of intravenous cyclophosphamide were the independent risk factors of ovarian failure, and that the presence of amenorrhea, regardless of its duration, was the risk factor of pregnancy failure. Pregnancy was possible with a favorable outcome after the withdrawal of intravenous pulse therapy, unless amenorrhea developed (Park et al., 2004). Although intravenous cyclophosphamide has been advocated as the 'golden' standard of therapy for patients needing prolonged treatment, the available data indicate that there is no hard evidence to support the superiority of long-term intravenous over oral cyclophosphamide in term of gonadal toxicity (Wetzels 2004). Suppression of ovulation by a gonadotropin releasing hormone agonistic analog (leuprolide) may be utilized concomitantly with cyclophosphamide to protect the ovary against cyclophosphamide-induced damage.

Dermatologic effects Alopecia is a well known dose-related side effect of cyclophosphamide. Hair growth will usually return after stopping the drug, but the newly grown hair may be curly and 'kinky.' Mucosal ulcerations, transverse riding of the nails, and increased skin pigmentation can also develop.

Gastrointestinal effects Nausea and vomiting are common, particularly after intravenous high-dose administration. These symptoms usually occur 6–10h after infusion. A chronic, fastidious nausea may also occur in some patients with oral administration. Concomitant administration of anti-motility and anti-emetic drugs, such as metoclopramide, can reduce this disagreeable side effect.

Hepatotoxicity Cyclophosphamide can induce an increase in serum transaminases and, rarely, jaundice and hepatitis. These disorders are usually reversible after the discontinuation of the drug. Hepatotoxicity is more likely to occur in patients with low serum cholinesterase levels. As cyclophosphamide induces a reduction of cholinesterase activity, the drug should be discontinued if cholinesterase activity is lower than 200U/L.

Cardiac toxicity High-dose cyclophosphamide can, rarely, lead to cardiac necrosis, myocarditis, and/or pericarditis. Cardiac involvement may be checked by measurement of brain natriuretic peptide and endothelin levels, which rise before cardiomyocyte necrosis. These parameters are much more sensitive indicators of myocardial injury than functional tests—such as echocardiography—whereas diastolic functional parameters are more sensitive predictors of early

cyclophosphamide-induced cardiotoxicity. Mild functional mitral regurgita-
tion may also develop in patients given high-dose cyclophosphamide therapy
(Zver et al., 2007). However, with the oral doses used in renal patients cardiac
complications are extremely rare.

Lung toxicity When given at high doses and for prolonged periods, cyclophosphamide can induce lung fibrosis. This side effect is unusual with the
dosages used in clinical nephrology, but some cases of pulmonary reactions
can occur within 3–6 weeks after the initiation of therapy. Exceptionally, a
fulminant interstitial pneumonitis may develop after short courses of cyclophosphamide. These cases are thought to be hypersensitivity reactions, as
shown by the presence of aggregates of histiocytes at lung biopsy. It is also possible that acrolein may decrease the antioxidant defense system of the lung.
However, the role of antioxidants such as acetylcysteine in preventing this rare
complication is still unclear.

Neoplasia Cyclophosphamide is included among the single agents which
have been recognized to have a carcinogenic effect. Bladder cancer can occur
more frequently in patients given cyclophosphamide than in the general population. In a Swedish study on patients with Wegener's granulomatosis treated
with cyclophosphamide a matched case–control study was performed to estimate the association between cyclophosphamide and *bladder cancer*. The
median cumulative doses of cyclophosphamide among cases and controls
were 113g and 25g, respectively. The risk of bladder cancer doubled for every
10g increment in cyclophosphamide. Treatment duration longer than 1 year
was associated with an eightfold increased risk. The absolute risk for bladder
cancer reached 10% 16 years after diagnosis of Wegener's granulomatosis
(Knight et al., 2004). In another Scandinavian study on patients with Wegener's
granulomatosis the risk of bladder cancer was 3.6 times greater for patients
who received > 36 g of cyclophosphamide than for those given less than 36 g
or no cyclophosphamide at all (Faurschou et al., 2008). The pathogenesis of
this cancer is probably related to the chronic mucosal inflammation and irritation caused by acrolein although it is not possible to rule out a direct oncogenic effect of cyclophosphamide or its metabolites on the urothelium. All
cyclophosphamide-treated patients who receive long-term treatment should
have urinary cytologic evaluation, even after cyclophosphamide treatment has
been stopped. In the case of hematuria a cystoscopic evaluation is mandatory.

The data are more uncertain about the risk of *hematological malignancies* in
patients receiving prolonged administration of cyclophosphamide. Small-
sized studies reported conflicting results with some of them outlining an
increased incidence of leukemia and non-Hodgkin's lymphoma, while others

could not find a higher incidence of tumors than in general population. In the largest study undertaken to ascertain the incidence of cancer in SLE, which is usually treated with cyclophosphamide, 9547 SLE patients with an average follow-up of 8 years were compared with the general population. An increased risk of cancer was found among patients with SLE. The standardized incidence ratio was 2.75 for all hematological malignancies and it was 3.74 for non-Hodgkin's lymphoma. The data also suggested an increased risk of lung cancer and hepatobiliary cancer with a standardized incidence ratio of 1.37 and 2.60 respectively. However, the study could not define whether the increased risk for these malignancies was mediated by genetic factors or exogenous exposures (Bernatsky et al., 2005). In Wegener's granulomatosis a dose of cyclophosphamide $\geq$ 100mg/day for more than 1 year had a standardized incidence ratio of acute myeloid lekemia of 59 compared to general population (Faurschou et al., 2008).

With the exception of these types of cancer, the relative risk of developing other neoplasias does not seem to be increased with cyclophosphamide. However, most of the available data come from patients with systemic diseases. We lack information for patients with primary glomerulonephritis. Anecdotal cases of leukemia and solid tumors in cyclophosphamide-treated patients have been reported, but there is not a systematic study on this problem. Theoretically it is possible that the peculiar immune status of primary glomerulonephritides makes patients more susceptible to neoplastic diseases and that cytotoxic therapy may further increase this risk. Prior to the elucidation of the problem, it would be prudent not to use cyclophosphamide for more than 6–12 months. In the case of prolonged administration, transient discontinuation of the drug might reduce the risk of bladder cancer.

Pregnancy Cyclophosphamide has both mutagenic and teratogenic effects. Measuring the sister chromatid exchanges may be a valuable parameter for assessing the chromosome damage. Cytogenetic studies of chromosme 5q may also reveal the alkylating agent damage. Cyclophosphamide is contraindicated in pregnancy. All women contemplating its use *must* have a negative pregnancy test before commencing on the drug and at least two methods of contraception should be used by sexually active women in the reproductive age group during the administration of the agent.

Chlorambucil

Chlorambucil is an *N, N*-bis (2-chloroethyl)-amino-phenyl-butyric acid. The drug has been widely used in the therapy of chronic lymphocytic leukemia, polycythemia vera, Waldenström's macroglobinemia, and as an adjuvant therapy for various types of cancer. This drug has also been used in autoimmune diseases. In primary glomerulonephritis chlorambucil has been mostly used in minimal change nephropathy and in membranous nephropathy. The drug is supplied in tablets that should be kept at 4°C.

Clinical pharmacology

Chlorambucil is passively absorbed in the upper gastrointestinal tract. The absorption is adequate and reliable with peak levels occurring 15–30min after oral administration. The oral bioavailability is close to 100% and is not influenced by food. After absorption, chlorambucil rapidly disappears from plasma, with a half-life of 1h, but has a delayed onset of action. The drug is beta-oxidized in the liver to phenylacetic acid mustard, which seems to have cytotoxic properties similar to those of its parent compound. The uptake into cells is unaffected by metabolic inhibitions and does not take place against a concentration gradient. Chlorambucil and its metabolites may be fixed in several tissues, including adipose tissue, from which they are removed very slowly. This might account for some delayed effects of chlorambucil. There are large inter- and intraindividual variations in the pharmacokinetics of chlorambucil, which are even more pronounced for the cytotoxic metabolite phenylacetic acid mustard. At any rate, both this metabolite and its parent compound are almost completely metabolized, as shown by their extremely low urinary excretion of less than 1%.

Mechanisms of action

The pharmacological and cytotoxic actions of chlorambucil are similar to those of cyclophosphamide.

Toxic-effects

Although most side effects of chlorambucil are similar to those of cyclophosphamide, chlorambucil is neither a vesicant nor does it produce urothelial damage and bladder toxicity.

Bone marrow toxicity The myelosuppressive effects of chlorambucil are clearly dose-dependent. With a dosage of 0.2mg/kg per day, leukopenia can occur. This complication is less frequent and milder with doses of 0.1mg/kg per day. As for other immunosuppressive agents along with chlorambucil, we do not seek leukopenia, but rather we halve the dose if the leukocyte count decreases below 5000/cumm and we stop the drug if leukocytes fall below 3000/cumm. Chlorambucil is reintroduced at half of the previous dosage only when leukocytes are above 5000/cumm. The bone marrow of elderly and uremic patients is particularly vulnerable. In these instances the administration of chlorambucil should be very careful with frequent monitoring of blood cells. It must be pointed out that leukopenia can develop late—sometimes after chlorambucil treatment has already been stopped. This is probably due to the tissue accumulation of the drug, with slow release.

Ocular complications Diplopia, papillary edema, and keratitis are possible, although rare, side effects.

Neurological complications Hallucination, seizures, and electroencephalographic changes have been reported in children with idiopathic nephrotic syndrome treated with chlorambucil. In a meta-analysis of studies with cytotoxic drugs in children with idiopathic nephrotic syndrome, seizures were reported in 3.6% of children treated with chlorambucil (Latta et al., 2001).

Dermatological effects The skin may become darkened and dry under treatment with chlorambucil. Alopecia is exceptional.

Gonadal toxicity Chlorambucil appears to be more gonadal toxic than cyclophosphamide in males (Latta et al., 2001). It is difficult to fix a threshold cumulative dose, because of different individual sensitivities. A pediatric study reported that children who developed oligo- or azoospermia received a mean cumulative dose of chlorambucil of 17mg/kg, but two patients developed azoospermia after receiving respectively 9.3 and 11.6mg/kg (Callis et al. 1980). It is not known whether the post-pubertal testis is more or less resistant than the pre-pubertal testis to chlorambucil. At any rate, whenever a young male is scheduled to receive a cumulative dose of chlorambucil of more than 10mg/kg, it is advisable to collect his sperm in a semen bank before beginning chlorambucil therapy. During treatment, the monitoring of plasma follicular stimulating hormone, which increases in cases of testicular germinal epithelium damage, may be useful for deciding when to discontinue the drug.

Little is known about the toxic effects on the ovary at the doses used for glomerular diseases. Amenorrhea rarely occurs; most girls have normal pubertal development, a normal menarche, and regular menstruation (Callis et al. 1980).

Gastrointestinal effects In some patients anorexia, nausea and vomiting may occur, leading to treatment being stopped in 1–2 % of cases. Rarely a mild and reversible increase of liver transaminases can occur.

Malignancy Chlorambucil has been recognized by the International Agency for Research on Cancer as a potential human carcinogen, with bone marrow specificity. Chlorambucil has highly reactive electrophilic centers that react with DNA to form mutagenic adducts and cross-linking. This effect is dose-dependent and cumulative.

A marked increase of *acute leukemia* has been noted in patients given long-term chlorambucil. This risk is particularly high for patients treated with chlorambucil because of polycythemia vera, breast cancer, or ovarian cancer (Kaldor et al. 1990). However, patients with primary neoplasia (polycythemia is considered to be a pre-leukemic condition) are particularly exposed to the hazard of a second cancer. Moreover patients who developed malignancy had been given chlorambucil for many months or years.

In rheumatic patients no cases of leukemia were seen in patients who received <1g of chlorambucil and in whom the duration of treatment was <6 months. We have little information about the leukemogenic effect of chlorambucil in renal patients. Cases of acute myeloid leukemia have been reported in patients with Wegener's granulomatosis who received high cumulative doses of chlorambucil often in association with other cytotoxic agents over treatment periods up to 43 months.

The relative risk for the other types of cancer seems not to be increased by treatment with chlorambucil, at least in rheumatic patients. As for other immunosuppressive agents we lack solid data about the oncogenicity of chlorambucil in renal diseases. In the meta-analysis of Latta et al. (2001) out of 1504 children who received cytotoxic therapy for idiopathic nephrotic syndrome, 14 cases of malignancy occurred (0.9%) in patients treated with high doses of either cyclophosphamide or chlorambucil. In adults with idiopathic membranous nephropathy who received chlorambucil for 3 months the risk of cancer was similar to that reported in general population (Ponticelli et al., 1998). Since the oncogenic effect depends on the dose and the duration of treatment, it is prudent not to prolong cumulative therapy for more than 3–6 months and not to re-expose to the drug those patients who developed agranulocytosis or chromosomal abnormalities.

Pregnancy Chlorambucil can induce gene mutations which are dose-dependent and cumulative. Like cyclophosphamide the drug is contraindicated in pregnancy.

Clinical use in glomerulonephritis

Because of their potential toxicity, alkylating agents should be used only in selected cases, using clear cut indications and by experienced clinicians. The cumulative doses should be as low as possible in order to prevent disquieting toxicity. Repeated courses should be avoided whenever possible as the toxicy is cumulative. Several precautions should be taken to minimize the potential side effects (Table 2.4).

The choice between cyclophosphamide and chlorambucil is open and subject to several variables. However, the majority of nephrologists prefer the use of cyclophosphamide as they are more familiar with this drug, which is also easier to use than chlorambucil. At present there is no firm evidence that one

Table 2.4 Prevention of side effects of alkylating agents

Leukopenia	The risk is dose-related being higher with daily doses ≥ 3mg/kg for cyclo-phosphamide (Cyc) and ≥ 0.2mg/kg for chlorambucil (Chl).
	Daily doses ≤ 2mg/kg for Cyc and ≤ 0.1mg/kg for Chl are better tolerated.
	Warnings: in elderly patients or patients with renal failure the doses should be further decreased to 1mg/kg and 0.05mg/kg respectively.
	The dose should be halved if white blood cells (WBC) are <5000 per mm^3. Stop the drug if WBC <3000 per mm^3 and start again only after WBC are >5000 per mm^3
Bladder toxicity	It is related to the urinary excretion of acrolein, a metabolite of Cyc. To prevent bladder toxicity frequent voiding and forced diuresis are recommended.
	If high dose of intravenous cyclophosphamide are given, patients should receive intravenous MESNA.
	Courses of oral acethycysteine, 600mg/d, may be useful in patients who receive prolonged administration of Cyc.
	Urinary sediment should be periodically screened in patients under Cyc.
	Warning: patients with hematuria should receive a cystoscopy. Chl does not cause bladder toxicity.
Tumor	Do not administer Cyc or Chl to patients with previous neoplasia or poly-cytaemia vera. The higher the cumulative dose of alkylating agents, the higher the risk of neoplasia.
	Warnings: cumulative doses ≥ 36g with Cyc or ≥ 2g with Chl should not be exceeded whenever possible.
	The risk of haematological neoplasia is increased in patients who developed agranulocytosis.
	It is advisable to stop transiently the administration of an alkylating agent whenever leucocytes fall under 3000/cmm.
Gonadal toxicity	In males a cumulative dose ≥ 250mg/kg for Cyc and ≥10mg/kg for Chl can cause azoospermia.
	Sperm collection is advisable if long-term treatment with either alkylating agent is scheduled.
	In females the risk of ovarian failure is more frequent in women aged more than 30 years. Suppression of ovulation with leuprolide may protect from ovarian failure.

agent is superior to the other in terms of efficacy. However, although the mechanisms of action are similar for cyclophosphamide and for chlorambucil, their metabolism, excretion, interference with other drugs, and toxicities are different. The characteristics of each agent may influence the choice at least in some instances. For example, gonadal toxicity in males is probably more severe for chlorambucil; therefore in boys cyclophosphamide may be preferred.

On the other hand, in older adult patients it may be better to give chlorambucil, which does not cause bladder toxicity. Epileptic patients should not be given cyclophosphamide, as barbiturates and other antiepileptic drugs stimulate the microsomal liver enzymes which activate cyclophosphamide and can therefore cause unexpected toxicity. On the other hand, chlorambucil may also cause seizures in 3–4% of children, but very rarely in adults.

Some studies in lupus nephritis have shown that high-dose intravenous pulses of cyclophosphamide given intermittently may show fewer and less severe long-term effects than conventional daily oral cyclophosphamide. In particular, there may be a lower risk of infections, hemorrhagic cystitis, or neoplasia in patients treated with monthly or quarterly pulse doses of intravenous cyclophosphamide. However, these data have been challenged by a comprehensive review of the literature which did not find hard evidence to support the superiority of long-term intravenous cyclophosphamide in terms of complications (Wetzels 2004). There is little experience with intermittent pulse cyclophosphamide in primary glomerular diseases, so any comments regarding efficacy or safety must be regarded as preliminary. Small controlled trials in patients with focal and segmental glomerulosclerosis or with membranous nephropathy did not report favorable results (see Chapters 6 and 7).

In summary, in spite of their potential toxicity, alkylating agents still may play a role in the management of primary glomerular diseases. They proved to be able to prolong remission in steroid-dependent patients with minimal change disease or focal segmental glomerular sclerosis; in association with glucocorticoids they may obtain remission and protect renal function in patients with membranous nephropathy; and they are an important component of the aggressive treatment for crescentic glomerulonephritis. However, patients under treatment with these cytotoxic drugs should be strictly monitored and these drugs should be replaced with less toxic immunomodulating agents as soon as the renal disease is stabilized.

Ifosfamide

Ifosfamide is a bifunctional alkylating agent, used as a racemic mixture by intravenous route in the treatment of various tumors. It is an oxazaphosphorine derivative with a structural formula similar to that of cyclophosphamide. As a prodrug it requires activation in the liver by a cytochrome mixed-function oxidase system. Among various metabolites, ifosfamide mustard probably represents the most important cytotoxic compound able to produce irreparable cross-links between DNA strands. Pharmacokinetics is markedly influenced by route of administration and duration of treatment, age, co-medication, liver and renal function.

Ifosfamide is known by nephrologists because it may be responsible for severe acute and chronic nephrotoxicity probably caused by chloroacetaldehyde. Hemorrhagic cystitis is another frequent side effect, caused by acrolein. MESNA can prevent urotoxic effects but not nephrotoxicity or neurotoxicity. The drug is not indicated in any of the primary glomerulonephritides.

Calcineurin inhibitors

Cyclosporine

Cyclosporine A (CsA) is a powerful immunosuppressive drug derived from the Norwegian fungus *Tolypocladium inflatum*, is an undecapeptide of molecular weight 1203kDa, with a cyclic sequence of 11 amino acids. The compound has several N-methylated amino acids and one novel C9 amino acid. The amino acids in positions 1, 2, 3, and 11 form a hydrophilic active immunosuppressive site. CsA crystallizes from acetone to give white prismatic needles which dissolve easily in most organic solvents, but only poorly in water. The drug is now available as oral solution, capsules, and intravenous infusion. It is stabilized with olive oil vehicles for oral administration and with castor oil (Cremophor®) for intravenous infusion. The relative bio-equivalence of oral to intravenous doses is 1:3. A microemulsion formulation of CsA (Neoral®) is also available. It is a preconcentrate that, upon contact with aqueous gastrointestinal fluids, immediately forms a microemulsion, making CsA available for absorption. CsA is usually administered twice-daily.

Clinical pharmacology

After oral administration, CsA is absorbed from the upper small intestine into the vascular compartment via a bile-dependent process. In blood, almost 60% of CsA is bound to erythrocytes, 33% is distributed in the plasma, mainly bound to high-density and low-density lipoproteins, while only a small fraction circulates free. CsA is extensively metabolized by cytochrome-P450 3A (CYP3A) enzymes in the liver and intestine including the CYP3A5 isoenzyme which is also expressed in the kidney. The metabolites are primarily excreted in the bile and to a small extent (about 6%) in the urine. CsA is extensively distributed to the tissues. Liver accounts for most of the body stores, but CsA can also be found in ectodermic tissues (skin, gingiva, central nervous system) and mesodermic tissues (Kahan and Kelly 2000).

There are differences between the old formulation of CsA and the new microemulsion. With the old formulation the gastrointestinal absorption is slow, incomplete, and variable. The average bioavailability widely ranges between 5–89%, with a mean of 30%. Peak concentrations in blood also vary considerably between 1–8h, with a mean of 3.8h. With the microemulsion the absorption is more rapid (time to maximum concentration 1.5 vs. 2.1h) and complete (almost 1/3 higher area under the curve). With the old formulation of CsA the area under the curve is about 60% higher when the drug is given with food than without food. The blood levels increase even more after introduction of olive oil, corn oil, or grapefruit. Instead eating does not influence absorption when the microemulsion (Sandimmune®, Neoral®) is used. In summary, the new oral microemulsion has a better bioavailability, with reduced inter- and intraindividual variability and more predictable pharmacokinetics (Kovarik et al., 1996).

Other variables can influence the bioavailability and the pharmacokinetics of CsA:

◆ Bile deficit impairs the absorption of CsA, which is a lipophilic drug.

◆ Patients with diarrhea or with short-bowel syndrome show poor absorption and lower than expected blood levels.

◆ The clearance of CsA is accelerated in children and slowed in elderly patients, possibly as a consequence of the different lipoprotein levels.

◆ Hypercholesterolemia can reduce blood levels of CsA.

◆ Coadministration of drugs that interact with the cytochrome P-450 system may affect CsA metabolism and interfere with blood levels (Table 2.5).

◆ Variations in the ABCB1, ABCC2, SLCO1B1, CYP3A4, CYP3A5, or NR1I2 gene polymorphism may be associated with variations on the bioavailability and the pharmacokinetics of CsA. Although the effect of single nucleotide polymorphisms in the MDR1/ABCB1 and CYP3A5 genes on the pharmacokinetics of immunosuppressant has been widely examined, some contradictions have been emerged (Masuda and Inui 2006). Further studies are required to evaluate the predictive role of genotyping for individualization of CsA.

Mechanisms of action

Most of the immunosuppressive effects of CsA result from the inhibited transcription of IL-2, and other cytokines by T-helper cells.

After entering the blood circulation CsA easily diffuses through the cell membrane. Within cells, CsA binds to a specific protein receptor, called cyclophilin, a 17kDa ubiquitous isomerase which catalyses a rate-determining isomerization in protein folding in vitro. Cyclophilin mediates the cis–trans-isomerization of proline imino bonds and so allows the slow refolding phase in which proteins fold to their native three-dimensional structure which is necessary for their function as enzyme or structural protein. CsA inhibits the function of this particular isomerase by forming an active complex with cyclophilin.

Table 2.5 Main factors interfering with the pharmacokinetics of calcineurin inhibitors and potentiating their renal toxicity

Increase blood levels	Decrease blood levels	Potentiate renal toxicity
Elderly age	Pediatric age	Elderly age
Eating (old CsA formulation)	Fasting (old CsA formulation)	Renal insufficiency
Macrolide antibiotics	Barbiturates	Hypertension
Azole antifungal agents	Carbamazepine	Amphotericin B
Calcium channel blockers	Isoniazid	Anti-inflammatory drugs
HMG-CoA reductase inhibitors	Rifampin	Cidofovir
High-dose steroids	Rifabutin	Aminoglycosides
Acetazolamide	Nafcillin	Dehydration
Grapefruit	Bile deficit	Diuretics
Gene polymorphism (?)	Hypercholesterolaemia	Sulphonamides

This complex binds to and inhibits calcineurin, a calcium-dependent phosphatase which has a key role in T-cell activation. Calcineurin removes phosphates from the nuclear factor of activated T cells (NF-AT). Dephosphorylation allows this cytosolic factor (NF-ATc) to enter the nucleus, where it dimerizes with another protein (induced by a signal from T-cell receptors), NF-ATn, to form a heterodimeric active nuclear factor. This binds to and activates the gene for IL-2, ultimately resulting in IL-2 secretion.

Being its dephosphorylation inhibited by CsA, NF-AT cannot enter the nucleus and cannot encode and synthesize IL-2 and other cytokines produced by T-helper-1 cells. As a consequence of the inhibited production of IL-2, the proliferation and differentiation of cytotoxic and other effector T cells that destroy target cells by interaction with the antigen, are both inhibited. Moreover, as the secretion of IL-2 by TH1 cells activates B cells to secrete antibodies, the production of humoral antibodies is also reduced.

Other important mechanisms of action are represented by the inhibited synthesis of IFNγ, colony-stimulating factor, and macrophage-activating factor, which provide signals activating macrophages and monocytes and play an important role in inflammatory processes. All these effects are rapid in onset, dose-dependent, and often quickly reversible after stopping treatment (Kahan, 2000).

CsA also has a direct anti-proteinuric action on glomerular capillary wall perm-selectivity that is *unrelated* to its immunosuppressive properties, as demonstrated by various human studies and animal models with no immunologic background. Thus, the rationale for using CsA in idiopathic nephrotic syndrome may be twofold; CsA reduces proteinuria through an immunosuppressive effect, possibly through the inhibition of a lymphokine secretion and perhaps also through a direct, non-immunologic effect on glomerular permeability (Cattran et al., 2007).

Toxic effects

Most of the side effects of CsA have been observed in organ transplant recipients who are usually given higher doses than patients with glomerulonephritis. Since the toxicity of CsA is dose- related, side effects may be prevented by the use of relatively low doses.

Arterial hypertension Hypertension represents a frequent complication of CsA. The drug increases sympathetic nervous activity, activates the renin–angiotensin system, increases the production of renal thromboxane A_2, reduces the expression of vasodilating prostaglandins, increases the renal synthesis of endothelin, and reduces the expression of nitric oxide (Olyaei et al., 2001). As a result, CsA causes systemic vasoconstriction and increases the peripheral vascular resistances. In turn, the vasconstrictive effect on afferent preglomerular arterioles enhances the proximal resorption of sodium chloride with consequent volume expansion and increased cardiac output leading to a volume-dependent hypertension. Although the plasma renin levels are often normal they may be inappropriately elevated in front of volume expansion, and may concur in causing hypertension.

Calcium channel blockers are probably the most effective drugs for treating CsA-induced hypertension. It should be reminded, however, that non-dihydropyridinic calcium channel blockers (such as diltiazem and verapamil) may substantially increase the blood levels of CsA.

Nephrotoxicity Nephrotoxicity is usually dose-dependent and includes different individual sensitivities and various additional risk factors. The increased renal vascular resistance caused by CsA may induce an acute renal dysfunction characterized by reduced GFR and by an even more profound decrease of renal blood flow with a consequent increased filtration fraction. These hemodynamic abnormalities may cause histological changes which are initially but can eventually lead to severe and irreversible renal damage.

Tubular toxicity of CsA includes appearance of giant mitochondria predominantly in the convoluted part of the proximal tubule, isometric vacuolization in the straight part of the proximal tubule and microcalcifications of tubular cells caused by calcification of Tamm–Horsfall protein casts. Although highly characteristic, these changes are not specific for CsA toxicity. The clinical findings of tubular toxicity are comparable to those associated with mild renal insufficiency from various causes, although the decrease in GFR is more profound than that of the blood renal flow. No signs of proximal tubular dysfunction are seen: hypouricemia is absent (there is, rather, hyperuricemia), and lysozymuria and N-acetyl glucosamidase excretion are within normal limits. The Fanconi syndrome has never been described. The fractional excretion of magnesium is slightly higher and that of calcium is lower than pretreatment values. CsA administration results in a decrease in the rate of hydrogen ion secretion by the collecting tubule, which combined with a hyporeninemic hypoaldosteronism induced by the drug, may lead to hyperkalemic acidosis. Tubular toxicity is usually dose-related, but can also develop in patients with normal trough blood levels of CsA, either in the presence of additional risk factors (see Table 2.5) or in patients with individual sensitivity to CsA. The presence of tubular toxicity is a sign of general cytotoxicity, which can also occur in endothelial cells. It should lead the clinician to modify the doses of CsA or to stop the use of concomitant nephrotoxic therapies.

Cyclosporin nephropathy: the two principal inter-related lesions that characterize CsA nephropathy are represented by arteriolar changes and interstitial fibrosis. The vascular lesions predominate in afferent arterioles, while interlobular and arcuate arteries are usually spared. CsA-related arteriolopathy may be characterized by circular nodular protein deposits which permeate the arteriolar wall and/or by a mucinoid thickening of the intima which result in narrowing of the lumen. Early arteriolopathy may be reversible if CsA is stopped or reduced; otherwise these lesions lead to scarring. The consequent vasoconstriction and ischemia may lead to irregular foci or stripes of interstitial fibrosis with atrophic tubuli in the renal cortex. A sparse mononuclear infiltration is often seen in the fibrotic areas. Clinically, CsA-associated chronic nephropathy is characterized by progressive deterioration of renal function and arterial hypertension.

Some stabilization and even amelioration of lesions can be obtained if CsA is stopped when early arteriolar lesions occur. However, severe vascular lesions, focal interstitial fibrosis, and tubular atrophy are irreversible and usually lead to progressive renal failure. A common lesion seen in kidneys of those who develop progressive CsA nephrotoxicity is focal and segmental glomerulosclerosis.

Dermatologic complications The skin is one of the principal sites of accumulation of CsA. The drug, which is highly lipophilic, may partly be eliminated through the sebaceous glands. This could explain the frequent pilosebaceous lesions observed in CsA-treated patients.

A frequent complication of CsA is represented by *hypertrichosis*, which is more frequent and severe in children. Hypertrichosis is characterized by thick and pigmented hair appearing over the trunk, back, shoulder, arms, neck, forehead, helices, and malar areas. This complication is particularly disturbing not only in children but also in black-haired women. A possible mechanism for CsA-induced hypertrichosis is the increased activity of α-reductase, an enzyme that transforms androgens into dihydrotestosterone in peripheral tissues. If so, treatment with finasteride, an inhibitor of α-reductase successfully used in patients with idiopathic hirsutism, may be helpful.

Alopecia areata and universalis and accelerated male-pattern balding may occur. Skin hyperpigmentation and bullous or vegetative lesions have also been reported in CsA-treated patients. Sebaceous hyperplasia, epidermal cysts, and pilar keratosis may occur more rarely.

Gingival hyperplasia Gum hypertrophy occurs in about one-third of patients treated with CsA. It is caused by hyperplasia of epithelial and connective tissue components as well as by altered extracellular metabolism. This complication generally occurs after 3 or more months of treatment and can be worsened by the concomitant administration of calcium channel blockers or phenytoin. Gingival overgrowth is at least partially preventable with careful oral hygiene. Initially, a hyperplasia of the anterior interdental papillae occurs which subsequently spreads to the whole gum also involving the inner side. A 5-d treatment with azithromycin, a macrolide antimicrobial agent, may improve the subjective symptoms and the clinical picture. The most severe cases require gingivectomy.

Severe lip enlargement associated with CsA is less recognized and has seldom been reported in the literature. This complication may be severe enough to lead to social, physical, and psychological stress, especially in the older childhood and adolescent age groups.

Gastrointestinal complications About 10% of patients complain of some gastric symptoms, namely anorexia, nausea, and vomiting. These side effects are rarely severe.

Hepatotoxicity CsA alters calcium fluxes across hepatocyte cell membranes *in vitro*, elevates serum bile acids, and decreases bile flow. As a consequence, a slight increase in the bilirubin level unaccompanied by abnormalities in transaminases is common. An increased incidence of cholelithiasis and choledocolithiasis may also occur.

Neurologic complications Tremor, burning paresthesias, headache, flushing, depression, confusion, and somnolence have been reported in about 20% of renal transplant recipients treated with CsA. These complications respond slowly to dose reduction. A few cases of convulsions have also been reported, more often in transplanted children. Seizures may be favored by an increased water content in the brain because of hypertension, by hypomagnesemia, or by concomitant therapy with intravenous methylprednisolone, all of which would enhance the distribution of CsA into the nervous system (Ponticelli and Campise 2005).

A reversible *posterior leukoencephalopathy* can develop even at levels of CsA within the normal range, being that occipital white matter is particularly vulnerable to the adverse effects of CsA and tacrolimus. Children are more susceptible to this cerebral complication. The clinical symptoms include headache, vomiting, confusion seizures, cortical blindness, and other optic abnormalities. Neuroimaging studies typically show low density white matter lesions suggestive of edema in the posterior areas of cerebral hemispheres but abnormalities may also involve other cerebral areas, the brain stem, or the cerebellum. The pathogenesis of this complication is still unclear. It has been suggested that an enhanced nitric oxide production may inhibit the drug-efflux pump causing disruption of the blood–brain barrier that could facilitate the passage of calcineurin inhibitors into the cerebral interstitium (Wijdicks et al., 2001).

Other rare complications are hearing loss, tinnitus, or otalgia. These symptoms are often reversible with the reduction or withdrawal of the offending drug.

Glucose intolerance CsA can induce an acquired insulin sensitivity defect. This diabetogenic effect is strongly enhanced by the concomitant administration of glucocorticoids. Older patients, obese patients, the carriers of hepatitis C virus, and those with a familial history of diabetes are at increased risk of developing diabetes.

Hyperlipidemia CsA may increase LDL and VLDL cholesterol levels, VLDL triglyceride levels, as well as apolipoprotein B and lipoprotein (a). CsA may inhibit the enzyme 26-hydroxylase, so decreasing the synthesis of bile acids from cholesterol and the transport of cholesterol to the intestines. CsA also binds to the LDL receptor, which results in increased serum levels of LDL-cholesterol and impairs the clearance of VLDL and LDL by decreasing lipoprotein lipase activity (Kobashigawa and Kasiske 1997). HMG-CoA reductase inhibitors (statins) are the drugs of choice for treating hypercholesterolemia. Although previous studies reported an increased CsA exposure under statin treatment, other studies found that the area under the curve of CsA is only slightly influenced by simvastatin pravastatin, or atorvastatin (Asberg 2003).

Hyperuricemia Most patients develop hyperuricemia under treatment with CsA. In some patients plasma urate levels considerably increase, and may even lead to the development of severe acute gouty arthritis and chronic tophaceous gout. Although the mechanisms of CsA-related hyperuricemia are still unclear it is likely that decreased urate clearance, caused by reduced GFR and impaired renal handling of urate, have a major role. It can be aggravated by concomitant diuretic therapy, as urate reabsorption is very sensitive to circulating plasma volume.

Electrolyte abnormalities The most noticeable change in electrolyte handling is the decreased reabsorption of magnesium, with consequent *hypomagnesemia*. There is a decreased secretion of potassium and hydrogen ions by the distal tubules, leading to mild *hyperkalemia* and *acidosis*.

Thromboembolic complications Increased concentrations of factor VIII, fibrinogen, antithrombin III, and protein C have been reported in renal transplant recipients treated with CsA. Moreover, CsA may alter ADP-induced platelet aggregation and mononuclear cell procoagulant activity.

It is still disputed whether CsA-treated patients are exposed or not to an increased risk of thromboembolic complications as a consequence of these hemostatic changes. It is possible, however, that activated coagulation and uncontrolled platelet aggregation may contribute to the development of CsA-related arteriolopathy and even to thrombotic microangiopathy.

Musculoskeletal pain Isolated musculoskeletal pain may develop during therapy with CsA. The pain mainly involves the joints, but tendons may also be affected. Rare cases of tendon rupture may occur. An increased risk of myopathy and exceptional cases of rhabdomyolysis have been reported in patients given CsA and statins. As both drugs are metabolized by the P450 cytochrome enzymatic system, there are bilateral pharmacokinetics interactions that can increase the area under the curve of statins. However, the relevance of these interactions has been differently estimated. At any rate, to prevent any possible side effect, when given to CsA- treated patients the doses of statins should not exceed 10–20mg/d for simvastatin, atorvastatin, and pravastatin, 20–40mg/d for fluvastatin.

Neoplasia CsA can lead to an increased risk of cancer, which is dose- and time-dependent. In transplant patients the incidence of *de novo* neoplasms seems to be as high with CsA as with azathioprine (Penn 1991). However, patients treated with CsA seem to develop neoplasia earlier, and are more prone to lymphoproliferative diseases and to Kaposi's sarcoma.

Pregnancy In transplant patients who are being treated with CsA the risk of premature births is increased. Limited number of observations in children exposed to CsA *in utero* is available, up to an age of approximately 7 years. Renal function and blood pressure in these children were normal.

The incidence of birth defects with CsA is low and the pattern is extremely variable. According to the National Transplantation Pregnancy Registry the prevalence of major structural malformations ranges between 4–5% in new-borns from transplanted mothers versus a 3% observed in newborns from mothers without diseases (McKay and Josephson 2006). Meta-analysis studies in rheumatic patients could not see any significant difference in birth defects between pregnancies with pre-natal exposure to CsA and controls (Chambers et al., 2006).

Clinical use in glomerulonephritis

CsA has been mainly used in patients with minimal change nephropathy, focal segmental glomerulosclerosis, or membranous nephropathy. In these diseases CsA should be considered as a second treatment in case of failure, bad tolerance, or contraindications to the standard primary treatment.

Recommendations for the use of CsA in idiopathic glomerular diseases have been provided by a workshop of experts (Cattran et al., 2007). CsA should be given at the smallest effective dose for at least 6 months. If proteinuria is not reduced by 50% by the end of this time frame, an alternate therapy should be considered. Treatment targets should include complete or partial remission of proteinuria, maintenance of stable GFR (not more than 30% of pre-treatment level), avoiding hypertension. Measuring blood levels is not strictly necessary but some random check may be useful to verify the adequacy of doses. We try to keep C_0 (trough) levels <150ng/mL and C_2 (2h after drug administration) levels between 400 and 600ng/mL. If complete remission occurs, CsA should be tapered off over 3–4 months. For partial remission, CsA should be given at full dose for an additional 1–2 years and perhaps maintained at a non-toxic level indefinitely if renal function is stable and the case has been a particularly difficult one to manage and/or the patient has previously failed alternate forms of treatment. Alternatively CsA could be tapered slowly over 2–3 years and increased as required following any relapses. If there is no response to CsA or if a response occurs with adverse effects, an alternative therapy should be considered. In order to minimize the risk of renal toxicity some guidelines should be respected (Table 2.6).

Unfortunately most patients who attain complete disappearance of proteinuria with CsA show early relapse of proteinuria after CsA is stopped or even reduced. However, the rate of relapses may be reduced if CsA is given for a prolonged period and then tapered off gradually.

Table 2.6 Suggested guidelines for the use of calcineurin inhibitors (CNI) in primary glomerulonephritis

◆ Patients with a stable creatinine clearance < 60mL/min or with severe uncontrolled hypertension or advanced tubulointerstitial lesions at renal biopsy should not receive CNI.

◆ Caution is recommended in patients with creatinine clearance between 60–90mL/min and/or moderate tubulointerstitial lesions at renal biopsy. In hypertensive patients it is advisable to start CNI only when blood pressure has returned to normal with therapy.

◆ The initial dose with cyclosporine Neoral® should not exceed 4mg/kg/d in adults and 125mg/m^2/d in children. The initial dose of tacrolimus should be 0.1–0.2mg/kg/d.

◆ If there is no response at all within 6 months CNI are probably ineffective—possible exception membranous nephropathy which may respond later.

◆ In case of response the dose should be slowly reduced until reaching the minimal effective dose.

◆ Regularly check serum creatinine. If levels increase >30% over the baseline, CNI doses should be reduced until creatinine returns to basal levels. Stop treatment if creatinine increases >50% over the baseline.

◆ Sporadic checks of trough blood levels may be useful. Keep them <150 ng/mL with cyclosporine <6 ng/mL for tacrolimus.

◆ Factors that may interfere with CNI pharmacokinetics or may enhance nephrotoxicity should be taken into account (see Table 2.5).

Tacrolimus

Tacrolimus (TAC; also known as FK-506) is a macrolide immunosuppressant derived from the fungus *Streptomyces tsukubaensis*. It has a molecular mass of 822kDa and is poorly soluble in water, while it is very soluble in ethanol, methanol, propylene glycol, and polyethylene glycol. The drug inhibits cellular immune responses and humoral immune responses to a less extent. TAC is available for intravenous and oral administration. The pills are given in a twice-daily administration but recently the FDA approved a new formulation of TAC that can be given once a day. Phase III studies with a once-daily new oral formulation are under way.

Clinical pharmacology

After oral administration TAC is rapidly, but incompletely, absorbed in the gastrointestinal tract. Peak plasma concentrations are usually reached within 1h but sometimes up to 4h. The oral bioavailability is poor and ranges widely ranges, from 6–56%, with a mean of 25%. Its half-life is also variable ranging from 3.5–40.5h with a mean value of 11.3h. TAC is highly distributed into red blood cells. Plasma protein binding approaches 99% with the majority of the drug binding to α1-acid glycoprotein and albumin. TAC is almost completely metabolized by the cytochrome P450 (CYP)3A4 isoenzymes in the liver.

Intestinal mucosa also concurs to metabolize the parent drug by P450 (CYP)3A4 isoenzymes and P-glycoprotein. Most metabolites do not show immunosuppressive properties. Tacrolimus and its metabolites are primarily eliminated by biliary tract and excreted in feces, less than 2% of the drug is eliminated unchanged in the urine.

TAC has a large inter- and intraindividual variability. African-Americans and Hispanics have a poorer bioavailability than Caucasians. Children have a higher clearance of TAC than adults, while the clearance is reduced in patients with liver dysfunction. Also in view of its low therapeutic index, the doses of the drug should be adjusted in these particular subsets of patients. Whole blood drug monitoring can help in optimizing treatment.

Mechanisms of action

TAC shares a number of immunosuppressive properties with CsA. Through the inhibition of calcineurin, both the drugs strongly inhibit the induction of the synthesis of IL-2 and other cytokines and it has been assumed that this may be the key to their action. As CsA also TAC is a lipophilic drug and easily enters the cell where it binds to a cytoplasmic receptor, called FK-binding protein, which is structurally different from cyclophilin. The drug-receptor complex undergoes an allosteric conformational change which allows it to bind to calcineurin. In turn this binding inhibits the activity of calcineurin, which, as outlined above, is a complex of phosphatases particularly important for the entry into the nucleus of cytosolic factors which can promote transcription of cytokine genes. Thus both cyclophilin and FK-binding protein represent part of a signal transduction pathway used during T-cell activation which is important for the activation of select lymphokine genes. FK-binding protein and cyclophilin are related and one may be transformed into the other by the enzyme rotamase. TAC interacts with its binding protein with greater affinity than CsA binds to cyclophilin.

Toxic effects

Despite major differences in the chemical structure, TAC and CSA seem to have many effects in common. This phenomenon can be explained by the inhibition of the calcineurin pathway characteristic for both drugs. Patients treated with TAC may suffer from the same potential adverse events that may occur with CsA. Some differences can be found in the prevalence and intensity of clinical side effects. Most of side effects are dose-dependent.

Nephrotoxicity The prevalence of nephrotoxicity is similar with TAC and CsA. In particular, morphologic changes associated with toxic drug effects in the kidney are indistinguishable from one another, i.e., tubular lesions, arteriolopathy, microangiopathic changes in glomeruli and vessels (Mihatsch et al., 1998).

Hypertension Arterial hypertension is less pronounced with TAC than with CsA.

Diabetes mellitus One of the most frequent and severe complications of TAC is the onset of a dose-dependent *de novo* diabetes mellitus. There is agreement that TAC is more diabetogenic than CsA probably because it also exerts a direct toxicity on islet cells

Dermatological effects Hypertrichosis and gingival hyperplasia usually are not observed with TAC while *alopecia* can occur.

Gastrointestinal symptoms Gastrointestinal troubles, particularly diarrhea, are more frequent with TAC.

Neurological complications These complications are more frequent and more severe with TAC. Tremors, paresthesias, insomnia are common. Convulsions, aphasia, and paralysis can also occur. *Hearing loss* is more frequent with TAC than with CsA.

Hypercholesterolemia Hypercholesterolemia is significantly less frequent in patients given TAC than in those treated with CsA.

Electrolyte disturbances About one-third of patients show an increase of *potassium* in the blood, *hypomagnesemia* is also frequent.

Malignancy The risk of malignancy is similar to that of CsA. However, a higher incidence of lymphoproliferative disorders has been reported with TAC in transplanted children (Smith et al., 2003).

Pregnancy The FDA classifies TAC, as well as CsA, as category C, meaning that human risk can not be ruled out, because the human studies are lacking and the experimental studies are either positive for risk or lacking. The incidence of major malformations is low, similar to that reported for CsA. The pattern of defects is so variable that it is difficult to define either drug as teratogen or foetotoxic (McKay and Josephson 2006).

Clinical use in glomerulonephritis

There are no formal indications for TAC in the treatment of primary glomerulonephritis. Some few non-randomized studies reported a good response of proteinuria in patients with minimal change nephropathy or focal segmental glomerular sclerosis. A small-sized randomized trial also reported good results in membranous nephropathy. As for CsA, however, most patients suffered from relapse of nephrotic syndrome, when TAC was interrupted. At present, TAC may be considered to have the same role and the same limits than CsA in treating glomerular diseases. Recommendations with the use of TAC in glomerulonephritis are similar to those given for CsA (see Table 2.6). The initial doses may range between 0.1–0.2mg/kg per day, with gradual reduction; treatment should be interrupted if no change in proteinuria is seen after 6 months of therapy. Checking blood levels is not strictly needed in adults (although some sporadic check may be useful to control the bioavailability and the adherence to prescription). In children it is recommended to check the trough blood levels, at least in the first period, being the bioavailability and the pharmacokinetics of TAC variable and unpredictable.

mTOR inhibitors

There are two drugs, sirolimus (rapamycin) and its derivate everolimus (not available in the US) which inhibit the mammalian target of rapamycin (mTOR). They are very similar for mechanisms of action and potential toxicity, but differ in pharmacokinetics.

Clinical pharmacology

Sirolimus is macrolide lactone naturally produced by *Streptomyces hygroscopicus* containing a diketoamide moiety similar to that present in tacrolimus. The compound is insoluble in water. The drug has a long half-life, about 62h, and a high concentration in the brain. Its derivate *everolimus* has a similar chemical structure but a covalently-bound 2-hydroxyethyl group was introduced at position 40 to improve bioavailability and reduce the half-life to about 26h.

The compounds are absorbed rapidly with a peak concentration 1–2h after an oral dose. The steady state is achieved after 4d with everolimus and after 8d with sirolimus. The drugs are actively and reversibly taken up by erythrocytes. The oral bioavailability of both drugs is minimal and is affected by food with a reduction of 60% with high-fat meals in comparison to fasting state. Both sirolimus and everolimus are metabolized by the hepatic P450(CYP) enzymes. The metabolites do not exert immunosuppressive activity. The clearance ranges around 8–9 L/h, but is reduced in patients with hepatic impairment. There is a strong interaction with other drugs metabolized by hepatic cytochrome enzymes, as for calcineurin inhibitors (Table 2.5).

Mechanisms of action

After oral administration mTOR inhibitors enter the cells and bind to a specific cytoplasmic receptor, FKbinding protein 12, the same receptor of TAC.

However, differently from TAC the complex drug-receptor does not inhibit the enzymatic activity of calcineurin but blocks a serine-threonin kinase called mTOR, which exists in two complexes, MTOR 1 and 2. This kinase is the downstream effector of phosphatydilinositol-3-kinase (PI3k), which together with a protein-kinase B (Akt) governs several signal pathways by phosphorylating a cascade of other kinases that provide the signals for cell proliferation. A number of different stimuli - including IL-2, IL-15, oncogenic proteins, vascular endothelial growth factor (VEGF), and CMV may activate PI3-k. In response to IL-2 and/or IL-15 the PI3k activates a cascade of kinases that provide the signal for T cell proliferation. Sirolimus and everolimus inhibit mTOR-1 so interfering with the signals leading to T cell proliferation. Apart from the immunosuppressive activity these agents are showing protective effects on the endothelium by inhibiting the VEGF that stimulates the endothelial cell proliferation and angiogenesis through the family of kinases governed by PI3-k. Of importance, mTOR antagonists can exert anti-tumor activity in cancers caused either by an overactivity of PI3-k, or deficiency of PTEN the physiological inhibitor of PI3-k, or overexpression of mTOR.

Both sirolimus and everolimus have important immunosuppressive properties and may synergize with calcineurin inhibitors. While CsA and TAC interfere with the synthesis of IL-2 and other cytokines, mTOR antagonists inhibit the response to IL-2 and IL-15. Calcineurin inhibitors interfere with cell cycle between G0 and G1, while mTOR antagonists inhibit the cell cycle between G1 and S. There are also pharmacological interactions between CsA and mTOR inhibitors. CsA increases the area under the curve of mTOR inhibitors but not vice versa. The interference between TAC and mTOR inhibitors is still poorly investigated but TAC does not seem to increase the exposure to mTOR inhibitors.

Toxicity

The side effects of mTOR antagonists are mainly related to their anti-proliferative activities.

Hyperlipidemia

It is the most frequent side effect of mTOR-inhibitors. These drugs may increase the serum levels of total cholesterol, LDL-cholesterol, triglycerides, and Apo C-III. Lipid abnormalities are probably the result of complex interferences of the class of m-TOR inhibitors on lipid metabolism. Experimental and clinical studies showed that mTOR inhibitors may upregulate apolipoprotein C III, reduce the catabolism of VLDL apoB100-containing lipoproteins, alter the insulin signaling pathway with increased hepatic synthesis of triglycerides and increased secretion of VLDL, and/or impair the bile salt synthesis with consequent hypercholesterolemia. Statins should be part of the drug regimen in patients with hypercholesterolemia

Bone marrow toxicity

Thrombocytopenia and anemia may occur in patients treated with mTOR inhibitors but they are usually mild.

Renal toxicity

In experimental animals mTOR inhibitors can cause tubular toxicity characterized by tubular collapse, vacuolization, and nephrocalcinosis. These drugs may protect from the development of interstitial fibrosis in animals with obstructive uropathy and worsen the progression of sclerosis in the remnant glomeruli after 4/5 nephrectomy. The opposite results not only depend on the different models but even more on the extension of underlying lesions. In the presence of initial lesions mTOR inhibitors may exert a protective role against interstitial fibrosis while they can enhance the development of irreversible lesions in the presence of severe chronic damage.

Up to 30% of renal transplant recipients may develop proteinuria within 1 year after conversion from CsA or TAC to an mTOR inhibitor. The mechanisms responsible for proteinuria are still under investigation. After conversion from CsA there is probably an increase in intraglomerular pressure which might explain proteinuria, at least partially. Due to their apoptotic mechanisms mTOR inhibitors may interfere with the protein endocytosis in the tubular epithelial cell leading to impaired tubular resorption of albumin. On the other hand they could induce apoptosis of podocytes which cannot regenerate. Precipitous decrease of renal function with an increase in proteinuria has been observed in patients with FSGS treated with sirolimus (Cho et al., 2007).

Cases of *de novo* hemolytic uremic syndrome caused by thrombotic microangiopathy have been reported in transplant patients given mTOR inhibitors in the context of contemporaneous or contiguous administration of calcineurin inhibitors. It may be hypothesized that, by downregulating VEGF, mTOR inhibitor may induce anti-angiogenic activity with late repair of endothelial lesions caused by calcineurin inhibitors, rejection, or virus infection. Usually the withdrawal of the offending drug may obtain resolution of the disease, if the diagnosis is made early.

Wound healing

Retarded wound healing after surgery has been noted in patients treated with mTOR inhibitors probably as a consequence of their antiproliferative activity.

Interstitial pneumonia

A number of cases of interstitial pneumonia caused by sirolimus have been reported. Patients present with cough and dyspnea followed by fatigue and fever. Chest x–ray and computed tomography may show bilateral patchy or diffuse alveolo-interstitial infiltrates. The differential diagnosis with lung infection can be difficult. Sirolimus discontinuation or reduction leads to resolution within 3 weeks in most cases.

Mouth ulcers

The development of mouth ulcers seems to be dose-related as they can improve after dose reduction. Painful oral ulcers seem to be particularly frequent and severe in patients given an association of sirolimus and MMF. This may either depend on over-immunosuppression or on the use of sirolimus in form of oral emulsion rather than in form of tablets.

Joint pain

Joint pain may occur in up to 25% of patients given high doses of mTOR inhibitors. Pain may be disabling, but usually may resolve with dose reduction or drug withdrawal in more severe cases. It is possible that pain is caused by changes of circulation in the bone.

Edema

Eyelid and/or leg edemas may occur. These edemas are dose dependent. They are usually mild to moderate and may reverse with low-dose furosemide.

Pregnancy

mTOR inhibitors increased the mortality of fetus in experimental animals. However no teratogenic effects have been seen either in rats or rabbits. There is insufficient information about pregnant women treated with these drugs. The FDA classifies sirolimus (everolimus is not available in US) as category C (teratogenic risk cannot be ruled out because of lack of information).

Neoplasia

Sirolimus and everolimus are believed to posses anti-neoplastic properties. Both drugs and the derivate temsirolimus are currently under investigation in different types of cancer.

Clinical use in glomerulonephritis

Both mTOR inhibitors have been tested in several models of experimental glomerulonephritis with different results, according to the model and the doses employed. These drugs worsened glomerular pathology in a model of mesangioproliferative disease due to inhibition of endothelial cell proliferation (Daniel et al., 2005) but at subimmunosuppressive levels inhibited mesangial cell proliferation and extracellular matrix production (Lock et al., 2007). Favorable results were observed in a model of Heymann nephritis (Naumovic et al., 2007) and beneficial effects on the time course of chronic anti-Thy1 nephritis have been reported (Wittmann et al., 2008), but it has also been demonstrated that they can elicit the development of *de novo* focal segmental glomerular sclerosis in man when given at high doses (Letavernier et al., 2007).

With the exception of one study (Tumlin et al., 2006) the few attempts of treating human primary glomerulonephritis with mTOR inhibitors proved to be unsuccessful. Whether they may be of some utility when given at low doses in combination with other drugs is still unknown. It should be pointed out, however, that these drugs can worsen two important component of the nephrotic syndrome, namely proteinuria and hypercholesterolemia. As, when given at very low doses in mice, they can inhibit both proliferation and extracellular matrix production in mesangial cells (Lock et al., 2007), they could find, at the utmost, some therapeutic role in non advanced glomerular diseases with mild proteinuria and normal serum lipid levels (i.e., some cases of IgA nephritis).

Biological immunomodulators

Rituximab

Rituximab is a chimeric human/murine monoclonal antibody with a high affinity for the CD20 antigen, a membrane protein expressed on a subset of B cells (Table 2.7). The main indication of rituximab is follicular non-Hodgkin's B cell lymphoma, but it has been also used off-label in organ transplantation and in a number of autoimmune diseases, including rheumatoid arthritis, SLE, and some forms of primary glomerular diseases. It is available in vials. The usual dosage is $375mg/m^2$ to be repeated at different intervals according to the clinical response and the count of B cells (as assessed by a monoclonal antibody to CD-19 whose expression on B-cells is not affected by anti-CD20 administration). A recent auto-immune protocol involves giving 1000mg at two intervals 2 weeks apart. Either course virtually assures nearly complete elimination of circulating CD19+ and CD20+ B cells, but has no effect on mature plasma cells which lack the CD20 antigen. Because of the risk of allergic reactions and massive lymphocyte destruction the first dose should be given very slowly, with antihistamines and small doses of hydrocortisone, under surveillance of a doctor or a specialized nurse.

Table 2.7 Main characteristics of rituximab

- *A chimeric monoclonal antibody* with high affinity for the CD20 antigen expressed on a subset of B lymphocytes

- *Possible mechanisms of action in autoimmune diseases:* depletion of memory cells, abolition of antigen presentation by B cells, increase of number and function of regulatory T cells

- *Administration:* given intravenously (slow infusion!) at doses of 375mg/m² at different intervals according to the clinical response

- *Lysis syndrome:* the first injection may cause fever, hypotension, arrhythmias, bronchospasm which may be quenched by the pre-emptive administration of antihistamines or glucocorticoids

- *Potential side effects:* anemia, thrombocytopenia, severe and long-lasting lymphopenia, viral infection, interstitial pneumonia, posterior leukoencephalopathy(?)

- *Use in primary glomerulonephritis:* good results in minimal change nephropathy, in membranous nephropathy and in rapidly progressive glomerulonephritis but no controlled study is available. Uncertain results in steroid-resistant focal segmental glomerular sclerosis

Clinical pharmacology

Following intravenous injection, serum levels and the half-life of rituximab are proportional to dose. A more rapid disappearance may be seen in patients with nephrotic syndrome, due to loss of the antibody in the urine. Such patients may have less complete eradication of circulating B cells. In patients with non-Hodgkin's lymphoma given 375mg/m² as an intravenous infusion for 4 weekly doses, the mean serum half-life is 76.3h (range: 31.5–152.6h) after the first infusion and 205.8h (range: 83.9 –407.0h) after the fourth infusion. The wide range of half-lives may reflect the variable tumor burden among patients and the changes in CD20-positive (normal and malignant) B-cell populations upon repeated administrations (Cvetkovic and Perry 2006).

Mechanisms of action

Rituximab induces a rapid elimination of B cells, The Fab domain of Rituximab binds to the CD20 antigen on B lymphocytes, and the Fc domain recruits *immune* effector functions to mediate B-cell *lysis* in vitro. Possible mechanisms of cell lysis include complement-dependent cytotoxicity, antibody-dependent cell mediated cytotoxicity, and stimulation of the apoptotic pathway. In autoimmune diseases the effect of rituximab on circulating levels of auto-anti-bodies (presumably being secreted by mature plasma cells unaffected by the anti-CD20 antibody) are minor and rather inconsistent. Probably additional mechanisms of action may operate, including depletion of memory cells, abolition of antigen presentation by B cells, and increase of number and function of regulatory T cells.

Toxicity

Lysis syndrome The first dose of rituximab can cause a massive lysis of B cells with release of cytokines and can be associated with fever, chills, rigor, orthostatic hypotension, irregular heart rhythms, and bronchospasm. This reaction correlates with the number of circulating CD20 cells and is more frequent in patients with tumor while it is milder in patients with autoimmune disease. In patients with pre-existing cardiac morbidity, arrythmias, angina, and acute respiratory distress syndrome have been reported. Infusion should be interrupted in case of severe bronchospasm. Pre-medication with glucocorticoids or anti-histamine agents can reduce the intensity of symptoms.

Infection Rituximab abates CD20 lymphocytes and decreases the serum levels of immunoglobulin M but usually has little short term effect on immunoglobulin G levels. Nevertheless, its use may be associated with an increase in susceptibility to infection, particularly in patients who are heavily immunosuppressed. The majority of infections are caused by bacterial or opportunistic viral agents (such as herpesvirus) and generally develop 30d to 11 months after the end of therapy The most common respiratory system adverse events experienced are cough, rhinitis, bronchospasm, dyspnea, and sinusitis. In both clinical studies and post-marketing surveillance, there have been a limited number of reports of *bronchiolitis obliterans* presenting up to 6 months postrituximab infusion and a limited number of interstitial pneumonitis presenting up to 3 months post-rituximab infusion. The pathogenesis of interstitial pneumonitis is unknown. Prompt and aggressive treatment with glucocorticoids may lead to resolution of the disease. Patients who worsen despite glucocorticoids have a poor outcome. The safety of resumption or continued administration of rituximab in patients with pneumonitis or bronchiolitis obliterans is unknown.

Other serious infectious events include sepsis, and hepatitis B virus (HBV) reactivation with related fulminant hepatitis. A few cases of universally fatal PML, probably caused by reactivation of JC virus, have also been reported in patients with SLE and rhuematoid arthritis. These patients were also receiving other immunomodulating drugs and were severely immunosuppressed. Rituximab should be avoided in the presence of active significant infections and in carriers of HBV infection.

Hematologic events Severe decreases in red or white blood cells and platelets may occur rarely with rituximab therapy. Lymphopenia usually resolves within 14d but may last up to 20 months.

Immunogenicity The incidence of antibody positivity in an assay is highly dependent on the sensitivity and specificity of the assay and may be influenced by several factors including sample handling, concomitant medications, and underlying disease. For these reasons, the incidence of human anti-chimeric antibody antibodies (HACA) to rituximab may be misleading. In clinical studies of patients with low-grade or follicular non-Hodgkin's lymphoma receiving rituximab as a single therapy, HACA were detected in 1.1% patients.

Hypersensitivity reactions As a chimeric protein, rituximab may be associated with serum sickness-like reactions and, rarely, by anaphylaxis.

Pregnancy Rituximab has not been shown to be teratogenic in animal studies. In women only seven cases of rituximab administration during pregnancy were reported. No adverse events are described for fetus and neonate. However, rituximab passes the placenta and inhibits neonatal B-lymphocyte development for many months (Klink et al., 2008). According to the FDA a teratogen risk cannot be excluded for rituximab (category C). The administration of rituximab to a pregnant woman should be discouraged unless the benefits outweigh the potential risk for the fetus. Offspring of mothers receiving rituximab during pregnancy often have profoundly reduced CD19 levels at birth but they usually achieve full immunologic reconstitution by 2–4 months after delivery.

Clinical use in glomerulonephritis

Due to the role of antibodies in some glomerular diseases and to the strict interaction between B cells and T cells it is not surprising that rituximab is being used in several forms of primary glomerulonephritis. Sporadic non-controlled studies have reported good results in minimal change nephropathy, focal segmental glomerular sclerosis, and membranous nephropathy. Anecdotal reports also pointed out the possibility of inducing remission (usually partial) in cases of glomerulonephritis recurring after transplantation. Unfortunately, apart from the drawbacks of the non-controlled nature of the studies and the lack of comparison with historical controls, the short-term nature of follow-up precludes any definitive evaluation of overall, long-term benefits, especially regarding relapses and the need for repeated therapy. Randomized clinical trials in patients with minimal change nephropathy and focal segmental glomerulosclerosis are underway and hopefully will show the actual role of rituximab in treating these diseases.

Alemtuzumab

Alemtuzumab (Campath 1H®) is an unconjugated, fully humanized, monoclonal antibody directed against the cell surface antigen CD52 on lymphocytes and monocytes. The drug is approved for use in lymphocytic leukemia but it has also been used off-label in multiple sclerosis, rheumatoid arthritis, and for induction therapy in organ transplantation. Alemtuzumab is available as a white powder which must be dissolved in water and slowly infused intravenously, usually at a dose of 30mg/day three times weekly. The drug can also be administered by subcutaneous injections.

Clinical pharmacology

Only a small amount of pharmacokinetic data is available (Frampton and Wagstaff 2003). The peak plasma concentration and the area under the curve show relative dose proportionality. The average half -life after a single dose administration is 12d. Steady state has a large interpatient variability. Details about metabolism and excretion are unavailable but no dose adjustment is required in patients with renal or hepatic failure.

Mechanisms of action

CD52 is a cell surface glycoprotein expressed on more than 95% of peripheral blood lymphocytes. Alemtuzumab is a monoclonal antibody which targets the CD52 antigen. After binding its target alemtuzumab causes cell death through complement-dependent cytolysis, antibody-dependent cellular cytotoxicity, and apoptosis.

Toxic effects

Allergic reaction The injection may cause cutaneous erythema and pruritus. Rarely dyspnea, bronchospasm, and hypotension may also occur. Antihistamine agents or glucocorticoids are usually administered before the first administration to reduce the risk and the severity of allergic reaction.

Cytokine release syndrome Chills, fever, headache, sweating, bronchospasm, muscle and joint pain may occur during the infusion. These symptoms are almost constant with intravenous infusion while are less frequent and severe with subcutaneous injection. The syndrome is more frequent with the first administration and may be mitigated by pre-medication with glucocorticoids. The symptoms usually remit spontaneously in a few hours.

Hematological toxicity Thrombocytopenia, anemia, and neutropenia are frequent but tend to resolve within 3–4 weeks. Lymphocytes completely disappear after infusion and a profound lymphocytopenia may last for many months.

Infections The profound, long-lasting lymphopenia may increase the susceptibility to infection. Prophylaxis with sulfamethoxazole/trimethoprim as well as a careful control for viral or bacterial infection is recommended.

Pregnancy It is not known if alemtuzumab can harm a developing baby when given during pregnancy. However, as the drug can cross the placenta and attack the blood cells of the fetus, women and their partners should use effective methods of contraception both during treatment and for at least 6 months after stopping treatment.

Clinical use in glomerulonephritis

B cells and their products, antibodies, may play an important role in the pathogenesis of primary glomerular diseases. Specific B-cell directed therapy with alemtuzumab might theoretically influence the outcome of glomerulonephritis which do not respond to standard treatment. However, the clinical value of specific B-cell subset targeting/depletion in these diseases has not been addressed. As alemtuzumab may cause adverse events related to depletion of non-pathogenic B-cell populations, well conducted clinical trials are needed before using it in primary glomerulonephritis.

Eculizumab

Eculizumab is a monoclonal antibody approved for the treatment of paroxysmal nocturnal hemoglobinuria (PNH). Due to its particular mechanism of action eculizumab might find a role in the treatment of some primary glomerular diseases. In paroxysmal hemoglobinuria eculizumab is given intravenously over 25–45min every week for 4 weeks and then every 2 weeks.

Clinical pharmacology

Eculizumab is a fully humanized monoclonal antibody directed against the complement protein C5. The monoclonal antibody has a molecular weight of 148 kD. The clearance of eculizumab for a patient weighing 70kg is 22mL/h and the volume of distribution is 7.7 L. The estimated half-life ranges between 8–15d (mean 11d). There are not pharmacokinetics studies in patients with impaired renal function and the disappearance rate of the antibody may be increased in the presence of nephrotic syndrome, due to urinary losses of the infused antibody.

Mechanisms of action

Patients with PNH have a somatic genetic mutation in the X-linked gene PIG-A. This leads to the absence of a complement regulatory protein and to a generation of abnormal red blood cells that are deficient in terminal complement inhibitors. These erythrocytes are particularly sensitive to persistent terminal complement-mediated destruction. Intravascular hemolysis is a prominent feature of PNH. Excessive or persistent intravascular hemolysis causes anemia, hemoglobinuria, and complications related to free hemoglobin such as thrombosis, abdominal pain, and pulmonary hypertension.

Eculizumab is directed against the protein C5, a terminal component of the complement cascade. By binding to C5, eculizumab inhibits its cleavage to C5a and C5b and prevents the generation of the inflammatory terminal complement complex C5b-9 which exerts hemolytic activity.

Toxic effects

Meningococcal meningitis Eculizumab increases the risk of meningococcal infections perhaps due to the reduction in the levels of C5 activity. Patients should be vaccinated or revaccinated with a meningococcal vaccine at least 2 weeks prior to receiving the first dose of eculizumab. Patients should also be monitored closely for early signs of meningococcal infections and evaluated immediately if infection is suspected, and treated with antibiotics if necessary.

Non-specific symptoms Headache, nasopharyngitis, back pain, cough, and nausea may occur in the period following injection.

Pregnancy In animals eculizumab crosses the placenta and causes increased rates of development abnormalities. Rare cases of retinal dysplasia have been reported in newborns from mothers treated with eculizumab. Some reports outlined an increased mortality in males. The drug should be administered to pregnant women only if benefits may justify the potentially increased risk for the fetus.

Indications in primary glomerulonephritis

The mechanism of action of eculizumab renders this monoclonal antibody potentially attractive for treating patients with membranous nephropathy, as the terminal components of the complement, C5b-C9, play a prominent role in mediating the inflammation and the damage of podocytes and GBM (see Chapter 7). A preliminary trial of eculizumab for idiopathic membranous nephropathy was negative, but the doses employed may not have been sufficient to maintain a low level of C5 activity. It is also a possible therapeutic option in dense deposit disease (MPGN type II—see Chapter 9), which is sustained by a defective complement regulation (see Chapter 9), but no trials have yet been conducted (Nurmohamed and Dijkmans 2005).

Anti-tumor necrosis factor agents

Tumor necrosis factor (TNF) is a naturally occurring cytokine that is involved in normal inflammatory and immune responses. TNF-targeted therapies are increasingly used for a rapidly expanding number of rheumatic and autoimmune diseases. There are three drugs that interfere with TNF. *Etanercept* is a soluble fusion protein that binds specifically to TNF, *infliximab* and *adalimumab* are monoclonal antibodies directed against TNFα but not TNFβ. These drugs are approved by regulatory authorities for treatment of rheumatoid arthritis, ankylosing spondylitis, plaque psoriasis, and psoriatic arthritis. Etanercept and adalimumab are administered by subcutaneous injection while infliximab is injected intravenously.

Clinical pharmacology

After a single subcutaneous injection of 25mg of *etanercept* the mean half-life is 102 ± 30 h and the time to maximal concentration is 69 ± 34 h. After 6 months of twice weekly administration of 25mg there is a two- to sevenfold increase in peak serum concentrations and approximately a fourfold increase in the area under the curve. Pharmacokinetic parameters are not different between men and women and do not vary with age in adult patients.

Infliximab is an antibody with high affinity to both membrane bound and soluble TNFα. It has a bioavailability of 100%, being administered intravenously. Its half-life is 9.5 h. It is metabolized by the reticulo-endothelial system. Little is known about its excretion.

Adalimumab is a complete human antibody against TNFα. It has a volume of distribution of 4.7–6.0 L and an average bioavailability of 65%. Its pharmacokinetics were linear over the dose range of 0.5–10.0mg/kg following a single dose. The mean terminal half-life is approximately 2 weeks, ranging from 10 to 20d across studies. No gender-related pharmacokinetic differences were observed after correction for a patient's body weight.

No pharmacokinetic data are available for these drugs in patients with hepatic or renal impairment or nephrotic syndrome.

Mechanisms of action

Etanercept binds specifically to TNF and blocks its interaction with cell surface TNF receptors. Two distinct receptors for TNF, a 55 kDa protein (p55) and a 75 kDa protein (p75), exist naturally as monomeric molecules on cell surfaces and in soluble forms. Biological activity of TNF is dependent upon binding to either cell surface TNF receptor. Etanercept is a dimeric soluble form of the p75 TNF receptor that can bind to two TNF molecules. It inhibits the activity of TNF *in vitro*.

Infliximab and adalimumab are in the subclass of 'anti-TNFα antibodies' (they are in the form of naturally occurring antibodies), and are capable of neutralizing all forms (extracellular, transmembrane, and receptor-bound) of TNFα. These monoclonal antibodies have high specificity for TNFα, and do not neutralize TNFβ, a related but less inflammatory cytokine that utilizes the same receptors as TNFα. They neutralize the biological activity of TNFα by binding with high affinity to the soluble (free floating in the blood) and transmembrane (located on the outer membranes of T cells and similar immune cells) forms of TNFα and inhibit or prevent the effective binding of TNFα with its receptors. The anti-TNFα antibodies have the capability of lysing cells involved in the inflammatory process, whereas the receptor fusion protein apparently lacks this capability. However, the clinical significance of these differences has not been absolutely proven (Nurmohamed and Dijkmans 2005).

Toxic effects

Injection site reactions About 14–37% of patients may complain of mild-to-moderate reactions (erythema and/or itching, pain, or swelling) at the site of injection of etanercept. Injection site reactions generally occur in the first month and subsequently decrease in frequency. The mean duration of injection site reactions is 3–5d. Systemic side effects are headache, rash, nausea, and stomach upset.

Infections The risk of infection of anti-TNFα agents is difficult to evaluate as most patients receiving these drugs are also treated with glucocorticoids or immunosuppressive agents. However, the rate of serious infections such as tuberculosis, sepsis, and fungal infections appears to be increased in anti-TNF treated subjects compared to the expected rate. Some of these infections can be severe and life-threatening. Individuals with active infections should not be treated with anti-TNFα agents.

Neurologic toxicity Optic neuritis, polyneuropathy, Guillain–Barré syndrome may seldom occur. Exceptional cases of demyelinating disease have been reported in patients treated with etanercept.

Malignancies Theoretically, drugs that block the activity of TNFα may increase the risk of malignancy. Once again, however, it is difficult to assess the oncogenic risk of anti-TNF agents, as patients given these agents have also been treated with other immunosuppressive drugs often given at high doses and for prolonged periods of time. Moreover, patients with rheumatoid arthritis have a higher rate of cancers than the general population, the connection between cancer and use of anti- TNFα agents is unclear.

Immunogenicity Antibodies to the TNFα receptor portion or other protein components of the drug product may be detected in sera of adult patients treated with anti-TNFα agents. These antibodies were all non-neutralizing. No apparent correlation of antibody development to clinical response or adverse events was observed.

Induction of autoimmune disease Through a Medline search Ramos-Casals et al. (2007) identified 233 cases of autoimmune diseases (vasculitis in 113, lupus in 92, interstitial lung diseases in 24, and other diseases in 4) secondary to TNFα-targeted therapies in 226 patients. Leukocytoclastic vasculitis was the most frequent type of vasculitis, and purpura was the most frequent cutaneous lesion.

Pregnancy The few available data about pregnancy mainly come from case-reports or retrospective studies. From the small numbers available there was no excess of birth defects with etanercept or infliximab. However, exposed newborns were more likely to be born prematurely and to be lower in body weight than other newborns from mothers with rheumatoid arthritis (Chambers et al., 2006). The FDA includes all the three anti-TNFα agents in the category B (no documented increased risk for structural defects).

Clinical use in glomerulonephritis

Anti-TNFα agents have been used successfully in some cases of vasculitis and lupus nephritis. Experimental studies and clinical observations support a role for TNFα in the pathogenesis of acute and chronic renal disease. It has been showed, for example, that TNFA2 and TNFd2 alleles are strongly associated with occurrence/initiation of idiopathic membranous nephropathy and these should be considered as *susceptibility* genes for this disease. However, caution should be used before considering anti-TNFα agents for treatment of primary glomerulonephritis. In fact, given their dual functions in inflammation and immune regulation, TNF may mediate both proinflammatory as well as immunosuppressive effects, particularly in kidney diseases. As pointed out above blockade of TNF may lead to the development of autoantibodies, SLE, or vasculitis in patients affected by other auto-immune diseases. These data raise concern about using TNFα-blocking therapies in renal disease because the kidney may be especially vulnerable to the manifestation of autoimmune processes. On the other hand, there are sporadic reports emphasizing good results with the use of anti-TNFα agents in lupus nephritis and vasculitis, exactly the same diseases that may be triggered by their administration. Thus, further studies are needed to better understand the actual role of TNFα in glomerular diseases. In this context, it is possible that the two TNF receptors may exert different activities in mediating local inflammatory injury in the kidney and systemic immune-regulatory functions as suggested by experimental studies.

Miscellaneous immunomodulating agents

Intravenous immunoglobulins

Intravenous immunoglobulins (IVIg) are purified IgG extracted from the plasma of thousands of blood donors. IVIg are mainly used in primary immune deficiencies, infections, inflammatory and autoimmune diseases. The commercially available products include certain characteristics:

* They should be prepared out of at least 1000 different human donors.
* All four IgG subgroups (1–4) should be present.
* The IgG should maintain biological activity and lifetime of at least 21d.
* The product can not contain samples which are HIV, hepatitis B, hepatitis C positive.
* The product must be screened and treated in a manner that destroys viruses.

IVIg are administered by infusion. Dosage of IVIg is dependent on indication. In renal diseases IVIg are usually given at a dose of 400mg/kg of body weight every 3–4 weeks.

Mechanisms of action

The precise mechanism by which IVIg suppress harmful inflammation has not been definitively established but is believed that they can exert multiple functions. Acceleration of the rate of IgG catabolism is the most plausible unifying explanation for the beneficial action of high doses of IVIg. Such a process would eliminate individual IgG molecules in direct proportion of their relative concentration in plasma.

Another possibility is that IVIg exert inhibitory effects on a Fcγ receptor, by a competitive blockade of the Fcγ receptor and of the effector function and/or by modulating the expression of Fc receptors (up-regulation of inhibitory receptors and downregulation of activating receptors). Recent studies have localized the anti-inflammatory and immunomodulating effects of IVIg to a highly sialylated subfraction of IgG where the terminal sialic acid is linked to an asparagine residue (Asp297) of the constant Fc domain of IgG (Kaneko et al., 2006; Kaveri et al., 2008). Preparations of Ig enriched for this subfraction may eventually come into broad clinical use as therapeutic agents for autoimmune diseases (Kaveri et al., 2008)

Additionally, IVIg may immunoregulate the anti-idiotype antibodies, by neutralizing the activity-inhibition of the binding to the respective autoantigen.

They may also prevent the lytic effects of the terminal complement complex C5b-9 (the membrane attack), by scavenging complement components and diverting membrane attack from cellular targets. Finally, IVIg may modulate cytokines by triggering the production of IL-1 receptor antagonist; may interact with the membrane molecules of antigen-presenting-cells, T cells, and B cells; and may inhibit the differentiation and maturation of dendritic cells.

Toxic effects

Undesirable effects from IVIg occur in less than 5% of patients.

Influenza-like syndrome The most common adverse effects occur soon after infusions and can include headache, flushing, chills, myalgia, wheezing, tachycardia, lower back pain, nausea, and hypotension. If this happens during an infusion, the infusion should be slowed or stopped. If symptoms are anticipated, a patient can be premedicated with antihistamines and intravenous hydrocortisone.

Allergic reaction IVIg can induce reactions in patients with IgA deficiency. This occurs in 1 out of 500–1000 patients. Serious anaphylactoid reactions occur soon after the administration of IVIg. Anaphylaxis associated with sensitization to IgA in patients with IgA deficiency can be prevented by using IgA-depleted immune globulin. The presence of IgG anti-IgA antibodies is not always associated with severe adverse reactions to IVIg.

Acute renal failure An uncommon but life-threatening and potentially irreversible adverse event is acute renal failure. Acute renal failure with IVIg therapy occurred with the sucrose-stabilized formulation, but not with the D-sorbitol–stabilized formulation (Vo et al., 2006). The issue of potential IVIg nephrotoxicity should be fully considered when prescribing IVIg to a renal patient. Products containing sucrose as a stabilizer have an elevated osmolality and are mainly associated with such injury through the mechanism of osmotic nephrosis. Apart from unmodifiable risk factors such as pre-existing renal disease and old age, another important risk factor for such toxicity is represented by volume depletion. A correct level of hydration is therefore mandatory before or during the infusion of IVIg.

Thrombosis IVIg may cause rare cases of thrombosis. Cases of strokes, transient ischemic attacks, myocardial infarction, deep venous thrombosis (DVT), and retinal artery infarct have been reported. These complications are more frequent when products with high osmolality are used (Vo et al., 2006) and in patients with underlying risk factors such as hypertension, hypercholesterolemia, atrial fibrillation, history of vascular disease and stroke, and DVT. It is recommended to be vigilant about the possibility of thromboembolic complications and to be judicious with the use of IVIg in patients with underlying risk factors.

Pregnancy IVIg have been largely used in pregnancy. The tolerance is usually good. No adverse impact on the fetus has been reported.

Clinical use in glomerulonephritis

There are anecdotal encouraging reports on the efficacy of prolonged IVIg in primary glomerulonephritis, mainly membranous nephropathy, resistant to conventional therapy. However, the exact success rate, optimal dosage, and clinical indications remain undetermined. Treatment with IVIg is expensive and is not devoid of side effects. Patients with glomerulonephritis for whom a treatment with IVIg is prescribed should be closely monitored and receive an adequate hydration to correct volume depletion, which together with renal disease represents a risk factor for nephrotoxicity. It is likely that the discovery of a recombinant form of sialylated Fc IgG that recapitulates the anti-inflammatory activity of whole IVIg preparations will stimulate activity in this area pharmacotherapeutics (Anthony et al., 2008).

Levamisole

This agent is asynthetic imidazothiazole derivative that has been used for many years as an anti-helminthic drug. After levamisole was shown to have immunomodulatory properties it has been used as a steroid-sparing agent in patients with minimal change nephropathy and frequent relapses of the nephrotic syndrome. The drug is available in form of tablets. Levamisole is not available or approved for use in glomerular disease in the USA but is available in Canada, Europe, and in Asia.

Clinical pharmacology

Levamisole is a levo-isomer of tetramisole. After administration by mouth it is rapidly and completely absorbed with a plasma peak after 2–4h. The drug is metabolized by the liver. The opening of the thiazolic ring produces the metabolite DL-2-oxy-3 (2-mercaptoethyl)-5 phenylimidazoline, which has immunomodulating effects. The drug is mainly excreted by the kidney and by the gastrointestinal tract. The plasma half-life is about 4h. Only 5% of the drug is excreted unmodified in the urine.

Mechanisms of action

Levamisole enhances the specific immune response and restores immunity in immune-deficient hosts. The drug stimulates the differentiation of T cells, restores the function of T cells, and increases the activity of macrophages when the immune system is depressed, so amplifying the immune response. It also increases the motility of neutrophils.

The exact mechanism of action in renal disease is still poorly defined. It has been hypothesized that the sulphur contained in levamisole may release a factor that would interfere with T-cell function, in a way similar to thymic hormone. Moreover the imidazolic group increases the cellular content of GMP. The consequent increased intracellular ratio GMP/AMP stimulates the immunological response and enhances the production of cellular clones.

Toxic effects

Adverse reactions are usually mild and consist of fatigue, arthralgias, and fever often associated with nausea, diarrhea, and metallic taste.

Allergic reactions Cutaneous complications are a cause of discontinuation of the drug. Allergic reactions can also be responsible for difficulty in breathing, closing of the throat, and swelling of the lips, tongue, or face.

Hematological tolerance Significant neutropenia may occur in about 10% of nephrotic patients.

Vasculitis Cases of leukocytoclastic vasculitis have been reported.

Neurological complications Rarely the drug may be responsible for tremors, agitation, seizures, and confusion.

Pregnancy Levamisole has not been studied for use by pregnant women. It is unknown whether Levamisole may be dangerous for the fetus. Although it is unlikely that the drug produces teratogenic effects, it has been classified in category C (insufficient information) by the FDA. It is better to avoid the use of levamisole during pregnancy.

Clinical use in glomerulonephritis

Levamisole has been used in children with minimal change nephropathy, on the assumption that the drug might restore abnormal T-cell function. The drug is mainly used in children with frequent relapses of idiopathic nephrotic syndrome as a steroid-sparing agent. At doses of 2.5mg/kg twice a week (from 6 to 12 months) the drug is well tolerated. Non-controlled studies emphasized the effectiveness of levamisole but the results of randomized trials are less optimistic. In patients not able to take or tolerate other therapies it may have a role. At present the drug is not commercially available in many Western countries.

Deoxyspergualin

15-Deoxyspergualin (DSG). is a synthetic analog of spergualin, a natural product of the bacterium *Bacillus laterosporus*. DGS has been initially developed as an anti-cancer drug, but strong immunosuppressive properties were later discovered in several animal models of transplantation, and of autoimmune disease. DGS has been successfully used in patients with recurrent kidney transplant rejections. DGS comes in the form of white powder and is easily dissolved in water. The drug is supplied for intravenous or subcutaneous injection. The European Commission has assigned to DGS the status of *orphan drug* treatment of Wegener's granulomatosis..

LF 15-0195, an analog of DGS, also has powerful immunosuppressive properties and has been shown to be able to prevent rejection and to induce operational tolerance in mouse cardiac allograft models.

Clinical pharmacology

DGS is a 1-amino-19-guanidino-11-hydroxy-4, 9, 12-triazanona-decane-10, 1–3-dione with a molecular weight of 497. A small fraction of DSG is excreted unmetabolized in the urine. The amount of DSG in the urine correlates strongly to renal function. Pharmacokinetics are otherwise not affected by the degree of renal function. Therefore, the drug can safely be given to patients with impaired renal function.

Mechanisms of action

DGS binds to an immunophilin, Hsc 70, involved in the refolding and allosteric changes of proteins but the mechanism of action is not well understood. DGS can inhibit several immunologic functions, such as the development of plaque-forming cells, but, in particular, it inhibits lysosomal enzyme release and superoxide production by monocytes. It has, therefore, been suggested that DGS may be immunosuppressive via a predominantly antimonocyte-macrophage effect. The drug may also inhibit lymphocyte proliferation in response to mitogenic and allogenic stimuli and antibody production by B cells.

Toxic effects

Leukopenia Neutropenia is frequent but it is usually transient and reversible. In contrast to neutrophil counts, lymphocyte and monocyte counts are less affected by DSG. However a slight decrease in absolute lymphocyte counts of approximately 20% below the normal range may be observed.

Infections Infections, mostly of the upper respiratory tract, may occur. They usually resolve quickly with the use of antibiotics, without further consequences.

Opportunistic infections are rare but may develop in patients taking concomitantly other immunosuppressive drugs.

Gastrointestinal troubles Some patients complain of gastric discomfort and flushing.

Pregnancy There is no information about the use of DGS in pregnant women.

Clinical use in glomerulonephritis

Experimental studies showed the efficacy of DGS in animal models of lupus nephritis, mesangial proliferative glomerulonephritis, and crescentic glomerulonephritis. From preclinical and clinical data, DSG appears to be a potent immunosuppressant with a favorable side effect profile exerting no renal, liver, or diabetogenic toxicity

The drug has been successfully used in few patients with vasculitis or lupus nephritis, although the available reports refer to only short-term follow-up. Hotta et al. (1999) demonstrated that DSG shows therapeutic efficacy in patients with crescentic proliferative glomerulonephritis, but no randomized controlled comparative trials with other effective treatments in this or other primary glomerulonephritis are available.

Imatinib

Imatinib mesylate is a protein-tyrosine kinase inhibitor approved for treatment of chronic myeloid leukemia, gastrointestinal stromal tumors, and some brain tumors. The drug may also exert favorable effects in some rheumatic diseases. It is available in form of rigid capsules that should be taken in a single daily administration during a meal with a glass of water.

Clinical pharmacology

Imatinib is well absorbed after oral administration with a peak in plasma concentration achieved within 2–4 h post-dose. Mean absolute bioavailability is 98%. Following oral administration in healthy volunteers, the elimination half-lives of imatinib and its major active metabolite, the N-demethyl derivative, are approximately 18 and 40 h, respectively. At clinically relevant concentrations of imatinib, binding to plasma proteins in *in vitro* experiments is approximately 95%, mostly to albumin and a1-acid glycoprotein.

CYP3A4 is the major enzyme responsible for metabolism of imatinib. Other cytochrome P450 enzymes play a minor role in its metabolism. The main circulating active metabolite in humans is the N-demethylated piperazine derivative, which shows *in vitro* potency similar to the parent imatinib. The plasma protein binding of N-demethylated metabolite CGP74588 is similar to that of the parent compound. Approximately 81% of the dose is eliminated mostly as metabolites within 7d, in feces (68%) and urine (13%). Unchanged imatinib accounts for 25% of the dose.

Mechanisms of action

Imatinib is a 2-phenylaminopyrimidine derivative that functions as a specific inhibitor of a number of tyrosine kinase enzymes. It occupies the *TK* active site, leading to a decrease in activity. In particular, imatinib inhibits the bcr-abl tyrosine kinase, the constitutive abnormal tyrosine kinase created by the Philadelphia chromosome abnormality in chronic myeloid leukemia. Imatinib inhibits proliferation and induces apoptosis in bcr-abl-positive cell lines as well as fresh leukemic cells from Philadelphia chromosome positive chronic myeloid leukemia. Imatinib inhibits colony formation in assays using *ex vivo* peripheral blood and bone marrow samples.

Imatinib is also an inhibitor of the receptor tyrosine kinases for platelet-derived growth factor (PDGF) and stem cell factor (SCF), c-kit, and inhibits PDGF-and SCF-mediated cellular events.

Toxic effects

Hepatotoxicity Cases of acute hepatitis with five to more than twenty times upper normal levels of transaminases or four times upper normal values of bilirubin have been reported in 0.4–3.5% of patients. Data about liver histology varies between reports from focal periportal necrosis with mixed lymphocyte, neutrophil, and plasmocyte infiltration to massive hepatic necrosis or cytolytic acute hepatitis. The time between beginning treatment and development of liver toxicity varies from 11d to 49 weeks. Hepatotoxicity is usually resolved with imatinib dose reduction or interruption. Yet permanent imatinib discontinuation for hepatic toxicity may be required in 0.5% of patients. Exceptionally, deaths from hepatic failure have been reported (Ridruejo et al., 2007).

Edema Most patients present with periorbital and leg edema. Sometimes fluid retention may be severe with pleural and/or pericardial effusion.

Gastrointestinal side effects Nausea, vomiting, diarrhea may occur in 40–70% of patients.

Pain Musculoskeletal or abdominal pain is common but mild. They may be managed with medication without reducing the prescribed dosage.

Cardiac complications Severe congestive cardiac failure is an uncommon but well recognized side effect of imatinib. Mice treated with large doses of imatinib show toxic damage to their myocardium.

Bone marrow toxicity Anemia and cytopenias have been rarely described. A very few case reports of bone marrow aplasia following imatinib therapy have been reported so far.

Pregnancy Imatinib has been found to be teratogenic in rats and is not recommended for use during pregnancy. There is a paucity of data regarding patients on imatinib mesylate becoming pregnant and completing pregnancy. Only a few pregnancies in women with chronic myeloid leukemia proceeded to term; most of them had normal infants, one infant had hypospadias.

Clinical use in primary glomerulonephritis

Experimental studies showed that imatinib may reduce mesangial cell proliferation, may block a non-Smad TGFβ pathway so reducing renal fibrogenesis (Wang et al., 2006), and may obtain an amelioration of disease in NZB/W lupus mice probably due to its interference with platelet derived growth factor (Zoja et al., 2006). These data may render imatinib of potential interest for treating primary glomerulonephritis (such as IgA nephropathy) and lupus nephritis, but the serious side effects of therapy remain a significant concern.

References

Anthony KM, Nimmerjahn F, Ashline DJ, Rheinhold VN, Paulson JC, Ravetch JV (2008). Recapitulation of IVIg anti-inflammatory activity with a recombinant IgG Fc. *Science* **320**:373–6.

Appenzeller S, Blatyta PF, Costallat LT (2008). Ovarian failure in SLE patients using pulse cyclophosphamide: comparison of different regimes. *Rheumatology International* **28**:567–71.

Asberg A (2003). Interactions between cyclosporine and lipid-lowering drugs: implications for organ transplant recipients. *Drugs* **663**:367–78.

Atanasov AG, Odermatt A (2007). Readjusting the glucocorticoid balance: an opportunity for modulators of 11beta-hydroxysteroid dehydrogenase type 1 activity? *Endocrinological. Metabolic Immune Disorders Drug Targets* **7**:125–40.

Barnes PJ (2006). Corticosteroids the drugs to beat. *European Journal Pharmacology* **533**: 2–14.

Behrend M, Braun F (2005). Enteric-coated mycophenolate sodium: tolerability profile compared with mycophenolate mofetil. *Drugs* **65**:1037–50.

Berg AL, Rafnsson AT, Johannsson M, Dallongeville J, Arnadottir M (2006).The effects of adrenocorticotrophic hormone and an equivalent dose of cortisol on the serum concentrations of lipids, lipoproteins, and apolipoproteins. *Metabolism* **55**:1083–7.

Bernatsky S, Ramsey-Goldman R, Clarke AE (2005). Revisiting the issue of malignancy risk in systemic lupus erythematosus. *Current Rheumatological Reports* **7**:476–81.

Boumpas DT, Tassiulas IO, Fleisher TA, et al. (1999).A pilot study of low-dose fludarabine in membranous nephropathy refractory to therapy. *Clinical Nephrology* **52**:67–75.

Callis L, Nieto J, Vila A, and Rende J (1980). Chlorambucil treatment in minimal lesion nephrotic syndrome: a reappraisal of its gonadal toxicity. *Journal of Pediatrics* **97**: 653–6.

Casetta I, Iuliano G, Filippini G (2007). Azathioprine for multiple sclerosis. *Cochrane Database Systematic Review* **4**:CD003982.

Cattran DC, Alexopoulos E, Heering et al. (2007). Cyclosporin in idiopathic glomerular disease associated with the nephrotic syndrome: workshop recommendations. *Kidney International* **72**:1429–47.

Chambers CD, Tutunku ZM, Johnson D, Jones KL (2006). Human pregnancy safety for agents used to treat rheumatoid arthritis: adequacy of available information and strategies for developing post-marketing data. *Arthritis Research Therapy* **8**:215–25.

Cho ME, Hurley JK, Kopp JB (2007). Sirolimus therapy in focal segmental glomerular sclerosis is associated with nephrotoxicity. *American Journal Kidney Diseases* **49**: 310–17.

Chocair PR, Duley JA, Sabbaga E, Arap S, Simmonds HA, and Cameron JS (1993). Fast and slow methylators: do racial differences influence risk of allograft rejection? *Quarterly Journal Medicine* **86**:359–63.

Cvetkovic RS, Perry CM (2006). Rituximab. *Drugs* **66**:791–820.

Daniel C, Renders L, Amann K, Schulze-Lohoff E, Hauser IA, Hugo C (2005). Mechanisms of everolimus-induced glomerulosclerosis after glomerular injury in the rat. *American Journal Transplantation* **5**:2849–61

Fardet L, Kassar A, Cabane J, Flahault A (2007). Corticosteroid-induced adverse events in adults. *Drug Safety* **30**:861–81.

Faurschou M, Sorensen IJ, Mellemkjaer L, et al. (2008). Malignancies in Wegener's granulomatosis: incidence and relation to cyclophosphamide therapy in a cohort of 293 patients. *Journal of Rheumatology* **35**:100–5.

Filaretova L, Bobryshev P, Bagaeva T, Podvigina T, Takeuchi K (2007).Compensatory gastroprotective role of glucocorticoid hormones during inhibition of prostaglandin and nitric oxide production and desensitization of capsaicin-sensitive sensory neurons. *Inflammopharmacology* **15**:146–53.

Frampton JE, Wagstaff AJ (2003). Alemtuzumab. *Drugs* **63**:1229–43.

Harris M, Hofman PL, Cutfield WS (2004). Growth hormone treatment in children: review of safety and efficacy. *Paediatric Drugs* **6**:93–106.

Heitzer MD, Wolf IM, Sanchez ER, Witchel SF, Defranco DB (2007).Glucocorticoid receptor physiology. *Endocrinology and Metabolism Disorders* **8**:321–30.

Hirayama T, Athanasou NA (2002). Effects of corticosteroids on human osteoclast formation and activity. *Journal of Endocrinology* **175**:155–63.

Hirsch HH, Knowles W, Dickenmann M, et al (2002). Prospective study of polyomavirus type BK replication and nephropathy and renal transplant recipients. *New Engl J Med* **347**:488–96.

Hotta O, Furuta T, Chiba S, Yusa N, Taguma Y (1999). Immunosuppressive effect of deoxyspergualin in proliferative glomerulonephritis. *American Journal Kidney Diseases* **34**:894–901.

Imbasciati E, Gusmano R, Edefonti A et al. (1985). Controlled trial of methylprednisolone pulses and low oral dose prednisone for minimal change nephrotic syndrome. *British Medical Journal* **291**:1305–8.

Iuchi T, Akaike M, Mitsui T, et al. (2003).Glucocorticoid excess induces superoxide production in vascular endothelial cells and elicits vascular endothelial dysfunction. *Circulation Research* **92**:81–7.

Kahan BD (2000). Immunosuppressive drugs: molecular and cellular mechanisms of action. In BD Kahan and C Ponticelli (eds) *Principles and Practice of Renal Transplantation*, pp.315–48. Martin Dunitz, London.

Kahan BD, Kelly P (2000). Immunosuppressive drugs: Pharmacology. In BD Kahan and C Ponticelli (eds) *Principles and Practice of Renal Transplantation*, pp.251–314. Martin Dunitz, London.

Kaldor JM, Day NE, Pettersson F, et al. (1990). Leukemia following chemotherapy for ovarian cancer. *New England Journal of Medicine* **322**:1–6.

Kaneko Y, Nimmerjahn F, Ravetch JV (2006). Anti-inflammatory activity of immunoglobulin G resulting from Fc sialylation. *Science* **313**:670–3.

Kaveri SV, Lacroix-Desmazes, Bayry J (2008). The anti-inflammatory IgG. *New England Journal of Medicine* **359**:307–9.

Klink DT, van Elburg RM, Schreurs MW, van Well GT (2008). Rituximab administration in third trimester of pregnancy suppresses neonatal B-cell development. *Clinical and Developmental Immunology* **271**:363–9.

Knight A, Askling J, Granath F, Sparen P, Ekbom A (2004).Urinary bladder cancer in Wegener's granulomatosis: risks and relation to cyclophosphamide. *Annals Rheumatic Diseases* **63**:1307–11.

Kobashigawa JA, Kasiske BL (1997). Hyperlipidemia in solid organ transplantation. *Transplantation* **63**:331–8.

Korkmaz A, Topal T, Oter S (2007). Pathophysiological aspects of cyclophosphamide and ifosfamide induced hemorrhagic cystitis; implication of reactive oxygen and nitrogen species as well as PARP activation. *Cell Biology Toxicology* **23**:303–12.

Kovarik JM, Mueller EA, Niese D (1996). Clinical development of a cyclosporine microemulsion in transplantation. *Therapeutic Drug Monitonitoring* **18**:429–34.

Lamche HR, Silberstein PT, Knabe AC, Thomas DD, Jacob HS, Hammerschmidt DE (1990). Steroids decrease granulocyte membrane fluidity, while phorbol ester increases membrane fluidity. Studies using electron paramagnetic resonance. *Inflammation* **14**:61–70.

Latta K, von Schnakenburg C, Ehrich JH (2001). A meta-analysis of cytotoxic treatment for frequently relapsing nephrotic syndrome in children. *Pediatric Nephrology* **16**:271–82.

Lee MJ, Wang Y, Ricci MR, Sullivan S, Russell CD, Fried SK (2007). Acute and chronic regulation of leptin synthesis, storage, and secretion by insulin and dexamethasone in human adipose tissue. *American Journal Physiology Endocrinology Metabolism* **292**:E858–64.

Letavernier E, Bruneval P, Mandet C, et al. (2007). High sirolimus levels may induce focal segmental glomerulosclerosis de novo. *Clinical Journal American Society Nephrology* **2**:326–33.

Lock HR, Sacks SH, Robson MG (2007). Rapamycin at subimmunosuppressive levels inhibits mesangial cell proliferation and extracellular matrix production. *American Journal Physiology Renal Physiology* **292**:F76–81.

Lou T, Wang C, Chen Z, et al. (2006). Randomised controlled trial of leflunomide in the treatment of immunoglobulin A nephropathy. *Nephrology* (Carlton) **11**:113–16.

Löwenberg M, Stahn C, Hommes DW, Buttgereit F (2008). Novel insights into mechanisms of glucocorticoid action and the development of new glucocorticoid receptor ligands. *Steroids* **73**:1025–9.

Lu NZ, Cidlowski JA (2004). The origin and functions of multiple human glucocorticoid receptor isoforms. *Annals New York Academy Science* **1024**:102–23.

Masuda S, Inui K (2006). An up-date review on individualized dosage adjustment of calcineurin inhibitors in organ transplant patients. *Pharmacology Therapeutics* **112**:184–98.

McKay DB, Josephson MA (2006). Pregnancy in recipients of solid organs – effects on mother and child. *New England Journal of Medicine* **354**:1281–93.

Mihatsch MJ, Kyo M, Morozumi K, Yamaguchi Y, Nickeleit V, Ryffel B (1998).The side-effects of ciclosporine-A and tacrolimus. *Clinical Nephrology* **49**:356–63.

Naumovic R, Jovovic D, Basta-Jovanovic G, et al. (2007). Effects of rapamycin on active Heymann nephritis. *American Journal Nephrology* **27**:379–89.

Nurmohamed MT, Dijkmans BA (2005). Efficacy, tolerability and cost effectiveness of disease-modifying antirheumatic drugs and biologic agents in rheumatoid arthritis. *Drugs* **65**:661–94.

Olyaei AJ, de Mattos AM, Bennett WM (2001). Nephrotoxicity of immunosuppressive drugs: new insight and preventive strategies. *Current Opinions Critical Care* **7**:384–9.

Park MC, Park YB, Jung SY, Chung IH, Choi KH, Lee SK (2004). Risk of ovarian failure and pregnancy outcome in patients with lupus nephritis treated with intravenous cyclophosphamide pulse therapy. *Lupus* **13**:569–74.

Penn, I. (1991). The changing pattern of posttransplant malignancies. *Transplantation Proceedings* **23**:1101–3.

Ponticelli C, Altieri P, Scolari F, et al. (1998). A randomized study comparing methylprednisolone plus chlorambucil versus methylprednisolone plus cyclophosphamide in idiopathic membranous nephropathy. *Journal American Society Nephrology* **9**:440–50.

Ponticelli C, Campise R (2005). Neurological complications in kidney transplant recipients *Journal Nephrology* **18**:521–8.

Ponticelli C, Passerini P, Salvadori M, et al. (2006).A randomized pilot trial comparing methylprednisolone plus a cytotoxic agent versus synthetic adrenocorticotropic hormone in idiopathic membranous nephropathy. *American Journal Kidney Diseases* **47**(2):233–40.

Ramos-Casals M, Brito-Zerón P, Muñoz S, et al. (2007). Autoimmune diseases induced by TNF-targeted therapies: analysis of 233 cases. *Medicine* (Baltimore) **86**:242–51.

Ransom RF, Lam NG, Hallett MA, Atkinson SJ, Smoyer WE (2005). Glucocorticoids protect and enhance recovery of cultured murine podocytes via actin filament stabilization. *Kidney International* **68**:2473–83.

Ridruejo E, Cacchione R, Villamil AG, Marciano S, Gadano AC, Mando OG (2007). Imatinib-induced fatal acute liver failure. *World Journal Gastroenterology* **13**:6608–11.

Saviola G, Abdi Ali L, Shams Eddin S, et al. (2007). Compared clinical efficacy and bone metabolic effects of low-dose deflazacort and methylprednisolone in male inflammatory arthropathies: a 12-month open randomized pilot study. *Rheumatology* (Oxford) **46**:994–8.

Schlesinger N (2008). Overview of the management of acute gout and the role of adreno-corticotropic hormone. *Drugs* **68**:407–15.

Smith LJ, McKeage K, Keam SJ, Plosker GL (2003). Tacrolimus. *Drugs* **63**:1247–97.

Tumlin JA, Miller D, Near M, Selvaraj S, Hennigar R, Guasch A (2006) A prospective, open-label trial of sirolimus in the treatment of focal segmental glomerulosclerosis. *Clinical Journal American Society Nephrology* **1**:109–16.

Vasudev B, Hariharan S (2007). Cancer after renal transplantation. *Current Opinion Nephrology Hypertension* **16**:523–8.

Vanrenterghem Y, Ponticelli C, Morales J et al. (2003). Prevalence and management of anemia in renal transplant recipients: A European Survey. *American Journal Transplantation* **3**:835–45.

Vo AA, Cam V, Toyoda M, et al. (2006).Safety and adverse events profiles of intravenous gammaglobulin products used for immunomodulation: a single-center experience. *Clinical Journal American Society Nephrology* **1**:844–52.

Wang S, Wilkes MC, Leof EB, Hirschberg R (2006). Imatinib mesylate blocks a non-Smad TGF-beta pathway and reduces renal fibrogenesis in vivo. *Federation American Societies for Experimental Biology Journal* **19**:1–11.

Wetzels JF (2004). Cyclophosphamide-induced gonadal toxicity: a treatment dilemma in patients with lupus nephritis? *Netherlands Journal Medicine* **62**:347–52.

Wijdicks EF. (2001). Neurotoxicity of immunosuppressive drugs. *Liver Transplantation* **7**:37–942.

Wittmann S, Daniel C, Braun A, et al. (2008). The mTOR inhibitor everolimus attenuates the time course of chronic anti-Thy1 nephritis in the rat. *Nephron Experimental Nephrology* **108**:45–56.

Xing CY, Saleem MA, Coward RJ, Ni L, Witherden IR, Mathieson PW (2006). Direct effects of dexamethasone on human podocytes. *Kidney International* **70**:1038–45.

Zoja C, Corna D, Rottoli D, Zanchi C, Abbate M, Remuzzi G (2006). Imatinib ameliorates renal disease and survival in murine lupus autoimmune disease. *Kidney International* **70**:97–103.

Zver S, Zadnik V, Bunc M, Rogel P, Cernelc P, Kozelj M (2007). Cardiac toxicity of high-dose cyclophosphamide in patients with multiple myeloma undergoing autologous hematopoietic stem cell transplantation. *International Journal Hematology* **85**:408–14.

Chapter 3

Evaluation of observational and controlled trials of therapy

Richard J. Glassock and Daniel C. Cattran

Introduction

The literature on the subject of treatment of glomerular disease is immense (over 15,000 articles in PubMed as of July, 2008). Negotiating this broad and complex panorama can be a difficult task, especially in relationship to the evaluation of the *best evidence for a particular treatment strategy for a specific disease entity occurring in an individual patient.* Perfection is not attainable in clinical trials of therapy and every report has some pitfall or limitation. Some studies, however, stand out as excellent examples of design and execution. Unfortunately, in the field of treatment of glomerular disease such studies are relatively uncommon. The good news is that well designed and executed studies of treatment of primary glomerular disease are being reported with increasing frequency in recent years. This has occurred in part because of increased collaboration among groups interested in furthering knowledge in this important area of inquiry, but also because of better recognition of the deficiencies of past efforts to study treatment of glomerular disease in clinical trials. Many interinstitutional collaborative studies have been aided by improvements in trial design and by more complete descriptions of the natural history of untreated disease. One of the main weaknesses of clinical studies of therapy in primary glomerular disease is the small numbers of subjects studied in individual reports. This increases the risks of confounding and of both false positive and false negative results.

The purpose of this chapter is to provide a concise analysis of the strengths and weakness of the various approaches to the study of therapeutic efficacy and safety of agents used in primary glomerular disease. The focus will be on observational studies, controlled clinical trials, and meta-analyses of published reports. The specific aims are to equip the discerning reader for improved understanding of the evidence-base for therapy of primary glomerular disease. The details of the specific reports and how they can be integrated into an 'evidence-based' approach to therapeutic decision-making are dealt with in the chapters devoted to specific disease entities which follow.

Observational studies

Strictly speaking, an observational study would include any examination of the efficacy or safety of a treatment strategy that does not include a prospectively selected, contemporaneous control group (placebo-treated or treated with a comparator agent or regimen, usually one chosen as a 'standard of care') (Shlipak and Stehman-Breen, 2005). Thus, observational studies are of several types:

- ◆ Individual case reports.
- ◆ Collection of case series (often accumulated retrospectively).
- ◆ Case–control studies in which both cases and controls are examined retrospectively.
- ◆ Cohort studies in which both cohorts are selected retrospectively.
- ◆ Studies in which an actively treated group are compared to non-concurrent (historical) controls.
- ◆ Post-hoc (secondary) examination of selected subset of observations from prospective, randomized controlled trials (see below).

Data acquired from renal biopsy registries (Lacut, et al., 2007; Cattran et al., 2008) can also be added to the list of observational studies. Observational studies are primarily 'hypothesis-generating'in that they cannot be used as definitive proof of efficacy or safety of a specific drug for a disease or group of diseases.

Strengths

Observational studies have utility in preliminary examination of treatment regimens in that they are relatively simple to design and execute. They can also involve large numbers of subjects representing diverse features of a given disease, and thus provide clues regarding differential responses to therapy or safety. Cohort and case–control studies are preferred to individual case reports or small case series. Case series with comparison to appropriately selected historical controls may also be useful when the selection of the control group is performed with great care to avoid confounding. Post-hoc examination of selected subgroups from randomized controlled trials may be particularly valuable in identifying potential candidates for other prospectively designed trials. Formal statistical analysis of data from observational trial often 'fails to increase the credibility of the postulated associations' (Ioannidis, 2008).

Pitfalls

The primary weakness of observational studies is that they can demonstrate an association with a studied effect only, which may or may not be casual. Epidemiological studies involving large databases are particularly vulnerable to this pitfall. The phenomenon of 'reverse-causality' where an observed effect (e.g., lowering of blood pressure) is not casually related to the intervention (e.g., a drug treatment), but the intervention is casually related to the effect can be encountered. Effects arising from the indications for intervention may also be observed. Here a benefit is falsely ascribed to a drug intervention when the real effect is the intrinsic behavior of patients selected for the intervention which respect to specific outcomes. Certain criteria may be used to enhance the likelihood that an observational (epidemiological) study is demonstrating a true effect. These criteria, often referred to as the *Bradford Hill* criteria (after Sir Bradford Hill who elaborated them in 1965) (Hill, 1965), include such items as biological plausibility, dose-effect relationships, strength and independence of the association, experimental studies, and consistency of the effect across studies. When many or most of the Bradford Hill criteria can be met the confidence that the observed effect is real is enhanced, but a true casual relationship for an intervention to a specified outcome can only be reliably tested in a randomized controlled clinical trial (see below).

Confounding

A confounding factor or factors may often be present in observational studies and randomized clinical trials are also not immune to this defect (see below) (Streiner and Norman, 1996). A confounding factor is a variable that is closely related to both the intervention being studied and the outcome examined When these confounding factors are not randomly distributed between two arms of an observational study they may distort the true relationships between the intervention and the effect in both positive or negative directions. Well-designed observational studies make a concerted effort to reduce these confounders, but they can never be completely eliminated in studies using an observational design. Confounders must meet three criteria to be considered important:

- They must be associated with the intervention.
- They must predict the outcome being measured.
- They must not be a consequence of the intervention itself.

Randomization of subjects with stratification for known confounders are methods used to minimize the effect of such confounding on the analysis of a study (see below). Statistical adjustment (multivariate analysis) for the effect of possible confounding factors is a frequently used strategy to overcome, at least partially, the effect of these factors on the outcome. The utility of these statistical adjustments is limited to the factors included, which may not be a complete listing of all possible confounding variables.

Lead-time bias

Differences in the stage of a progressive disease between a group undergoing an intervention and the group selected for comparison in observational studies (and randomized controlled trials as well) can give rise to a bias (a constraint on the validity of the study) (Geddes, et al., 2003). In this circumstance subjects enrolled in the intervention group may have had less (or more) time to reach a specified end point than the comparator group. Even if the treatment is totally ineffective the outcomes might be different in the two groups (or vice versa). Lead-time bias is a particular problem in the study of chronic disease having ill-defined starting points or in which the stage of progression is very difficult to accurately quantify in advance.

Equality of comparator groups

Perhaps the most difficult aspect of observational studies that include both an intervention and a comparator group (case–control, cohort, case series with historical controls) is whether the two groups are truly equivalent in all or most of the important elements likely to have an effect on the measured outcome. Balancing for demographic factors (age, sex, ancestry), clinical, and/or renal functional parameters (serum creatinine, urine protein excretion, blood pressure), or renal pathological findings prior to an intervention may not be sufficient to overcome inherent or hidden biases. Subtle differences between the two groups may have magnified effects, especially if the post-intervention periods are lengthy.

Hierarchal values of observational studies

Reports of observational studies are not all of equal value in determining the likelihood of a benefit or harm from a specific intervention. Individual case reports usually have little overall merit for several reasons. First, publication bias leads to the fact that positive studies will be reported more often than negative studies. Nevertheless, dramatic effects in diseases thought to be totally unresponsive to therapy and having a very low frequency of spontaneous improvement cannot easily be disregarded. Whether short-term observation of this kind will translate into long-term benefits is always uncertain. Case series without any concurrent or historical controls showing a consistent trend towards benefit can have an important effect on generating a testable hypothesis, but should not be regarded as anything more than a 'proof of concept.'

These studies are subject to many pitfalls, some of which are outlined above. Case–control and cohort studies are helpful when randomized studies are not feasible and may also be useful when sample sizes available for controlled trials are limited. However, both types of these studies are subject to inherent biases and thus have only limited validity. When the differences between cases and control or between differentially exposed cohorts are small (hazard ratios of ≤2.0) suspicion regarding validity should be raised. Post-hoc analyses of subgroups enrolled in randomized clinical trials are perhaps the most powerful of the observational category of studies in terms of generating testable hypotheses, but as indicated below they cannot be used alone to prove efficacy or safety of a given therapeutic strategy.

Reporting of observational studies

Ideally, reports of observational studies should conform to generally agreed upon guideline. The Strengthening The Reporting of Observational Studies in Epidemiology (**STROBE**) is one such guideline (von Elm, et al., 2007)

Evaluating harms in observational studies

The potential for harm must always be a part of the balancing act of determining the overall desirability of a particular therapeutic regimen or strategy. Observational trials are very important in identifying potential signals for harmful effects; however, small sample sizes may limit the ability to detect uncommon events. The characteristics of the patients studied will likely have an important bearing on the frequency of these harmful effects of therapy (Chou and Helfand, 2005). The age of the patient and the baseline renal function are two obvious elements in this formulation. It is hazardous to extend safety estimations beyond the population examined or the duration of treatment reported in the study. Studies that encompass a broad range of subjects will likely have more meaning in terms of assessment of safety.

Randomized, controlled clinical trials

The randomized controlled trial (RCT) is considered the 'gold-standard' for the testing of the efficacy and safety of therapeutic agents (Streiner and Norman, 1996; Mathews and Farewell, 1996). Its major feature, in comparison to observational studies is that subject allocation to treatment is under the control of the investigator.

Its main advantages are:

- The groups being studied are more comparable (versus observational studies) because potentially confounding variables are more likely to be balanced.

- Investigators, study assessors, and the patients can be masked to treatment allocation.

- The standard statistical tests used for analyses were developed based on random patient allocation.

The main disadvantages of the RCT design are:

- They are expensive to conduct in terms of both time and money.

- The patients that agree to participate (after informed consent) may not represent the full spectrum of the disease.

- Potentially effective treatment is withheld from some subjects (by design).

- Patients may be exposed to potentially dangerous agents without their (or the investigators') knowledge.

- The final results can be delayed for years, during which time new developments may invalidate the trial design.

- They are very inefficient for the detection of safety signals, expect for very common adverse events. The trial is usually designed to evaluate efficacy using stringent statistical criteria. Such statistical evaluation of safety is often not possible, due to the relative infrequency of events.

Reporting guidelines

It has long been recognized that the reporting of RCT should be standardized. The **CONSORT** statement (Consolidated Standards Of Reporting Trials; see Table 3.1) was first published in 1996 with an overarching objective of improving reporting of clinical trials; a checklist and flow diagram that focused on producing a set of standards that can be used by readers (and study designers) and their evaluation of published trials (Begg et al., 1996). The original checklist consisted of 21 items that pertained to all elements of the RCT, including methods, results, and discussion sections. It also identified key pieces of information to help the reader in the evaluation of both the internal and external validity of the report. A flow diagram provided standardized information that should be reported during the progress of patients throughout a parallel design trial, the most common published type of RCT. The most recent update of CONSORT has added that, depending on the design, every study should include how the randomization allocation sequence was generated (e.g., by computer random allocation), and concealed (e.g., opaque sealed envelope) up to the precise point the patient was randomized (Altman et al., 2001). Each of these areas is highly relevant to the evaluation of the quality and reliability of the RCT. This was emphasized by the observation that on review of

Table 3.1 The CONSORT statement for reporting of randomized clinical trials—
22 items in five major categories*

Title/abstract	
Introduction/ background	Rationale and purpose of the trial
Methods	Eligibility, exclusion, study sites
	Interventions
	Objectives/null hypotheses
	Pre-specified primary and secondary outcomes (including adjudication)
	Sample size (and power)
	Randomization (sequence allocation, concealment, stratification)
	Blinding
	Statistical evaluation
Results	Flow of participants (diagram)
	Protocol deviations, withdrawals and discontinuations
	Recruitment
	Numbers analyzed (intention-to-treat, absolute number of events)
	Ancillary and subgroup analysis
	Adverse events (serious and non-serious)
Discussion	Interpretation (potential biases, errors from multiplicity of analyses of outcomes)
	Generalizability (external validity)
	Overall evidence in context of existing evidence
	Conclusions

*Adapted with permission from Altman DG, Schulz KF, Moher D et al. (2001). The revised CONSORT statement for reporting randomized trials: explanation and elaboration. *Ann Intern Med* **134**:663–94.

published RCT data, an allocation sequence with inadequately concealment yielded larger estimates of treatment effects when compared to trials with adequate concealment. The revised CONSORT statement suggests five new subheadings in any RCT trial to allow the reader to better assess the quality of the trial (Altman et al., 2001). Three of these subheadings would fall within the methods section and include specifics of the protocol, assignment, and masking. The protocol would include, for instance, the planned study population together with inclusion/exclusion criteria; the assignment would include the unit of randomization (e.g., individual, cluster or geographic); and the details of masking would include the specific characterization of the therapeutic options (e.g., the similarity in appearance and taste of both the active agent and placebo). The overall objective of the revised CONSORT statement was to minimize the length, optimize the readability of the trial description, and to enhance the clarity through the organization of the actual report of the trial. Its ultimate purpose was to provide the reader with enough valid and meaningful information concerning design, conduct, and analysis of the RCT for the reader to assess its validity. The CONSORT statement process has been expanded, updated and revised over the last decade and these updates are available through their web site at http://www.consort-statement.org.

Study design

Important variations in design need to be considered in evaluating the results of any RCT. However, it is worth noting that even for well-designed clinical trials to succeed, they should be focused on answering an interesting question (for the investigator, sponsor, reader, and, most importantly, the patient).

Placebo control

Typically in a RCT, the comparison group is prescribed conventional (also called 'standard-of-care') therapy that may vary from no treatment at all to a complex array of interventions believed at the time of trial planning to be the best available. To ethically justify any study there should be a reasonable probability that the comparison group, even if on no therapy (placebo), will prove to be as good as, or superior to, the therapy under study, and will not expose the participant to an undue risk of adverse events. If a placebo is to be used it should be totally innocuous. Sometimes the comparison may involve agents, which by virtue of their different routes of administration or other characteristics (IV drugs for example) make the true 'masking' of active agents impossible.

Superiority trial

This is the typical two-group clinical trial with outcomes of either success or failure where the investigators are interested in finding out whether an innovative treatment reduces the frequency of failure relative to standard therapy. This question can be answered by testing the null hypothesis of equal efficacy against the alternative hypothesis of superiority. If the null hypothesis can be rejected in favor of the alternative hypothesis we conclude that the new therapy is superior. This is the classic design of a superiority trial. This is the most common type of clinical trial use in studies of glomerular diseases when a new therapy with no track record in humans appears and there is no recognized alternative therapy for the disease in question except conservative measures.

Active control trial (equivalence trial)

When an effective standard-of-care therapy exists, a new experimental treatment may be investigated because of potentially less toxicity, lower cost, or some other characteristic that would make it the treatment of choice assuming equal efficacy to the standard option. This type of design has been designated an active control trial or equivalence (non-inferiority) trial and the statistical evaluation cannot be based on the usual significance tests because failure to reject the null hypothesis of no treatment difference in a clinical trial does not establish the equivalence of the two treatments compared (Piaggio et al., 2006). This is becoming an increasingly common trial design published in the literature. When a treatment has been shown to be beneficial for a serious medical conditions (e.g., some of the glomerular diseases), it is considered unethical to conduct a subsequent trial with a placebo-control or with any control therapy that is less effective than the best available one. If a superiority trial is conducted under these conditions and the null hypothesis is not rejected, the temptation of the investigators (and reader) is to interpret this as meaning that the two treatment options examined in the study are therapeutically equivalent (Sackett, 2004). This interpretation can be *seriously* flawed for a number of reasons. The study may have insufficient number of patients (i.e., inadequate power) to detect the possibility that one or the other of the tested therapies is clinically better. Fundamentally, demonstrating equivalence reverses the role of the null and alternative hypotheses. This type of design mandates that the trial specify *in advance* the difference between the innovative treatment and the standard therapy (δ in epidemiological terms) that is clinically acceptable. Then, the innovative therapy is judged *not to be equivalent* to standard therapy if the null hypothesis is accepted (true) and to be *equivalent* if the alternative hypothesis holds. Statistically, this commonly translates into using a one-sided test of the null hypothesis at a specified type 1 error rate (α). An essentially identical approach to the design of such a trial uses the one-sided $1 - \alpha$ confidence intervals for the difference between the innovative therapy and the standard therapy and concludes that treatments are equivalent if the upper limit of the confidence interval is less than δ, which is the maximum difference previously determined to be acceptable between the two treatments being tested. An additional component of the equivalence trials is that the study must include a sample size sufficient to yield a power (β) of 0.8 or greater.

The question of choosing a superiority versus non-inferiority (equivalency) trial design (in advance of initiating the trial, not after the trial is concluded) is very important. When a potentially effective new therapy presents itself, the most common question of the clinician is whether it is better than current therapy (i.e., superior) and if not superior is it just as good (non-inferior) but preferable for some other reason (e.g., fewer side effects, better tolerated, less toxic, or less expensive). This type of question is best examined by a superiority trial design that uses the traditional two-sided test of statistical significance requiring rejection of the null hypothesis to prove superiority. However, such a study often results in 'statistically non-significant differences' between the study groups leading to the interpretation by the investigators (and the reader) that the two therapies are therefore equal rather than the *real conclusion* that the results of the study are indeterminate or uncertain. Two-sided p-values tell us the probability that the results are compatible with the null hypothesis. When this probability is small (i.e., standard p of <0.05), we feel safe in rejecting the null hypothesis and accept that the differences between the two therapies are real although the results do not tell us the direction (i.e., whether the new treatment is better or worse than the standard therapy). In this standard interpretation of two-sided p-values, authors report studies as 'negative' statistically (the null hypothesis was not rejected) but occasionally they (erroneously) go on to conclude that the absence of proof of a difference between two treatments constitutes prima facie proof of equivalency or of non-inferiority. In truth, one can never claim the treatments have no effect or that there is no difference in the effects of treatment when this statistical approach is used since there will always be some uncertainty based on the estimate of the treatment effects and therefore small differences can never be excluded. The idea of using one-sided t-test relates to this situation. Even the CONSORT statement (see above) omits any requirement for two-sided significance testing and many prominent journals have accepted and published one-sided non-inferiority trials. However, it must be remembered that an essential element for applying the one-sided testing is the specification of the exact non-inferiority value (δ) in the design phase of the RCT. This is one of the major reasons for the need to register all RCT in their design stage and for publishing the protocols in open-access journals. It is not appropriate to use this type of analysis when the preliminary analysis indicates that conventional two-sided test have generated indeterminate results.

The value of δ can be very difficult to define. It is usually thought of as the smallest value that would present an important clinical difference or the largest value that would not present an important difference between the two treatment options being tested. One option that has been suggested is to use a value that is one half that of the 'value that is of undisputed clinical importance' for δ. It must be obvious that the value of δ is not easily quantified and that each physician, and certainly most patients, will have a different concept of 'an important difference.' If an equivalence limit is chosen based on a clinically meaningful difference, it is important that the authors present not only the hypothesis test results but also the *confidence interval* estimate (95% confidence interval between the mean or median) of the true difference when discussing the study, with a note to the new reader that they must ultimately decide whether the difference is meaningful. Using p-values to reject null hypothesis in RCT may ultimately be replaced by a Bayesian approach hypothesis conditional on the data. Many statisticians prefer the Bayesian analysis over traditional frequent test on p-value methods.

Entry and exclusion criteria

Strict entrance and exclusion requirements for enrollment into any RCT are done to generate a maximally homogeneous patient population and to minimize adverse events by eliminating subjects at higher risk of complications from the drugs under study (e.g., pregnancy, active infection, bleeding disorders, etc.). They are generally created to facilitate treatment comparisons with smaller number of patients. This is a common approach used in the glomerular diseases given the overall low numbers of patients with these disorders. In contrast, larger studies and/or those that consist of a more heterogeneous population would have more meaning to the practicing physician. In epidemiological terms this is considered the question of *external validity*; do the results of this particular treatment trial have relevance to the individual patient seeking advice regarding care? This is in contrast to the other issue of credibility termed the *internal validity*. The assessment of whether the trial results, in the patient population studied, are correct and do not have systematic bias, such as improper and/or unbalanced allocations to the comparison groups or chance error determined by the reader by examination of the p value, study power, and confidence intervals in the paper being reviewed.

Power calculations

Despite the difficulties in determining whether the study has the proper sample size, it is unwise to ignore this element of a trial. It is not widely appreciated that the failure to detect a treatment difference is more often related to *inadequate* sample size than the actual lack of a real difference in the treatment options of the study. The importance of sample size calculations is demonstrated by the fact that they provide information about two important design questions (Mathews and Farewell, 1996a):

- How many subjects should participate in the study?
- Is the study worth doing if only a limited number end up participating in the trial?

The calculations concerning sample size depend on the question of the study. Since sample size calculations depend on the proposed method of analysis, some tentative assumptions must be made. In a trial where the effectiveness of a particular treatment is being compared, the primary question usually relates to the clinically relevant treatment difference (e.g., improved renal survival). This harkens back to whether the null hypothesis is accepted as true. Although this statistical convention may be inappropriate at the time of analysis, it is convenient to invoke at the design stage.

If no treatment difference exists, then α represents the probability of obtaining an unlikely positive outcome in that situation and therefore deciding (incorrectly) that the data contradicts the null hypothesis, by convention a false positive conclusion or type 1 error. If a real treatment difference exists (i.e., the null hypothesis is false and is rejected), the probability that the investigator will make the right conclusion is 1–β. But, if the investigators incorrectly conclude that the null hypothesis is true, this results in a false negative conclusion or type 2 error. This probability depends largely on the total sample size but also on the actual magnitude of the treatment differences. Increasing the sample size (or alternatively the event rate by the use of composite outcomes, see below) is therefore viewed as a way of decreasing the false-negative rate when a real treatment differences exist.

It is beyond the scope of this chapter to give the details involved in performing sample size calculations. These are available in standard statistical manuals (Mathew and Farewell, 1996). It is however essential for a reader to understand the relationship between α and β since both represent the probabilities of making an erroneous decision. In the best of all possible worlds we would like both α and β to be close to zero. Unfortunately if α is decreased without changing the total sample size then β necessarily increases. Conversely, if β must decrease without changing the total numbers involved, then α must necessarily increase. Only by increasing the sample size (or event rate) can a reduction in both these elements in any study design be achieved.

Typically the value of α is fixed by the designer of the trial (usually at p <0.05) since it is the p value and the one that will determine whether the study outcome is positive. The decision regarding adequate sample size for any study will necessarily be a compromise, balancing what can be achieved statistically, and by a sample size that is practical and attainable.

The probability, 1–β, of detecting a specified difference, δ, is called the power of the study. The higher the probability of detecting an important treatment difference the more powerful the study. It has been proposed that if the study fails to reject the null hypothesis, that it is important to state the power of the study. Although this might aid in the interpretation of the conclusion of the study there is some concern that this is an inappropriate use of power calculations. Sample size (or power) calculations are relevant at the time of study design not analysis. A confidence interval should be provided for an estimated treatment difference at the analysis stage and if it is, the power estimates of the study will provide no additional information.

All of these elements need to be considered by the reader of all RCT. The statistician will require, for example, that the study investigators estimate the difference in renal survival they expect between the two groups and as well hopefully comment on what they expect in terms of the clinically relevant difference at the design stage. In addition the investigators should include the value of α, i.e., the probability of false-positive results they are willing to accept. A table of sample sizes can then be generated and the corresponding values of β, i.e., the probability of a false-negative result, obtained and included in the manuscript for the reader to review.

These calculations will provide and specify total sample size requirement. The reader however, should examine the specifics of the study including the therapies offered, the duration of the study and the adverse effects profile, (both in terms of quantity and quality), to help them assess whether a reasonable number of cases have been added by the investigators to this total to adjust for the expected number of dropouts, withdrawals, and non-compliance (nonadherence) to the protocol. Although classically an additional 10–15% of the calculated total is added, any or all of these particular issues can substantially alter this percentage.

Stratification

Although random sampling is the classic way of assigning patients to treatment groups there are certain circumstances where it is important to consider alternate methods (Streiner and Norman, 1996). This is most commonly done in the selection phase of the study to ensure that the final sample has certain desired characteristics. The most common reasons for stratification are to match the population for certain key variables and to include sufficient number of subjects in all strata to permit sub-analyses.

If a stratification of randomized patients is noted in the methods section, there should be an explanation as to the justification for such stratification. Often this is done to try to prevent—at the end of the study—ending up with too few people in a particular subgroup. For instance, in a particular glomerular disease trial, ancestry may be felt to be an important issue affecting the response to therapy, therefore the patients are best stratified at the time of randomization by ancestry in order to avoid the possibility at the end of the study that the sub-group size is unbalanced in the randomization process and thereby reduce the power of the statistical tests to be applied. Another reason might be that the investigators are aiming for a study population that is more similar in distribution of specified characteristics to the general population, such as age of onset of the disease and/or certain histological features (e.g., diffuse proliferative lupus nephritis). Although random sampling ensures that the two groups will be well matched in the long run, this may requires a much larger sample than seen in most glomerular disease trials (where the numbers are often fewer than 200 subjects). This small sample size substantially increases the likelihood of over- or under-sampling of subjects from a particular age group or those with a particular pathologic feature if intentional stratification is not carried out as a part of the prospective trial design.

Stratified allocation

This is a somewhat separate issue and is done when it is believed that the stratification variables may affect the outcome of the study if the groups are not balanced on this particular item (Streiner and Norman, 1996). The concern is that if this is not accounted for in the design of the study, at the end of the trial the differences that are determined may relate to variations in the allocation of this element rather than the intervention. The reader must be aware of this possibility. For instance, the sex of the individual might be critical to the response to the drug, so the therapeutic and the control groups must not differ in relationship to this particular factor. It is often impractical, for logistic reasons, to have more than two or three stratified variables unless the available study population is very large. If there are more than two variables that are felt likely to affect the outcome, the one that is more strongly associated with the outcome should be the variables chosen for stratification.

Number needed to treat

Taking the inverse of the absolute risk reduction (ARR) of a particular study is how the number needed to treat (NNT) is derived (Streiner and Norman, 1996; Laupacis et al., 1988). Although the value for the ARR is appropriate for displaying how much improvement is due to the intervention, as compared to the competing therapy or placebo, conceptually it is difficult to translate directly into the issue of patient care. For example, suppose a glomerular disease trial determined that the renal survival rate in the treatment group was 90% (90 of 100 patients treated) and the renal survival in the control group was 80% (80 of 100 patients) over a 10-year period. This would give a risk reduction of renal failure of 50% (10/100 divided by 20/100). However, the reader often wants to know the actual increase in renal survival attributable to the treatment (the attributable risk [AR] to the patients not treated). In the case above, this would be 20/100 −10/100 or 10 per 100 cases. The ARR in this case would be 10%. The NNT in this case would be its reciprocal i.e., 1/0.10 which is equal to 10 (10 patients would need to be treated in order to avoid one case of renal failure at 10 years). The NNT is easier to comprehend for the clinician and the patient and is potentially helpful in deciding whether the benefit of preventing renal failure in one patient over a 10-year period is worth the side effects and costs of the drug to the other nine (who receive no benefit for renal survival and only the risks of therapy).

Primary and secondary end points

All RCTs must have a primary end point selected in advance. The primary end point (or end points if a composite of several end points is used) should be as objective as possible and preferably have some immediate clinical relevance (such as renal failure, dialysis or death). However, *surrogate* end points may be used (see below) so long as their limitations are recognized (Prentice, 1989; Mathews and Farewell, 1996a; Molenberghs, et al., 2002). Often an independent Event Adjudication Committee (EAC) is used to verify that a protocol defined primary end point has been unequivocally reached. Obviously, it is essential that the EAC be 'blinded' to the treatment assignment and use pre-specified and consistently employed criteria for making their decisions.

Secondary end points may also be included in the protocol but they often cannot be statistically analyzed due to the power calculations being primarily determined by the primary event considerations. They are often included to provide clues for future randomized trials and are not used to determine the overall efficacy or safety of a drug. Thus, they are often considered as 'exploratory' end points.

Study duration

This facet must be carefully considered by a reader attempting to evaluate the quality of any RCT. This factor comes into play regardless of whether a drug effect is being assessed in terms of superiority or equivalency. Study duration is a particularly crucial item in terms of the end points being assessed in most glomerular disease trials. In these studies, most of the 'hard' end points, such as survival from renal failure or doubling of baseline serum creatinine (or reduction by 50% from baseline creatinine clearance) are difficult to achieve, given the relatively small sample sizes available, the slow progression of these diseases, and the funding-related restrictions of most clinical RCT. One potential answer to the problem is the use of *composite end points*. Although this feature in the design is likely to increase the number of end points and thereby reduce both sample size and duration of the study, the question of whether each of the components of the composite end points are truly equivalent is critically important. For example, in a glomerulonephritis trial where the two components of a composite end point may both relate to renal progression and therefore appear equal, it is possible that they represent completely different severity of disease states. For example, one of the composite end points might be the requirement for dialysis and the other, a 50% reduction in creatinine clearance. In one patient this might represent a change in creatinine clearance from 20mL/min to 10mL/min over the study duration compared to the alternate end point reached by a second patient whose creatinine clearance changed from 100 to 50mL/min over the same time frame. The latter represents a loss of 50mL/min, the former 10mL/min a fivefold difference in *absolute* progression rate, likely indicating a major difference in terms of disease severity. This example emphasizes the need for the reader to very carefully scrutinize the specific values of each of the individual endpoints when composite end points are used in an RCT, to ensure their equality. If the composite end points are not equal or if one or more can be influenced by events external to the study (such as a subjective choice to intervene in some way) then the validity of the results of the study should be questioned.

Surrogacy

In most glomerular diseases there is a long time delay between the initiation of treatment and the 'hard' outcomes which might be chosen for the evaluation of the effect. This fact stands in sharp contrast to the frequent need to keep the trial duration short (the latter an important goal from the patients', investigators', and funding agencies' point of view). Hence there is an increasingly compelling desire for the use of surrogate end points by all of the above stakeholders. Prentiss defines a valid *surrogate* marker as 'a response variable for which a test of the null hypothesis of no relationship to the treatment groups under comparison is also a valid tests of the corresponding null hypothesis based on the true end point'(Prentice, 1989). Although potentially a useful definition this is very restrictive and rarely satisfied in practice. The study duration can often be substantially foreshortened by the use of surrogate end points (e.g., using reduction in proteinuria or rate of decline in renal function (in GFR as mL/min/year) instead of the more clinically (and patient) relevant end point of renal survival (need for dialysis or transplantation) or mortality. Certainly measuring an outcome that is continuous such as decline in renal function (or slope of creatinine clearance or eGFR) will require fewer subjects in a trial compared to endpoints that are dichotomous events i.e., renal failure versus no renal failure but it is fraught with its own problems in relationship to how closely it parallels the kidney structural change, the problems of reliability of serial laboratory measurements, and how to account for potential normal biologic variation in kidney function. Any surrogate end point, despite being more efficient in terms of trial construction (smaller sample size), must have been proven to track closely with the true outcome since reliance on their validity based on theory or clinical acumen alone, will be insufficient to convince the discriminating reader and certainly fail to impress most peer reviewers, editors or regulatory agencies. In general, a time-to-event analysis is preferred to an analysis of rates of changes in a continuous variable such as eGFR or proteinuria, in surrogate end point trials.

Ancestry

The ancestral background of an individual is a variable that could potentially alter outcome and has implications as a potential source of bias in trials of glomerular disease. There is reasonable evidence in lupus nephritis, for instance, to indicate that ancestry is relevant to progression, being worse in the African-American population versus Caucasians and the latter in turn worse than in the Asian population. Ancestral factors may also come into play in studies examining the efficacy and safety of treatment of primary glomerular disease. However, variations in outcome may also be influenced by factors completely independent of the individual's ancestral background. The African-American population in general may be socially disadvantaged and/or have less access to medical care and hence the lack of adequate funds and/or education results in poor blood pressure control, the major reason for the more rapid deterioration in renal function rather than their ancestral background. In contrast, it may be the different diet in the Asian population compared to North American Caucasian population that explains the benefit that accrues in this ancestral group versus a specific immunomodulating response to the therapy. Furthermore, the pharmacokinetics and pharmacodynamics of individual drugs may be greatly influenced by genetic background and genetic polymorphisms may influence both the response to drugs and their side effects. The reader when examining results of an RCT that contains multiple ancestral groups must consider each of these factors. This potential association between two variables, when none truly exists, is called *confounding* (Streiner and Norman, 1996). It is often caused by a third variable, the *confounder*, which is correlated with the first two, for example poor hypertension control resulting from inadequate health coverage that results in the more rapid deterioration in renal function and hence increasing the end points in this ancestral population group but is not truly related to it.

Adverse event recording and analysis

The increasing recognition by regulatory agencies of the importance of the adverse events associated with the exploding number and variety of available drugs has promoted the development of standardized reporting of adverse events in all clinical trials. Most RCT also have a mandated provision for an independent body (The Data Safety and Monitoring Board or DSMB, also called the Data Monitoring Committee or DMC) charged with reviewing blinded or unblinded data during the progress of a trial to assure that the safety of the participants is protected (Ellenberg, et al., 2002). Such monitoring may involve interim examination of unblended data bearing on efficacy so that the balance between safety risk and efficacy (equipoise) can be periodically evaluated during the conduct of the trial. If the results of this analysis indicate 'futility' of therapy or possible danger to the subjects then the trial may be prematurely stopped before it has reached its efficacy evaluation milestones.

Adverse events arising in a trial (treatment emergent adverse events, TEAE) are commonly broken down into major (serious adverse events or SAE) and minor (non-serious) categories by preset definitions. They may be also categorized as to whether they are thought be drug-related or not (even if the investigator is 'blinded' to treatment assignment) and whether they resulted in participant study discontinuance. It is however, up to the reader to critically evaluate the relevance of the categories as well as the patient care implications rather than merely reading the bottom line that may indicate that there were no major differences in adverse events between the two arms of the trial. An SAE such as a bacterial pulmonary infection that responded quickly and completely to antibiotic treatment will not have the same implication as a similar pulmonary infection but caused by an opportunistic virus or parasite resistant to therapy. Other scenarios include the development of a malignancy secondary to an immunosuppressive drug and which may be significantly delayed beyond the time frame of the trial. This risk must somehow be accounted for in the assessment of therapeutic risk especially when it is being compared to a drug whose adverse effects may be severe but reversible and occurs concurrent with the therapy. A RCT of small size that show important differences in efficacy may be completely inadequate to evaluate the risks for TEAE or SAE, especially for relatively uncommon events since such studies are 'powered' by efficacy considerations not adverse event risks.

Primary analyses

Most RCT are analyzed according to the intent-to-treat (ITT) principle (Brittain and Lin, 2005). In the ITT approach, patient outcomes (primary and secondary end points) are based on the group to which the subjects were originally randomized, regardless of whether they actually received the planned intervention. In the ITT principle all subjects randomized are followed for events (primary and secondary end points) until the planned end of the study, irrespective of whether they actually took the study medication or its comparator drug, and whether they met all of the study objectives for appropriate follow-up during the conduct of the trial. Withdrawal from a trial (by patient's or physician's request) still requires that follow-up data relative to the primary end points of the trial be obtained, unless the Informed Consent to Participate has been rescinded by the patient. If the drop-out (withdrawal) rates are high in a study (greater than 5%), its validly may be questioned. Sometimes an evaluation on a per-protocol (PP) basis may be instructive. In this analysis only those subjects who adhered to the protocol (took the medications as required by the protocol) are included in the analysis. This type of analysis has much less validity as it introduces serious confounding into the interpretation of the trail results. Such analyses should not be used for proof of efficacy.

Secondary analyses

Classically, the primary question of the study and the analyses that are to be undertaken given the results should be specified before the data is collected. Additional data analysis is often undertaken beyond this primary objective. In general, if one continues to look at subsets of the data, it is likely, from a probabilistic perspective that something interesting will be found. There is virtual certainty that one of twenty such examinations will be positive, if one uses a α of p = 0.05. As a 'hypothesis generating' activity and/or in order to suggest further research questions, secondary analyses are valuable but the nature of this activity tends to undermine the probabilistic ideas of formal significance testing. All results of secondary analyses should therefore be treated with great caution. *They should never be used to justify a claim of efficacy for a particular form of therapy.* Although it is not inappropriate to include such secondary analyses in published papers, the nature of the analysis, which led to these results, should be clearly indicated in the manuscript. It is also important for the reader to consider when such secondary analyses are reported to look for the appropriate 'discounting' of the reported significant levels. Statistical methods are available for the 'discounting' procedure (Mathews and Farewell, 1996).

Meta-analyses and systematic reviews

A *meta-analysis* is a quantitative method of analysis in which the results of several studies are combined into a single pooled or summary estimate of the effects (Strauss et al., 2005; Zwahlen M et al., 2008). A *systematic review* involves a critical assessment of reported studies utilizing approaches that reduce the occurrence of bias. Both forms of analyses are critically dependent on the quality of the reports included in the review. Accumulating many trials into a single analysis can greatly improve the power of identifying a true effect (by greatly increasing sample size) and can also provide information on the variations (confidence limits about the mean) for reported trials. The output of the analysis should be expressed as a weighted average of the treatment differences and confidence limits about the average observed in each study. Summary effects sizes (hazard ratios) in meta-analyses in which the 95% confidence limits do not exceed or fall below 1.0 can be regarded as inconclusive or not supportive of a significant effect. Both forms of analysis can include observational as well as randomized clinical trials, but the greatest reliability and validity can be obtained when such analyses are limited to randomized clinical trials. Various methods can be used to assess the quality of the trials included in meta-analyses but the most popular is the Jadad Score (Moher et al., 1995).

Methods to improve the reliability and validity of meta-analysis and systemic reviews have been agreed upon (see Quality Of Reporting Of Meta-analysis of Randomized Clinical Trials; QUOROM criteria, Table 3.2) (Moher et al., 1996). Meta-analysis and systematic reviews conducted by the Cochrane Collaboration (see http://www.cochranelibrary.com) have an excellent track-record of accuracy and reliability and should be used for the best resource for latest meta-analysis of randomized clinical trials. For best results, the meta-analyses should include all available material from an exhaustive and comprehensive search of the published literature and should attempt to verify findings or add critical points by direct questioning of the authors of the included papers.

Table 3.2 The QUOROM statement on reporting of meta-analyses and systematic reviews: 21 items in five major categories*

Title/abstract	
Introduction/ background	Explicit statement of purpose and rationale of the meta-analysis
Methods	Search (databases, languages, dates of publication)
	Selection criteria (inclusion and exclusion)
	Validity assessment
	Study characteristics (including formal assessment of study heterogeneity)
	Quantitative synthesis (statistical evaluation, relative risks, weighted mean differences)
Results	Trial flow (diagram): inclusions and exclusions
	Study characteristics (for each included study)
	Quantitative synthesis: confidence intervals, statistical evaluation, forest plots, funnel plots
Discussion	Major findings/hypotheses generated
	Clinical inferences
	Validity assessment
	Bias (including publication bias, study heterogeneity)
	Future research needed to confirm hypotheses generated

*Adapted from Moher D, Cook DJ, Eastwood S, et al. (1999). Improving the quality of reports of meta-analyses of randomized controlled trials: The QUOROM statement. *Lancet* **354**:1896–1900, with permission from Elsevier.

Several critical requirements must be met for a meta-analysis to have validity:

- The included studies must be independent of each other.
- The analysis should examine identical or very closely similar outcomes of an intervention.
- The type, the doses, and the duration of treatment used in the single trials should be as homogeneous as possible (it is difficult to consider equivalent a treatment with prednisone 2mg/kg/every other day for 2 months and a treatment based on prednisone 1mg/kg/daily for 2–3 months then gradually tapered off over 1 year).

Even with all of the efforts to assure accuracy, meta-analyses tend to be valid only for short periods of time (usually 5 years or less) due to the constant additional of new material to the available literature (Shojania et al., 2007). In some very rapidly evolving fields the period of validity may be significantly less. In addition to the problem of a rapidly evolving literature, meta-analysis may suffer from the effects of 'publication bias.'

Publication bias

Publication bias arises from the inclusion of studies of differing size and standard error is a significant shortcoming of meta-analyses (Hayashino et al., 2005; Dwan K et al., 2008; Peters et al., 2008). The inclusion of small studies with wide standard errors of the differences can contribute to false conclusion. The use of '*funnel plots*' help to evaluate the presence or absence of publication bias. Funnel plots are scatter plots of the treatment effect (odds ratio) on the X axis and the sample size (or standard error) on the Y axis. Any asymmetry of these plots indicates that publication bias is operative (Sterne and Egger, 2001; Souza et al., 2007; Ho, 2007).

'*Forest plots*' which examine the estimated relative risks and the 95% confidence intervals about the mean effects size for all studies is another way to evaluate the quality of meta-analysis (Lewis and Clarke, 2001; Ho, 2007). One must be very cautious in interpreting meta-analyses when one very large trial dominates the statistical evaluation of the effect size, as shown in a forest plot.

Heterogeneity

Heterogeneity of the studies included in the analysis should always be tested by formal statistical methods (such as a chi square test or the Q-statistic) (Biggerstaff and Jackson, 2008). Analyses which have a high degree of heterogeneity should be interpreted with great caution (i.e., considering patients with the same disease at renal biopsy, but with wide difference in the amount of proteinuria or in serum creatinine).

In summary, meta-analyses and systematic reviews are primarily '*hypothesis-generating*' rather than providing proof of efficacy or safety. Nevertheless, a high quality meta-analysis can provide a substantial evidence-based rationale for a particular therapeutic regimen, at least until additional trials require a reassessment of the findings of the analysis. The meta-analysis should always conform to the quality and reporting requirements of *QUOROM* (see Table 3.2).

Summary and practical recommendations

The application of the literature to the formulation of 'evidence-based' guidelines is an exacting task. The quality of the available literature may be very deficient, particularly for uncommon disorders where the organization of RCT may be difficult or impossible. Even when RCT are available, the power of the study to evaluate differences in outcome with interventions can be limited, especially for subgroups pre-specified as being important variables. Most randomized trials are not adequately powered to examine safety, most importantly for uncommon adverse events. Inclusion and exclusion criteria may lead to study populations which are quite different than the population encountered in everyday practice. This generalization of a specific study to another population may be difficult and potentially hazardous. Nevertheless, a hierarchy of studies with respect to their overall value for an evidence-based recommendation has been developed. In descending order of value these are:

- A properly designed and executed prospective randomized controlled trial.
- A high-quality meta-analysis of reported randomized trials.
- A large observational study with well-matched but non-randomized controls.
- A large observational study without controls.
- A case-series.
- A case report.

This hierarchy has been adapted to a system of grading of evidence (Grades of Recommendation Assessment, Development and Evaluation, *GRADE*—see Table 3.3) (GRADE Working Group, 2004; Uhlig et al., 2006). The citation of the quality evidence underlying any evidence-based recommendation should be specified using this system. Weakness in individual studies (threats to validity) used as a basis for evidence-based guidelines should be specified (e.g., limited power, short-term follow-up, unequal composite end points, imbalanced characteristics at randomization, potential confounding, etc.).

Table 3.3 Grading evidence from the published literature for development of evidence-based practice guidelines and clinical decision making*

Quality of evidence	**High (A):** further research is unlikely to change the confidence in the evidence of the effect (high quality RCT without major limitations, plausible confounders, or threats to validity)
	Moderate (B): further research is likely to have an important impact on confidence in the estimate of the effect and may change the estimate (observational study without inconsistencies showing a dose-response effect size)
	Low (C): further research is very likely to have an important impact on the confidence in the estimate of the effect and may change the estimate (small case series, other evidence)
	Very low (D): any estimate of an effect is very uncertain (case reports)
Strength of recommendation	**Strong (1):** the quality of evidence is *high (A)* and supported by other considerations. The recommendation may be 'positive' ('we recommend that you do it') or 'negative' ('we recommend that you not do it'), depending on the quality of the evidence and an assessment of the risks and benefits support a net health benefit or hazard.
	Weak (2): the quality of the evidence is *high (A)* or *moderate (B)* but other considerations support a lower level of recommendation. The recommendation is to *suggest* that an action, either positive or negative be taken, indicating some weakness in the quality of the evidence or some uncertainty in the balance of health benefits and risks.
	Unclear (3): the quality of the evidence is *low (C), very low (D), or absent.* No recommendation can be made because of the poor or insufficient quality of evidence and/or serious uncertainties exist regarding the balance of health benefits and risks. (An alternative is to develop *consensus-based* recommendations in which an unbiased 'expert-opinion' is developed by analysis of potential health benefits and risks. Such consensus-based recommendations are not evidence-based but often have broad public support. There is an expectation that consideration should be given to follow the recommendation statement, at least until the quality of the evidence base changes.)

*Adapted with permission from GRADE Working Group (2004). Grading quality of evidence and strength of recommendations. *BMJ* **328**:1490–4 and Uhlig K, MacLeod A, Craig J, et al. (2006). Grading evidence and recommendations for clinical practice guidelines in nephrology: A position statement from Kidney Disease: Improving Global Outcomes (KDIGO). *Kidney Int* **70**:2058–65.

Application of evidence-based guidelines arising from analysis of observational and controlled studies involving specific intervention to the *individual* patient should always be carried out with caution. The nuances of individual patient's diseases and their responsiveness (sometimes genetically predetermined) to specific interventions may not be accurately reflected in the outcome of trials which aggregate many patients into supposedly 'homogeneous' groups. In addition, it is seldom practical to study the effects of therapy of diseases which have a very indolent nature without relying on 'surrogate' markers for efficacy. Such studies are subject to well-known limitations. Most studies will not be able to detect or analyze relatively uncommon adverse event of treatment and the physician should always be alert to unexpected side-effects. Indeed, the hazards of treatment may not be appreciated until large numbers of patients are treated for longer periods of time well after the first report appears.

As pointed out by Uhlig et al. (2006) one must be careful in extrapolating evidence from non-renal diseases to renal diseases and also to consider the importance of high incremental cost and low incremental benefit in creating recommendations.

Finally, as we learn more about the genetic underpinnings of disease susceptibility and the response to pharmacological interventions it may be possible to devise evidence-based guidelines which are more individually specific and employ the emerging disciple of pharmacogenomics. This new approach has the prospect of individual optimization of the desired beneficial effects while simultaneously avoiding many of the adverse ones.

References

Altman DG, Schulz, KF, Moher D, et al. (2001). The revised CONSORT statement for reporting randomized trials: explanation and elaboration. *Ann Intern Med* **134**:663–94.

Begg C, Cho M, Eastwood S, et al. (1996).Improving the quality of reporting of randomized controlled trials: the CONSORT statement. *JAMA* **276**:637–9.

Biggerstaff BJ, Jackson D (2008). The exact distribution of Cochran's heterogeneity statistic in one –way random effects meta-analysis. *Stat Med* **27**:6093–110.

Brittain E, Lin D (2005).A comparison of intent-to-treat and per-protocol results in antibiotic non-inferiority trials. *Stat Med* **24**:1–10.

Cattran DC, Reich HN, Beanlands HJ, et al. (2008). The impact of sex in primary glomerulonephritis. *Nephrol Dial Transplant* **23**:2247–53.

Chou R, Helfand M (2005). Challenges to systematic reviews that assess treatment harms. *Ann Intern Med* **142**:1090–9.

Dwan K, Altman DG, Arnaiz JA, et al. (2008). Systematic review of the empirical evidence of study publication bias and outcome reporting bias. *PLoS ONE* **3**:e3801.

Ellenberg SS, Fleming T, DeMets DL (2002). *Data Monitoring Committees in Clinical Trials: A practical perspective.* Wiley and Sons, New York.

Geddes CC, Rauta V, Gronhagen-Riska C, et al. (2003). A Tricontinental view of IgA nephropathy. *Nephrol Dial Transplant* **18**:1541–48.

GRADE Working Group (2004). Grading quality of evidence and strength of recommendations. *BMJ* **328**:1490–4.

Hayashino Y, Noguchi Y, Fukul T (2005). Systematic evaluation and comparison of statistical tests for publication bias. *J Epidemiol* **15**:235–43.

Hill AB (1965). The environment and disease: association or causation? *Proc R Soc Med* **58**:295–300.

Ho KM (2007). Forest and funnel plots illustrated the calibration of a prognostic model: a descriptive study. *J Clin Epidemiol* **60**:746–51.

Ioannidis JP (2008). Effect of statistical significance on the credibility of observational associations. *Am J Epidemiol* **168**:374–83.

Lacut K, Le Gai G, Mottier D (2007) Do observational studies have a role in assessing treatment. *Presse Med* **36**:536–40.

Laupacis A, Sackett DL, Roberts AS (1988). An assessment of clinically useful measures of the consequences of treatment. *N Engl J Med* **318**:1728–33.

Lewis S, Clarke M (2001). Forest plots: trying to see the wood from the trees. *BMJ* **322**:1479–80.

Mathews DE, Farewell VT (1996) *Using and understanding medical statistics,* 3rd edn. Karger Publishing, Basal Switzerland.

Moher D, Jadad AR, Nichol G, et al. (1995). Assessing the quality of randomized controlled trials: an annotated bibliography of scales and checklists. *Control Clin Trials* **16**:62–73.

Moher D, Cook DJ, Eastwood S, et al. (1999). Improving the quality of reports of meta-analyses of randomized controlled trials: The QUOROM statement. *Lancet* **354**:1896–1900.

Molenberghs, G, Buyse, M, Geys H, et al. (2002). Statistical challenges in the evaluation of surrogate endpoints in randomized trials. *Control Clin Trials* **23**:607–25.

Peters JL Sutton AJ, Jones DR, et al. (2008). Comparison of two methods to detect publication bias in meta-analyses. *JAMA* **295**:676–80.

Piaggio G, Elbourne DR, Altman DG, et al. (2006). Reporting of non inferiority and equivalence randomized trials: An extension of the CONSORT statement. *JAMA* **295**:1152–60.

Prentice RL (1989). Surrogate endpoints in clinical trials: definitions and operational criteria. *Stat Med* **8**:431–40.

Rawlins M (2008). De testimonio: on the evidence for decisions about the use of therapeutic interventions. *Lancet* **372**: 2152–61.

Sackett DL (2004). Superiority trials, non inferiority trials, and prisoners of the 2-sided null hypothesis. *ACP J Club* **140**:A11.

Shlipak M, Stehman-Breen C (2005). Observational Research Databases in Renal Disease. *JASN* **16**:3477–84.

Shojania KG, Sampson M, Ansari MT, Ji J, et al. (2007). How quickly do systematic reviews go out of date? A survival analysis. *Ann Intern Med* **147**:224–33.

Souza JP, Pileggi C, Cecatti JG (2007). Assessment of funnel plot asymmetry and publication bias in reproductive health meta-analyses: an analytic survey. *Repro Health* **4**:3.

Sterne JA and Egger M (2001). Funnel plots for detecting bias in meta-analyses: guidelines on choice of axis. *J Clin Epidemiol* **54**:1046–55.

Strauss SE, Richardson WS, Glasziou P, et al. (2005). *Evidence-Based Medicine.* 3rd edn. Elsevier, Churchill, Livingstone, Edinburgh.

Streiner DL, Norman GR (1996) *PDQ Epidemiology*, end edn. Chapter 3, Research Methodology. Mosby, St. Louis, MO.

von Elm E, Altmanb DG, Egger M, et al. (2007). The strengthening the reporting of observational studies in epidemiology (STROBE) statement: guidelines for reporting observational studies. *Lancet* **370**:1453–57.

Uhlig K, MacLeod A, Craig J, et al. (2006). Grading evidence and recommendations for clinical practice guidelines in nephrology: A position statement from Kidney Disease: Improving Global Outcomes (KDIGO). *Kidney Int* **70**:2058–65.

Zwahlen M, Renehan A, Egger M (2008). Meta-analyses in medical research: Potentials and limitations. *Urol Oncol* **26**:320–29.

Chapter 4

Acute post-infectious glomerulonephritis

Gabriella Moroni and Claudio Ponticelli

Introduction and overview

Definition

Acute post-infectious glomerulonephritis (APIGN) is a primary glomerular disease characterized by intra-glomerular inflammation and cellular proliferation resulting from immunological events triggered by a variety of bacterial, viral, and protozoal infections. We use the term 'primary' to describe this disease since the kidney is the only organ directly involved in the disease, and extra-renal manifestations are generally the consequence of disturbed kidney function. The prototype of APIGN is post-streptococcal glomerulonephritis (PSGN) which most often occurs in children following a pharyngeal infection caused by a particular strain of streptococci and has a favorable outcome.

However in the last few decades the spectrum of APIGN has changed. The incidence of PSGN, particularly in its epidemic form, has progressively declined in industrialized countries. In many cases APIGN is caused today by other Gram-positive bacteria such as staphylococci or by Gram-negative bacteria. Moreover the disease tends to affect more and at a higher frequently adults with an immunocompromised background, due to alcoholism, diabetes, drug addiction, and/or viral hepatitis. Finally, while spontaneous recovery within few weeks is still the rule in children affected by the typical PSGN, the prognosis in immunodeficient adults is often severe and the response to treatment is uncommon. Therefore we will treat separately these two sub-types of acute glomerulonephritis.

Post-streptococcal glomerulonephritis

The disease usually develops after upper respiratory tract or skin infections and is caused by β-hemolytic streptococci of group A. PSGN predominantly affects children in epidemic or sporadic forms while it is rare (<10% of cases)

Table 4.1 Main features of acute post-streptococcal glomerulonephritis

Pathology:	Hypercellularity of the glomeruli secondary to proliferation of resident cells and infiltration of inflammatory cells. At immunofluoresecence there are IgG and C3 deposits in the mesangial cells and along the glomerular capillary walls. On electron microscopy there are subepithelial deposits.
Pathogenesis:	It is an immune-complex disease. Antibodies directed against streptococcal antigens either may cross-react with some component of the GBM or may attack the antigens planted on the glomerular basement membrane (GBM), eliciting an inflammatory response.
Etiology:	The disease is triggered by infections caused by nephritogenic strains of β-hemolytic group A streptococci.
Clinical presentation:	The disease may be asymptomatic (only microscopic hematuria) or may present with a nephritic syndrome with microscopic or macroscopic hematuria, proteinuria, hypertension and rarely renal failure (see Table 4.2).
Epidemiology:	The disease is more frequent in children and in males. May occur in an epidemic or sporadic form. It tends to be less and less frequent in developed countries.
Prognosis:	The prognosis is generally favourable, particularly in children, as glomerulonephritis spontaneously recovers in a few days. Some adults presenting with nephritic syndrome or renal insufficiency may show persisting urinary abnormalities in the long term or may even develop renal failure.
Treatment:	Salt and water restriction is recommended in the first days particularly in oliguric patients. Diuretics, anti-hypertensive drugs, and anti-streptococcal antibiotics may be required in the early phases.

in adults. The clinical manifestations may vary from subclinical forms with mild urinary abnormalities to the acute forms characterized by the abrupt onset of macroscopic hematuria, decrease in glomerular filtration rate (GFR), fluid retention with consequent edema, and hypertension (Table 4.1).

Pathology

In the acute phase, light microscopy shows a pattern of exudative glomerulonephritis, characterized by a diffuse and global involvement of the glomeruli. Hypercellularity, due both to cellular infiltration and endogenous cellular proliferation with consequent enlargement of the glomerular tuft, is the main characteristic. The cellular composition depends on the stage of the disease. In the acute phase the prevailing proliferating cells are endothelial cells, while polymorphonuclear granulocytes are the predominant infiltrating cells (see Atlas plate 1). Proliferation of mesangial cells, infiltrating macrophages, and lymphocytes are also present. Helper T cells are in higher proportion in early stages of the disease while the amount of suppressor T cells remains constant throughout the course of the disease. As a consequence of the hypercellularity occlusion of the capillary lumens is not infrequent. Necrosis of the glomerular tufts is infrequent. Few glomeruli may show extra-capillary proliferation with segmental crescents. The glomerular basement membrane (GBM) is generally normal. In some cases, with the trichrome stain, using oil immersion lens, it is possible to recognize tiny subepithelial deposits, the so called *humps* (see Atlas plate 2). Macrophages and lymphocytes are also present in the tubulo-interstitial areas. In few cases an arteriolar fibrinoid necrosis may be seen.

In the resolving phases of the disease, proliferation of mesangial cells and matrix are predominant, the number of neutrophils diminish progressively while few mononuclear cells may still be present in the capillary lumens. During this phase the capillary lumen are patent. The residual mesangial hypercellularity usually slowly resolves within months.

At immunofluorescence granular immune deposits of IgG and C3 are present in mesangial areas and along the glomerular capillary walls. IgG is present only in the acute phase of the disease while C3 is present in the early and in the late phases of the disease. IgM may be present in small amount and at lower intensity as well as IgA. Sorger et al. (1982) described three distinct immunofluorescent patterns. *The starry sky pattern*, which may be seen in the first weeks of the disease, is characterized by finely granular immune deposits in the capillary walls and to a lesser degree in the mesangium (see Atlas plate 1). In the *garland pattern* there are heavy confluent deposits of IgG and C3 along the capillary walls that correlate with a large number of subepithelial humps at electron microscopy. This pattern is usually associated with persistence of heavy proteinuria and worse long-term prognosis (Sorger et al. 1987). The *mesangial pattern* is defined by the presence of granular deposition of C3 in the stalk region of the glomerulus, immunoglobulins are not always present. This pattern is associated with mesangial hypercellularity and is most often found in the resolving phases of the disease (see also 'Mesangial proliferative glomerulonephritis' in Chapter 11).

On electron microscopy, the most characteristic feature in the acute phase of the disease is the presence of subepithelial electron dense deposits called *humps* as they resemble camel humps (see Atlas plate 2). Humps usually resolve within 4–6 weeks leaving translucent or electron-lucent areas. Mesangial, subendothelial and intramembranous deposits are also present in variable amounts, subendothial deposits predominating.

Pathogenesis

On the basis of the clinical course of the disease together with constant evidence of the deposition of immunoglobulins and complement within the glomeruli, acute PSGN is classified as an *immune-complex disease*. However, in spite of decades of investigations the sequence leading to immune-complex formation and activation of complement and inflammation has not been completely clarified.

A first hypothesis suggested that some antibodies produced against streptococci antigens may cross-react with GBM antigens or with antigens planted on the glomerular cells surface. This hypothesis was supported by experimental studies showing that soluble glycoproteins of streptococcal nephritogenic strains were able to induce nephritis, that the injection of the antiserum of the affected animals induced nephritis in normal animals, and that antibodies against streptococcal cell membranes were able to cross-react with glomeruli in tissue section or isolated glomeruli (reviewed in Lange, 1980). In addition, in serum of patients with PSGN, antibodies to type IV collagen, heparan sulphate, and laminin have been detected (Kefalides et al., 1993).

Alternatively, it has been hypothesized that nephritogenic streptococci can produce and release in the circulation proteins that have a particular affinity for normal glomerular sites. After lodging into the sites of the glomerulus, for which they have intrinsic affinity, the nephritogenic proteins would attract properdin and activate the alternative pathway of complement. On the other hand, the nephritogenic proteins deposited in the glomerulus could act as planted antigens and bind to circulating antistreptococcal antibodies with subsequent immune complex formation in situ, activation of complement, and recruitment of inflammatory cells and of inflammatory mediators including chemoattractans, proteases, cytokines, oxidants, and growth factors that together with proliferating resident cells can damage the glomerulus (Couser and Johnson, 1997). The involvement of other factors, such as local generation of terminal complement components, cell-mediated immunity, and apoptosis (Oda et al., 2007), has also been suggested but their role in the pathogenesis of PSGN has not been completely clarified.

During the last decades several streptococcal proteins have been investigated as possible nephritogenic antigens. A first candidate was a complex of intracellular anionic proteins called *endostreptosins*. Antibodies against *endostreptosins* were present in high titers in patients with PSGN and were able to react with glomeruli of affected patients. However, elevated titers of these antibodies have been documented also in patients with streptococcal infection but without glomerulonephritis. Further studies of the group of Treser isolated among the endotreptosins complex an antigen termed *preabsorbing antigen* (Yoshizawa et al., 1992). Antibodies to *preabsorbing antigen* were present in 30 out of 31 patients with PSGN and only in 1 out of 36 patients with streptococcal infection but without nephritis. This protein was the only one detected in the glomeruli of affected patients and was able to activate the alternative pathway of complement. *Nephritis strain-associated protein* (NSAP) is another potential antigen isolated from strains of streptococci derived from patients with PSGN. Anti-NSAP antibodies were found both in sera and in biopsy specimens from patients with PSGN. An extracellular plasmin-binding protein secreted by nephritis-associated Group A streptococci identical to *streptococcal pyrogenic exotoxin B* (SPEB) and to a streptococcal proteinase has also been identified (Poon-King et al., 1993). The titers of anti-SPEB antibodies were found to be significantly higher in children with PSGN than in normal children or in those with acute rheumatic fever or scarlet fever. In kidney biopsy specimens stained for SPEB, 67% of PSGN were positive versus only 16% of non post-streptococcal GN. Anti-SPEB titers tended to rise rapidly after the onset of the disease reaching a peak after 2 weeks and decreased slowly without returning to baseline after one year (Cu et al., 1998). Thus a single attack can confer a long-term immunity, so explaining why recurrence of PSGN is extremely rare. The more recent described nephritogenic antigen isolated from Group A streptococcus is the *nephritis-associated plasmin receptor* (NAPlr) whose nucleotide sequence shows high homology as well as similar functions to that of the plasmin receptor (Plr) of group A streptococcus. Significant glomerular deposition of *NAPlr* was documented in the early phases of PSGN, suggesting that the deposited *NAPlr* can entrap and maintain plasmin in the active form inducing glomerular damage (Yoshizawa et al., 2004). Further studies showed that glomerular plasmin activity was absent or weak in normal controls and in patients with rapidly progressive glomerulonephritis, while it was prominent in patients with PSGN and positive glomerular *NAPlr*, suggesting that *NAPlr* upregulates the glomerular plasmin activity and has nephritogenic activity (Oda et al., 2005). By a comparison between the nephritogenic activity of SPEB and plasmin receptor, glyceraldehyde-3-phosphate-dehydrogenase (Prl GAPDH) Batsford et al. (2005) concluded that SPEB is probably the major nephritogenic antigen involved in the pathogenesis of PSGN. By reviewing the above mentioned pathogenetic hypothesis Rogriguez-Iturbe and Batsford (2007) concluded that nephritogenicity probably acts with two different mechanisms: i) inflammation resulting from plasmin-binding entrapment and sustained activity due to *NaPlr*; and ii) glomerular-immune complex formation due to the co-localization of the putative antigen with complement and immunoglobulins as has been suggested for streptococcal SPEB.

Etiology

Based on a bulk of clinical and laboratory evidence accumulated during the last decades it has been ascertained that both specific nephritogenic strains of streptococci and a specific immune response by the host are required for the development of acute PSGN. Group A streptococci nephritogenic strains M types 1, 2, 4, and 12 are involved in upper respiratory tract infections while M type 25, 45, 47, 49, 55, and 57 are involved in the skin infections (Rodriguez Iturbe and Parra, 2001). Rarely also non-group A streptococci may be involved in the pathogenesis of glomerulonephritis. However only a minority of patients infected with a nephritogenic streptococcal strains develop overt disease. The possibility of a genetic predisposition may be suggested by a higher incidence of HLA-DRB1*03011 in patients with PSGN (Ahn and Ingulli, 2008) and by prospective family studies showing the development of PSGN in 38% of the siblings in cases of sporadic disease (Rodriguez-Iturbe et al., 1981).

Clinical presentation and features

The typical PSGN is generally preceded by infection of nephritogenic group A streptococci in throat or skin. Exceptionally the disease may occur following circumcision or spider bites. Throat streptococcal infection may be characterized either by sore throat alone or by a more severe disease with fever, cervical lymphadenopathy, and tonsillar exudate. Scarlet fever may be recognized by the rash due to an erythrogenic toxin which blanches on pressure which is more intense along antecubital fossae and axillae and is accompanied by enanthema consisting of punctuate erythema and petechiae on the soft palate. Streptococcal impetigo is characterized by grouped small vesicles, localized in exposed areas generally associated with regional lymphadenopathy. Vesicles cause intense itching, rapidly break, and become covered with thick crusts and heal without scarring.

After a latent period of 1–2 weeks for upper respiratory tract infection and 3–6 weeks for skin infection the symptoms and signs of glomerulonephritis develop. During the latent period one-third of patients develop microscopic hematuria.

Glomerulonephritis may present in a sub-clinical form or in an acute form. The sub-clinical forms are more frequent, exceeding the symptomatic cases by 4–5 times. Sub-clinical disease manifests with microscopic hematuria and a reduction of serum complement associated or not with an increase in blood pressure. At renal biopsy intracapillary proliferation is present.

The typical clinical presentation of the acute forms is an acute nephritic syndrome without significant differences in the frequency of presentation between sporadic and epidemic forms (Rodriguez-Iturbe, 1984). Acute nephritic syndrome is characterized by the abrupt onset of oliguria, proteinuria, hematuria, edema, and hypertension. The typology of clinical presentation may be variable with the age. Edema of the face is sudden and very frequent, being present in >50% of patients; in some cases edema involves the legs and sacrum. Anasarca is more common among young children. Transient oliguria of 1–2 weeks duration is described in about 50% of patients, but anuria is rare. Hypertension commonly occurs in children, adults, and elderly. It is more frequent and more severe in adults and in the elderly but not all patients require drug treatment. Hypertensive encephalopathy is a rare complication which may be associated to seizures. Congestive heart failure is the presenting symptoms in some patients, being more frequent in adults and older patients. Rare cases of posterior leukoencephalopathy and autoimmune hemolytic anemia have also been reported in patients with PSGN. Oliguria and fluid retention are partly due to decreased GFR resulting from the inflammatory glomerular reaction that progressively reduces the area of the glomerular capillaries. Renal blood flow is normal and as a consequence the filtration fraction is depressed. The reduced GFR is not the only factor responsible for the sodium retention observed in these patients as severe sodium retention can occur even in presence of mild reduction of GFR, probably as a consequence of an increased salt and water tubular reabsorption. In the acute phase of PSGN sodium retention persists in spite of increased plasma levels of atrial natriuretic peptide, suggesting an impaired response of the kidney to this peptide (Ozdemir et al., 1992). Salt and water retention often results in dilutional anemia, hypertension, and congestive heart failure (Glassock, 1988). The increased plasma levels of endothelin may also contribute to arterial hypertension and to the lack of response to atrial natriuretic peptide (Ozdemir et al., 1992). *Plasma renin activity* is severely depressed during acute episodes.

Hematuria is a constant finding in acute GN being macroscopic in one-third of the patients and microscopic in the remaining patients. Macroscopic hematuria rapidly disappears with the increase in the urine output, while dysmorphic microscopic hematuria usually persists longer. In addition to red blood cells, the urinary sediment is characterized by the presence of leukocytes (polymorphonuclear in the acute phases, mononuclear in the resolving phases), tubular cells, and granular, erythrocyte, and leukocyte casts.

Mild proteinuria is frequent but nephrotic syndrome is rare in children being present in around 4% of cases while it is around 20% in adults and elderly. Constitutional symptoms including anorexia, malaise, nausea, vomiting, and back pain are common at presentation.

The clinical presentation is more severe in adults and in elderly in comparison to that of children (Table 4.2). Dyspnea, congestive heart failure, oliguria, massive proteinuria, and renal insufficiency are more frequent in adults and in older patients than in children. Rarely the dominant picture is that of rapidly progressive renal insufficiency and these cases are generally associated with

Table 4.2 Clinical presentation of acute post-streptococcal glomerulonephritis

	Children (Potter et al., 1982; Clark et al., 1988)	**Adults** (Baldwin., 1977; Lien et al., 1979; Vogl et al., 1980)	**Elderly** (Melby et al., 1987; Washio et al., 1994)
Hematuria	97–100%	86%	100%
Macroscopic hematuria	30%	NA	NA
Proteinuria	47–80%	56–99%	92%
Nephrotic syndrome	4%	20–32%	20%
Renal failure	25–40%	38–51%	72–83%
Hypertension	50–60%	63–89%	81–86%
Cardiac failure	<5%	46%	43%

diffuse crescents. This rapidly progressive course to end-stage renal disease (ESRD) occurs in <0.5% of the sporadic forms and is even rarer in the epidemic forms.

During the first 2 weeks of active disease, C3 and total hemolytic complement levels are significantly depressed in >90% of patients; C4 and C2 levels are usually normal or only mildly depressed. Marked reduction of C4 suggests an alternative diagnosis such as systemic lupus erythematosus (SLE). A role for the terminal cascade C5b–C9, the membrane attack complex, in the pathogenesis of the disease has also been suggested (Matsell et al., 1994). In the majority of patients, complement normalized within 4 weeks; however, occasionally it may take months. The level of serum complement has no prognostic value but persistent hypocomplementemia may suggest a different diagnosis. Rheumatoid factor is demonstrated in about one-third of patients and most patients show polyclonal cryoglobulinemia (composed by IgG and IgM) in the acute phases of the disease. Hypergammaglobulinemia is present in about 90% of patients. Anemia is frequent in the early phases of the disease, due to dilutional phenomenon in the great majority of cases although cases of hemolytic anemia have also been reported.

Cultures for streptococcus in patients with post-streptococcal glomerulonephritis are frequently positive in epidemic forms (around 70%), while in sporadic forms they are positive only in 25% of patients. Increasing titer of one or more antistreptococcal serum antibodies suggest recent infection. Antistreptolysin O titers are more frequently elevated in throat infection than in skin infection. Parra et al. (1998) found elevated antistreptolysin O titers only in one-third of patients with skin infections, whilst anti-DNA titers were elevated in around 70%. Antibody titers increase during the first week of infection and reach the peak at 1 month, then progressively reduce over many months. Patients who are treated with antibiotics early in the course of infections or elderly patients may not have significant rise in antibodies titers.

Epidemiology

Acute PSGN most commonly affects children and young adults. The peak of incidence is in the first decade of life; however, the disease may also occur in adults and is not so infrequent in old patients. Males are affected more commonly than females, the ratio often being 2:1. Pharyngitis and tonsillitis are more frequent in spring and in winter in temperate climates, while impetigo is more frequent in summer and in tropical areas.

As already described, the disease may present in epidemic or in sporadic forms.

Five decades ago a number of epidemic cases of acute PSGN had been documented worldwide. During the last decades epidemics are becoming rare in developed countries but continue to be reported from underdeveloped countries where they tend to occur in close communities with poor hygienic conditions (Rodriguez-Iturbe et al., 1984). The epidemics tend to be cyclic in certain areas with low socioeconomic status such as in the Red Lake, Port of Spain, Trinidad, Venezuela. Isolated outbreaks have been described in Australia (Muscatello et al., 2001), in rugby team members due to infected skin lesions (Ludlam and Cookson, 1986), and more recently in Nova Serrana, Brazil, following the ingestion of unpasteurized cheese infected with *Streptococcus zooepidemicus* from bovine mastitis (Balter et al., 2000).

Also the incidence of the sporadic forms of PSGN is decreasing in developed countries. Simon et al. (1994) documented a progressive decrease until virtually the complete disappearance of post-streptococcal GN in the French region of Bretagne since 1976 to 1990. Roy et al. (1990) observed a decrease in the hospitalization in Memphis from 25–37 cases per year over the years 1961–70 to 8–10 cases during 1980–88. At the Florida University of Jacksonville, Ilyas and Tolaymat (2008) compared a recent cohort of children with PSGN between 1999–2006 with an earlier cohort of patients admitted between 1957–73. The average incidence was 6.4 patients per year versus 10.9 patients per year respectively. In the recent cohort, 64% of patients had antecedent pharyngitis and milder symptoms of GN at presentation, and all cases recovered. Instead in the earlier cohort 66% of patients had an antecedent pyoderma and mortality was reported in 1.3% of children. A decreasing incidence of the disease has also been reported in urban areas of Australia, and in many countries of Central Europe. Today the global burden of severe group A streptococcal disease is concentrated largely in developing countries and Indigenous populations such as Aboriginal Australians (Steer et al., 2007).

Natural history

The prognosis is excellent for patients with sub-clinical forms of PSGN. For patients presenting with an acute nephritic syndrome the short-term prognosis is generally favorable in children. Less than 1% of children die of complications caused by renal failure and the risk of death is further decreased in the last years in developed countries. More uncertain are the results in the long term. Excellent prognosis was reported in studies published around 1940, but the follow-up of patients was too short to draw firm conclusions. Subsequent studies reported contrasting results. Most studies with long-term follow-up showed that the majority of children and patients with an epidemic form of PSGN had an excellent prognosis. In a 12-year follow-up study after the onset of epidemic PSGN in Trinidad, Nissenson et al. (1979) reported two cases of death due to renal insufficiency and ten other deaths from unrelated causes out of 722 patients (of them only 38 were aged more than 20 years). At the last observation three patients had serum creatinine >1.2mg/dL, nineteen had proteinuria, three hematuria, three proteinuria plus hematuria, and six lordotic proteinuria. Adding those patients to the two deaths due to renal insufficiency the percentage of patients with renal abnormalities was 1.4%. Hypertension was present in 2.3% of patients, being more common in adults, but did not exceed that found in Trinidad people. Although in a subsequent follow-up study of the same cohort extended up to 17 years the proportion of patients with abnormal urine increased to 3.6% (Potter et al., 1982) the outlook remained generally good. Garcia et al. (1981) reported the long-term outcome for 71 patients who had a PSGN during an epidemic outbreak in Maracaibo. After a follow-up of 11–12-years a reduction in GFR was observed in 11.2% patients, proteinuria in 9.8%, hematuria in 4.2%, arterial hypertension in 1.4%. Altogether 16% of children and 55% of adults had one or more urinary abnormalities but only one patient reached ESRD.

More controversial are the results in the sporadic forms. The early literature on this subject (pre-1968) is confounded by the fact that some case of 'clinically apparent' PSGN may have actually been examples of an acute exacerbation of IgA nephropathy (see also Chapter 8). Baldwin et al. (1977) reported a reduction of GFR in 38% of 174 patients (mainly adults) followed for 2–12 years, proteinuria in 46%, and arterial hypertension in 42%. Taken together these data, 60% of patients had renal abnormalities. In a Japanese study Kasahara et al. (2001) followed 138 children with non-epidemic PSGN admitted to the hospital between January and December 1997. The diagnosis was based on the presence of hematuria, transient hypocomplementemia, and evidence of group A beta-hemolytic streptococcal infection. None of the patients had renal insufficiency. In all patients serum complement normalized within 12 weeks, hematuria disappeared within 4 years, and proteinuria within 3 years. The authors concluded that the prognosis of PSGN is good in children when the disease is adequately diagnosed. In summary, in children with PSGN the risk of mortality in the acute phase is extremely low and there is little evidence of progression to chronic renal failure in the long term. Some differences among studies may be due to different diagnostic criteria (pathological versus clinical) different typology of patients (not all the studies separated the outcomes in children and in adults), different severity of the acute episode (hospitalized versus outpatients). There is agreement however that patients with nephrotic syndrome at presentation (Chugh et al., 1987; Sorger et al., 1987), those with crescentic glomerulonephritis and those with acute renal failure tend to have a worse prognosis (Nissenson et al., 1979; Askenazi et al., 2006).

In adults the prognosis is less favorable than in children both for epidemic and sporadic forms. As mentioned above, the percentage of patients with persisting urinary abnormalities was higher for adults than for children in the epidemic outbreak of Venezuela (Garcia et al., 1981). In Brazil, Balter et al., (2000) reported that during an outbreak of PSGN resulting from consumption of cheese contaminated with *Steptococcus zooepidermicus* 3.7% of adults entered ESRD. Sesso et al. (2005) reported the 5-year follow-up of this epidemic nephritis in 56 patients (96% adults) and found that half of them had a creatinine clearance <60mL/min; increased microalbuminuria (>20mcg/min) was documented in 22% although only 8% of patients had proteinuria (one plus or more) by dipstick; 30% of patients had arterial hypertension. Concerning sporadic cases in adults, Vogl et al. (1986) reported a complete recovery only in 59% of adults with PSGN after a mean follow-up of 4.8 years. In India, Chugh et al. (1987) reported the development of irreversible renal insufficiency in 40 out of 142 adults (28%) followed for 4–10 years, the majority of whom had progressed to ESRD.

Specific treatment

In patients with sub-clinical disease no specific or symptomatic treatment is required, but patients should be advised to follow a moderate salt restriction and their blood pressure and body weight should be checked regularly.

In patients with symptomatic acute nephritic syndrome, bed rest is usually prescribed, although there is no evidence that it is strictly necessary, with the exception of patients with congestive heart failure or severe hypertension with encephalopathy. Restriction of water and salt intake is recommended to prevent edema, hypertension, and congestive heart failure. Even more efficacious are loop diuretics that may easily reverse oliguria in the early phases of the disease. Although hypertension is generally attributed to sodium and water retention, diuretics alone may be insufficient to control hypertension and it is advisable to administer anti-hypertensive agents. Good results have been reported with ACE inhibitors, which should be used with caution in patients with hyperkalemia. In case of an emergency, oral nifedipine (0.25–0.5mg/kg) or intravenous labetolol (0.2–1mg/kg) may be administered and repeated if necessary to control hypertensive spikes. Intravenous diazoxide (1–3mg/kg) and intravenous nitroprusside (0.5–1mcg/min up to a maximum of 8mcg/kg/min) should only be given in Intensive Care Units. Penicillin, cephalosporin, or macrolides are usually prescribed to eliminate the antigen. These measures can resolve the streptococcal infection, but are of little help for reversing glomerulonephritis, as the glomerular lesions caused by immune complexes are already established. Anti-microbial therapy is indicated primarily to prevent the spread of the nephritogenic streptococcus among relatives or close contacts. Prophylactic antimicrobials are not indicated in long-term follow up.

Glucocorticoids and/or immunosuppressive agents are not indicated in the typical cases of acute PSGN. These drugs have been successfully used in a few cases with extensive glomerular crescents and rapidly progressive glomerulonephritis which may have a more severe prognosis. However, the evidence for their efficacy is weak. While a few anecdotal reports (Vijayakumar, 2002; Raff et al., 2005) supported a potential benefit of glucocorticoids in crescentic PSGN, in a small randomized trial conducted in children with crescentic PSGN, treatment with prednisone, azathioprine, cyclophosphamide, dypiridamole, and anticoagulants did not offer advantages over supportive therapy (Roy et al., 1981).

Atypical post-infectious acute glomerulonephritis

Definition

While the frequency of typical PSGN in children is progressively declining at least in developed countries, an *atypical* APIGN is increasing, particularly in adults and in the elderly. Non-streptococcal bacterial infections, such as staphylococcal and Gram-negative infections, and viral or prototozoal infections (such as parvovirus, cytomegalovirus, and toxoplasmosis) and atypical sites of bacterial infections (pneumonia, endocarditis, ostemyelitis, urinary tract infections, phlebitis, deep-seated abscess) characterize these new described forms of post-infectious glomerulonephritis. Many patients with atypical AIPGN are immunocompromised subjects with a background of alcoholism and drug addiction, or with underlying diseases such as malignancies, diabetes, or liver cirrhosis. The clinical presentation is often more severe than in PSGN with a high frequency of acute renal insufficiency and nephrotic syndrome; renal biopsy shows necrotizing glomerular lesions, crescents, and glomerular and interstitial infiltrations of mononuclear cells in a larger number of patients. At immunofluorescence C3 is the dominant protein deposited in many cases, but dominant IgA is frequent in acute post-staphylococcal GN, particularly in diabetic patients (thus this form of post-infectious GN may closely resemble primary IgA nephritis). The prognosis is poor in many patients who may develop ESRD, in spite of antibiotics and/or steroids therapy (Table 4.3).

Pathology

At light microscopy, an endocapillary glomerulonephritis is observed in 92–98% of patients. Glomerular infiltration with monocytes is common in the viral-associated forms (especially parvovirus). A membranoproliferative pattern accounts for the remaining cases. Extracapillary proliferation in >20% of glomeruli may be seen in 3.5–36% of renal biopsies, associated with segmental tuft necrosis in 16–22% of cases. Interstitial mononuclear infiltration is present in about one-third of patients associated with a variable amount of tubular necrosis (from 18–61% of cases). A correlation analysis in our cohort revealed that the number of patients with moderate/severe interstitial nephritis significantly increased over the years. The percentage of patients with interstitial nephritis was 12% between1979–84; 28% between 1985–89; 42% between 1990–94; and 55% between 1995–99 (p<0.02) (Moroni et al., 2002).

At immunofluorescence C3 is the dominant immune deposit, being present in 93- 100% of glomeruli, followed by IgG in about half of cases, and by IgA which has been found in 28-44 % of cases in two large series (Moroni et al., 2002; Nasr et al., 2008). In particular IgA was the dominant or the co-dominant immunoglobulin deposited in 22 cases of *Staphylococcus*-associated glomerulonephritis reported in the English literature; of note acute nephritis was superimposed to diabetic glomerulosclerosis in eight of these patients (Reviewed by Nasr et al., 2007).

On electron microscopy subepithelial dense deposits with a hump-shaped appearance are present almost in all patients, subendothelial deposits, generally small, are seen in around 50% of cases and mesangial deposits in 33–90% of cases.

Pathogenesis

The pathogenetic mechanisms of atypical APIGN have been poorly investigated, with the exception of post-staphylococcal GN with dominant or co-dominant

Table 4.3 Atypical acute post-infectious glomerulonephritis

Pathology:	Endocapillary proliferation of the glomeruli is a constant finding.
	Extracapillary proliferation may be seen in up to 1/3 of cases and an interstitial nephritis is present in more than 1/2 of cases in recent series.
	C3 is the prevailing deposit at immunofluorescence, IgA deposits are also frequent.
Pathogenesis:	In cases following a *S. aureus* infection, a staphylococcal enterotoxin could operate as a superantigen and cause a massive T-cell activation with large production of cytokines.
	An increased production of immune complexes containing IgA has also been postulated in diabetic patients with post-staphylococcal GN.
Etiology:	Most cases are elicited by Gram-positive bacteria (in particular *S. aureus* and *S. epidermidis*), more rarely by Gram-negative bacteria.
	The disease may often develop in patients with bacterial endocarditis or shunt nephritis. More rarely the disease is caused by viruses or parasites.
Clinical presentation:	Patients usually present with a nephritic picture, characterized by decreased GFR, oliguria, hypertension.
	Hematuria is constant, often macroscopic. Leukocytes and erythrocyte casts are present in the urine sediment.
	A number of patients may present with nephrotic syndrome or severe renal failure (see Table 4.4).
Epidemiology:	This atypical form is more frequent in adults.
	The upper respiratory tract represents the most frequent site of infection but most cases are triggered by infections located in different sites.
	About half of patients have an immunocompromised background.
Prognosis:	The outcome may be severe, particularly in adults with an underlying disease or an immunocompromised background.
	Some 10% of patients die in the acute phase. In the medium or long term about 25–50% of patients develop some degree of renal failure, with 10% of them requiring dialysis.
Treatment:	Patients with atypical acute GN require hospitalization and appropriate symptomatic treatment.
	Although there is not good evidence that glucocorticoids may be of benefit, a course with high-dose intravenous methylprednisolone followed by oral prednisone may be tried in cases with a rapidly progressive course and crescents at biopsy.

deposition of IgA in glomeruli. Arakawa et al. (2006) found elevated titres of serum IgA against *S. aureus* cell membrane antigen and hypothesized that staphylococcal enterotoxin could act as a superantigen triggering glomerulonephritis. A superantigen can bind on antigen presenting cells and then may interact with T cells causing massive T-cell activation and production of large amount of cytokines including those with IgA class-switching functions (Koyama et al., 1995). In diabetic patients the pathogenesis of post-staphylococcic GN may be also related to increased serum levels of IgA and circulating immune complexes containing IgA as a consequence of subclinical mucosal infections (Eguchi et al., 1995).

Etiology

Recent series reported that streptococcal infections accounted for only 10–28% of acute glomerulonephritis (Montseny et al., 1995, Moroni et al., 2002; Nasr et al., 2008). *S. aureus* and *S. epidermidis* represent now the most frequent Gram-positive bacteria responsible of APIGN, being isolated in 12–24% of cases. Gram-negative bacteria account for 3.3–22 % of cases. Bacterial endocarditis and shunt infections are frequently associated with an acute GN. Viruses and parasites can also cause atypical APIGN. However, in around 50% of the recently reported cases of APIGN no infective agent was isolated. Inapparent viral infection (such as parvovirus) may account for some of these cases.

Clinical presentation and features

As in PSGN, hematuria is the most frequent clinical manifestation in APIGN, being present in 88–100% of patients. Macroscopic hematuria occurs in a variable percentage of cases, from 20% (Nasr et al., 2008) to 73% (Keller et al., 1994). The most impressive difference with PSGN is the high frequency of nephrotic syndrome and/or impaired renal function in atypical APIGN. Nephrotic syndrome was reported in about 50% of patients, with proteinuria exceeding 10g/d in about 20% of cases (Moroni et al., 2002). Impairment of renal function ranged between 56–92% in the different series. Serum creatinine was >3.5mg/dL in one-third of patients (Moroni et al., 2002) and 13–18% of patients required dialysis at presentation (Keller et al., 1994; Montseny et al., 1995). Acute renal failure is the presenting manifestation in the majority of patients with acute post-staphylococcus GN and IgA deposits are dominant or co- dominant at immunofluorescence (Satoskar et al., 2006). Around 60% of patients have arterial hypertension, C3 and C4 levels are usually depressed (Table 4.4).

Epidemiology

A review of the literature shows that, excluding allograft biopsies, atypical APIGN accounts for only 0.6–4.6% of the total amount of renal biopsies performed during the last 20 years (Keller et al., 1994; Montseny et al., 1995;

Table 4.4 Clinical presentation of 'atypical' post-infectious glomerulonephritis

	Keller et al. (1994)	Montseny et al. (1995)	Moroni et al. (2002)	Nasr et al. (2008)
Hematuria	NA	88%	100%	90%
Macroscopic hematuria	73%	NA	54%	24%
Proteinuria	70%	NA	76%	100%
Nephrotic syndrome	50%	35%	52%	41%
Renal insufficiency	80%	56%	82%	92%
Hypertension	57%	67%	66%	63%
Low C3	NA	35%	68%	64%
Low C4	NA	NA	15%	49%

Moroni et al., 2002; Nasr et al., 2008). The median age of patients with atypical APIGN ranges between 49–58 years but age is significantly increasing over the years. In a study, a correlation analysis showed that the mean age of patients was 10 years in the period between 1979–84, 28 years between 1985–89, and 55 years between 1990–99 (p<0.01) (Moroni et al., 2002). Males are affected more commonly than females, with a ratio ranging between 1.5:1–3:1. In all series the majority of patients were Caucasian. The most frequent sites of infections were upper respiratory tract infections (23–42%), dental infections (13–23%), skin infections (1.3–25 %), pneumonia (6.6–18%), urinary infections (5–12%), endocarditis (3.3–13%), osteomyelitis (3.3–5%), deep-seated abscess (2–3.3%), and phlebitis (1.2–4%). A typical feature in the cases of APIGN recently described was the presence of an underlying condition causing an immunocompromised background in about 50% of affected patients; the more frequent were alcoholism, diabetes, drug addiction, malignancies, and liver cirrhosis. In our Renal Unit the number of immunocompromised patients significantly increased over the years. No patients had immunocompromised background between 1979–84, versus 19% between 1985–89, 55% between 1990–94, and 63% between 1995 and 1999 (p<0.01) (Moroni et al., 2002).

Natural history

The prognosis of sporadic forms of atypical APIGN in adults seems to have worsened during the last four decades. In the 1970s, complete remission was reported in 70–80% of adults (Hinglais et al., 1974; Lien et al., 1979).

More recently, Montseny et al. (1995) found complete remission in only 26% of adults, half of them having an underlying disease. This data should be interpreted with caution because the short follow-up of the study (mean 9 months) may have precluded the observation of later recoveries. As a matter of fact it has been reported that complete remission may occur after a median follow-up of 12 months (Lien et al., 1979; Moroni et al., 2002). However, a correlation analysis in our cohort of adults actually showed that the number of patients who achieved a complete remission significantly decreased over the years. More than 80% of cases diagnosed between 1979–84 achieved the remission in comparison to 40% of those diagnosed between 1985–89, 37% between 1990–94, and 30% between 1995–99 (p = 0.001). Altogether, after a mean follow-up of 90 months only 22 of our 50 patients were in complete remission. As expected, the outcome was poorer in patients with an immunocompromised background who had a rate of remission of 14% in comparison with 64% of remission in patients without other underlying diseases. Ten patients (20%) were in partial remission at the last follow-up without significant differences between patients with and without an immunocompromised background. Chronic renal insufficiency was present in 26% of patients and another 10% of patients were on regular dialysis. Once again renal insufficiency was more frequent in patients with an immunocompromised background. Five out of 50 patients, all with renal failure died. At multivariate analysis the absence of an underlying disease (relative risk 3.5) and the absence of interstitial infiltration at renal biopsy (relative risks 8.7) were predictive of complete remission (Moroni et al., 2002).

The outcome reported by Nasr et al. (2008) in 52 patients (with IgA-dominant or co-dominant lesions) after a mean follow-up of 25 months was even worse with 56% of patients having various degrees of chronic renal failure at the last follow-up. Of the eleven patients with diabetes included in that study all had renal insufficiency at presentation. None of them recovered renal function and nine progressed to ESRD. Eighteen out of 41 patients (44%) without diabetes had persistent renal dysfunction, and seven of them progressed to ESRD. The other eighteen patients were not included in the analysis because they had a follow-up <3 months; eight of them had persistent renal dysfunction, and other six were dialysis dependent. 12% of patients died. The only significant predictor on multivariate modeling of ESRD was an elevated serum creatinine at diagnosis. These data suggest that atypical APIGN should be considered a serious disease in adults, particularly in those with an immunocompromised background. The clinical course of the uncommon forms of atypical APIGN due to viral infection is less well understood.

Specific treatment

The supportive therapy is similar to that described for post-streptococcal GN and should be started early, particularly in immunocompromised patients. Control of infection is important and again it should be initiated as soon as possible.

The results reported with glucocorticoid therapy are difficult to evaluate. Anecdotal cases of good response to intravenous high-dose steroids in patients with a high percentage of crescents have been reported. We did not see significant differences in the remissions between patients treated with glucocorticoids (44%) and those given only symptomatic treatment (70%); however only patients with more severe disease received steroid therapy (Moroni et al., 2002). Nasr et al. (2008) treated 17 patients with glucocorticoids. The main indication for steroid therapy was renal insufficiency with or without crescents. Among treated patients twelve of seventeen (70%) had complete remission, 18% persistent renal dysfunction, and 12% progressed to ESRD. Among the other 23 patients who did not receive glucocorticoids, ten (43%) entered complete remission.

As specific treatment may be disappointing once the glomerulopathy is diagnosed, public health measures comparable to those applied to prevent bacterial endocarditis should be encouraged, especially in groups at risk such as alcoholics. A careful management of the underlying diseases, abstinence from alcohol and strict control of arterial hypertension may be useful in slowing the renal progression of these patients.

Practical recommendations

Whether a patient with a suspected acute glomerulonephritis should be hospitalized or followed as an outpatient depends on the severity of the disease. Asymptomatic patients do not need hospitalization, unless a renal biopsy is required in case of persistence of microscopic hematuria or development of heavy (nephrotic-range) proteinuria or uncertainties regarding the correct diagnosis. In case of children with edema, proteinuria, and hypertension the hospitalization is needed in case of poor response to diuretics and/or antihypertensive agents, the risk of hypertensive encephalopathy being higher in these patients. Adults with acute nephritic syndrome should be hospitalized, as they may have a poor prognosis, particularly in case of nephrotic syndrome and/or renal failure due to the high risk of congestive heart failure.

The diagnostic work-up includes a number of tests to determine the cause of the acute nephritic syndrome (Table 4.5). The diagnosis of acute GN is usually easy. However, if the etiological microorganism is not identified it may be difficult to recognize at the beginning whether it is a typical PSGN or an

Table 4.5 Diagnostic laboratory work-up for patients with acute nephritic syndrome

- ◆ Serum creatinine.
- ◆ Serum urea.
- ◆ Urinalysis with urine sediment and measurement of daily proteinuria (or protein/creatinine ratio (mg/mg).
- ◆ Anti-streptolysine O titer.
- ◆ Culture of throat and skin lesions.
- ◆ Blood culture (if endocarditis or sepsis).
- ◆ Serum complement (C3 and C4) levels
- ◆ Antinuclear antibodies.
- ◆ Perinuclear-staining antineutrophil cytoplasmic antibodies (pANCA).
- ◆ Cytoplasmic-staining antineutrophil cytoplasmic antibodies (cANCA).

atypical form. Moreover, a large number of other primary or secondary glomerular diseases may present with similar signs and symptoms. Acute GN and hypocomplementemia may be seen in many systemic diseases, such a SLE and cyroglobulinemia. The more frequent diseases that may make difficult the differential diagnosis are IgAN, lupus nephritis, membranoproliferative GN, cryoglobulinemic nephritis, and rapidly progressive GN. IgAGN is clinically characterized by hematuria, sometimes associated with arterial hypertension and some degree of renal dysfunction but the C3 levels are normal. Some patients may have episodes of macroscopic hematuria often associated with throat or respiratory infection. The differential diagnosis with APIGN may be difficult if hematuria occurs for the first time in a patient who is not known to be a carrier of IgA GN. Laboratory may orientate the diagnosis as hypocomplementemia plays for APIGN while increased levels of serum IgA play for IgAN. However these parameters may be normal in either disease, particularly if the patients with APIGN present late in the course of the disease, after C3 levels have returned to normal. Lupus nephritis, membranoproliferative type I and II, and cryoglobulinemic GN may all present with an acute nephritic syndrome associated with hypocomplementemia. However, patients with SLE may have a constellation of extra-renal symptoms and biological markers that make easier the diagnosis in the typical cases. More difficult may be the clinical diagnosis for patients with membranoproliferative GN. A nephrotic syndrome is more frequent in these patients but some of them may have only moderate proteinuria. On the other hand, nephrotic syndrome may occur also in atypical APIGN, particularly in adults. Cryoglobulinemic patients are often carrier of hepatitis C virus. Although some patients with APIGN may also show circulating cryoglobulins, the amount of cryoglobulins and the levels of 'cryocrit' are usually more elevated in patients with cryoglobulinemic GN. Finally, the differential diagnosis with a rapidly progressive GN can be difficult on clinical grounds alone, particularly for those patients with APIGN showing renal function deterioration. The determination of pANCA and cANCA may help the differential diagnosis in a number of cases. Viral forms of APIGN, such as parvovirus, may resemble lupus nephritis, including hypocomplementemia.

Since most of the above reported diseases may be difficult to recognize at the beginning, the nephrologist has to choose between two options i) to perform a renal biopsy to identify the underlying kidney disease; ii) to wait and see what is the short-term outcome (spontaneous remission or persisting disease). The first option includes a minimal risk of biopsy-related complications, but offers the advantage of a prompt diagnosis and of prompt specific therapeutic intervention. Moreover, the result of renal biopsy may also give prognostic information. The second option is less expensive and avoids the possible complication caused by the biopsy. However, in case of wrong diagnosis it exposes the patient to the risks of a delayed diagnosis and specific treatment (if any). Although any single decision should be taken on the basis of a patient's history, clinical characteristics, and pertinent laboratory investigations (such as serology and complement levels), we are in favor of renal biopsy in case of a suspected symptomatic APIGN in adults, while in young children we prefer to wait for a few days before taking a decision, unless the patient presents nephrotic proteinuria or renal dysfunction.

Treatment remains mostly conservative (Table 4.6). An early and aggressive symptomatic treatment is of paramount importance in severe cases to prevent life-threatening complications such as congestive heart failure, hypertensive encephalopathy, and hyperkalemia. Apart from the restriction of water, sodium, and potassium the generous use of loop diuretics should be encouraged. In treating hypertension the choice of the anti-hypertensive agent depends on the clinical conditions of the patient. ACE-inhibitors and angiotensin-receptor blockers (ARB) may be contraindicated in case of hyperkalemia, while in the presence of congestive heart failure the use of the old non-selective β-blockers should be replaced by selective β-blockers or mixed α1-β adrenergic antagonists, possibly in association with ACE-inhibitors or ARB if there is not concomitant hyperkalemia. Calcium-channel antagonists are particularly effective in case of severe hypertension. It is recommended to strictly monitor the blood pressure, particularly in edematous children who are more susceptible to hypertensive encephalopathy. Calcium-channel blockers, intravenous labetalol, diazoxide, or nitroprusside should be immediately administered if this complication develops. Kayexalate should be given in oliguric patients with serum potassium levels ≥6mEq/L.

Table 4.6 Practical recommendations for APIGN

Hospitalization:	In children it is recommended only for cases with loop-diuretic resistant oliguria or nephrotic syndrome.
	Hospitalization is always recommended for adult and elderly patients.
Renal biopsy:	It is usually avoided in children with epidemic forms of PSGN and in those with sporadic forms without nephrotic syndrome or signs of acute renal failure.
	It is recommended in children with persisting nephrotic syndrome and/or renal dysfunction.
	Renal biopsy is recommended in adult and elderly patients with PSGN. It is mandatory in adults and older patients with atypical APIGN.
Conservative treatment:	A course of antibiotics is recommended, particularly in cases of atypical APIGN, which are often caused by strains of *S. aureus* or by visceral infections.
	Water, sodium, and potassium restriction, and generous use of loop-diuretics should be administered to patients with edemas, congestive heart failure, and antihypertensive agents should be added to patients with arterial hypertension (caution with ACEi/ARB in case of hyperkalemia).
	Hypertensive emergencies should be treated with potent vasodilators (nifedipine, labetalol, diazoxide, nitroprusside).
Glucocorticoids:	The results with glucocorticoids are controversial.
	A short course of high-dose intravenous steroids, followed by 1–2 months with oral prednisone, should be restricted to patients with rapidly progressive course, and/or high percentage of crescents and severe interstitial lesions at renal biopsy.

There is no substantial body of evidence that glucocorticoids are useful in APIGN. Theoretically these agents may reduce inflammation and accelerate the recovery of the acute nephritic syndrome, but we do not recommend their use in children with typical PSGN, as the syndrome spontaneously recovers in a few days. In adults with extracapillary proliferation high-dose glucocorticoids may have at least a partial beneficial role. Unless an active infection is still present, a cycle of glucocorticoids (three intravenous high-dose methylprednisolone pulses followed by oral prednisone 1mg/kg/d for 1 month and then gradually tapered) may be tried in case of a rapidly progressive course of APIGN, although the results are still controversial.

Finally, we recommend that all patients, particularly adults, are monitored regularly in the long-term to evaluate whether the disease may result in progressive renal insufficiency.

Transplantation

At the best of our knowledge only 11 cases of *de novo* post-infectious acute GN have been reported in renal transplant recipients (Moroni et al., 2004; Plumb et al., 2006). In contrast with the typical PSGN, the location of infections was variable, ranging from skin abscess to mycotic aorta aneurysm. The etiological agents more often identified were staphylococci but *E. coli* and streptococci could be recognized as the etiological agents in a couple of patients. The clinical presentation was characterized by an acute decline of graft function in all but one patient. Acute renal dysfunction recovered in most patients, but in the long term three patients lost their graft function and one died. It is difficult to ascertain whether progression was due to chronic allograft nephropathy, to glomerulonephritis, or both. Five patients were treated with methylprednisolone pulse therapy and two of them eventually progressed to ERD. Six patients did not receive glucocorticoids, of them one died and another one needed regular dialysis.

It may be concluded that APIGN is a possible, although rare, complication in renal transplant recipients. It has an unusual presentation and may have a poor outcome in the long term. The role of therapy is still undefined.

References

Ahn SY, Ingulli E (2008). Acute poststreptococcal glomerulonephritis: an update. *Current Opinion in Pediatrics* **20**:157–62.

Arakawa Y, Shumizu Y, Sakurai H et al. (2006). Polyclonal activation of IgA against Staphylococcus aureus cell membrane antigen in post-methicillin-resistant *S. aureus* infection glomerulonephitis. *Nephrology Dialysis Transplantation* **21**:1448–9.

Askenazi DJ, Feig DI, Graham NM, Hui-Stickle S, Goldstein SC (2006). 3-5 year longitudinal follow-up of pediatric patients after acute renal failure. *Kidney International* **69**: 184–9.

Baldwin DS. (1977). Poststreptococcal glomerulonephritis. A progressive disease? *American Journal of Medicine* **62**:1–11.

Balter S, Benin A, Pinto SWL et al. (2000). Epidemic nephritis in Nova Serrana Brazil. *Lancet* **355**: 1776–80.

Batsford SR, Mezzano S, Mihatsch M, Schiltz E, Rodriguez-Ingelmo B (2005). Is nephritogenic antigen in post-streptococcal glomeruonephritis pyrogen exotoxin B (SPE B) or GAPDH? *Kidney International* **68**:1120–9.

Chugh KS, Malhotra HS, Sakhujia V et al. (1987). Progression to end stage renal disease in poststreptococcal glomerulonephritis (PSGN)–Chandighar Study. *International Journal of Artificial Organs* **10**:189–94.

Clark G, White RHR, Glasgow EF et al. (1988). Poststreptococcal glomerulonephritis in children: clinicopathological correlation and long-term prognosis. *Pediatric Nephrology* **2**:381–8.

Couser WG, Johnson RJ (1997). Postinfectious glomerulonephritis. In WG Couser (ed) *Immunologic renal disease*. Lippincott-Raven, Philadelphia, pp.915–43.

Cu GA, Mezzano S, Bannan JD, Zabriskie JB (1998). Immunohistochemical and serological evidence for the role of streptococcal proteinase in acute post-streptococcal glomerulonephritis. *Kidney International* **54**:819–26.

Eguchi EK, Kagame M, Suzuki D et al. (1995). Significance of high levels of serum IgA and IgA circulation immunecomplexes (IgA-CIC) in patients with non insulin dependent diabetes mellitus *Journal of Diabetes and its Complications* **9**:42–8.

Garcia R, Rubio L, and Rodriguez-Iturbe B (1981). Long-term prognosis of epidemic post-streptococcal glomerulonephritis in Maracaibo: follow-up studies 11–12 years after the acute episode. *Clinical Nephrology* **15**:291–8.

Glassock RJ (1988). Pathophysiology of acute glomerulonephritis. *Hospital Practice* **23**:163–9.

Hinglais N, Garcia-Torres R, Kleinknecht D (1974). Long-term prognosis of acute glomerulonephritis. *American Journal of Medicine* **56**:52–60.

Ilyas M, Tolaymat A. (2008). Changing epidemiology of acute post-streptococcal glomerulonephritis in Northeast Florida: a comparative study. *Pediatric Nephrology* **23**:101–6.

Kasahara T, Hayakawa H, Okabo S et al. (2001). Prognosis of acute poststreptococcal glomerulonephritis (APSGN) is excellent in children when adequately diagnosed. *Pediatrics International* **43**:364–7.

Kefalides NA, Ohno N, Wilson CB, Filit H, Zabriskie J (1993). Identification of antigenic epitopes in type IV collagen by use of synthetic peptides. *Kidney International* **43**:94–100.

Keller CK, Andrassy K, Waldherr R and Ritz E (1994). Postinfectious glomerulonephrtis. Is there a link to alcoholism? *Quarterly Journal of Medicine* **87**:97–102.

Koyama A, Kobayashi M, Yamaguchi N et al. (1995). Glomerulonephritis associated with MRSA infection a possible role of bacterial superantigen. *Kidney International* **47**:207–16.

Lange C (1980) Antigenicity of kidney glomeruli. Evaluation by antistreptococcal cell membrane antisera. *Transplantation Proceedings* **12**:82–7

Lien JWK, Mathew TH, Meadows R (1979) Acute post-streptococcal glomerulonephritis in adults. A long term study. *Quarterly Journal of Medicine* **48**:99–111.

Ludlam H, Cookson B (1986). Serum kidney epidemic pyoderma caused by nephritogenic streptococcus pyogens in rugby team. *Lancet* **ii**:331–3.

Matsell DG, Wyatt RJ, Gaber LW (1994).Terminal complement complexes in acute post-streptococcal glomerulonephritis. *Pediatric Nephrology* **8**:671–6.

Melby PC, Musick WD, Luger AM, Khanna R (1987). Poststreptococcal glomerulonephritis in the elderly. Report of a case and review of the literature. *American Journal Nephrology* **7**:235–40.

Montseny JJ, Meyrier A, Kleinknecht D, Callard P (1995). The current spectrum of infectious glomerulonephritis: Experience with 76 patients and review of the literature. *Medicine* **74**:63–73.

Moroni G, Pozzi C, Quaglini S et al. (2002). Long-term prognosis of diffuse proliferative glomerulonephritis associated with infection in adults. *Nephrology Dialysis Transplantation* **17**:1204–11.

Moroni G, Papaccioli D, Banfi G, Tarantino A, Ponticelli C (2004). Acute post-bacterial glomerulonephritis in renal transplant patients: description of three cases and review of the literature. *American Journal Transplantation* **4**:132–6.

Muscatello DJ, O'Grady KA, Neville K, McAnulty J (2001). Acute poststreptococcal glomerulonephritis: public health implications of recent cluster in New South Wales and epidemiology of hospital admission. *Epidemiology and Infection* **126**:365–72.

Nasr SH, Share DS, Vargas MT, D'Agati VD, Markowitz GS (2007). Acute poststaphylococcal glomerulonephritis superimposed on diabetic glomerulosclerosis. *Kidney International* **71**:1317–21

Nasr AH, Markowitz GS, Stokes MB, Said SM, Valeri AM, D'Agati VD (2008). Acute postinfectious glomerulonephritis in the modern era. *Medicine* **87**:21–32.

Nissenson AR, Baraff LJ, Fine RN, Knuston D (1979). Poststreptococcal acute glomerulonephrits: Fact and controversy. *Annals of Internal Medicine* **91**:76–80.

Oda T, Yamakami K, Omasu F et al. (2005). Glomerular plasmin-like activity in relation to nephritis-associated plasmin receptor in acute poststreptococcal glomerulonephritis. *Journal American Society of Nephrology* **16**:247–54.

Oda T, Yoshizawa N, Yamakami K et al. (2007). Significance of glomerular cell apoptosis in the resolution of acute post-streptococcal glomerulonephritis. *Nephrology Dialysis Transplantation* **22**:740–8.

Ozdemir S, Saatci U, Besbas N, Bakkaloglu A, Ozen S, Koray Z (1992). Plasma atrial natriuretic peptide and endothelin levels in acute post-streptococcal glomerulonephritis. *Pediatric Nephrology* **6**:519–22.

Parra G, Rodríguez-Iturbe B, Batsford S, et al. (1998). Antibodies to streptococcal zymogen in the serum of patients with acute glomerulonephritis a multicenter study. *Kidney International* **54**:509–17

Plumb TJ, Greenberg A, Smith SR, et al. (2006). Postinfectious glomerulonephritis in renal allograft recipients. *Transplantation* **82**:1224–8.

Poon-King R, Bannan J, Viteri A, Cu G, Zabriskie JB (1993). Identification of an extracellular plasmin binding protein from nephritogenic streptococci. *Journal of Experimental Medicine* **178**:759–63.

Potter EV, Lipschulz SA, Abidh S, Poon-King E, Earle DP (1982). Twelve to seventeen-year follow-up of patients with poststreptococcal acute glomerulonephritis in Trinidad. *New England Journal of Medicine* **307**: 725–9.

Raff A, Hebert T, Pullman J, Coco M (2005). Crescentic post-streptococcal glomerulonephritis with nephrotic syndrome in the adult: is aggressive therapy warranted? *Clinical Nephrology* **63**:375–80.

Rodriguez-Iturbe B, Rubio L, Garcia R (1981). Attack rare of poststreptococcal glomerulonephritis in families. A prospective study. *Lancet* **i**:401–3.

Rodriguez-Iturbe B (1984). Epidemic poststreptococcal glomerulonephritis. *Kidney International* **25**:129–36.

Rodriguez-Iturbe B, Parra G (2001). Poststreptococcal glomerulonephritis. In S Massry and RJ Glassock (eds) *Textbook of Nephrology*, IV edn. Lippincott Williams & Wilkins, Philadelphia, pp.667–72.

Rodriguez-Iturbe B, Batsford S (2007). Pathogenesis of poststreptococcal glomerulonephritis a century after Clemaes von Pirquet. *Kidney International* **71**:1094–104.

Roy S 3rd, Murphy WM, Arant BS (1981). Post-streptococcal crescentic glomerulonephritis in children: comparison of quintuple therapy versus supportive care. *Journal of Pediatrics* **98**:403–10.

Roy S 3rd, Stapleton FB (1990). Changing prospectives in children with poststreptococcal acute glomerulonephritis. *Pediatric Nephrology* **4**:585–88.

Satoskar AA, Nadasdy G, Plaza JA et al. (2006). Staphylococcus infection-associated glomerulonephritis mimicking IgA nephropathy. *Clinical Journal of the American Society of Nephrology* **1**:1179–86.

Sesso R, Pinto SWL (2005). Five-year follow-up of patients with epidemic glomerulone-phritis due to Streptococcus zooepidemicus. *Nephrology Dialysis Transplantation* **20**:1808–12.

Simon P, Ramee MP, Autuly V et al. (1994). Epidemiology of primary glomerular disease in a French region. Variation according to period and age. *Kidney International* **46**:1192–8.

Sorger K, Gessler U, Hubner FK et al. (1982). Subtypes of acute postinfectious glomerulonephritis. Synopsis of clinical and pathological features. *Clinical Nephrology* **17**:114–28.

Sorger K, Gessler U, Hubner FK et al. (1987). Follow-up studies of three subtypes of acute postinfectious glomerulonephritis ascertained by renal biopsy. *Clinical Nephrology* **27**:111–24.

Steer AC, Danchin MH, Carapetis JR (2007).Group A streptococcal infections in children. *Journal of Paediatrics and Child Health* **43**:203–13.

Vijayakumar M (2002). Acute and crescentic glomerulonephritis. *Indian Journal of Pediatrics* **69**:1071–5.

Vogl W, Renke M, Mayer-Eichberger D, Schmitt H, Bohle A (1986). Long- term prognosis of endocapillary glomerulonephritis of poststreptococcal type in children and adults. *Nephron* **44**:58–65.

Washio M, Katafuchi R, Oh T, Janase Y, Hori K, Fujimi S (1995). Poststreptococcal glomerulonephritis with the nephrotic range of proteinuria. *International Urology Nephrology* **27**:457–64.

Yoshizawa N Oshima S, Sagel I, Shhimizu J, Treser G (1992). Role of a streptococcal anti-gen in the pathogenesis of acute poststreptococcal glomerulonephritis. *Journal of Immunology* **148**:3110–6

Yoshizawa N, Yamakami K, Fujino M et al. (2004). Nephritis associate plasmin receptor and acute postreptococcal glomerulonephritis: characterization of the antigen and asso-ciated immune response. *Journal of American Society Nephrology* **15**:1785–93.

Chapter 5

Minimal change nephropathy

Rosanna Coppo and Claudio Ponticelli

Introduction and overview

Definition

Minimal change nephropathy (MCN), also called 'minimal change disease' in the USA, is chiefly characterized by episodes of nephrotic syndrome—presenting with massive proteinuria, hypoalbuminemia, generalized edema, hyperlipidemia—and no lesions or only minimal glomerular abnormalities in the renal biopsy examined by light microscopy.

Pathology

Glomerular size and architecture are almost normal on light microscopy (see Atlas plate 3). Mild changes including a slight increase in mesangial matrix and mesangial hypercellularity may be seen. In some cases these lesions are more evident. No immunoglobulin or complement deposits can be seen at immunofluorescence. However, a few patients may show scanty or more well developed IgM mesangial deposits. Whether diffuse mesangial proliferation or IgM mesangial deposits confer a worse outcome and a poor response to therapy is still controversial. (Meyrier and Niaudet, 2005). The only lesion detected in MCN is a diffuse effacement of the foot processes of the podocytes on electron microscopy (see Atlas plate 4), which, however, is also seen in other glomerular diseases with nephrotic syndrome, including the unaffected (by light microscopy) glomeruli in focal and segmental glomerulosclerosis (FSGS).

Pathogenesis

In spite of several researches devoted to investigate the pathogenesis of MCN, no definite conclusions have been drawn. A T-cell dysfunction was suggested decades ago on the basis of the association with lymphomas and remission by measles virus infection. More recently T lymphocytes have been thought to elaborate a non-immunoglobulin 'permeability' factor. Several cytokines and growth factors have been supposed to have this activity in MCN, including vascular endothelial growth factor (VEGF), which in experimental animals plays a role in maintaining the glomerular permeability, but data in humans with MCN are inconclusive. Other mediators, including the soluble immune suppressor repressor (SIRS) or a highly glycosylated, hydrophobic protein proposed by Savin, have never been fully identified; however, these studies underline the central role of T cells in the pathogenesis of MCN. The association with allergy has suggested a Th2 lymphocyte activation. However, no clear up-regulation of Th2 cytokines has been proven in patients with MCN, in spite of several models in animals suggesting a role for some cytokines, as for instance IL-13 (Lai et al., 2007). Selective Th2 cell activation is suggested by several studies, and increased expression of a CXC chemokine GRO-gamma (growth related oncogene), which is expressed under the effect of the nuclear transcription factor kappa B (NF-kB) has been reported. A role for activation in circulating lymphomononuclear cells of NF-kB has been suggested mostly in steroid-resistant nephrotic syndromes which in general belong to FSGS. Some interest has recently been focused on Th17 which acts on the development of regulatory T cells and produce IL-17 which was found to be increased in urine of MCN. The search for a permeability factor has included also toxic proteases, inducing proteinuria and podocyte flattening in rats. For instance, altered isoforms of plasma hemopexin with enhanced protease activity have been observed in patients with MCN in relapse (Bakker et al., 2005).

In conclusion, the pathogenetic mechanism/s of activation of T lymphocytes leading to production of circulating vascular permeability factors, the precise identity of which remains elusive, is still unresolved despite numerous studies. These factors are postulated to interfere on the functional activity of the podocyte or with some constituent of the slit-pore diaphragm. The podocyte is a highly specialized and differentiated visceral epithelial cell that forms the outermost layer of the glomerular capillary loop and is thought to play a critical role in the maintenance of the glomerular filtration barrier. The integrity of podocyte foot processes and slit diaphragms, as well as the glomerular basement membrane (GBM) charge guarantee that molecules greater than 42Å or 200kDa are not filtered in the pre-urine. In this event podocytes play the major role, even though a disruption of filtered protein retrieval by tubular cells seems to be also relevant in allowing a minimal physiological urinary protein loss (Russo et al., 2007). The relevance of podocyte proteins has been proved by the identification in children with familial nephrotic syndrome—usually FSGS, but sometimes MCN—of mutations in genes encoding podocyte proteins participating in the slit diaphragm structure (Tryggvason et al., 2006). It is of interest that relevant podocitary proteins including nephrin and podocin can be down-regulated in experimental models of MCN (Lai et al., 2007) and in podocyte cultures by factors present in sera of patients with MCN during relapses of nephrotic syndromes (Mathieson 2007). Transcriptional regulation of podocyte gene expression in MCN is thought to play a role in the pathogenesis of the disease, and in this process modification of podocyte redox state seems to be relevant. Renal infusion of H_2O_2 induces proteinuria in rats. Puromycin aminoglucoside (PAN) and adriamycin induce nephrosis via modification of redox state and reactive oxyen species have been recently detected *in vivo* by using electron paramagnetic resonance in the PAN model of MCN. Oxidative damage of podocytes induces podocyte detachment from GBM. Podocyturia is thought to be a marker of severe nephrotic syndrome, mostly associated with FSGS.

It remains possible that MCN is a 'phenotype' and that the underlying mechanisms responsible for the disease may be heterogeneous. Whether MCN and FSGS should be considered as a unique and related entity, in which common pathophysiological mechanisms operate with different intensity, or as distinct and separate entities with different pathogenetic mechanisms is still a matter of considerable controversy. However, there are clear histological and clinical differences between MCN and FSGS. At renal biopsy FSGS is, by definition, characterized by focal and segmental glomerular lesions at the level of light microscopy. These lesions may affect a small minority of the glomeruli, easily missed when the sample is small, or may involve a substantial majority of glomeruli. Confusion in the differential diagnosis of MCN may originate in the early stages by the fact that the lesions of FSGS can be seen initially only in juxtamedullary glomeruli in the core of the biopsy. Since FSGS also shows fusion of foot processes of epithelial cells on electron microscopy, even in glomeruli apparently unaffected by the sclerosing lesion by light microscopy, and mesangial IgM or complement deposition in glomeruli (usually focal and segmental in distribution) at immunofluorescence, some biopsies initially classified as MCN may in fact have been FSGS from the start. Larger glomeruli have been detected in FSGS in comparison to MCN, and low birth weight has been included among the responsible mechanisms. The 'evolution' of MCN to a lesion of FSGS has been observed on serial renal biopsies in individual patients. Whether this represents a true 'transformation' from one 'disease' to another, cannot be answered definitely due to the limitations of a purely morphological approach.

Etiology

No precipitating causes are identifiable in many cases. However, in a number of patients the onset of the nephrotic syndrome is preceded by upper respiratory tract infection, allergic reaction, or vaccinations. About 20% of patients

Table 5.1 Possible associations between MCN and tumors, drugs, or other diseases

Tumors	Infections	Other diseases	Drugs	Others
Hodgkin's lymphoma	Syphilis	Diabetes mellitus	Thiola	Bee stings
Non-Hodgkin's lymphoma	HIV	Dermatitis herpetiformis	NSAID	Other allergies
Leukemia	Schistosoma	Obesity	Gold	
Mesothelioma		Stem cell transplantation	Trimethadione	
Thymoma		Systemic lupus erythematosus	Paramethadione	
Carcinoma of colon, pancreas, prostate, lung, kidney			Mercury	
Nephroblastoma			Penicillamine	
Waldenström's macroglobulinaemia			Interferon	
Kimura's disease			Lithium	

who develop MCN have a history of bronchial asthma, contact dermatitis, or allergy to milk or other foods. Significantly increased levels of IgE have been detected in association with relapsing MCN. Although MCN is usually idiopathic in nature, rare cases occurring in association with other diseases have been reported (Table 5.1). The most frequent association with malignant disease is with Hodgkin's lymphoma (Audard et al., 2006). The association with non-Hodgkin's lymphoma or other solid tumors is rare (Glassock, 2003). Several drugs may precipitate a MCN. A number of cases have been reported after the consumption of non-steroidal anti-inflammatory drugs. Most frequently the nephrotic syndrome caused by these drugs is associated with an acute interstitial nephritis and acute renal failure, but some cases may exhibit only the lesion of MCN. Nephrotic syndrome usually reverses completely after discontinuation of the offending drug. Drug-induced MCN should always be considered in the differential diagnosis in view of the wide use of these agents.

Clinical presentation and features

Clinically, MCN is characterized by a 'full blown' nephrotic syndrome with urinary protein excretion ranging between 3–20g or more per day in adults (protein/creatinine ratio >3mg/mg), without 'nephritic' signs or symptoms. In children nephrotic syndrome is defined by proteinuria >40mg/m2/h or >50mg/kg/d or protein/creatinine ratio >3.0mg/mg and albuminemia <2.5g/dL (Table 5.2).

Table 5.2 Definitions used to describe nephrotic syndrome and responses and relapses in patients with MCN

Nephrotic syndrome	In adults, proteinuria >3.5g/day (protein/creatinine ratio >3.5mg/mg), without 'nephritic' signs or symptoms
	In children, proteinuria >40mg/m^2/h or >50 mg/kg/d or protein/creatinine ratio >3.0mg/mg and hypoalbuminemia (<2.5mg/dL)
Complete remission	Proteinuria <4mg/m^2/d in children or <0.2g/d in adults for 3 consecutive days
Partial remission	Proteinuria between 4–40mg/m^2/d in children or between 0.21–3.5g/d in adults for 3 consecutive days
Relapse of proteinuria	Proteinuria >4mg/m^2/d in children or 0.2g/d in adults for at least 1 week, in patients who were in complete remission
Relapse of nephrotic syndrome	Proteinuria >40mg/m^2/d in children or 3.5g/d in adults for at least 1 week, in patients who were in complete or partial remission
Frequent relapsers	Patients with two or more episodes of the nephrotic syndrome in 6 months or three or more episodes of the nephrotic syndrome in 12 months
Steroid-dependent nephrotic syndrome	Reappearance of the nephrotic syndrome within 2 weeks after reduction or discontinuation of glucocorticoids
Steroid-resistant nephrotic syndrome	Controversial (see text)

The onset of the nephrotic syndrome is typically abrupt rather than insidious, and patients may often be able to identify the day at which their disease was first manifest. In children 80% of the cases occur before the age of 6 years, the peak incidence being between the ages of 2–4 years. Pure MCN is very uncommon before the age of 2 years, since congenital and genetic forms at onset within the first year of age mostly have the histological features of FSGS or mesangial sclerosis. The incidence of MCN approaches that of adult levels after the age of 12 years. Severe hypoalbuminemia, sometimes out of proportion to the degree of proteinuria, and marked hypercholesterolemia are common. Proteinuria is typically 'selective,' with heavy loss of low molecular weight albumin while proteins of higher molecular weight are retained. Facial edema is often the major presenting symptom in children. Fluid retention increases, rapidly or gradually, often leading to a frank anasarca with impressive edema of legs, external genitals, and the peri-orbital area. Blood pressure is usually within normal values, but higher than controls in 10% of children with MCN, particularly in Afro-American children, whose renal arterioles exhibit significantly smaller lumens and thicker walls than white children. Such changes may contribute to the African-American predisposition to chronic renal disease and hypertension (Rostand et al., 2005). About one-third of young adults with MCN are hypertensive (Ritz et al. 1989). On the other hand, hypovolemia, postural hypotension, and even shock may sometimes occur as a consequence of sudden, massive loss of albumin in the urine and/or excessive administration of diuretics. Persistent microscopic hematuria is rare, although occasional positive tests occur in about one-third of cases; however, gross hematuria is exceptional. Renal function is usually normal at presentation but, especially in older patients, oliguric renal failure may be the presenting syndrome. During the height of disease manifestations marked depression of serum IgG levels, elevation of IgM and fibrinogen levels, and normal C3 and C4 levels are characteristic of MCN. These disturbances in the serum protein levels lead to marked elevation of the erythrocyte sedimentation rate.

As pointed out above, it may be difficult to distinguish at presentation whether the patient is affected by a true MCN or by a FSGS. Particularly in adults, the general outcome and response to therapy are usually quite different for patients with MCN and those with FSGS. However, some exception exists, and MCN non-responsive to treatment and progressing to renal failure have been reported. In children, it is generally thought that, even though MCN, mesangial proliferative nephropathy, IgM nephropathy, and FSGS are readily distinguished on biopsy, the clinical significance of the distinction is not clearly defined and it remains controversial. There is confusion in the literature, which often refers to steroid-sensitive nephrotic syndrome (SSNS) and steroid-resistant nephrotic syndrome (SRNS) other times to MCN and FSGS respectively. In children, regardless histopathology, SRNS have a poorer outcome than SSNS. On the other hand, it is true that in children most SRNS are FSGS and genetically conditioned nephrotic syndromes are mostly FSGS. Thus, we will follow current practice and will treat these two lesions having distinctive clinical entities separately (see Chapter 6).

Epidemiology

MCN accounts for about 85% of cases of apparently 'idiopathic' nephrotic syndrome in children and for about 20% of cases of apparently 'idiopathic' nephrotic syndrome in adults. The disease is ubiquitous, but it occurs more frequently in Asian than in Caucasian subjects, while it seems to be rare but with a more severe outcome in black children. There is a male:female ratio of 2:1 in children. Male preponderance is also observed in adults (Meyrier and Niaudet, 2005). In most Western countries, the incidence of nephrotic syndrome is estimated to be between 2 and 7 new cases per 100,000 children and the prevalence about 16 cases per 100,000 children.

There are some data indicating that over the last decade there has been an increase in the ratio between FSGS and MCN in children. In USA the race does not seem to influence the incidence of nephrotic syndrome, while it is likely to have an impact on the distribution of histological lesions, as African-American children have more frequently FSGS and SRNS.

Natural history

Since today most patients are given glucocorticoids or other effective drugs soon after the diagnosis has been made, it is difficult now to appreciate the true natural, untreated course of the disease. Studies conducted in the pre-glucocorticoid era indicated that early spontaneous remission is uncommon, and more frequently spontaneous remission may occur after several years of observation. Some studies showed spontaneous remission rates of about 40% after 1–2 years of observation. For reasons that are poorly understood, treatment-induced remissions are associated with a prominent tendency to relapse whereas spontaneous remissions are less likely to be followed by relapses. For the great majority of patients with MCN the clinical course is characterized by an initial remission, either spontaneous or induced by therapy. Remission may be followed by relapses of the nephrotic syndrome which may occur without apparent cause or after infections or allergic reactions. About 30–35% of children who respond to initial therapy do not ever have any relapses, 10–20% have infrequent relapses, and 45–60% have frequent relapses or become steroid dependent (see definitions in Table 5.2). About 65–75% of children may eventually develop a prolonged relapse-free interval or definitive remission several years after the diagnosis (usually after the onset of puberty), but some patients need 20–30 years or even more before entering definitive remission.

The prognosis for preservation of renal function is usually excellent if patients continue to respond to glucocorticoids. The risk of developing progressive renal dysfunction and end-stage renal disease (ESRD) is minimal (<5% at 25 years of follow-up in children), although some cases of acute tubular necrosis occurring in the older population of adult patients may result in irreversible renal failure.

Acute renal failure occurring in the course of MCN (usually in adults over 40 years of age) can be due to hypovolemia, acute (drug-induced) hypersensitivity interstitial nephritis, or, very rarely, acute bilateral renal vein thrombosis, but is most often caused by diuretics or hemodynamic factors. In a series of 95 adult patients with MCN, acute renal failure occurred in 24 patients; they tended to be older and hypertensive with lower serum albumin and more proteinuria than those without acute renal failure. A minority of patients (4.2%) progressed to ESRD (Waldman et al., 2007). Intravascular volume depletion in children may cause oliguria and sometimes acute renal failure, which regresses after successful glucocorticoid therapy.

Apart from renal failure, patients with MCN are exposed to all the infectious and thrombophilic complications of a severe nephrotic syndrome, such as bacterial peritonitis, cellulitis, septicemia, pneumonia, meningitis (all usually related to encapsulated organisms such as pneumococci), or deep venous thrombosis with or without pulmonary embolism, and spontaneous arterial thrombosis. Cerebral complications, including convulsions, hypertensive encephalopathy, and cerebral thrombosis (sagittal vein thrombosis) can also occur. Fatal events are rare but possible. In children followed for 5–10 years the mortality rate is <2% and may be caused by infection or acute hypovolemia (ISKDC, 1984). However, about 1% of deaths are related to treatment, particularly to glucocorticoid or cytotoxic drugs when used at high doses or for prolonged periods (Latta et al., 2001). In adults, the mortality rate is about 6–10% (Schena and Cameron 1988) while 35–45% of elderly patients die, usually within 3 years of the clinical onset (Lorca and Ponticelli 1995). The most frequent causes of death in adults and in elderly patients are related to the nephrotic syndrome per se (e.g., cardiovascular disease, pulmonary embolism, renal failure) or to its treatment (e.g., infections, malignancy). Death is particularly frequent in patients with renal dysfunction and in those untreated or refractory to treatment. Whether the hypercholesterolemia associated with MCN results in accelerated atherogenesis is controversial.

Prognostic factors

See Table 5.3.

Presentation

Patients without edema and identified by chance proteinuria tend to have less relapse than symptomatic patients. This is a quite uncommon presentation for MCN. The magnitude of the proteinuria at the time of presentation does not predict the subsequent response rate.

Age

The response to glucocorticoids is both lower in frequency and slower to develop in adults than in children with MCN (Nolasco et al., 1986) and among children, those aged below 6 years have a faster response, while in adults, those aged over 40 years respond more slowly than younger patients aged 18–39 years. While progression to chronic renal failure is quite exceptional in children, it may occur in about 14% of patients older than 60 years (Lorca and Ponticelli, 1995). On the other hand, the risk of relapses is inversely correlated with age, being higher in patients whose nephrotic syndrome started before age six than in older children and adolescents (Trompeter et al., 1981). The risk of relapse is lower in adults. Only 10 to 20% of adults develop multiple

Table 5.3 Factors which may influence the prognosis and the response to therapy in patients with MCN

Presentation	Asymptomatic proteinuria	Very little risk of progression
Age	Children	Better response to glucocorticoids. Lower mortality rate. Lower progression to chronic renal failure
	Adults	Slower and lower response to glucocorticoids. Lower risk of relapses
Sex	Males	Higher risk of relapses
Race	Black and Caucasian	Lower response to therapy
Response to glucocorticoids	Steroid responders	Good long-term outcome
Duration of initial treatment	Prolonged	Higher rate of response and less frequent relapses
Duration of remission	Remission for >1 year	Lower rate of relapse
Relapses	Early relapses	Higher probability of frequent relapses
	Repeated relapses in the first 6 months of treatment	Higher mortality rate
Glomerular lesions	Glomerular hypertrophy	Progression to focal glomerulosclerosis
	Mesangial proliferation	Debated poor prognosis
	IgM deposits	Debated poor prognosis
	IgG deposits	Irrelevant

relapses (Nolasco et al., 1986, Nakayama et al., 2002; Tse et al., 2003). Elderly patients have the lowest rate of relapses. In a review of the literature only 20% of elderly patients showed one or more relapses after initial remission (Lorca and Ponticelli, 1995).

Race/ethnicity

By reviewing data from the literature, Schena and Cameron (1988) found that the number of patients who did not respond to treatment or showed only partial remission was significantly higher in Caucasian than in Asian series. The steroid resistance is particularly elevated in African-American black patients (Kim et al., 2006). A higher prevalence of FSGS, 'misdiagnosed' as MCN in the original biopsy sample can be considered, besides genetic factors.

HLA antigens and other genetic influences

Children with idiopathic nephrotic syndrome and HLA DR3/DR7 or DQ2 are at risk of frequent relapses, steroid-dependence, or steroid-resistance, while children with HLA DR2, DR6, or DQ1 appear to be at lesser risk to develop relapses (Bouissou et al., 1995). SRNS is often associated with HLA-DR4 and DQ8 (Krasowska-Kwiecień et al., 2006).

Heterozygous amino acid changes in nephrin and podocin are seen in about one-third of patients with typical MCN, but no amino acid changes were observed for Neph1 and CD2AP in 104 adults with childhood-onset MCN. From this study it appears that MCN is a multifactorial disease, in which genetics play a minor role (Lahdenkari et al., 2005)

Response to glucocorticoids

A good long-term prognosis is generally observed in MCN with steroid-sensitive nephrotic syndrome. These patients do not progress to renal failure and most achieve a persisting remission. On the contrary, patient and kidney survival rates are poor in rare cases of MCN with steroid-resistant nephrotic syndrome, most of which eventually show an underlying FSGS at repeated biopsy.

Duration of initial treatment

As will be detailed later, the rate of response and of relapses is roughly proportional to the duration of initial treatment, both in children and in adults.

Duration of remission

The longer the remission (the relapse-free interval) the better the prognosis. After 1 year of remission relapses are uncommon. Shilliday et al. (1993) reported that 97% of patients who relapsed did so within 36 months after the initial remission. The authors concluded that patients who have been in remission without steroids for 36 months might be considered 'cured.' However, occasionally relapses may occur after 20 or more years. We have seen patients with a relapse of full blown nephrotic syndrome due to MCN after 30 years of complete remission.

Spontaneous versus treatment induced remission

Limited data suggest that a spontaneous remission is followed by a longer relapse-free interval that in treatment induced remissions, but in the absence of prospective controlled observations this is difficult to verify.

Relapses

An early relapse, occurring within 6 months after remission, is often followed by a frequent relapsing course. The number of relapses during the first 6 months in patients who were given a standard glucocorticoid regimen is highly predictive of the subsequent clinical course. Old studies, such as the International Study of Kidney Diseases in children (ISKDC, 1984) reported a mortality rate of 0.4% in 283 children with MCN who were not early relapsers versus 6.3% in 63 patients who had relapse during the initial 8 weeks' treatment. Most deaths were caused by infection. Relapse-free survival rates increases with the cumulative dosage of cytotoxic agents and are higher in children with frequently relapsing than steroid-dependent patients (Latta et al., 2001).

Variations in glomerular lesions

The presence of *glomerular hypertrophy* on morphometric analysis is considered as a good predictor of evolution from MCN to FSGS on serial renal biopsy and has therefore a bad prognostic significance. Whether *mesangial hypercellularity* is associated with a decreased response to glucocorticoids, steroid-dependency, and poorer prognosis or does not have any impact on these variables is still a matter of controversy. Some patients with otherwise typical MCN may show *mesangial IgM deposition* with or without a slight increase in mesangial matrix. Some investigators think that this IgM nephropathy represents a separate entity bearing a poor prognosis while others feel that patients with IgM deposits neither can be differentiated clinically from MCN nor have different outcome and response to treatment. The presence of *mesangial deposits of IgG* is usually considered to be non-specific. The presence of *tip lesions* in otherwise normal glomeruli at light microscopy has been considered as a distinct entity within MCN/FSGS spectrum (Stokes et al., 2004). These lesions however do not influence a response to steroids similar to what observed in patients with classic MCN.

Qualitative aspects of proteinuria

Most patients with MCN have highly selective proteinuria, with a low level of urinary excretion of higher molecular weight proteins such as IgM or IgG. If non-selective proteinuria is present this should raise the suspicion that a lesion of FSGS is present and that steroid non-responsiveness is more likely. Future studies of urinary proteomics may yet define a pattern of urinary protein excretion in MCN that is highly correlated with the response or non-response to therapy.

Specific treatment

Goals and objectives of treatment

The three main objectives in treating MCN are:

♦ To induce a complete remission of the nephrotic syndrome as soon as possible in order to prevent the severe complications related to the nephrotic state.

♦ To avoid relapses of nephrotic syndrome.

♦ To minimize iatrogenic side effects in a disease which can run a long relapsing course.

Several drugs, used alone or in combination with others, and overall therapeutic strategies may be used to achieve these objectives in the majority of patients.

Glucocorticoids

Glucocorticoids (prednisone, prednisolone, dexamethasone, methylprednisolone) are universally considered as the drug class of choice for the initial treatment of MCN in both children and adults. It must be recognized that this dogmatic statement is primarily based on evidence from numerous uncontrolled observational trials, as the number of published randomized controlled trials involving a comparison of glucocorticoids to a placebo is very limited and inconclusive due to the small numbers of patients observed.

Initial regimen

See Table 5.4.

Children Approximately 95% of children with 'true' MCN can obtain a complete disappearance of proteinuria with high-dose oral predniso(lo)ne, while the rate of response is lower with lower doses. Today, a widely used schedule consists of oral predniso(lo)ne 60mg/m^2/d or 2mg/kg/d (up to a maximum dose of 80–100mg/d) given in a single morning dose for 4 weeks, followed by 40mg/m^2 or 2mg/kg every other day for 4 further weeks and then abruptly discontinued. Dividing the dosage of steroids among the daytime hours or administering the dose after 10 a.m. should not be done. The once-a-day and then alternate-day schedule is usually well tolerated and couples the advantages of a high response rate with those of a relatively long therapy which may prevent relapses. If the glucocorticoids have been administered on a once a morning or every other morning dosage regimen the risk of adrenocortical–pituitary–hypothalamic axis deficiency upon abrupt discontinuance of therapy is minimal.

Table 5.4 Suggested approach for initial treatment in MCN

Children	Prednisone 60mg/m²/d (or 2 mg/kg/day) for 4 weeks (6 weeks in case of no remission), then 40mg/m² /48h (or 2 mg/kg/48h) for 8 weeks, then reduce by 5–10 mg/m²/48h (or 0.5mg/Kg/48h) every 2 weeks
Adults	Prednisone 1mg/kg/d until remission or for 6 weeks (alternate-day regimen does not offer advantage for initial treatment in adults). In case of no remission continue with 1mg/kg /day for additional 2 weeks and at progressively reduced doses for other 3–5 months. In case of early remission reduce the doses to 1.6mg/kg/48h for 1 month, then reduce by 0.2–0.4mg/kg/48h every 2 weeks until complete discontinuation.
Elderly	Prednisone 1mg/kg/d until remission or for 4 weeks, then 0.8 mg/kg/d for 2 weeks, then 1.6mg/kg/48h for 2 weeks, then reduce by 0.4 mg/kg/48h every 2 weeks. If no remission continue with 1.2 mg/kg/48h for another 4 weeks then reduce
Contraindications to prednisone	Cyclophosphamide 2mg/kg/d or chlorambucil 0.15mg/kg/d for 8–12 weeks

Complete remission of proteinuria occurs in about half of children within 1 week, in 75% within 2 weeks, and in approximately 90% within 4 weeks. Those children who do not respond within 4 weeks were defined as 'steroid resistant' in the past (ISKDC, 1984). However, this definition is now applied to children with no response after 6 weeks of full doses of oral steroids, and some authors (Meyrier and Niaudet, 2005) include in the definition also the lack of response to additional three intravenous methylprednisolone pulses (10mg/kg each). The major problem in children is represented by the risk of relapse. The abrupt discontinuance of glucocorticoids after obtaining remission may favor relapses. Of great importance, a longer duration of initial treatment not only can obtain remission in some late responders but can also reduce the rate of relapses without increasing the risk of side effects. Using data from systematic reviews and randomized controlled trials in SSNS, Hodson et al. (2001) found that 6 months of prednisone for the initial treatment was significantly more effective than 3 months (relative risk [RR] 0.57; 95% confidence interval [CI] 0.45–0.71). Higher prednisone doses given for the same duration reduced the risk of relapse (RR 0.59; 95% CI 0.42–0.84) suggesting that both dose and duration of prednisone therapy lead to prolonged remission.

Adults The initial dose of predniso(lo)ne is usually 1mg/kg/d (100mg/d maximum), rather lower in proportion to body weight than that given to children. Some clinicians prefer to administer glucocorticoids every other day from the outset of initial therapy to reduce side effects. However, in a retrospective study no difference in the rate of remissions and in the risk of relapses was found between adults treated with an initial prednisone dosage of 1mg/kg on the daily regimen and approximately 2mg/kg on alternate day (Waldman et al., 2007). There were also no differences in side effects. As with children the glucocorticoid dosage should always be administered in the morning between 8–10 a.m.

Very differently from children, only 50–60% of adults become free of proteinuria within 8 weeks of therapy, regardless of the schedule of administration. However, if glucocorticoid therapy is continued for 16 weeks or more, complete remission of proteinuria may be obtained in about 80% of adult patients with MCN (Nolasco et al., 1986; Korbet et al., 1988). It is difficult to establish whether this slower response is due to a genuine lower sensitivity of adults to glucocorticoids, or to the fact that the effective doses of glucocorticoids given to adults are proportionally lower (as assessed by pharmacokinetics of the glucocorticoid of the area under the curve of the serum concentration of the glucocorticoid after oral administration) than those given to children. In adults, as observed in children, the duration of initial treatment influences the subsequent risk of relapses.

Treatment of infrequent relapses

Relapses are usually as responsive to glucocorticoids as the initial episode of nephrotic syndrome. Unlike the first episode of the nephrotic syndrome, however, the duration of treatment of relapses does not seem to influence the subsequent rate of additional relapses. Spontaneous remission can occur within 4–14d after onset of a relapse, but it is impossible to predict in advance which patients will remit spontaneously and which will not. Some clinicians recommend starting treatment of relapses early if proteinuria of more than 2–3g/d (2–3g/g protein/creatinine on spot urine samples, 3+ to 4+ on dipstick) persists for 3 consecutive days, in order to prevent a full-blown nephrotic syndrome. Others prefer to wait 7–10 days to avoid a useless glucocorticoid therapy in those patients who may remit spontaneously.

For children with infrequent relapses treatment is with prednisone or prednisolone 60mg/m^2/d until the urine is protein-free for 3 consecutive days; this is followed by 4 weeks of alternate-day prednisone at a dose of 40mg/every other day (Brodehl, 1991). A similar regimen, with lower doses of prednisone (1mg/kg/d for the relapse and then 0.8mg/kg every other day for 4 weeks), may be used in adults.

Other protocols suggest adopting in children with infrequent relapses who have been steroid-free for months or years the same protocol used for the initial treatment.

Treatment of frequently relapsing/ steroid-dependent patients

The management of patients with frequent relapses of the nephrotic syndrome represents a challenge for the clinician. These patients usually remain steroid-responsive but repeated courses of high-dose glucocorticoids may induce severe

Table 5.5 Possible options for steroid treatment of frequently relapsing/steroid dependent patients

- Wait for relapse, then treat with either a 2-month course with alternate-day prednisone or with three intravenous infusions high-dose methylprendisolone pulses, followed by oral prednisone at moderate doses (0.5 mg/kg/d) for 4 weeks.
- Give prophylaxis with low-dose predniso(lo)ne (<0.5 mg/kg/d or <1 mg/kg/48h)

hypercorticism (exogenous Cushing syndrome) and even an increased risk of life-threatening complications (see Chapter 2). Some strategies may be adopted to reduce the toxicity of prolonged glucocorticoid treatment. One such strategy is a 6-month course of alternate-day therapy or a treatment based on three intravenous pulses of high-dose methylprednisolone followed by oral prednisone at moderate doses ($30mg/m^2$ in children, 0.5mg/kg in adults, gradually tapered).

The two somewhat opposing strategies more frequently adopted (Table 5.5) are: (i) to wait for relapse (which will almost certainly occur in the frequently relapsing patient) and then treat it as described above or (ii) to use continuous 'prophylaxis' with low-dose preniso(lo)ne (usually ≤0.5mg/kg every other day).

A meta-analysis of three randomized trials (Palmer et al., 2008) did not find a difference between intravenous methylprednisolone plus oral prednisone compared with oral prednisone alone for complete remission. Prednisone, compared with short-course intravenous methylprednisolone, increased the number of subjects who achieved complete remission (RR 4.95). On the other hand, a short-course approach may be preferable in steroid-dependent and frequently relapsing patients, in order to exploit the benefits of steroid-free periods, reducing steroid-related complications, providing that the intervals without proteinuria are not too short.

Growth retardation is a significant problem for the continuous use of glucocorticoids in children. Although some patients may tolerate these treatments without side effects others develop important steroid toxicity. The longer the treatment the higher is the risk of severe toxicity. Thus, alternative treatments designed to reduce the overall exposure to the adverse effects of glucocorticoids are required in many frequent relapsing and steroid-dependent patients

Immunomodulating agents

Several immunomodulating drugs have been used in patients with MCN. The two more popular agents are cyclophosphamide and chlorambucil.

Alkylating agents

Cyclophosphamide

The efficacy of daily oral cyclophosphamide in preventing relapses of the nephrotic syndrome has been known for more than 30 years and proven by suitably designed randomized clinical trials, mostly carried out in children with doses of 2–2.5mg/kg/d for 8–12 weeks. A systemic review confirmed the superiority of cyclophosphamide over prednisone alone in preventing relapses in children (Hodson et al., 2008). Less information about overall efficacy and safety of cyclophosphamide based regimens is available in adults. After treatment with cyclophosphamide, the cumulative rate of sustained remissions may range from 50–78%. Several factors can influence the response to cyclophosphamide (Table 5.6):

- An important variable is the duration of cyclophosphamide treatment. Only few patients enter a complete remission with a 4-week treatment. For those patients who do not respond to a course of 8 weeks, treatment may be prolonged to 12 weeks.

- Steroid-sensitive patients usually have an excellent rate of response to cyclophosphamide, independent of kidney histopathology, while in general steroid-resistant children do not respond to an 8-week therapy with cyclophosphamide (ISKDC 1984).

- Frequently relapsing patients have a higher rate of sustained remission than steroid-dependent patients. About 70% of frequently relapsing children versus <30% of steroid-dependent children with MCN treated with 8 weeks of oral daily cyclophosphamide maintain stable remission. When steroid-dependent children were given daily oral cyclophosphamide for 12 weeks about two-thirds of them remained in remission after two years (Brodehl, 1991).

Table 5.6 Factors influencing the response to cyclophosphamide in MCN

Duration of initial treatment:	An 8 or 12 week course gives better chances of complete remission than shorter courses in preventing relapses
Steroid sensitivity:	The probability of remission is better in steroid-sensitive patients than in steroid-resistant patients
Frequent relapses:	Frequently relapsing patients are more likely to respond with sustained remission than steroid-dependent patients
Age:	In responders a prolonged remission is more frequent in adults than in children

◆ The age at onset of MCN correlates inversely with relapse rate. In adults some 60% of patients still enjoyed remission 15 years after a course of cyclophosphamide treatment in the experience of Guy's Hospital in London (Nolasco et al., 1986).

The major problem with the use of cyclophosphamide concerns its toxicity. Side-effects of this agent have been detailed elsewhere in this book (see Chapter 2). In a meta-analysis on 1504 children treated with oral daily cyclophosphamide or chlorambucil for MCN the fatality rate of the treatment was approximately 1% (Latta et al., 2001). The four most important side effects of the alkylating agent class of cytotoxic drugs (including cyclophosphamide, chlorambucil, and nitrogen mustard) are bladder toxicity (hemorrhagic cystitis, induction of transitional cell metaplasia, and neoplasia), bone marrow toxicity (agranulocytosis, pancytopenia), gonadal toxicity (premature ovarian failure, aspermatogenesis/azoospermia), and oncogenicity (mainly induction of lymphomas and leukemias).

Bladder toxicity is rare (but always possible!) with the oral doses and duration used in MCN. To reduce the risk further it is advisable to put patients into remission first using corticosteroids and then to give cyclophosphamide only after diuresis has been induced. MESNA should be prescribed if cyclophosphamide has to be given for a prolonged period.

Bone marrow toxicity depends on the dose used. Leukopenia may occur in about one-third of patients. At a daily dose not exceeding 2mg/kg every 24h for 8–12 weeks leukopenia may develop but it is usually reversible by decreasing the doses. Pancytopenia is rare at conventional doses of oral cyclophosphamide.

The risk of *azoospermia* is related to the *cumulative* dosage of cyclophosphamide. In a meta-analysis study no safe threshold for a cumulative amount of cyclophosphamide was found in males, but there was a marked increase in the risk of oligo- or azoospermia with higher cumulative doses (Latta et al., 2001). Thus, dosages of 3mg/kg body weight per day for 8 weeks or 2mg/kg for 12 weeks may be recommended, not to exceed a cumulative dose of cyclophosphamide >200mg per kg, as the standard scheme. Females rarely develop gonadal toxicity with the oral administration of cyclophosphamide in conventional dose or duration.

The *oncogenic risk* also depends on the cumulative dosage. Transitional cell carcinoma of the bladder or uro-epithelial tract or acute myelogenous leukemia have an increased incidence in patients who were given several grams of cyclophosphamide over many months (see Chapter 2). In the meta-analysis of Latta et al. (2001), fourteen cases of malignancies were observed in 1504 (0.9%) children treated years ago with high doses of either cyclophosphamide or chlorambucil. The oncogenic risk using 2–3 months of therapy is minimal. An impairment of

T-helper cells can occur in patients treated with cyclophosphamide. The immune function reverts to normal within 6–12 months in patients treated for 8 weeks.

In summary, an 8–12 week course of cyclophosphamide at a dose of 2mg/kg/d (<200mg/kg as a cumulative dose) is generally well tolerated both in the short and long term. Further subsequent courses, however, can increase the risk of gonadal toxicity, neoplasia, and prolonged immune dysfunction and should be avoided whenever possible. To be on the safe side leuprolide may be administered in females during cytotoxic treatment, and sperm banking may be recommended to males requiring more than one course of cyclophosphamide. Intravenous pulses of cyclophosphamide may also reduce the cumulative dosage of this agent, but the experience in MCN is limited.

It should be reminded that both cyclophosphamide and chlorambucil are absolutely contraindicated in pregnancy and all sexually active females receiving the drug should have a negative pregnancy test before starting the agent and be advised to use at least two contraceptive measures during its use or to entirely avoid intercourses while receiving the drug. Caution should be recommended with the use of alkylating agents in very young children with no prior history of varicella or who have negative anti-varicella antibody tests.

Chlorambucil

Good results have been reported with oral daily chlorambucil, although there is considerably less experience with this agent than with cyclophosphamide. The dosage more frequently used in patients with MCN is 0.2mg/kg/d for 8 weeks, but to be on the safe side it is probably better to administer doses of 0.10-0.15mg/kg/d. In an analysis of 26 studies including 1173 children Hodson and Craig (2008) found that chlorambucil (RR 0.15, 95% CI 0.02–0.95) significantly reduced the relapse risk at 6–12 months compared with prednisone alone. There was no difference in relapse risk at two years between chlorambucil and cyclophosphamide (RR 1.31, 95% CI 0.80 to 2.13).

It is likely that oral daily chlorambucil has lower bladder toxicity and a higher risk for azoospermia and other severe adverse events than cyclophosphamide. In the meta-analysis of Latta et al. (2001) severe infections were more frequent in children treated with chlorambucil than in those treated with cyclophosphamide (6.8% versus 1.5%) and seizures occurred in 3.6% of patients given chlorambucil versus none with cylcophosphamide. To prevent disquieting side effects we suggest not to exceed a cumulative dosage of 10–20mg/kg with chlorambucil. The leukemogenic effect of chlorambucil is related to the cumulative dosage of the drug (see Chapter 2), but the risk with the doses usually employed in MCN should be low.

In summary, an 8-week course of chlorambucil is relatively safe. However, there is a substantial risk for azoospermia and the drug should be used with great caution in males with MCN. The daily dose should not exceed 0.2mg/kg. Probably a dose of 0.15mg/kg/d is equally effective and certainly less toxic. More prolonged or repeated courses should be discouraged as they entail an increased risk of long-term side effects. The same precautions in sexually active females pertain to chlorambucil use (Table 5.7).

Table 5.7 Alternative treatments to glucocorticoids/alkylating agents

Azathioprine:	Little experience
	No evidence of benefits
Mycophenolate salts:	No controlled trials available either with MMF or myfortic
	Good rate of response with MMF in non-controlled trials
	Side effects mild
	Proposed doses in adults: 2g/d until complete remission, tapered to 1g/d for 1–2 years (for mycophenolate sodium 1440mg/d tapered to 720mg)
Cyclosporine:	Controlled trials available
	High rate of remission
	Frequent relapses at discontinuation
	Dose-dependent adverse events (see Table 5.8)
	Proposed initial dosage with Neoral®: 100mg/m²/d in children, 4 mg/kg/d in adults
Tacrolimus:	Non-controlled trials available
	Good efficacy in small studies
	Frequent relapses at discontinuation
	Dose-dependent adverse events (nephrotoxicity, diabetes, neuro-logical complications)
	Proposed dosage: 0.1mg/kg
Levamisole:	Conflicting results with randomized trials (as effective as cyclophosphamide in some studies, ineffective in others)
	Frequent relapses in responders
	Adverse events: neutropenia, cutaneous lesions
	Proposed dosage: 2.5mg/kg three times a week
Rituximab:	Little experience
	Small series reported efficacy in preventing relapses
	Usually well tolerated
	Fever, chills with the first dose
	Little is known about long-term effects
	Proposed dosage: 375mg/m2 weekly for 4 weeks

Calcineurin inhibitors

Cyclosporine

The efficacy of cyclosporine (CsA) in reducing the risk of relapse in children with MCN was reported more than 20 years ago, and was confirmed by a large number of studies, including randomized controlled trials. A review found that overall 78% of adults and 85% of children with steroid-sensitive MCN achieved complete remission following CsA therapy. Remission of proteinuria usually developed within the first 3–4 months of treatment and was maintained with continued administration of CsA; however, relapse occurred when the drug dose was reduced or stopped (Ponticelli and Passerini 1999), a manifestion of 'CsA-dependency.'

Randomized controlled trials provided clear evidence of the efficacy of CsA in MCN. In a French study (Niaudet and the French Society of Pediatric Nephrology, 1992) 40 children were randomized to receive CsA (6mg/kg/d for 12 weeks then tapered off over a further 12 weeks) or chlorambucil (0.2mg/kg/d for 40 days). Excellent and comparable remission rates were achieved with both treatments but at drug withdrawal, the relapse rate was higher in children receiving CsA. The actuarial remission rate at two years was only 5% for CsA versus 45% for chlorambucil. Ponticelli et al. (1993a) randomly assigned 73 frequently relapsing or steroid-dependent patients, stratified for adults and children, to receive either cyclophosphamide (2.5mg/kg/d) for 8 weeks or the old formulation of CsA (5–6mg/kg/d in children) for 9 months, then tapered off within the year. At 9 months 64% of patients on cyclophosphamide and 74% of patients on CsA entered complete remission. However, after drug interruption many patients given CsA had relapses of nephrotic syndrome. At 2 years 25% of patients assigned to CsA versus 63% of patients assigned to cyclosphosphamide were still in remission. A German trial compared glucocorticoid monotherapy prednisone 60mg/m^2 per day for 6 weeks tapered to 40mg/m^2 for a further 6 weeks) with glucocorticoid/CsA combination therapy in children (prednisone as in the other arm plus CsA,150mg/m^2 per day, commenced upon remission of proteinuria and given for 8 weeks). Those assigned to glucocorticoid monotherapy had higher relapse rates during the first 18 months of follow-up than those receiving glucocorticoid/CsA; however, relapse rates in the two groups were virtually equal by 24 months of follow-up (Hoyer and Brodehl, 2006). A Japanese trial in children with frequently relapsing nephrotic syndrome, compared different CsA doses to maintain remission and found that targeting CsA to keep trough blood levels between 60–80ng/mL obtained more remissions and less relapses than a fixed dose of CsA of 2.5mg/kg/d; however blood levels <40ng/mL were not effective (Ishikura et al., 2008).

Table 5.8 List of the most frequent adverse reactions and side-effects requiring discontinuation of the drug in 661 patients treated with cyclosporine for various types of glomerular diseases[*]

Clinical adverse reactions		Side effects requiring discontinuation	
Hypertrichosis	18%	Renal dysfunction	3.7%
Gingival hyperplasia	16%	Infection	1.1%
Gastrointestinal symptoms	11%	Gastrointestinal symptoms	0.8%
Hypertension	9%	Malignancies	0.7%
Paresthesias	6%	Hypertension	0.6%
Tremor	4%	Cardiac infarct	0.2%
Headache	3%	Hypertrichosis	0.2%

[*]Data collected from the Collaborative study group of Sandimmun in nephrotic syndrome (1991). *Clinical Nephrology* **35**(Suppl.1): S48-60.

The rapid recurrence of nephrotic syndrome following cessation of CsA therapy led to the concept of 'cyclosporine-dependency,' and the prospect of indefinite patient exposure to a potentially nephrotoxic drug. However, some patients with a long duration of uninterrupted treatment (>12 months) followed by progressive and gradual tapering of drug dose may maintain remission even after interruption of CsA therapy. On the other hand, durable remission can also be maintained with quite low doses of CsA, ranging around 1–2mg/kg/d (Meyrier et al., 1994).

Hypertrichosis, gingival hyperplasia, and arterial hypertension are the most frequent side effects of CsA (Table 5.8). Hyperuricemia is rarely checked in children but is frequent in adults. These adverse events are mostly dose- dependent. With the CsA microemulsion (Neoral®, Novartis Basel) the doses used in MCN rarely exceed 100mg/m² in children and 4mg/kg in adults. With such a dosage side effects are mild and reversible. They may be further reduced by administering the drug in a single morning dose that proved to have the same efficacy and lower toxicity than the standard double daily administration (Chishti et al., 2001). If the above mentioned dosages are respected, CsA-related nephrotoxicity is rare and usually mild in patients with MCN. Meyrier et al. (1994) reported the results of repeat biopsy in 22 adults with MCN treated with CsA (not Neoral®) for a mean period of 19 months at a mean dose of 5.5mg/kg/d because of idiopathic nephrotic syndrome. Mild-to-moderate tubulo-interstitial lesions were observed only in the 7 patients in whom the second biopsy revealed a FSGS. Other studies confirmed that at the dosages usually employed, CsA does not cause nephrotoxicity in MCN. In children with MCN and SDNS, CsA given in mean for 5 years failed to manifest CsA toxicity at renal biopsy (Kranz et al., 2008). However, it is possible that a long duration of therapy may increase the risk for nephrotoxicity. A recent workshop suggested that it is prudent to perform regular renal biopsies in patients receiving long-term (i.e. >2 years) CsA therapy (Cattran et al., 2007).

In summary, CsA is effective and reasonably safe in maintaining remission in multi-relapsing or steroid-dependent patients, both adults and children. This agent can be considered as an alternative to glucocorticoids and alkylating agents for treating difficult-to-manage patients. When using CsA Neoral® we suggest doses no greater than 100mg/m^2/d in children or 4mg/kg/d in adults. At these dosages the drug is well tolerated and does not cause severe renal damage. The main disadvantage is represented by the need for prolonged treatment. It is likely that many responders can maintain remission also with low doses (around 2mg/kg/d in adults and less than 100mg/m^2/d in children), which reduces further the risks of renal toxicity and of other side effects. Some patients may maintain remission after stopping CsA, provided that treatment was prolonged for 2 years or more. Monitoring the blood levels of CsA may be useful to check the compliance to treatment and to prevent over- or under-dosage.

Tacrolimus

Some small-sized non-randomized studies reported that tacrolimus (TAC) either given alone or associated with small doses of prednisone may obtain a quick remission of the nephrotic syndrome and maintain remission when given as mono-therapy in MCN. However, steroid resistant patients usually did not respond to TAC and, like CsA, relapses were frequent after interruption of TAC, even when the doses were lowered gradually. The results seem to be particularly good in Asian patients. A high rate of complete remission (85%) has been reported in 22 Indian children (nine with MCN) with SRNS treated with TAC for a mean period of 290 days (Gulati et al., 2008). A small prospective study in 26 Chinese adult patients with SDNS, TAC given for 6 months at doses able to keep blood levels between 4–8ng/mL was compared with cyclophosphamide pulses (Li et al., 2008). All patients also received prednisone; 91% of patients achieved complete remission in the TAC group, versus 77% in the cyclophosphamide group. During a follow-up of 23 months, remission was maintained in 60% and 50% of cases respectively.

In patients with MCN TAC may be given at doses of 0.1mg/kg/d that may be gradually tapered in responders. The risk of nephrotoxicity is presumably low at these dosages, but serum creatinine levels should be regularly checked. The side effects of TAC are similar to those observed with CsA, however glucose intolerance is more frequent with TAC. Gingival hyperplasia and hypertrichosis do not occur with TAC but a few patients may develop alopecia.

TAC alone (monotherapy) may be as effective as when it is combined with steroids, but this is not well established and any differences observed could be due to differing plasma TAC levels. It is not known if regular monitoring of plasma trough or peak TAC levels is needed to provide optimum results in terms of safety and/or efficacy, but such assays would considerably increase the overall cost of such treatment.

Inhibitors of purine synthesis

Azathioprine

It is difficult to assess the role of oral azathioprine in patients with MCN. From the few available observational and controlled studies performed one might conclude that short-term treatment of MCN with azathioprine is of little benefit while long-term administration may obtain remission in at least some patients. Differentiating spontaneous from treatment-induced remissions is difficult from the available literature. However, although azathioprine is generally considered to be less oncogenic than alkylating agents, a treatment prolonged for 4 years or more is not completely devoid of neoplastic risk (see Chapter 2). While waiting for further definitive information it is probably better to reserve the long-term use of azathioprine as adjunctive therapy for the very few patients who do not respond to more conventional treatments.

Mycophenolic acid derivatives

A number of non controlled studies conducted on few patients followed for a short period indicated that mycophenolate mofetil (MMF) may be of benefit in the treatment of patients with steroid-sensitive or steroid-dependent MCN (Sepe et al., 2008). In severe steroid-dependent cases, MMF 30mg/kg/d for 2 years associated with low tapering doses of prednisone were effective as steroid-sparing agent, with prednisone dose reduction from 0.7 to 0.3mg/kg/d (Bagga et al., 2003). The frequency of relapses was significantly reduced from 6.6 to 2 each year. Side effects were usually mild and mostly gastrointestinal in nature but some severe infections such as varicella and herpes zoster were reported. Unfortunately, the doses used and the duration of treatment were variable in the few studies available and no randomized trials have yet been conducted. With these limitations in mind, oral MMF may be considered as a useful adjunctive therapy in difficult patients with frequently-relapsing MCN who have developed steroid toxicity and who refuse treatment with cyclophosphamide or chlorambucil (on account of fears of side effects) or who have some contraindication for their use (such as a history of bladder cancer or prior herpes zoster). We suggest to start with a daily dose of 30mg/kg/d in children (2g in adults) to be kept until complete remission is obtained followed by 20–25mg/kg/d (1.5g in adults) for 2 months and then 15mg/kg/d (1g in adults). Treatment may be continued for more than 2 years if well tolerated. MMF withdrawal after 1–2 years of treatment was followed by relapse in 68% of the cases. Enteric coated sodium mycophenolate may also be used, but less data is available on efficacy and safety.

No data is yet available, on the utility of monitoring of the plasma level of mycophenolic acid for optimizing efficacy and safety of MMF or mycophenolate sodium therapy of MCN.

Miscellaneous

Levamisole

A number of studies reported that oral levamisole at doses ranging from 2.5mg/kg twice weekly to 2.5mg/kg per day allows complete or partial steroid-sparing in many children with frequently relapsing MCN, although this beneficial effect disappeared when the drug was stopped. Randomized trials gave different results, from no difference in duration of remission between patients assigned to receive levamisole and those assigned to placebo (Dayal et al., 1994) to efficacy similar to cyclophosphamide in preventing relapses in steroid dependent nephrotic syndrome (Donia et al., 2005). A systematic review of the available controlled trials found that levamisole was more effective than steroids alone (RR 0.43, 95% CI 0.27–0.68) in reducing the risk of relapses at 6 and 12 months, but the effects were not sustained once treatment was stopped (Hodson et al., 2008).

The clinical impression is that the drug may be helpful in milder cases of MCN. It is possible that higher doses and more prolonged courses might obtain better results but there are no solid data supporting this hypothesis. The drug is usually well tolerated, with the exception of neutropenia and of cutaneous lesions which may occur in some patients. The clinical interest with this drug is vanishing as it is not commercially available any more in many Western countries.

Rituximab

Francois et al. (2007) reported a young adult with multi-relapsing MCN who eventually entered a prolonged remission after rituximab in 4 weekly doses of 375mg/m². Since then, an increasing number of anecdotal reports pointed out the successful use of rituximab on steroid-dependent and frequently relapsing MCN, suggesting the possibility that this drug might replace Cyclophosphamide and CsA in SDNS (Dotsch et al, 2008); however, a report bias to publish only favorable results has to be considered.

In a multicenter series 22 patients, aged 6–22 years with severe SDNS or SRNS but CsA-sensitive, were treated with 2–4 infusions of rituximab. Seven patients were nephrotic at the time of treatment, and three went into remission. Peripheral B cells were depleted in all subjects. Immunosuppressive treatments could be withdrawn in nineteen patients (85%), with no relapse of proteinuria. Rituximab was effective in all patients when administered during a proteinuria-free period in association with other immunosuppressive agents. When relapses occurred, they were always associated with an increase in CD19 cell count. Adverse effects were observed in 45% of cases, but most of them were mild and transient (Guigonis et al., 2008). Although the mechanism of action of rituximab in MCN is still a matter of speculation, the most likely explanation is that B cells may play an important role in MCN, possibly by regulating T-cell function. No randomized trials of rituximab in MCN have yet been reported. Waiting for the results of ongoing randomized trials in France and in Italy, cost and acute adverse events of rituximab are to be considered, and its long-term efficacy and safety have still to be evaluated.

Quinolones

Anecdotal reports pointed out that pefloxacin was effective in both steroid-dependent and steroid-resistant patients. However, disappointing results and a high rate of tendon complications were reported by other reports (Meyrier and Niaudet, 2005)

Treatment of steroid-resistant minimal change nephropathy

Some 10% of all patients with an initial histological diagnosis of MCN (about 5–7% of children and 10–12% of adults) do not respond to glucocorticoids given in conventional dosages as outlined above. In children in this condition, methylprednisolone pulses (10–30mg/kg) on alternate days for 2 weeks and then at reduced frequency, but with pulses maintained for 2 years, have been proposed by Mendoza et al. (1990) with up to 75% of remissions; however, the side effects of this protocol are very high and it is used in a minority of cases.

The clinical impression is that in these patients the adjunctive use of oral cyclophosphamide does not show any important benefit. Most of these cases had FSGS on further renal biopsies. In a few studies good results have been reported in such patients using intravenous infusions of cyclophosphamide at a dose of 500mg/m^2 given every month for 6 months. Remission was obtained, but the possible side effects do not favor this schedule.

Discordant results have been reported with CsA in uncontrolled studies. Some investigators reported a good rate of remission, particularly when CsA was associated with intravenous methylprednisolone pulse therapy, while other studies could not find any benefit with CsA either alone or associated with glucocorticoids. In an Italian controlled trial, nephrotic patients (with either MCN or FSGS) who did not respond to a 6-week course of prednisone were randomly assigned to be, given CsA (5mg/kg/d for adults and 6mg/kg/d for children) for 6 months then tapered off by 25% every 2 months until complete discontinuation (Ponticelli et al., 1993b). Of the treated patients 32% entered complete remission and 27% partial remission versus a 16% partial remission rate in untreated controls (see also Chapter 4). Good results have been reported by Niaudet et al. (1994) in steroid-resistant children with a histological picture of MCN. Patients were given CsA (150mg/m^2/d) plus prednisone (30mg/m^2/d tapered to alternate-day administration) for 6 months. Of 45 children, 21 (47%) entered complete remission and two (4%) had partial remission for an overall remission rate of 51%. More recently, Plank et al. (2008) reported the results of a controlled multicenter randomized open label trial comparing CsA versus cyclophosphamide pulses in the initial therapy of children with newly diag-nosed idiopathic SRNS. Patients were randomized either to receive CSA at doses able to achieve trough levels of 120–180ng/mL, or intravenous cycophos-phamide pulses at a dose of 500mg/m^2 per month. All patients were on alter-nate prednisone therapy. At week 12, 60% of the CsA patients showed at least partial remission. In contrast, 17% only of patients receiving cyclophosph-amide responded (p <0.05) and the study was stopped. After 24 weeks, complete remission was not significantly different in the two groups.

Good results have also been reported with TAC in children. In a prospective but uncontrolled study, nine consecutive children with steroid-resistant MCN were examined. TAC was initiated with a dose of 0.10mg/kg/d, and the dose was increased to attain a trough level of 5.0–10.0mcg/L. These patients were treated with concomitant prednisone, which was subsequently tapered off and stopped. Complete remission was seen in eight children (89%), two (22%) within 2 months (Gulati et al., 2008). Small numbers of cases of remission in patients with MCN resistant to glucocorticoids with the use of MMF have also been reported (Mendizábal et al., 2005).

In summary, the results of treatment in the uncommonly seen steroid-resistant nephrotic patients with MCN are often disappointing but variable. The difference may be accounted for by the fact that some few series consid-ered only patients who maintained a histological picture of MCN while most other papers also included patients who developed FSGS later. It is also possi-ble that the diagnosis of MCN was incorrect in the patients included as steroid-resistant, most likely due to the under-diagnosis of FSGS from a 'sampling error' in the original diagnostic renal biopsy. Moreover, the definition of steroid-resistance varied considerably in the different studies, introducing another bias which makes it difficult to assess the effects of treatment. Finally, even when the same drug was used, the doses and durations of treatment varied considerably. For all these reasons a reappraisal of the overall effectiveness of any form of treatment in so-called steroid-resistant patients with MCN is impossible at present. The use of angiotensin converting enzyme inhibitors and angiotensin receptor blockers is recommended as these drugs not only allow reducing proteinuria but may also be protective on renal function. Statins are also recommended not only to lower lipid levels but also because they may have a protective role against cardiovascular disease and may even reduce proteinuria (see Chapter 1).

Practical recommendations

Although MCN is idiopathic in the large majority of cases, a careful medical history is important to exclude the few cases secondary to drug exposure or to other diseases. An underlying lymphoma should be suspected in patients with adenopathy, fever, sweating, and/or pruritus.

Idiopathic MCN may develop a spontaneous remission but it usually takes a long time (months or years), thus exposing the patient to the undesirable and potentially dangerous effects of an untreated nephrotic state. A simple measure which may be effective in a few children is search and elimination of allergens (cows' milk) in those with a strong history of allergies. However, most patients will remain nephrotic. In the face of the potential risks of prolonged, full-blown nephrotic syndrome, we are in favor of an aggressive approach, the main reasons for which have been summarized by Glassock (1993):

- Prolonged heavy proteinuria may result, of itself, in irreversible glomerular lesions.
- Hyperlipidemia, hyperfibrinogenemia and serum protein deficiencies have undesirable and potentially harmful effects (such as favoring thrombosis or atherogenesis.)
- The side effects of aggressive therapy are minimal, controllable, and reversible when the treatment is brief and the dosage not excessive.

While in favor of aggressive treatment not only in children but also in older patients with nephrotic syndrome, we recommend a 'wait-and-see' policy for the few patients with symptomless proteinuria, unless they develop full nephrotic syndrome.

Initial treatment

Since the duration of initial treatment influences the rate of subsequent relapses, we suggest prolonged administration of glucocorticoids as a first approach. It is also advisable to taper off the glucocorticoids gradually, in order to prevent a 'rebound' effect which may precipitate relapses.

In *children*, we start with 60mg/m²/d (or 2mg/kg/d) of prednisone (or equivalent doses of another analogue) as a single dose given between 8–10 a.m. for 4 weeks, prolonged, in cases of no remission, for 2 additional weeks. Then the child is switched to alternate-day prednisone, 40mg/m² or 2mg/kg/d every 48h, for at least 8 weeks, with subsequent tapering off of prednisone by 5–10mg/m² (0.5mg/kg) per 48h every 2 weeks. We conscientiously avoid the rapid discontinuance of steroid therapy as it may precipitate a relapse. Alternate-day administration of the dosage may be preferred since it may reduce the severity of side effects of more prolonged therapy.

We treat *adults* with prednisone, 1mg/kg/d as a single dose between 8–10 a.m. There is no objection to initiating therapy with alternate day regimen of 2mg/kg every other day (maximum dosage 150mg every other day), although there is no evidence that this regimen actually reduces the risk of side effects in comparison with daily treatment in adults (Waldman et al., 2007). Initial treatment is given for at least 6 weeks or until complete remission. In case of early response with disappearance of proteinuria, we continue prednisone at a dose of 1.6mg/kg every 48h, and reduce the dose by 0.2 to 0.4mg/kg per 48h every fortnight until complete discontinuation. In case of poor response, we continue the initial treatment for at least 6–8 weeks. Then, we switch the patient to alternate-day prednisone, 1.6mg/kg/48h. If there is no remission after 3–4 months of therapy, we give alternate day prednisone in decreasing doses for a total of (6–8months if tolerated) before considering an adult steroid-resistant. In patients older than 65, who are at major risk for iatrogenic side effects and are less prone to relapses, we taper off the prednisone more rapidly. This schedule is not rigid, but is tailored to an individual patient's needs. We reduce the glucocorticoid doses or stop treatment earlier if any sign of severe hypercorticism or any steroid-related complication occurs. In both children and adults we administer prednisone in a single morning dose, between 8–10 a.m. or 7–9 a.m. which is better, in order to reduce the side effects (see also Chapter 2).

For patients who may have contraindications to high-dose prednisone (i.e., diabetes mellitus, massive obesity, overt cardiovascular disease, severe dyslipidemia, peripheral obliterative vascular disease, psychiatric disorders, osteoporosis, etc.) we start treatment with cyclophosphamide, 2mg/kg/d for 8–12 weeks, or chlorambucil, 0.15mg/kg/d, for 8 weeks. Such an approach may be effective in adults and in elderly patients (Nolasco et al., 1986). The white blood cell count must be checked every 2 or 3 weeks. If it is <5000/mm³ the dosage of either cyclophosphamide or chlorambucil is reduced by 50%. If the white blood cell count is <3000/mm³ the drug is temporarily withdrawn. Usually lymphopenia precedes total leukopenia, so a differential count is useful.

Alternatively to cytotoxic drugs, CsA or TAC may be used for *primary* therapy of MCN in older adults at high risk of complications from steroids or alkylating agents or in patients who refuse cytotoxic agents, being concerned about their adverse effects..

Relapses may be triggered by infectious episodes and sometimes spontaneously remit after infection has been treated and cured. Whether to treat the relapse immediately in order to prevent the complications of a full nephrotic syndrome, or whether to wait for a spontaneous remission in order to avoid unnecessary glucocorticoid administration, is debatable. We prefer to wait for 7–10d before starting prednisone, but if severe proteinuria with intractable edema is present or appears we start treatment earlier. The standard therapy consists of $60mg/m^2$ (or 2mg/kg) per day for children and of 1mg/kg/d for adults. This dosage is given until the urine is protein free for 3 consecutive days. Then we give prednisone every other day for 4 weeks, at a dose of $40mg/m^2/48h$ for children and of 0.75mg/kg/48h for adults. The maximum duration of prednisone for patients who do not respond early is similar to that of the first episode.

Frequently relapsing and steroid-dependent patients

These patients can be maintained in remission with glucocorticoids in varying dosage but prolonged treatment may expose them to disabling and even life-threatening complications of steroid-related toxicity (exogenous Cushing syndrome). A few steroid non-responders can be kept in remission with relatively low doses of prednisone, but for those patients who need high-dose prednisone (i.e. >0.4mg/kg/d) to maintain remission we feel justified in administering a short course of an alkylating agent, which is usually well tolerated and can obtain a sustained remission in a number of patients.

In young males we give oral cyclophosphamide, at a dose not exceeding 2mg/kg/d, because this agent is probably less gonadotoxic than chlorambucil. In older males and in females (the ovary is less prone to the toxic effects of alkylating agents) we give chlorambucil, at a dose of 0.15mg/kg/d, mainly because this drug is less toxic to the bladder.

Since the duration of treatment influences the response, we are now in favor of extending cytotoxic therapy in all patients in whom it is used up to 12 weeks, not only in steroid-dependent patients but also in frequently relapsing patients. With a daily dose of 2mg/kg, the cumulative dosage of cyclophosphamide is 168mg/kg, which is below the estimated threshold of gonadal toxicity in males (200–250mg/kg). The cumulative dose of chlorambucil with daily dose of 0.15mg/kg would be 12.6mg/kg, an amount which could result in azoospermia in a few male patients, since the estimated threshold of testicular toxicity is

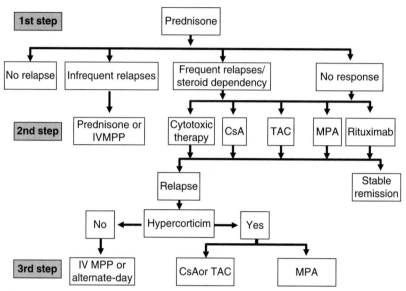

Fig. 5.1 Suggested therapeutic approach for patients with MCN. MPA: mycophenolic acid derivates; MPP: methylprednisolone pulses; CsA: cyclosporine; TAC: tacrolimus; MPA: mycophenolic acid.

between 10–20mg/kg. Thus when using chlorambucil it is safer to limit the period of treatment to 8 weeks.

If the nephrotic syndrome relapses, in our opinion the patient should not be treated again with alkylating agents, since their toxicity is cumulative. If the patient has no sign of hypercorticism he/she can be treated with glucocorticoids again (Fig. 5.1). However, instead of high-dose oral prednisone we prefer to administer three pulses of intravenous methylprednisolone (10–15mg/kg each) followed by prednisone, 0.5mg/kg/d until remission. This schedule exposes the patient, in fact, to fewer side effects than high-dose prednisone (Imbasciati et al., 1985). After remission, we continue prednisone 0.5mg/kg/d for 2–4 weeks and then switch to alternate-day prednisone (1mg/kg/48h). We reduce the dose by 0.1mg/kg/48h trying to identify the minimal effective dose. In our experience, a few patients maintained remission with doses as low as 0.3–0.4mg/kg/48h, having a relapse when the dosage was further lowered. Clearly at these dosages prolonged glucocorticoid therapy usually does not pose any particular problem. Other patients tolerate well repeat administrations of intravenous methylprednisolone pulses followed by alternate-day prednisone.

However, a number of patients develop signs of hypercorticism and others, psychologically depressed by the frequent relapses, ask for a 'more powerful' drug. After obtaining remission with corticosteroids we give cyclosporine Neoral® to these patients, at a dose of 100–125mg/m²/d in children <6 years of age; 100mg/m²/d for children between 6–16 years; and 4mg/kg/d for patients >16 years. We check through whole-blood levels after 2–4 weeks initially and then every 2–3 months both to verify the compliance of the patient and to keep blood levels below an arbitrary threshold of 120ng/mL, as assessed by the monoclonal assay or with the HPLC method. If the patient remains in remission, CsA may be reduced after 6–12 months by 25% every 2 months, to determine the minimal effective dose. If a patient maintains remission with CsA doses of 2–3mg/kg/d or less, therapy may be continued for years with low risk of side effects. However, these patients should be regularly monitored and some authorities recommend they receive a renal biopsy every 2– years to check for histological evidence of nephrotoxicity (Cattran et al., 2007). In the other cases, we prefer to stop CsA gradually after 2 years. A few patients may maintain remission without any therapy. In the other cases alternative drugs (including glucocorticoids, mycophenolic acid, or alkylating cytotoxic agents if not already used) may be rotated.

If the patient relapses, we treat her/him again with glucocorticoids for 6–12 months and then again with CsA for a further 1–2 years, in order to prevent the potential toxicity of prolonged administration of either drug. Before beginning a second course of CsA we advise the patient of her/his relatives about the utility of a renal biopsy which may detect the presence of CsA-related lesions. For those patients who develop hypertrichosis CsA may be replaced by TAC. Rituximab should be reserved to those patients who show intolerance to other treatments. On the basis of the little experience with this drug it is better first to induce remission with glucocorticoids and then administer rituximab in order to maintain a stable remission.

Steroid resistant patients

Patients with a histologic 'diagnosis' of MCN who do not respond to a sufficiently prolonged course of high-dose glucocorticoids (orally and/or intravenously), as described above, almost always show, sooner or later, focal and segmental glomerulosclerosis in a more careful examination of the original renal biopsy or upon a repeat renal biopsy and should be treated accordingly (see Chapter 6). In the very few cases showing only minimal abnormalities at the initial or repeat renal biopsy an attempt at therapy with CsA, TAC, mycophenolic acid, or rituximab may be tried. Repeat renal biopsies are almost never indicated in patients who display an initial pathological diagnosis of MCN and who pursue a glucocorticoid treatment-responsive, though relapsing course. Even if a lesion of FSGS were to be discovered in such repeat biopsies, the course of treatment recommended would not be altered as a result of this finding.

Transplantation

Occasional cases of 'de novo' MCN in renal transplants meeting strict clinical-pathologic criteria for this diagnosis have been reported. Nephrotic syndrome is the usual presentation (Zafarmand et al., 2002) but reversible acute renal failure may also occur. The disease develops early after transplantation, usually within 4 months. Steroids, ACE-inhibitors and angiotensin receptor blockers have been used. A sustained remission of proteinuria can be achieved in most cases within a year, but some patients may enter remission after 3 or more years (Zafarmand et al., 2002). Rarely, MCN may recur in the transplanted kidney (in a patient with MCN as the original disease leading to ESRD), but because typical MCN so rarely produces ESRD, the opportunity to observe such a recurrence is exceedingly uncommon.

References

Audard V, Larousserie F, Grimbert P, et al. (2006). Minimal change nephrotic syndrome and classical Hodgkin's lymphoma: report of 21 cases and review of the literature. *Kidney International* **69**:2251–60.

Bagga A, Hari P, Moudgil A, Jordan SC (2003). Mycophenolate mofetil and prednisolone therapy in children with steroid-dependent nephrotic syndrome. *American Journal of Kidney Diseases* **42**:1114–20.

Bakker WW, van Dael CM, Pierik LJ, et al. (2005). Altered activity of plasma hemopexin in patients with minimal change disease in relapse. *Pediatric Nephrology* **20**:1410–5.

Bouissou F, Meissner I, Konrad M, et al. (1995). Clinical implications from studies of HLA antigens in idiopathic nephrotic syndrome in children. *Clinical Nephrology* **44**:279–83.

Brodehl J (1991). Conventional therapy for idiopathic nephrotic syndrome in children. *Clinical Nephrology* **35**(Suppl.1):S8–15.

Cattran DC, Alexopoulos E, Heering P, et al. (2007). Cyclosporin in idiopathic glomerular disease associated with the nephrotic syndrome: Workshop recommendations. *Kidney International* **72**:1429–47.

Chishti AS, Sorof JM, Brewer ED, Kale AS (2001). Long-term treatment of focal segmental glomerulosclerosis in children with cyclosporine given as a single daily dose. *American Journal of Kidney Diseases* **38**:754–60.

Dayal U, Dayal AK, Shastry JCM, and Raghupathy P (1994). Use of levamisole in maintaining remission in steroid-sensitive nephrotic syndrome in children. *Nephron* **66**:408–12.

Donia AF, Ammar HM, El-Agroudy Ael-B, Moustafa Fel-H, Sobh MA (2005). Long-term results of two unconventional agents in steroid-dependent nephrotic children. *Pediatric Nephrology* **20**:1420–5.

Dotsch J, Muller-Wiefel DE, Kemper M (2008). Rituxibam: is replacement of cyclophos-phamide and calcineurin inhibitors in steroid-dependent nephrotic syndrome possible? *Pediatric Nephrology* **23**:3–7.

François H, Daugas E, Bensman A, Ronco P (2007).Unexpected efficacy of rituximab in multirelapsing minimal change nephrotic syndrome in the adult: first case report and pathophysiological considerations. *American Journal of Kidney Diseases* **49**:158–61.

Glassock RJ (1993). Therapy of idiopathic nephrotic syndrome in adults. A conservative or aggressive therapeutic approach? *American Journal Nephrology* **13**:422–8.

Glassock RJ (2003). Secondary minimal change disease. *Nephrology Dialysis Transplantation* **18**(Suppl.6):S52–8.

Guigonis V, Dallocchio A, Baudouin V, et al. (2008). Rituximab treatment for severe steroid- or cyclosporine-dependent nephrotic syndrome: a multicentric series of 22 cases. *Pediatric Nephrology* **23**:1269–79.

Gulati S, Prasad N, Sharma RK, Kumar A, Gupta A, Baburaj VP (2008). Tacrolimus: A New Therapy for Steroid-Resistant Nephrotic Syndrome in Children. *Nephrology Dialysis Transplantation* **23**:910–13.

Hodson EM, Craig JC (2008). Therapies for steroid-resistant nephrotic syndrome. *Pediatric Nephrology* **23**:1391–4.

Hodson EM, Knight JF, Willis NS, Craig JC (2001). Management of the initial episode of steroid-responsive nephrotic syndrome. *Pediatric Nephrology* **16**:526–7.

Hodson EM, Willis NS, Craig JC (2008). Non-corticosteroid treatment for nephrotic syndrome in children. *Cochrane Database Systemic Review* **23**(1):CD00229.

Hoyer PF, Brodehl J (2006). Initial treatment of idiopathic nephrotic syndrome in children: prednisone versus prednisone plus cyclosporine A: a prospective, randomized trial. *Journal American Society Nephrology* **17**:1151–7.

Imbasciati, E., Gusmano R, Edefonti A, et al. (1985). Controlled trial of methylprednisolo-ne pulses and low dose oral prednisone for minimal change nephrotic syndrome. *British Medical Journal* **291**:1305–8.

Ishikura K, Ikeda M, Hattori S, et al. (2008). Effective and safe treatment with cyclosporine in nephrotic children: a prospective, randomized multicenter trial. *Kidney International* **73**:1167–73.

ISKDC (International study of kidney diseases in children) (1984). Minimal change nephrotic syndrome in children: deaths during the first 5 to 15 years of observation. *Pediatrics* **73**:497–501.

Kim JS, Bellew CA, Silverstein DM, Aviles DH, Boineau FG, Vehaskari VM (2006). High incidence of initial and late steroid resistance in childhood nephrotic syndrome. *Kidney International* **68**:1275–81.

Korbet S, Schwartz MM, Lewis EJ (1988). Minimal-change glomerulopathy of adulthood. *American Journal of Nephrology* **8**:291–7.

Kranz B, Vester U, Büscher R, Wingen AM, Hoyer PF (2008).Cyclosporine-A-induced nephrotoxicity in children with minimal-change nephrotic syndrome: long-term treat-ment up to 10 years. *Pediatric Nephrology* **23**:581–6.

Krasowska-Kwiecień A, Sancewicz-Pach K, Moczulska A (2006). Idiopathic nephrotic syn-drome in Polish children–its variants and associations with HLA. *Pediatric Nephrology* **21**:1837–46.

Lahdenkari AT, Suvanto M, Kajantie E, Koskimies O, Kestilä M, Jalanko H (2005). Clinical features and outcome of childhood minimal change nephrotic syndrome: is genetics involved? *Pediatric Nephrology* **20**:1073–80.

Lai KW, Wei CL, Tan LK, et al. (2007). Overexpression of interleukin-13 induces minimal-change-like nephropathy in rats. *Journal American Society Nephrology* **18**:1476–85.

Latta K, von Schnakenburg C, Ehrich JH (2001). A meta-analysis of cytotoxic treatment for frequently relapsing nephrotic syndrome in children. *Pediatric Nephrology* **16**:271–82.

Li X, Li H, Chen J, et al. (2008).Tacrolimus as a steroid-sparing agent for adults with steroid-dependent minimal change nephrotic syndrome. *Nephrology Dialysis Transplantation* **23**:1919–25.

Lorca E, Ponticelli C (1995). Idiopathic nephrotic syndrome in the elderly. *Geriatric Nephrology and Urology* **4**:189–95.

Mathieson PW (2007). Minimal change nephropathy and focal segmental glomerulosclerosis. *Seminars Immunopathology* **29**:415–26.

Mendizábal S, Zamora I, Berbel O, Sanahuja MJ, Fuentes J, Simon J (2005). Mycophenolate mofetil in steroid/cyclosporine-dependent/resistant nephrotic syndrome. *Pediatric Nephrology* **20**:914–19.

Mendoza SA, Reznik VM, Griswold WR, Krensky AM, Yorgin PD, Tune BM (1990). Treatment of steroid-resistant focal segmental glomerulosclerosis with pulse methyl-prednisolone and alkylating agents. *Pediatric Nephrology* **4**:303–7.

Meyrier A, Niaudet P (2005). Minimal change and focal-segmental glomerular sclerosis. In Davison A, Cameron JS, Grunfeld JP, et al. (eds) *Oxford Textbook of Clinical Nephrology*, 3 vol, pp.439-468, Oxford University Press, Oxford.

Meyrier A, Noel H, Auriche P, Callard P, Collaborative group of the Société de Néphrologie (1994). Long-term renal tolerance of cyclosporin A treatment in adult idiopathic nephrotic syndrome. *Kidney International* **45**:1446–56.

Nakayama M, Katafuchi R, Yanase T, Ikeda K, Tanaka H, Fujimi S (2002). Steroid responsiveness and frequency of relapse in adult-onset minimal change nephrotic syndrome. *American Journal of Kidney Disease* **39**:503–12.

Niaudet P, French Society of Pediatric Nephrology (1992). Comparison of cyclosporin and chlorambucil in the treatment of steroid-dependent idiopathic nephrotic syndrome: a multicentre randomized controlled trial. *Pediatric Nephrology* **6**:1–3.

Niaudet P, French Society of Pediatric Nephrology (1994). Treatment of childhood steroid-resistant idiopathic nephrosis with a combination of cyclosporine and prednisone. *Journal of Pediatrics* **125**:981–6.

Nolasco F, Cameron JS, Heywood EF, HicksJ, Ogg CS, Williams DG (1986). Adult-onset minimal change nephrotic syndrome: a long-term follow-up. *Kidney International* **29**:1215–23.

Palmer SC, Nand K, Strippoli GF (2008). Interventions for minimal change disease in adults with nephrotic syndrome. *Cochrane Database Systemic Review* **23**(1):CD001537.

Plank C, Kalb V, Hinkes B, et al. (2008). Cyclosporin A is superior to cyclophosphamide in children with steroid-resistant nephrotic syndrome-a randomized controlled multicentre trial by the Arbeitsgemeinschaft für Pädiatrische Nephrologie. *Pediatric Nephrology* **23**:1483–93.

Ponticelli C, Passerini P (1999). The place of cyclosporin in the management of primary nephrotic syndrome. *BioDrugs* **12**:327–41.

Ponticelli C, Edefonti A, Ghio L, et al. (1993a). Cyclosporin versus cyclophosphamide for patients with steroid-dependent and frequently relapsing idiopathic nephrotic syndrome: a multicentre randomized controlled trial. *Nephrology, Dialysis and Transplantation* **8**:1326–32.

Ponticelli, C, Rizzoni G, Edefonti A, et al. (1993b). A randomized trial of cyclosporine in steroid-resistant idiopathic nephrotic syndrome. *Kidney International* **43**:1377–84.

Ritz E, Rambausek M, Hasslacher C, Mann J, (1989). Pathogenesis of hypertension in glomerular disease. *American Journal of Nephrology* **9**(Suppl. 1):89–90.

Rostand SG, Cross SK, Kirk KA, Lee JY, Kuhlmann A, Amann K (2005). Racial differences in renal arteriolar structure in children with minimal change nephropathy. *Kidney International* **68**:1154–60.

Russo LM, Sandoval RM, McKee, et al. (2007). The normal kidney filters nephrotic levels of albumin retrieved by proximal tubule cells: retrieval is disrupted in nephrotic states. *Kidney International* **71**:504–13.

Schena P, Cameron JS (1988). Treatment of proteinuric idiopathic glomerulo-nephritides in adults: a retrospective study. *American Journal of Medicine* **85**:315–26.

Sepe V, Libetta C, Giuliano MG, Adamo G, Dal Canton A (2008). Mycophenolate mofetil in primary glomerulopathies. *Kidney International* **73**:154–62.

Shilliday IR, Simpson K, Jackson R, McLay AL, Boulton-Jones M (1993). Minimal change nephropathy in the West of Scotland: a review of sixty-four patients. *Scottish Medical Journal* **38**:70–2.

Stokes MB, Markowitz GS, Lin J, Valeri AM, D'Agati VD (2004). Glomerular tip lesion: a distinct entity within the minimal change disease/focal segmental glomerulosclerosis spectrum. *Kidney International* **65**:1690–702.

Trompeter RS, Evans PR, Barratt TM (1981). Gonadal function in boys with steroid responsive nephrotic syndrome treated with cyclophosphamide for short periods. *Lancet* **i**:1177–80.

Tryggvason K, Patrakka J, Wartiovaara J (2006). Hereditary proteinuria syndromes and mechanisms of proteinuria. *New England Journal Medicine* **354**:1387–401.

Tse KC, Lam MF, Yip PS, et al. (2003). Idiopathic minimal change nephrotic syndrome in older adults: steroid responsiveness and pattern of relapses. *Nephrology Dialysis Transplantation* **18**:1316–20.

Waldman M, Crew RJ, Valeri A, et al. (2007). Adult minimal-change disease: clinical characteristics, treatment, and outcomes. *Clinical Journal American Society Nephrology* **2**:445–53.

Zafarmand AA, Baranowska-Daca E, Ly PC, et al. (2002). De novo minimal change disease associated with reversible post-transplant nephrotic syndrome. A report of five cases and review of the literature. *Clinical Transplantation* **16**:350–61.

Chapter 6

Focal and segmental glomerular sclerosis

Francesco Scolari and Claudio Ponticelli

Introduction and overview

Definition

Focal and segmental glomerular sclerosis (FSGS) is a glomerular lesion which is associated with distinctive clinical features. Because it may be pathogenetically heterogeneous, it is not yet appropriate to call it a *disease*, yet its discovery in a renal biopsy in a patient with the nephrotic syndrome does have important connotations with respect to response to treatment and to long-term outcome. By light microscopy the characteristic finding is segmental areas of sclerosis (and hyalinosis) involving only some glomeruli. Patients with the FSGS lesion typically have proteinuria which is usually in the nephrotic range (>3.5g/d in an adult), accompanied by the typical constellation of signs and symptoms of the nephrotic syndrome and arterial hypertension. A minority of patients may have only asymptomatic proteinuria and these patients usually do not progress to end-stage renal disease (ESRD) but the natural course of FSGS is ominous in most patients with nephrotic syndrome. However, numerous observational studies have shown that about 50–70% of patients may respond completely or partially to prolonged glucocorticoid therapy or other 'immunosuppressive' treatments and thus have a fair outcome in the long term.

Pathology

At light microscopy the lesions of FSGS initially affect only a few glomeruli and are characterized by sclerosis (collapse and solidification) limited to a portion of the glomerulus, either at hilum or at the tip of the tuft, or at both levels. In the classic form, most often observed, the sclerotic lesions are randomly distributed among the capillary loops. Glomeruli unaffected by sclerosis may appear quite normal by light microscopy. The percentage of glomeruli affected is quite variable, but juxta-medullary glomeruli may be preferentially affected at least initially. If only small numbers of glomeruli are affected with the sclerosing lesion, the process of focal sclerosis may go undetected, particularly when the number of glomeruli in the specimen is small (e.g., <10 glomeruli), and the biopsy sample contains only superficial glomeruli. Immunofluorescence studies may be negative but IgM and C3 deposits are commonly found in the areas of sclerosis. On electron microscopy there is diffuse effacement of the foot processes of podocytes and no or only scanty electron dense deposits in the mesangium. In the primary form of FSGS the foot process effacement is diffuse and generalized, affecting even those glomeruli which are not affected by a sclerosing lesion. In secondary forms of FSGS, such as those occurring in oligonephronic states, the foot process effacement is less noticeable, and usually affects <50% of the glomerular capillary surface area. Frequently the podocyte will show features of vacuolization, degeneration, hypertrophy, and detachment for the underlying glomerular basement membrane (GBM). Special studies, of a research nature, will demonstrate that the podocyte has undergone de-differentiation to a more primitive state and has lost many cell-surface antigens characteristic of the differentiated state (e.g., podocalyxin, synaptopodin). Such de-differentiation of podocytes does not usually occur in the lesion of minimal change nephropathy (MCN). Thus, electron microcopy is a very important part of the evaluation of renal biopsies showing FSGS by light microscopy. Other ultramicroscopic findings are capillary collapse, mesangial expansion and hypercellularity, and visceral epithelial cell proliferation. Hyalinosis, sometimes containing lipid, is another feature of FSGS. These latter lesions represent the non-specific accumulation of proteins on the subendothelial side of the capillary lumen.

As mentioned above the early histological lesions predominate in the juxtamedullary glomeruli but progressively spread to the outer cortex. The lesion starts with hyalinosis of few capillary loops then the focal and segmental hyaline changes spread in the capillary tufts. Focal areas of podocyte detachment are followed by adhesion of the denuded GBM to the parietal layer of Bowman's space ('synechia'). The process of segmental sclerosis and capillary collapse progresses to sclerosis gradually obliterating the glomeruli. The completely sclerosed glomeruli may subsequently undergo complete 'reabsorption' leaving behind non-functioning aglomerular tubules (Kriz and LeHir, 2005). The lesions that initially affect only few glomeruli progressively involve an increasing larger fraction of the glomerular population and this progression is associated with a progressive form of interstitial fibrosis, tubular atrophy and vascular changes. In some cases, the lesion of FSGS can already be seen at renal biopsy at the onset of proteinuria, while in other patients initial biopsy shows only minimal changes (see also Chapter 5) and a full histological picture of FSGS may be seen only in repeat biopsies.

These observations indicating a possible evolution of MCN into FSGS led to a dispute as to whether FSGS should be considered as a separate clinico-pathological entity, or as a particularly severe subset of MCN that progresses to FSGS. Obviously, until we have complete understanding of the etio-pathogenesis of both FSGS and MCN, this dispute cannot be fully resolved. It is very clear that lesions of FSGS may be so focal in the early stages that they are easily 'missed' in an initial renal biopsy, even with an adequate number of glomeruli in the sample. Some subtle features in a renal biopsy, such as focal areas of interstitial fibrosis, extensive podocyte vacuolization and detachment, and evidence of a de-differentiated state for podocytes, may be clues to an underlying FSGS even when biopsies fail to reveal the typical sclerosing lesions. For the moment, we prefer to consider separately MCN and FSGS, as they have different pathological features, clinical presentation and outcome, and response to therapy.

More recently, emphasis has been placed on the variation in patterns of injury observed in renal biopsies demonstrating FSGS lesions. A working classification system (D'Agati et al., 2004) recognized five morphologic variants (based on light microscopic observations):

- The common, generic form of FSGS not otherwise specified—also known as 'classic' FSGS (see Atlas plate 5).
- A perihilar variant, with perihilar hyalinosis involving most of the glomeruli with segmental lesions (see Atlas plate 6).
- A cellular variant, with segmental endocapillary hypercellularity (see Atlas plate 7).
- A tip variant, with segmental lesion involving the tip domain.
- A collapsing variant (see Atlas plate 8), characterized by global collapse of glomerular capillaries of at least 20% of glomeruli, marked epithelial cell proliferation and de-differentiation, severe proteinuria, and rapid progression to end-stage renal failure.

However, the true clinical significance of this new classification of FSGS remains uncertain. Some investigators have suggested that the finding of certain variants connotes a particular pathogenesis and leads to an expectation of certain outcomes and responses to therapy. For example, the uncommon hilar form of FSGS may be more often seen in 'secondary' forms of FSGS, such as those seen in oligonephronic states and the collapsing form of FSGS may be seen more often in viral-associated (HIV) or drug-induced forms (pamidronate) of

FSGS. The 'classic' pattern of FSGS is most often seen in patients presenting with the features of primary or idiopathic FSGS.

Pathogenesis

There is general agreement that the *podocyte* is the major player in the genesis of FSGS and FSGS and is now categorized as a 'podocytopathy.' This highly differentiated and specialized cell type has essential roles in maintaining the integrity of glomerular architecture, resisting endocapillary hydraulic pressure and hindering egress of proteins into the urinary space. As a fully differentiated cell the resting podocytes are unable to replicate and even the damage of a single podocyte may initiate a sequence of events eventually leading to the degeneration of the whole glomerulus. Experimental studies show that the typical lesions of FSGS are preceded by podocyte detachment from the GBM and effacement of foot processes, followed by adhesion to the parietal layer of Bowmans'space (adhesions or synechiae). Moreover, it has been demonstrated that the podocyte is the first glomerular resident cell involved in cases of recurrence of FSGS after renal transplantation. Once initiated, podocyte lesions promote excess synthesis of extracellular matrix comprising collagen, proteoglycans, and glycoproteins that eventually lead to ensuing sclerosis (Meyrier, 2005). Injury to podocytes may also interfere with processes involving the cell-cycle and lead to an undifferentiated state capable of extensive proliferation (replication) of podocytes.

The question of what is the *primum movens* leading to podocyte injury in the primary or idiopathic form of the disorder remains very unanswerable at the present time. The experience with kidney transplantation showed that a number of patients with FSGS may have a very rapid recurrence of proteinuria almost immediately after transplantation, suggesting that some circulating factor (or factors) may be responsible for an increased glomerular permeability and FSGS recurrence. However, until now the nature of these factors has not been identified. There could be an excess of agents directly promoting of permeability or a deficiency of inhibitors of permeability promoting agents or both.

Etiology

FSGS is most commonly idiopathic in nature. However, reports of cases of familial FSGS associated with genetic mutations expressed in podocytes suggest a potential role of genetic abnormalities influencing the susceptibility to FSGS. Sporadic, apparently idiopathic, FSGS has also been associated with podocyte mutations, more frequently in children than in adults (see later). In addition to mutations affecting the structural genes for specific proteins,

Table 6.1 Diseases and conditions associated with the possible development of secondary glomerular segmental sclerosing lesions

Renal diseases	Other diseases/conditions	Drugs
◆ Vesico-ureteric reflux	◆ Familial dysautonomia	◆ Pamidronate (collapsing form)
◆ Reduced renal mass	◆ Morbid obesity	
◆ Vasculitis	◆ Elderly	◆ Cyclosporine
◆ Membranous nephropathy	◆ HIV/AIDS	◆ Tacrolimus
◆ IgA nephritis	◆ Diabetes mellitus	
◆ Chronic pyelonephritis	◆ Sickle-cell anemia	
◆ Proliferative glomerulonephritis	◆ Pre-eclampsia	
◆ Renal transplantation	◆ Arterial hypertension	
◆ Alport syndrome	◆ Polycytemia vera	
◆ Analgesic nephropathy	◆ Bartter syndrome	
◆ Obstructive uropathy	◆ Glycogen store disease	
	◆ Primary hyperaldosteronism	

functional variants of promoter regions, such as *NPHS2*, may also alter the level of their respective podocyte protein (Di Duca et al., 2006). It has also been suggested that heterozygous mutations for recessive genes may induce a 'vulnerable podocyte' phenotype—leading to abnormal glomerular permeability under states of cellular-stress or in the presence of sub-threshold injury.

A number of patients with proteinuria may also show segmental sclerosing lesions that can be associated with several clinical circumstances, including other primary glomerular diseases, such as membranous nephropathy (Table 6.1). This has led to nosologic confusion since many authors used the term FSGS not only to indicate the classic idiopathic form but also for any form of segmental sclerosing lesions, including those superimposed on another primary glomerular disease process, associated with other systemic diseases (e.g., angiitis), caused by functional hyperfiltration or triggered by massive proteinuria and/or systemic arterial hypertension.

In contradistinction to primary FSGS, these secondary forms of FSGS are associated with a lower frequency of hypoalbuminemia, particularly when sclerotic lesions are related to glomerular hyperfiltration, as in the case of vesico-ureteric reflux nephropathy, morbid obesity, renal hypoplasia, and reduced renal mass (oligonephronia). Edema is quite infrequently seen in the so called 'secondary' forms of FSGS, perhaps because the foot process effacement is more segmental than diffuse, and the more normal nephrons can excrete the sodium and water 'retained' by the more abnormal nephrons, thus maintaining homeostatic balance of fluid valumes (Rennke, personal communication).The progression to renal failure is also much less frequent and usually slower in the forms secondary to glomerular hyperfiltration than in primary FSGS. Such progression, if present, may be further delayed by the use of drugs interfering with the renin–angiotensin system and by weight loss in the obesity related glomerulopathy (Praga and Morales, 2006) (see also Chapter 1).

Genetics

In the last decade, molecular genetic studies uncovered several genes responsible for hereditary forms of nephrotic syndrome. These inherited podocytopathies are usually steroid-resistant and do not recur in the renal allografts; pathologic lesions consist of diffuse mesangial sclerosis (DMS) and, more frequently, of FSGS. Genetic forms of FSGS can be categorized as renal-limited disease or as part of a syndrome. For the aims of this chapter, we will review only renal-limited genetic FSGS, where genome-based defects affect assembly of podocyte structures, including slit diaphragm and actin-based cytoskeleton (Table 6.2). Additional genetic causes of FSGS involve mitochondrial gene mutations.

NPHS1 was the first disease gene identified as the cause of Finnish congenital nephrotic syndrome, a recessive disorder characterized by nephrotic syndrome at birth and ESRD within the first year of life. Nephrin, a key structural protein of podocytes, is the major constituent of the slit-diaphragm. Renal pathology is characterized by glomerular DMS. An overlap in the genes encoding nephrin and podocin (NPHS1/NPHS2) mutation spectrum has been documented in patients with congenital FSGS. In these cases, a specific di-genic inheritance of NPHS1 and NPHS2 resulting in a triallelic hit was associated with a modification of the phenotype from Finnish nephropathy to FSGS, providing evidence of a functional relationship between these two genes (Niaudet, 2004).

NPHS2 was identified later as the disease gene for a recessive form of FSGS linked to chromosome 1q25–31, characterized by steroid-resistant nephrotic syndrome and low risk for recurrent FSGS following renal transplantation. Podocin acts as a scaffold protein to recruit nephrin and CD2AP to the lipid rafts at the slit diaphragm. Recessive NPHS2 mutations are an important cause of childhood-onset FSGS, accounting for 26–34% of familial and 11–19% of sporadic steroid-resistant nephrotic syndrome, respectively. On the contrary, recessive NPHS2 mutations seem to be rare in adult, white FSGS patients. To date, >70 NPHS2 mutations have been reported that involve the whole length of the gene (Niaudet, 2004).

Mutations in the gene (ACTN4) encoding alpha-actinin4 an actin-binding protein associated with cytoskeleton and highly expressed in podocytes, cause

Table 6.2 Inherited (familial) renal-limited FSGS

Disease (OMIM)	Inheritance	Gene, protein, and function	Consequences
Finnish congenital NS	AR	*NPHS1*, nephrin. A key structural protein of podocytes	Diffuse mesangial sclerosis. Severe NS. ESRD within the first year
Steroid-resistant NS (OMIM 604766)	AR	*NPHS2*, podocin. A scaffold protein to recruit nephrin and CD2AP at the slit diaphragm	Steroid-resistant NS (25% of pediatric patients with FSGS)
Congenital NS	AR	*NPHS1/2*, nephrin + podocin	Coexistance with nephrin and podocin mutations
FSGS 1 (OMIM 603278)	AD	*ACTN4*, α-actinin4. A protein, highly expressed in podocytes associated to cytoskeleton	Subnephrotic proteinuria in the adolescence or adulthood. Slow progression
FSGS 2 (OMIM 603965)	AD	*TRPC6* channel which mediates Ca^{++} entry into the cell	Severe NS in the adulthood. Progression in >50% of patients
Nephrotic syndrome NPHS3 (OMIM 610725)	AR	Phospholipase Cε, an enzyme participating in intracellular signaling	Early onset of NS. Rapid progression to ESRD
FSGS 3 (OMIM 607832)	AR	CD2AP which forms a complex with nephrin and podocin with cell signaling properties	Increased susceptibility to glomerular diseases

NS=: nephrotic syndrome; ESRD: end-stage renal disease; AD: autosomal dominant; AR: autosomal recessive.

a rare dominant form of FSGS. The disease accounts for 3.5% of familial FSGS and <1% of sporadic FSGS, and is characterized by the onset of sub-nephrotic proteinuria during adolescence or early adulthood and slow progression to ESRD.

Mutations in the gene encoding TRPC6 were identified in families with dominant FSGS linked to 11q21. TRPC6, an ion channel mediating capacitative calcium entry into the cell, colocalizes to the slit diaphragm with nephrin, podocin, and CD2AP. To date, only six families with TRPC6 mutations have been reported. Most patients develop high-grade proteinuria and renal failure between 20–40 years of age. More than 50% of patients progress to renal failure within 10 years. It has been suggested that the TRPC6 mutations augment intracellular calcium influx into the podocyte, leading to FSGS through unclear mechanisms. Preliminary data revealed that tacrolimus can inhibit TRPC6 activity in vivo, suggesting that blocking TRPC6 channels within the podocyte might be of therapeutic benefit (Winn, 2008).

Mutations in *PLCE1*, which encodes an isoform of phospholipase C, an enzyme participating in intracellular signaling, have been described in seven families with early-onset nephrotic syndrome (NPHS3) and rapid progression to renal failure. NPHS3 is caused by a developmental rather than structural podocyte dysfunction. The histologic phenotype is that of DMS. However, a homozygous mutation in the catalytic domain of PLCE1 may cause FSGS. The monogenic forms of FSGS are usually considered to be resistant to treatment; however, two FSGS patients with PLCE1 mutations responded to steroids or cyclosporine, indicating that molecular causes of nephrotic syndrome may at least be modifiable (Hinkes, 2006).

CD2AP is an adapter protein which co-localizes to the slit diaphragm with nephrin and podocin, forming a complex with cell-signaling properties. The role of CD2AP in the kidney became apparent when CD2AP knockout mice developed proteinuria and kidney failure and CD2AP haplo-insufficiency was reported in patients with FSGS. In humans, two FSGS patients harboring heterozygous mutations in *CD2AP* have been reported. The role of a heterozygous loss of function mutation in the development of the FSGS phenotype is not clear. Trans-heterozygous mutations of *CD2AP* with another podocyte gene (di-genic inheritance) may provide an explanation. Alternatively, haplo-insufficiency of *CD2AP* may suggest that *CD2AP* can be viewed as a susceptibility gene for glomerular disease. Recently, however, a single patient with FSGS and a homozygous *CD2AP* mutation has been described. Both parents, free of disease, were proven to be heterozygous for this mutation, suggesting that not all heterozygous *CD2AP* mutations may be associated with the occurrence of FSGS.

Clinical presentation and features

The clinical presentation of FSGS is similar at any age although nephrotic syndrome is more frequent in children and hypertension is more frequent in adults (Korbet, 2003). The onset of the nephrotic syndrome is more often insidious than abrupt, different than that observed in MCN (see Chapter 3). About 70–90% of patients present with a full-blown nephrotic syndrome; patients who initially only have asymptomatic proteinuria may become frankly nephrotic at some time during their clinical course. Microscopic (dysmorphic) hematuria is found initially in about half of cases, while macrohematuria is quite rare. Some 30–40% of patients present with arterial hypertension. 'Malignant hypertension' is quite uncommon. Impaired renal function may be already present at the time of clinical discovery onset in about 20–25% of patients, implying slow steady progression even at an 'asymptomatic' stage of the disorder. Serum complement levels are normal, but lipid levels may be strikingly elevated. The fractional urinary excretion of IgG is often elevated and this may connote a treatment unresponsive and progressive lesion (Bazzi, 2003) (see also 'Prognostic factors').

Epidemiology

Primary (or idiopathic) FSGS accounts for 7–20% cases of nephrotic syndrome in children and for an even higher percentage in adults, depending on geographic and ancestral factors. There is a small predominance of FSGS in males over females in adults, while FSGS seems to be more frequent in girls in pediatric series (Boyer et al., 2007). The lesion of FSGS is far more commonly encountered in African-American blacks and in Hispanic than in Caucasian or Asian populations. There is also a variable ethnic distribution of the different morphologic variants of FSGS. While tip lesions are more common in Caucasian patients, the collapsing variant is more frequent among African-American blacks (Stokes et al., 2004).

In the recent decades an increased prevalence of FSGS lesion among renal biopsies performed for diagnosis of apparently idiopathic nephrotic syndrome has been reported in most Western countries (Kitiyakara et al., 2004; Dragovic et al., 2005), both in blacks and Caucasians. Of concern a Brazilian study reported an increased prevalence of FSGS also in children (Borges et al., 2007). The reasons for this exceptional growth in the frequency of FSGS are unknown. It is not due to the increased use of renal biopsy for diagnosis, and similar increases in prevalence have also been observed in predominantly Caucasian populations (Swaminathan et al., 2006). The involvement of a latent virus infection has been proposed but never proven. Some patients have signs of infection with polyoma virus or parvovirtus B-19.

Natural history

Primary FSGS is usually progressive and in the past about two-thirds of patients eventually developed end-stage renal disease (ESRD), usually within 10–15 years (Cameron, 1992). In a few cases, often called 'malignant' FSGS, the disease shows a rapidly progressive course associated with severe arterial hypertension, marked hyperlipidemia, and thrombotic complications. The prognosis for FSGS is much better today as most patients receive an adequate symptomatic (see Chapter 1) as well as specific treatment, after the demonstration that a large number of patients may benefit from glucocorticoids or other drugs which were previously considered to be rather ineffective. Although in a single patient proteinuria may have large day-to-day or month-to-month

Table 6.3 Variables that may influence the renal outcome of patients with FSGS (the most important factors are in bold).

Clinical parameters	Histological features
Age	Glomerular hypertrophy
Sex	Mesangial proliferation
Race	**Number of sclerotic glomeruli**
Proteinuria (amount duration)	Glomerular crescents
Response to therapy	**Histological variants**
Spontaneous remission	**Tubulo-interstitial changes** (chronic)
Arterial hypertension	Podocyte deficiency
Hyperlipidemia	
Genetic forms of FSGS	
Genetic polymorphism of RAS	

RAS= renin–angiotensin system.

fluctuations, spontaneous complete remission of the nephrotic syndrome is exceptional. A complete remission of proteinuria (as defined by urinary protein excretion <0.2g/d in timed urine samples or <0.2g protein per g of creatinine in a first morning 'spot' untimed urine samples) only occurs in 1.5–3% of untreated patients with nephrotic syndrome (Ponticelli, et al., 1999; Korbet, 2003).

Prognostic factors

A number of clinical and histological factors may influence the outcome of FSGS (Table 6.3). These factors are needed to be taken into account, both individually and collectively, in making treatment decisions.

Age

In patients with FSGS the *sclerosis index* (a semi-quantitative measure of the extent of the glomerular lesions) and the *chronicity index* (a semi-quantitative measure of the extent of cortical interstitial fibrosis and tubular atrophy) tend to increase in parallel with time. The glomerular filtration rate (GFR) also tends to be lower with advancing age (Hughson et al., 2007).On the other hand, the collapsing variant FSGS, which may portend a worse natural course, affects more frequently younger patients (Thomas et al., 2006). It is sometimes difficult to separate the morphologic effects of normal aging *per se* from the pathologic lesions engendered by superimposed FSGS.

Sex

In a Canadian retrospective review the mean levels of proteinuria at presentation and during follow-up were lower and the outcome was better in women with FSGS than in men (Cattran et al., 2008).

Race and ethnicity

In children, the rate of progression to renal failure is higher in African-American black than in white patients (Korbet et al., 1994). In adults, African-American blacks with FSGS have more severe disease than Caucasian patients as determined by the sclerosis index, the chronicity index, and estimated GFR. For approximately the same severity of disease, African-American black are 10 years or more younger than whites (Hughson et al., 2007). Black patients are also more frequently affected by collapsing glomerulopathy (absent HIV infection) which usually has a poor outcome and a natural course to ESRD (Stokes et al., 2004). The response to treatment is considerably poorer in African-American blacks than in Caucasian patients with FSGS (Crook et al., 2005).

Proteinuria

There is a general agreement that the level of proteinuria at presentation has very little diagnostic significance but that it has great prognostic importance. Patients with persisting nephrotic-range proteinuria in spite of therapy have generally a very poor prognosis, particularly when the amount of urine protein excretion exceeds 10g/d (Fig. 6.1). This may be explained by the fact that proteinuria not only is an indirect marker of the severity of renal lesions, but may also be directly involved in mechanisms favoring the progression of renal diseases. Exposure of the tubule to excess amounts of protein and the necessity for augmenting protein reabsorption can be a direct cause of phenotypic alteration in tubular behavior that promotes progressive interstitial fibrosis (Abbate et al., 2002).

The prognostic significance of the *quality* of proteinuria is still uncertain. Bazzi et al. (2003) found that in patients with FSGS, the fractional excretion of IgG (FE IgG) showed an excellent predictive value for remission, progression, and response to therapy (even independent of the *quantity* of proteinuria). However, in a preliminary study, Deegens and Wetzels (2007) showed that a high FE IgG is not invariably associated with a poor outcome in patients with primary FSGS, as about half of patients could obtain remission after therapy. Additional work is needed before one can accept the notion that examination of the *quality* of proteinuria per se, independent from the *quantity* of proteinuria (as exemplified by the FE IgG) should become a routine part of the evaluation of nephrotic patients with FSGS.

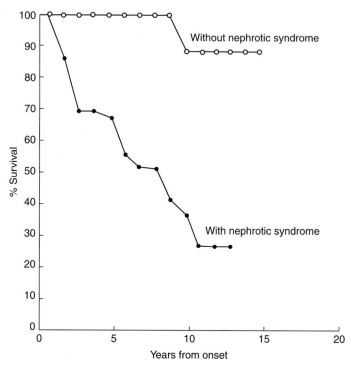

Fig. 6.1 Renal survival in patients with FSGS presenting without or with nephrotic syndrome. Adapted with permission from Cameron JS (1992). The long-term outcome of glomerular diseases. In RN Schrier and CW Gottschalk (eds), *Diseases of the kidney*, 2nd edn, pp.1895–958. Little Brown, Boston, MA.

Renal function

There is general agreement that impaired renal function at presentation indicates a poor prognosis. However, in assessing renal function in a nephrotic patient one should be aware of the fact that an increase in serum creatinine level does not necessarily reflect an already established chronic renal insufficiency. In a number of patients the serum creatinine level may increase temporarily because of hypovolemia, either caused by profound hypoalbuminemia or by diuretic therapy, and can completely reverse after hypovolemia has been corrected. However, in other cases objective signs of hypovolemia cannot be documented. In these cases the glomerular ultrafiltration coefficient may be reduced by as much as 50%, suggesting that severe reduction in GFR may result from an interaction between acute ischemic tissue injury and pre-existing intrinsic renal abnormalities or that diffuse foot process effacement may result in reduced hydraulic conductivity at the single nephron level. It is also worth remembering that the GFR as estimated from endogenous creatinine clearance or formulas predicting GFR from serum creatinine concentrations are often erroneously high due to augmented tubular secretion of creatinine in heavy proteinuric states.

Response to therapy

The response to therapy is considered by nearly all clinicians and investigators to be the *best* single clinical indicator of eventual outcome, even more important than the initial histological picture. Most patients who respond completely to glucocorticoid therapy maintain normal renal function over time (even when steroid-responsive relapses subsequently occur), while steroid-resistant patients often progress to ESRD. While there is also general agreement that a complete remission of proteinuria (usually defined by a daily proteinuria $\leq 200mg$) is associated with an excellent outcome in the long-term, it has also been demonstrated that a partial remission is a reliable predictor of good long-term renal survival (Troyanov et al., 2005).

Spontaneous remission

Although spontaneous complete remission of proteinuria is very exceptional, partial remission may occur in some patients. Spontaneous complete or partial remissions are usually associated with a significant improvement in the overall natural history of FSGS both in terms of progression to ESRD and of nephrotic syndrome related complications.

Arterial hypertension

It is well known that arterial hypertension contributes to the development of renal failure in renal diseases. FSGS does not represent an exception, although little attention has been paid to the prognostic role of hypertension in the available retrospective surveys. Recent data suggest that arterial hypertension may cause or aggravate glomerular sclerosis with two principal modes of glomerular sclerosis—ischemic and hypertrophic—the risk being higher in patients with severe hypertension and in black patients (Hill, 2008).

Hyperlipidemia

Elevation of plasma lipids and an abnormal partition of the lipid fractions is highly prevalent in nephrotic patients with FSGS (see also Chapter 1) and may contribute to an elevated cardiovascular risk as well as to the progression of kidney disease (Grone and Grone, 2008). Research has shown that HMG-coA-reductase inhibitors ('statins') may affect the expression of inflammatory elements, curtail oxidative stress, and enhance endothelial function.

Some preliminary data suggest that statin-mediated alterations in inflammatory responses and endothelial function may reduce proteinuria and the rate of progression of kidney disease (Campese and Park, 2007). The specific role of hyperlipidemia as an independent factor in determining the natural history of FSGS can only be inferred from larger studies of proteinuric renal disease in general.

Glomerular hypertrophy

Glomerular enlargement or 'glomerulomegaly' is frequent and pathogenetically important in secondary forms of FSGS (particularly in those conditions associated with hyperfiltration and oligonephronia) but its role in idiopathic FSGS is still unclear. A morphometric study reported that the mean glomerular area, the maximum glomerular area, the mean glomerular diameter, and the mean tangent diameter were all significantly greater in patients with primary FSGS who progressed to renal failure than in those who did not (Onetti Muda et al., 1994). These data suggest that glomerular hypertrophy might represent a compensatory change that could immediately precede a rapid decline in renal function as an expression of an adaptation to nephron loss that could itself maladaptively predispose to the future development of renal failure.

Mesangial proliferation

In a review of our own experience with FSGS we found by multivariate analysis that the presence of superimposed mesangial proliferation was significantly and independently associated with the risk of doubling of serum creatinine over time. Patients showing mesangial proliferation at renal biopsy had a relative risk of 4.6 for doubling their serum creatinine (Ponticelli et al., 1999). Such mesangial proliferation may also increase the risk of recurrent disease in the renal allograft (see below).

Number of glomeruli affected

Diffuse and multiple segmental lesions at initial biopsy (an increased sclerosis index) and even more an increase in the percentage of globally sclerotic glomeruli in a follow-up biopsy correlate highly with the development of chronic renal failure.

Glomerular crescents

True rather than 'pseudo' epithelial crescents are quite rare in FSGS. When present they may concur to a rapid progression of disease. When the podocyte undergoes marked de-differentiation and proliferation it can simulate a glomerular crescent ('pseudo-crescents' of FSGS).

Histological variants

The morphological variants of FSGS developed by D'Agati et al. (2004) may have prognostic and therapeutic significance, but it is not yet proven that this classification has value for prognostication or for predicting therapeutic outcomes independent of clinical features (such as serum creatinine level and proteinuria). All studies reported thus far are retrospective in nature and selection bias or other confounders could have significantly influenced the findings (see Chapter 3). For example, in a retrospective study on 87 nephrotic adults with biopsy-proven FSGS, Chun et al. (2004) found that the response to therapy was not significantly different in patients with classic FSGS lesions (53%; mean follow-up 73 months) and in those with cellular or collapsing lesion (64%; mean follow-up 52 months) or tip lesion (78%; mean follow-up 99 months). However, in a larger collaborative study comprising 197 patients, the group of Jennette (Thomas et al., 2006) found that the different histological variants of FSGS have substantial differences in renal outcomes. Patients with collapsing FSGS had a 3-year renal survival of 33% compared to a mean 3-year renal survival of 67% for the other variants. Patients with the tip lesion were more likely to receive glucocorticoids and thus more often achieved complete remission.

Tubulointerstitial changes

As in all other glomerular diseases, a very high correlation has been found between the severity of tubulointerstitial changes (chronicity index) and the final renal outcome in FSGS. The prognosis is particularly severe in patients showing diffuse interstitial fibrosis and tubular atrophy at renal biopsy (Banfi et al., 1991). This association merely reflects the fact that if chronic damage occurred in the past (as shown in the 'snapshot' of the renal biopsy at a particular time) it is most likely to continue into the future, all other things being equal.

Genetics

As reported above, most forms of genetic FSGS have a poor prognosis. This is true not only for familial cases but also for patients with sporadic FSGS and mutations of podocin, alpha-actinin4, and TRPC6. Anecdotal cases of response to therapy have been reported in patients with PLCE1 mutation. We also do not know whether or how single-nucleotide polymorphisms in the genes involved in hereditary forms of FSGS affect kidney function. These patients are good candidates to renal transplantation, as the risk of recurrence is very low.

There are discrepant views about the prognostic significance of genetic abnormalities of the renin–angiotensin-system (RAS). Frishberg et al. (1998)

found that homozygosity for the ACE insertion allele may have a protective effect in children with FSGS and can serve as a positive prognostic indicator at diagnosis. The D allele may exert a detrimental dominant effect on outcome. Neither the ACE gene polymorphism nor the other RAS polymorphisms studied are associated with disease prevalence. The AT1R and angiotensinogen gene polymorphisms are not associated with progression of renal disease in FSGS. Tabel et al., (2005) found that the angiotensinogen-235T allele was related with steroid resistance and progression to renal failure in nephrotic syndrome. In contrast, Dixit et al. (2002) found no association between the I/D polymorphism of the ACE gene and the presence of and rapidity progression of FSGS.

Specific treatment

Goals and objectives of treatment

The aims of treatment in FSGS should be clearly understood at the outset of a making a treatment decision and should also always balanced by an assessment of the potential risks both of specific and symptomatic therapy (see Chapters 1 and 2). The over-arching principles for the goals and objectives of specific treatment are: (i) to reverse, halt, or delay progression to end-stage renal failure; (ii) to favor a complete or partial remission of the proteinuria in order to prevent nephrotic syndrome-related complications; (iii) to render the patient as asymptomatic as possible within the constraints of undesirable side effects of therapy (e.g., to improve the overall quality of life).

Many different drugs and combinations of drugs have been and are now being used for the treatment of FSGS, showing that no single therapeutic approach has obtained ideal results. Unfortunately, any assessment of the validity of treatment is made difficult by the fact that most of the available studies are observational and retrospective and therefore contain the biases and potential confounding of non-controlled trials, namely ill-defined criteria of case inclusion and exclusion, different treatments for different periods, different follow-ups, poorly defined and heterogenous end points (see also Chapter 3). The lack of well-designed, adequately powered, appropriately controlled, long-term prospective studies coupled with the considerable underlying morphological and pathogenetic heterogeneity of the disorder explains many of the uncertainties about the optimum therapeutic approach to FSGS and the different attitudes held by nephrologists as a whole. We will attempt to sort out this confusing situation and offer our own advice regarding therapeutic approaches, adhering to the goals and objectives principles outline above.

Table 6.4 Recommendations for treatment of FSGS with nephrotic syndrome using glucocorticoids

Duration of therapy:	A short course (8–12 weeks) may obtain remission in about 25% of patients
	A prolonged course (≥6 months) may obtain complete or partial remission in at least 60% of patients
Dosages:	Start with 1mg/kg/day of prednisone (or equivalent doses of an analogue glucocorticoid) in adults and 1.5mg/kg/day in children for 12 weeks (if well tolerated)
	As an alternative prednisone can be given every other day in double dosage
	After 12 weeks (or before if a substantial reduction of proteinuria is obtained) reduce the daily dose by 5mg every week (or 10mg every other day)
	When a daily dose of 10mg (or 20mg every other day) is reached, the dose may be maintained until the 12th month if well tolerated
General:	Give the full dose in a single morning administration between 7–9 a.m., after breakfast
	Encourage physical activity (walking, swimming, aerobic)
	Recommend a low-salt normocaloric diet, avoiding excessive carbohydrate intake. Use about 0.8–1.0g high biologic value protein per kg dry body weight per day plus the amount of protein lost in the urine on a daily basis
	Regularly check blood pressure, glycemia, serum lipids levels. Maintain blood pressure at <130/80mmHg (with an ACE inhibitor or an ARB preferentially; add a 'statin' if total cholesterol >200mg/dL)
	Tailor the doses of the glucocorticoid according to the tolerance of the patient

Glucocorticoids (Table 6.4)

Since the prognosis of patients who attain complete remission of proteinuria is much better than that of patients who do not show any initial response, the most correct and most stringent way of interpreting the available retrospective studies is that of evaluating the rate of *complete remission*. The rate of complete response mainly depends on the doses and the duration of glucocorticoid treatment. By reviewing the pediatric literature before 1990, Cameron (1992) reported that only 112 of 389 (29%) of children with FSGS 'responded' to a prednisone treatment regimen given for 6–8 weeks at doses similar to those used in minimal change MCN (see Chapter 5). Many responders developed multiple relapses or became steroid-dependent and thus behaved similar to those with MCN. A retrospective review of 151 adults with FSGS showed that 16% of patients given a short course steroids obtained a complete remission and another 20% a partial remission, a 36% overall remission rate (Schena and

Cameron, 1988). It must be emphasized that in this review most adults received only short-term treatment with glucocorticoids, as patients were considered to be steroid-resistant if they did not achieve remission within 8–12 weeks.

A much more optimistic picture has evolved after the recognition that more prolonged administration of glucocorticoids was beneficial. Cattran and Rao (1998) conducted a retrospective study in 93 patients (55 adults and 38 children) with primary FSGS drawn from the Toronto Glomerulonephritis Registry. After an average follow-up of 11 years, the outcome of patients (adults versus children respectively) for complete remission was 22% versus 42%, and ESRD was 42% versus 34%. Most remissions were observed in patients receiving steroids for more than 6 months while shorter treatments did not appear to be beneficial either in children or adults. Long-term renal survival in both age groups was 100% for patients attaining complete remission. Among patients without a complete remission the 10-year survival rate was 62% in adults and 58% in children.

Ponticelli et al. (1999) in an uncontrolled study treated 53 adults with primary FSGS with prednisone at initial dose of 1mg/kg/d for 8 weeks then gradually tapered by 5–10mg/d until a maintenance of 10–15mg/d. The mean duration of treatment was 6 months. Twenty-one patients (39.6%) responded with a complete remission and another ten patients (18.8%) with a partial remission (overall remission rate of 58%). Of the 27 patients treated for 16 weeks or less only four (15%) entered a complete remission versus sixteen of the 26 (61%) treated for more than 16 weeks. Seventeen of the 31 patients who responded with complete or partial remission had one or more relapse. Only one responder progressed to ESRD after a mean follow-up of 86 months.

Chun et al. (2004), in another uncontrolled trial, gave an initial course of prednisone at a dose of 1mg/kg/d (up to 80mg) for 3–4 months. In patients who demonstrated complete or partial remission, the dose of prednisone was then tapered slowly over 2–3 months. Patients who were unresponsive to the initial therapy at 4 months were tapered off prednisone more rapidly, over 4–6 weeks. To minimize toxicity in the elderly, an alternate-day prednisone regimen (1–2mg/kg up to 120mg) was used for 4–5 months. With this regimen 63% of 87 nephrotic adults with biopsy-proven primary FSGS attained remission with a prolonged administration of glucocorticoids. The response to steroid therapy was similar among the different histological variants. The overall 10-year renal survival was significantly better for patients who entered remission compared with patients who did not enter remission (92% versus 33%) regardless of the variation in the underlying histologic lesion.

Although all observational, retrospective, and non-controlled, these studies have a high degree of consistency and strongly suggest that a course of prednisone for ≥ 4 months (usually 6 months in duration) may obtain complete remission of proteinuria in a reasonably high fraction of patients (about 50–60%). Thus regimens involving steroid treatment for <3 months (12 weeks) can be *considered inadequate* for FSGS, while it would be adequate for most children and at least some adults with MCN (see Chapter 5). This phenomenon leads one to conclude that a revision of the concept of *steroid resistance*, usually defined by a lack of response within 8 weeks of high-dose steroids, is needed. Today it is far more appropriate to define a patient with FSGS as *steroid-resistant* if he/she does not show any improvement of proteinuria after 4–6 months (16–24 weeks) of glucocorticoid therapy. It is doubtful that at this juncture a randomized, placebo controlled study of the efficacy and safety of glucocorticoid therapy for primary FSGS will ever be performed.

Among responders to glucocorticoid therapy, remissions seem to be more stable in adults than in children. Renal function also tends to be maintained at normal levels over time in most responders. Although it is not possible to exclude an effect of selection—only patients with a good tolerance to therapy and with some improvement of proteinuria continued glucocorticoids for a long period—a review of the available studies gives the strong impression that the more aggressive the glucocorticoid therapy is the higher is the rate of response.

Even if a prolonged course with glucocorticoids obtains remission in a substantial group of children and adults with FSGS, one cannot neglect the risks of adverse events with such a treatment. Unfortunately, not only remissions but also the incidence and the severity of side effects are proportional to the intensity and duration of steroid treatment. This may represent a problem for those patients who do not show an early (i.e., by 8–12 weeks of treatment) response (the majority unfortunately!) and even more so for those patients who have frequent relapses. On the other hand, it is very difficult to identify any clinical or pathological feature that can allow prediction of the response to glucocorticoids in nephrotic patients with sporadic (non-familial) FSGS (with the exception of genomic studies identifying a podocyte protein mutation in a sporadic form as discussed above). The value of identifying morphologic variants of FSGS for the selection of a specific treatment regimen has not yet been examined in a randomized controlled fashion. Thus, the only sure means to know whether a patient will or will not respond is to administer a full course (e.g., 4–6 months) of therapy with prednisone. Some measures should always be adopted to reduce the steroid-related morbidity likely to occur with this course of treatment. These include the administration of the daily steroid dose in a single morning administration (ideally between 7–9 a.m.) and the possible switch from a daily to an alternate-day administration for a maintenance treatment. The patient should also be encouraged to follow physical and dietetic measures to prevent increase in body weight, diabetes, myopathy, and osteoporosis. Blood pressure, lipidemia, and glycemia should be regularly checked and treated when necessary. The goal blood pressure should be 120–130/75–80mmHg, and the use of inhibitors of angiotensin II are preferred (see Chapter 1). However, the most important measure remains a strict control of clinical and psychological conditions by the regular monitoring of the patient by the physician and an adequate tailoring of the doses, according to the tolerance to treatment.

Alkylating agents (Table 6.5)

Cyclophosphamide and (less frequently) chlorambucil have been the alkylating agents most widely used as adjunctive therapy in patients with FSGS. Nitrogen mustard is no longer in use.

Cyclophosphamide

Good results have been reported with oral cyclophosphamide in FSGS but *only* in steroid-responsive or steroid-dependent patients About 65% of children and 75% of adults with a steroid-responsive form of FSGS responded with a complete or partial remission to a course of 8–12 weeks of cyclophosphamide at a mean dose of 2mg/kg/d (Ponticelli and Passerini, 2003). This response rate is comparable to that seen in steroid-responsive, relapsing MCN (see Chapter 5).

Table 6.5 Alkylating and antiproliferative drugs in FSGS

Alkylating agents:	When given as a first-line treatment the rate of response to an 8–12-week course of cyclophosphamide or chlorambucil is similar to that obtained with glucocorticoids (no added benefit)
	In steroid-sensitive patients either cyclophosphamide or chlorambucil may obtain a good response (partial or complete response)
	The longer is the treatment the higher is the rate of response but also the rate and severity of side effects
	In steroid-resistant patients the response to alkylating agents is poor or not existent
Antiproliferative agents:	*Azathioprine:* insufficient data—probably ineffective. Few uncontrolled studies suggest a benefit with long-term (>1 year) use. Not recommended for initial therapy
	Mycophenolate salts: possible benefit on proteinuria, but only few non-controlled trials available, with small number of patients and short-term follow-up. Not recommended for initial therapy

A good response may also be obtained when cyclophosphamide, either alone or in combination with glucocorticoids is given as a first treatment (before any knowledge is obtained regarding the potential for a response to steroids alone or for the potential for relapses), but usually treatment should be prolonged to obtain a complete or partial remission, just as with a steroid only course of treatment. A systematic review of non-controlled studies concluded that there is no clear evidence that an 8–12-week treatment with cyclophosphamide (plus steroids) is superior to steroids alone in inducing remission either in children or adults (Habashy et al., 2003). However, when compared to steroids alone cyclophosphamide *may* prolong the duration of remission in responders. Whether this benefit is sufficient to offset the additional risk imposed by the use of cyclophosphamide for initial therapy of FSGS is not well understood.

Contrariwise, the results of cyclophosphamide are uniformly poor in steroid-resistant cases. Long-term administration of cyclophosphamide may obtain a response only in a very few steroid-resistant patients. One should be remembered, however, that cumulative doses of cyclophosphamide higher than 200–300mg/kg can result in azoospermia or ovarian failure. Moreover, prolonged exposure to cyclophosphamide increases the risk of bladder toxicity or malignancy (see also Chapter 2).

Only one controlled study of the use of oral cyclophosphamide in children with steroid-resistant FSGS has been published (Tarshish et al., 1996). Sixty children, all with biopsy diagnosed FSGS and with unremitting nephrotic syndrome despite intensive therapy with glucocorticoids for at least 8 weeks (the old standard definition of *steroid-resistance*) were randomly allocated in a clinical trial comparing oral prednisone, 40mg/m^2 on alternate days for a period of 12 months (control group), with the same prednisone regimen plus a 12-week course of daily oral cyclophosphamide, 2.5mg/kg in a single morning dose (experimental group). One-quarter of the children in each group had complete resolution of proteinuria during follow-up. A Kaplan-Meier renal survival analysis revealed no significant differences between the two groups. On the basis of these data the authors concluded that cyclophosphamide therapy for children with steroid-resistant FSGS should not be recommended. No similar controlled data for the use of oral daily cyclophosphamide in adults with steroid-resistant FSGS is available.

A few uncontrolled and anecdotal studies have reported 'favorable' results with intravenous pulses of cyclophosphamide given monthly at a dose of 500mg/m^2 over 6 months together with high-dose oral prednisone. However, a meta-analysis found *no difference in* complete remissions between children treated with prednisone alone or with intravenous cyclophosphamide plus prednisone (Habashy et al., 2003). In sum, there appears to be absolutely no indication for the use of cyclophosphamide in the treatment of steroid-resistant adults or children. At most, the drug may have some use in controlling the frequency of relapses in steroid-responsive, frequently relapsing or steroid-dependent patients with FSGS.

Chlorambucil

Chlorambucil has also been used for FSGS but much less frequently than cyclophosphamide. Good results were reported in the distant past, but these are mainly anecdotes. Less encouraging have been the experiences in steroid-resistant FSGS that showed only little benefit for chlorambucil, similar to that observed with cyclophosphamide (Ponticelli and Passerini, 2003).

In a prospective randomized study Heering et al. (2004) compared two specific treatment protocols in children with steroid resistant FSGS. Fifty-seven patients were randomly assigned to receive steroids and cyclosporine (group 1; 34 patients) or steroids and chlorambucil for 6 months (group 2; 23 patients). When treatment was refractory to chlorambucil, the patients in group 2 were treated with cyclosporine. At the end of the chlorambucil therapy, patients had increased creatinine levels, from 1.5 to 1.8mg/dL, and a non-significant improvement in proteinuria (from 4.8 to 3.4 g/24h). After 4 years the mean creatinine level in group 1 was 1.7mg/dL and the proteinuria level was 2.5g/24h. In group 2, the mean creatinine level was 1.9mg/dL and the mean proteinuria level was 2.3g/24h. Neither difference was significant. Full remission occurred in 23% of the patients in group 1 and 17% of the patients in group 2. Partial remission was observed in 38% of the patients in group 1 and 48% in group 2 (p= n.s.). Four of 34 patients in group 1 and five of 23 patients in group 2 developed ESRD. The authors concluded that additional treatment with chlorambucil was found to be ineffective in FSGS.

In summary, the available studies show that a course with alkylating agents may favorably influence the renal outcome in nephrotic patients with FSGS who respond to steroids and may obtain results similar to those of glucocorticoids when given as a first-line therapy in untreated patients. In primary therapy the only advantage seen with these agents is a longer duration of remission. It is possible to speculate that with more long-term treatment the results may be improved. However, such prolonged therapy with alkylating cytotoxic agents exposes the patient to the risk of disquieting side effects such as bone-marrow toxicity, infection, gonadal toxicity, mutagenic effects, and neoplasia (see Chapter 2). The risk of severe toxicity and the limited benefits (if any) should greatly discourage the extensive use of long-term therapies with cyclophosphamide or chlorambucil in FSGS.

Inhibitors of purine synthesis

See also Table 6.5.

Azathioprine

More than 20 years ago, Cade et al. (1986) suggested that long-term administration of azathioprine might have value in 'steroid-resistant' MCN (most of these patients probably had FSGS). This has never been confirmed by a controlled trial. A good rate of remissions was reported in small uncontrolled studies in adults with FSGS when azathioprine associated with prednisone was administered for 2 years or more (Banfi et al., 1991). However, only a few patients received this form of treatment. Anecdotal successes with azathioprine in children with steroid-resistant nephrotic syndrome have also been reported in the past. The evaluation of this drug in FSGS is pending as it has been used more and more rarely to treat FSGS in recent years.

Mycophenolate mofetil (MMF)

Experimental studies in rat models of kidney disease showed that MMF has a favorable effect on glomerular scarring and interstitial fibrosis, but not on proteinuria or hypercholesterolemia.

There are only few preliminary observational clinical studies. The number of patients enrolled in these trials was too small and the follow-up was too short to draw any conclusions regarding efficacy or safety of MMF therapy in FSGS. In general, the results were not impressive, but some short-term benefit on proteinuria was reported in a few patients (Sepe et al. 2008). In a small randomized trial (Nayagam et al. 2008), 33 patients with FSGS were randomized to receive MMF (2g/d for 6 months) along with prednisone 0.5mg/kg/d for 8–12 weeks or prednisone 1mg/kg/d for 12–24 weeks followed by tapering over the next 8 weeks. After a mean follow-up of 16 weeks there was no difference in either complete remissions (10 versus 9) or partial remissions (2 versus 2).

Clearly, further studies should be conducted to better assess the role of MMF in FSGS. Well designed randomized trials comparing MMF with other treatments (such as cyclosporine or glucocorticoids, see below) have been and should continue to be organized. Such a trial sponsored by the NIH in the USA is currently in progress. These studies should also recruit a sufficient number of patients who should be followed for a minimum of 2 years to assess the impact of treatment, if any, on renal function. Moreover, the optimal dosage of MMF should be assessed, as the drug has been given in the few published studies at doses ranging between 0.5–2.5g/d. Finally it should be established whether MMF should be given as monotherapy or in association with steroids or a calcineurin inhibitor.

Combined immunosuppression

An aggressive approach has been proposed for steroid-resistant nephrotic children with FSGS by Mendoza and Tune. This regimen consists of intravenous methylprednisolone pulses, 20mg/kg each, three per week for 2 weeks, one per week for 8 weeks, one every other week for 8 weeks, and one per month for 10 months. Children were also given oral prednisone, 2mg/kg/48h for 78 weeks. When no response was obtained, cyclophosphamide (2mg/kg/d) or chlorambucil (0.2mg/kg/d) was added. At the end of a mean follow-up of 6.3 years, of 32 children treated with this regimen 21 were in complete and three in partial remission and had a normal creatinine clearance, five had reduced creatinine clearances, and three had progressed to end-stage renal failure (Tune et al., 1995). The Mendoza–Tune regimen as it has been called, was also used by Waldo et al. (1992) in thirteen children, eight African-American blacks and five Caucasians, ten with FSGS and three with MCN. Initially five patients had complete and two partial remission. Five of the responders relapsed under treatment; three were re-treated and two responded. After a mean follow-up of 47 months the three patients with MCN had protein-free urine. Of the ten patients with FSGS, six had ESRD, two renal insufficiency, and the other two were still nephrotic. Complications of treatment were minimal. Five patients developed mild hypertension which was easily treated. All patients experienced moderate weight gain. No other side effects were seen.

In summary, different results and tolerance have been obtained with the aggressive regimen of Mendoza–Tune. These discrepancies may be partly accounted for by the fact that African-American black children seem to be unresponsive to this treatment (Waldo et al., 1992). No other clinical or histological parameter predicting response could be identified in patients with FSGS. Taken together the results of Tune and Waldo, about two-thirds of children responded to Mendoza-Tune treatment regimen, most of them enjoying complete remission. The remaining patients progressed to renal insufficiency or to ESRD. It is a pity that after almost 20 years from the first data reported by Mendoza no randomized controlled trial has been performed to establish the role of this treatment in FSGS. Most importantly, it is not known if the results claimed by the Mendoza–Tune regimen can be achieved equally well (or not as well) by a regimen of a calcineurin inhibitor plus steroids (see below). The adverse event rate between a Mendoza–Tune regimen and a calcineurin inhibitor-steroid regimen (with or without combined MMF) also needs to be compared.

Table 6.6 Calcineurin inhibitors in FSGS

	General	Dosage	Recommendations
Cyclosporine	Randomized controlled trials showed that cyclosporine may obtain complete or partial remission of nephrotic syndrome in 50–60% of patients who did not respond to short courses of glucocorticoids.	Initial total daily doses (usually given in two divided doses daily about 12 hours apart) should not exceed 4mg/kg in adults and 100–150 mg/m2 in children when using the microemulsion preparation (Neoral®).	The association with small doses of prednisone (10–20mg daily) may increase the rate of responses. If there is no reduction of proteinuria after 3–4 months the treatment is probably ineffective. In case of response the treatment may be continued for 1–2 years at the minimal effective dosage. The drug should be tapered off slowly in case of discontinuation (risk of relapse).
			Chronic nephrotoxicity may appear on prolonged use (particularly with daily dosage exceeding 5mg/kg in adults).
			The valued of monitoring blood levels is uncertain, except to avoid toxicity.
Tacrolimus	No controlled trials available. Probably as effective as cyclosporine. Different profile of side effects. Equally nephrotoxic as cyclosporine.	Start with 0.1mg/kg/d	Same as for cyclosporine.

Calcineurin inhibitors (Table 6.6)

Cyclosporine (CsA)

An overview of retrospective studies in children and adults with FSGS indicated that about one-half of patients could be maintained in remission with CsA. In many cases proteinuria improved within 3 months and remission could be maintained with low doses of CsA. In some studies prolonged treatment with CsA was required to achieve remission. Many patients relapsed when CsA was stopped (Ponticelli and Passerini, 1999).

A few randomized controlled trials in patients with FSGS provided evidence in favor of CsA. Ponticelli et al. (1993) randomly assigned 45 patients (adults and children) with normal renal function and a nephrotic syndrome unresponsive to 6-week high-dose prednisone (actually too short to define steroid resistance by current standards) either to supportive therapy or to the old formulation of non-emulsified CsA (Sandimmune®) for 6 months at a dose of 5 mg/kg/d in adults and 6 mg/kg/d in children, with gradual tapering off over another 6 months. Of 22 patients receiving CsA seven obtained complete remission and six partial remission (total response 59%) compared with three partial remissions (14%) in the control group. Mean levels of serum protein, serum cholesterol, and urinary protein excretion significantly improved at 6 months in the CsA-treated patients. The mean levels of creatinine clearance did not differ at 6 months between the two groups. Patients were followed up to 2 years. One patient who received CsA and four in the control group developed a decrease in creatinine clearance >50%. Side effects were mild and reversible. No significant difference in blood pressure between the two groups was seen at any time. This study shows that a 1-year treatment course with CsA may obtain remission of the nephrotic syndrome in about 60% of patients with normal renal function who did not respond to short-term steroid treatment. Of interest, 38% of responders remained without a nephrotic syndrome for 1 year after CsA was stopped. No clinical or histological factor at presentation could predict the response to CsA or the occurrence of remission.

Cattran et al. (1999) assigned 49 adults with biopsy-proven FSGS who did not respond to an 8-week course with prednisone at a dose of 1mg/kg/d to receive CsA, at a dose of 3.5mg/kg/d for 26 weeks then tapered off during the next 4 weeks, or a placebo. Both groups also received low-dose prednisone, 0.15mg/kg/d. By week 26, complete or partial remission of proteinuria had occurred in 70% of patients assigned to CsA versus only 4% of the placebo group. Relapse after stopping CsA occurred in 40% of patients who entered remission by 52 weeks and in another 20% by week 78. Long-term renal function was better preserved in the CsA group. About 50% of patients in the placebo group versus 25% in the CsA group had their serum creatinine level doubled. A limit of these two randomized trials is represented by the definition of steroid-resistance, as patients were considered to be steroid-resistant if they did not respond to 6–8 weeks of intensive glucocorticoid treatment.

A further multicenter randomized trial compared CSA (at doses adjusted to achieve trough [Co] levels of 120–180ng/mL) versus intravenous cyclophosphamide (500mg/m^2 per month) in the initial therapy of children with steroid-resistant nephrotic syndrome and histologically proven MCN, FSGS, or mesangial hypercellularity (Plank et al. (2008). All patients were on alternate prednisone therapy. After 24 weeks, complete remission was reached in two of the fifteen (13%) patients receving CsA and one of the seventeen (5%) cyclophosphamide-treated patients (p = n.s.). Partial remission was achieved by seven of the fifteen (46%) CsA-treated patients and two of the fifteen (11%) cyclophosphamide-treated patients (p <0.05). Five patients in the CsA treated group and fourteen patients in the cyclophosphamide-treated group were withdrawn from the study, most of them during the non-responder protocol. The number of adverse events was comparable between both groups.

As already discussed, in a German study 23% of children achieved full remission and another 38% partial remission with steroids and CsA, while chlorambucil was found to be ineffective (Heering et al., 2004).

In a meta-analysis of randomized controlled trials in children, Habashy et al. (2003) found that CsA significantly increased the probability of complete remission, and reduced to 0.64 the relative risk for persistent nephrotic syndrome, when compared with placebo or no treatment.

The incidence of CsA side effects in patients with FSGS is comparable to that reported in MCN (see Chapter 5). One main concern with the use of CsA in FSGS is that the nephrotoxic effects of the drug may accelerate the progression of renal lesions. At least in a few patients, repeat biopsies disclosed worsening of the lesions of FSGS in spite of remission of proteinuria (Meyrier and Niaudet, 2005). However, the data suggest that the risk of CsA nephropathy is low if guidelines are followed and patients are monitored regularly (Cattran et al., 2007).

In summary, there is a high level of evidence that CsA can induce an antiproteinuric effect in about 50–60% of patients who have not responded to a short course of steroids and can be considered as an alternative treatment to glucocorticoids or immunosuppressive agents. Some of the patients enrolled in the trials mentioned above might have responded to a prolongation of the course of steroids, so the CsA responsiveness may have been over-estimated. Therefore, CsA may be a useful alternative therapeutic approach for patients with FSGS who display persistent nephrotic range proteinuria in spite of 8 weeks' treatment with high-dose oral prednisone with the addition of three intravenous methylprednisolone pulses (Meyrier and Niaudet, 2005). When using CsA microemulsion (Neoral®), the drug should be started at moderate doses (not greater than 100–150mg/m^2/d in children or 4mg/kg/d in adults). Long-term treatment (with the attendant potential risks of cumulative nephrotoxicity) is usually required. The association with alternate-day prednisone for the first 6 months (40mg/m^2/48h for 2 months, followed by 30mg/m^2/48h for 2 months, and then by 20mg/48h for 2 months in children) may significantly improve the results (Cattran et al., 2007).

We do not believe that regular monitoring of blood CsA levels is needed, but we periodically measure trough (Co) levels to verify the compliance to treatment and to reduce the dosage if CsA post-dosing trough blood levels exceed 150ng/mL. If a patient does not show any improvement within 3–6 months CsA is probably ineffective and should be withdrawn. In case of complete remission CsA may be gradually tapered off after 1–2 years of continuous therapy. A number of patients may subsequently relapse, but a long-term treatment with CsA reduces the probability of relapse. In case of relapse after discontinuation, CsA may be resumed and some patients may be maintained in remission by giving low-dose CsA for many years. Of course a continuous monitoring of renal function by GFR is required in these cases. A consensus conference recommended a repeat renal biopsy after 2–3 years of treatment with CsA (Cattran et al., 2007), although it may be difficult even for an expert pathologist to attribute increasing interstitial fibrosis and glomerular scarring to drug toxicity or natural progression of FSGS.

Tacrolimus

Although the experience with tacrolimus (also known as FK-506) in FSGS is more recent and limited in comparison with CsA, this drug proved to be able to induce remission in a number of small-series case reports of steroid-resistant patients with FSGS. No controlled trials in FSGS have been reported nor are there any head-to-head comparisons with CsA in FSGS.

In a prospective study (Bhimma et al., 2006) of 20 children with FSGS resistant to a short course of steroids, tacrolimus was administerd at doses adjusted to keep trough (Co) levels between 7–15ng/mL for 12 months in combination with low-dose steroids. At the end of the treatment period, eight (40%) children were in complete remission, nine (45%) were in partial remission, and three (15%) failed to respond. At last follow-up, in mean 27.5 months after cessation, five (25%) children were in complete remission, ten (50%) in partial remission, and two (10%) in relapse. Three children died from dialysis-related complications following cessation of tacrolimus treatment. Adverse events included sepsis (two), nausea (two), diarrhea (two), anemia (four) and worsening of hypertension (four).

In another prospective study (Gulati et al., 2008), 22 consecutive children with steroid-resistant nephrotic syndrome were given tacrolimus, adjusted to attain a trough (Co) level of 5–10ng/mL, and prednisone, which was subsequently tapered off and stopped. Of the 22 children, nine had MCN, eleven had FSGS, and the other two had diffuse mesangial hypercellularity on histopathology. Tacrolimus had to be withdrawn in three children because of side effects. Of the remaining nineteen children, complete remission was seen in

The Atlas

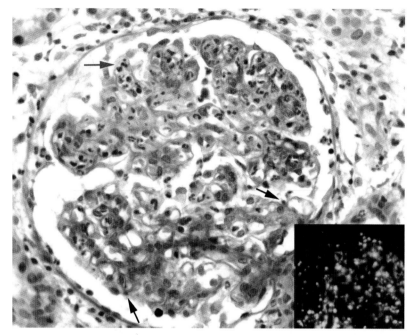

Plate 1 Acute post-infectious glomerulonephritis. Diffuse intracapillary hypercellularity with some small 'hump-like' deposit (black arrows) and polymorphs in the lumina (red arrow) (AFOG (aniline fucsin and orange G) stain × 63)). Insert: diffuse granular deposition of C3 ('starry sky') at immunofluorescence (× 50). *See also Chapter 4, p.154.*

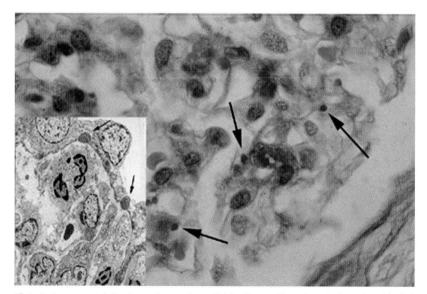

Plate 2 Acute post-infectious glomerulonephritis. 'Hump like' deposits in sub-epithelial position (arrows). (AFOG stain × 100). Insert. ovalar electrondense sub-epithelial deposits at electron microscopy (arrows) (× 9500). *See also Chapter 4, p.155.*

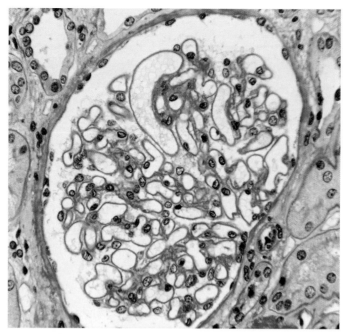

Plate 3 Minimal change disease. Light microscopy: the glomerulus is unremarkable; capillary lumina are patent, capillary walls are single contoured and there is no increase in cellularity (periodic acid-Schiff stain). *See also Chapter 5, p.179.*

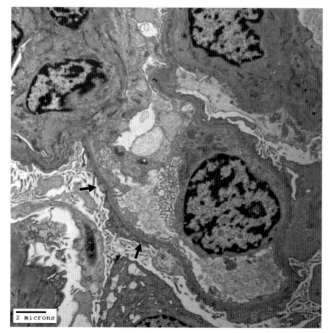

2 microns

Plate 4 Minimal change disease. Electron microscopy: glomerular capillaries with complete effacement of the processes of podocytes (arrows). Note microvillous transformation of the free surfaces of these cells. Basement membranes are normal. *See also Chapter 5, p.179.*

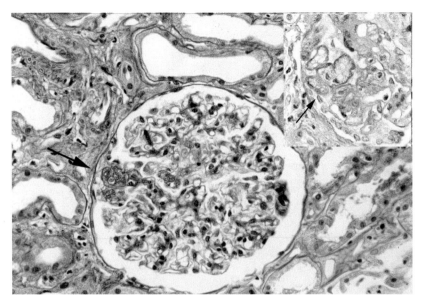

Plate 5 Focal segmental glomerulosclerosis ('classic' variant). Small area of capillary collapse and sclerosis at the periphery of an otherwise normal tuft (arrow) (AFOG stain × 63). *See also Chapter 6, p.217.*

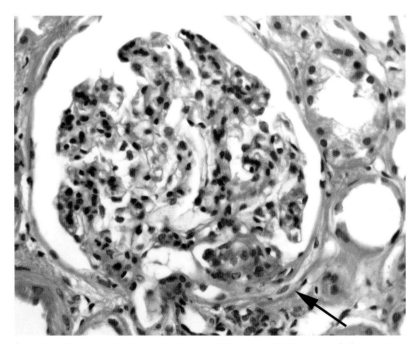

Plate 6 Focal segmental glomerulosclerosis ('hilar' variant). The area of glomerular sclerosis is adjacent to the vascular pole (arrow) (AFOG stain × 63). *See also Chapter 6, p.217.*

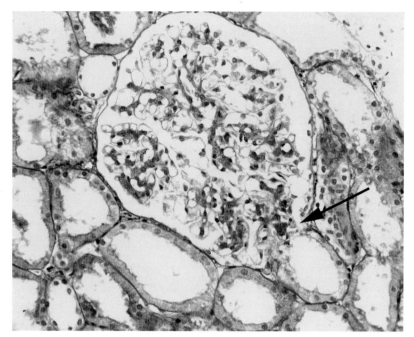

Plate 7 Focal segmental glomerulosclerosis ('tip' variant). Few collapsed capillaries adhere to swollen epithelial cells of the tubular pole of the glomerulus. (AFOG stain × 63). *See also Chapter 6, p.217.*

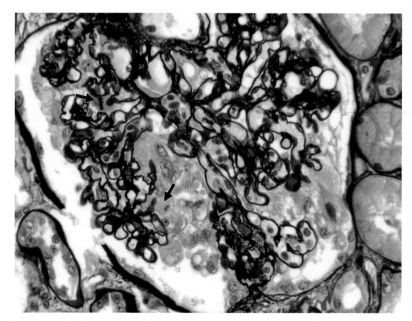

Plate 8 Focal and segmental glomerulosclerosis, collapsing type. Light microscopy: in this glomerulus, clusters of podocytes are enlarged, coarsely vacuolated and contain protein reabsorption droplets; mitotic figures are in several cells (arrows). Capillary walls in association. *See also Chapter 6, p.217.*

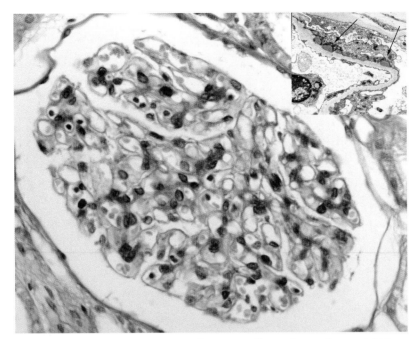

Plate 9 Membranous nephropathy. Initial stage. Capillary walls are of normal thickness (AFOG stain × 63). Insert: electron microscopy shows fine granular electrondense deposits in sub-epithelial position (arrows) (× 9100). *See also Chapter 7, p.261.*

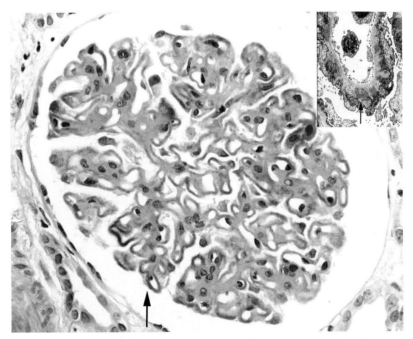

Plate 10 Membranous nephropathy. Later stage. Diffuse homogeneous thickening of capillary walls with coalescent granular (red) parietal deposits (AFOG stain × 63). Insert. sub-epithelial electrondense deposits are surrounded and partially covered by projections of newly formed basement membrane ('spikes') (× 7500). *See also Chapter 7, p.261.*

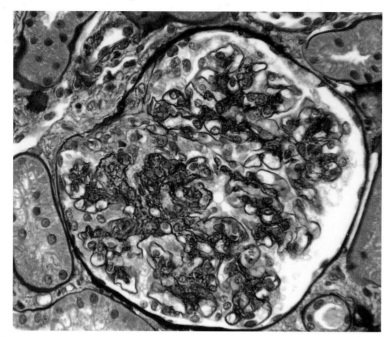

Plate 11 IgA nephropathy. Light microcopy: glomerulus with segmental increase in cellularity involving several mesangial regions. Capillary walls are single contoured. (periodic acid-methenamine silver stain). *See also Chapter 8, p.313.*

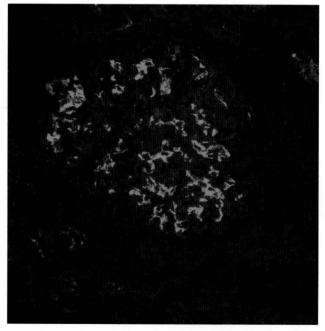

Plate 12 IgA nephropathy. Immunofluorescence: IgA deposits throughout mesangial regions of all lobules. *See also Chapter 8, p.314.*

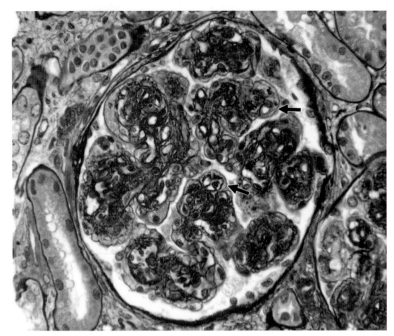

Plate 13 Membranoproliferative glomerulonephritis, type I. Light microscopy: the glomerulus has pronounced lobular architecture with increase in mesangial cellularity, leukocytes in some capillary lumina and many double-contoured capillary walls (arrows) (periodic acid-methenamine silver stain). *See also Chapter 9, p.377.*

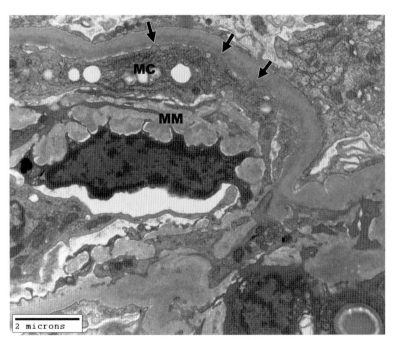

Plate 14 Membranoproliferative glomerulonephritis, type I. Electron microscopy: portion of glomerular capillary with thick wall because of interposition of mesangial cells (MC) and mesangial matrix (MM) between endothelial cell, the nucleus of which nearly fills the capillary lumen, and electron dense deposits (arrows) beneath the basement membrane. *See also Chapter 9, p.377.*

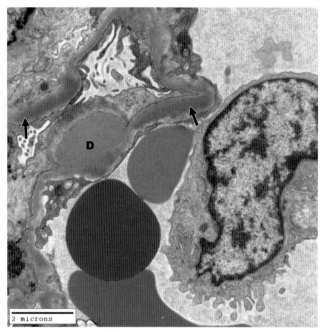

Plate 15 Membranoproliferative glomerulonephritis, type II (dense deposit disease). Electron micrograph with intramembranous elongated densities in several capillary walls (arrows); there is also a subepithelial hump shaped deposit (D). *See also Chapter 9, p.377.*

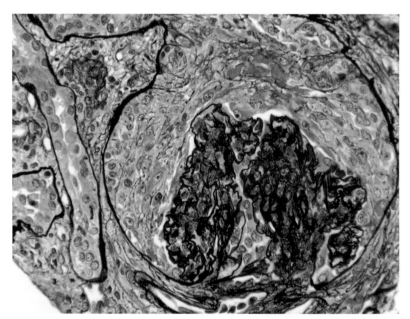

Plate 16 Crescentic glomerulonephritis. Light microscopy: glomerulus with extensive fresh crescent with cells and fibrin filling the urinary space and associated with compression and distortion of the capillary tufts (periodic acid-methenamine silver stain). *See also Chapter 10, p.399.*

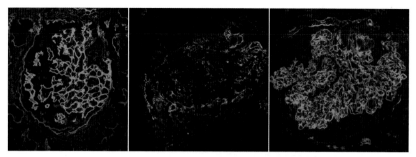

Plate 17 Crescentic glomerulonephritis. Immunofluorescence: this composite figure indicates the typical immunofluorescence patterns associated with crescentic glomerulonephritis.

A: linear IgG in all capillary walls, indicative of anti-glomerular basement membrane disease.

B: glomerulus with sparse and widely scattered granular deposits of C3, indicative of pauci-immune crescentic glomerulonephritis.

C: widespread granular deposits of C3 in mesangial regions and capillary walls, indicative of immune complex glomerulonephritis. *See also Chapter 10, p.401.*

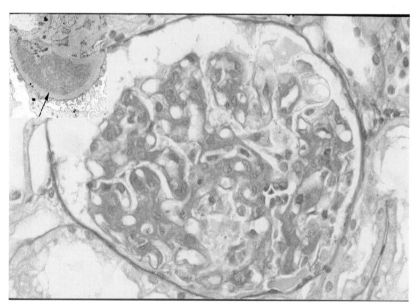

Plate 18 Fibrillary glomerulonephritis. Mesangisal areas and capillary walls are expanded by acellular material (PAS stain × 63). Insert: electron microscopy shows accumulation of non-branching, randomly arranged fibrils (× 16500). *See also Chapter 11, p.436.*

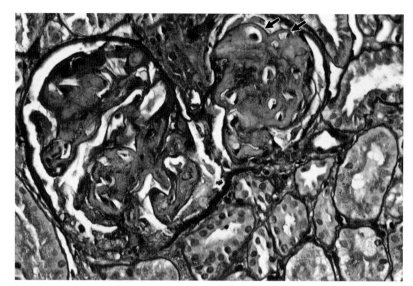

Plate 19 Collagenofibrotic glomerulopathy. Light microscopy: the glomeruli have widened mesangial regions with lighter staining material which is also present in the subendothelial aspects of capillary walls. Basement membranes are preserved (arrows) (periodic acid-Schiff stain). *See also Chapter 11, p.441.*

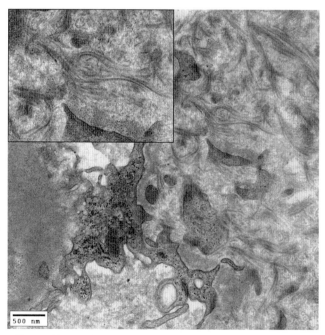

Plate 20 Collagenofibrotic glomerulopathy. Electron microscopy: the mesangium is replaced by collagen fibrils; some display defined periodicity and many are curved or frayed and are in irregularly-shaped bundles. The inset discloses these findings at higher magnification. *See also Chapter 11, p.441.*

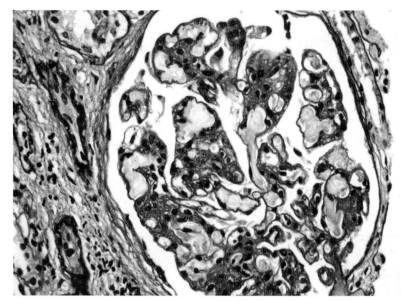

Plate 21 Lipoprotein glomerulopathy. Light microscopy: capillary lumina are filled with pale staining amorphous material forming 'thrombi.' There is widening and mild increase in cellularity of mesangial regions. Some capillary walls are double contoured (periodic acid-Schiff stain). *See also Chapter 11, p.450.*

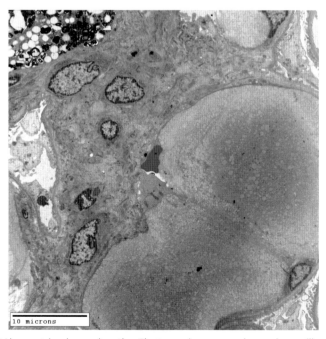

Plate 22 Lipoprotein glomerulopathy. Electron microscopy: glomerular capillary is filled with a mass of granular and finely vacuolated material. *See also Chapter 11, p.450.*

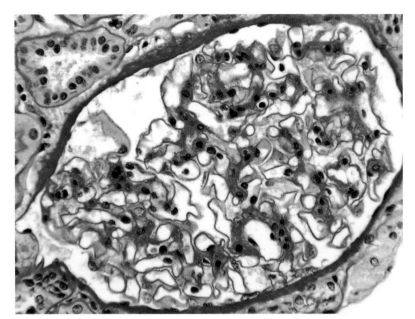

Plate 23 Mesangial proliferative glomerulonephritis. Glomerulus with mild widening of mesangial regions and mild increase in mesangial cellularity; there are no other abnormalities (periodic acid-Schiff stain). *See also Chapter 11, p.454.*

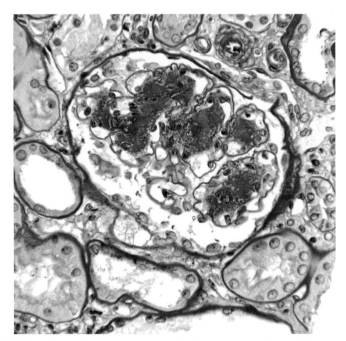

Plate 24 Idiopathic nodular glomerulosclerosis. The glomerulus has nodular appearance with increase in mesangial matrix and variable but mild increase in cellularity. Capillary basement membranes are of normal thickness and capillary lumina are patent. Note that there are no insudative lesions (hyalinosis) in the arterioles adjacent to the glomerulus (periodic acid-Schiff stain). *See also Chapter 11, p.465.*

sixteen (84%), two children (10.5%) attained partial remission and one was non-responsive. The mean time to achieve remission was 63.2 ± 44 days. The mean GFR values at the end of the study were similar to those prior to starting Tacrolimus.

Thus, observational studies show that tacrolimus may obtain a high rate of remissions but side effects are not rare and there is a high risk of relapse after withdrawal. There are no comparative trials to evaluate whether tacrolimus or CsA should be preferred for the treatment of patients who are resistant or intolerant to glucocorticoids. At present the indications and the recommendations for the use of tacrolimus in FSGS are similar to those of CsA. It should be reminded that the risk of nephrotoxicity and other major complications is mainly dose-related. Thus, we recommend that when tacrolimus is used for maintenance the mean dosage should be kept ≤ 0.1mg/kg/d (with the exception of small children who may require higher doses) and trough (Co) blood levels under 5–7ng/mL (or mcg/L) When compared to CsA, tacrolimus does not cause hypertrichosis or gum hypertrophy and has a minor impact on lipid profile but it is more diabetogenic and may cause alopecia or seizures (children only) in a few cases. The data in FSGS are insufficient to make any choice between CsA or tacrolimus. The decision would be more based on side-effect tolerance.

mTOR inhibitors

Sirolimus

The potential indications for sirolimus (rapamycin) in FSGS are controversial as a number of reports in kidney transplant recipients pointed out the onset of proteinuria, sometimes in a nephrotic range, in patients who were switched from calcineurin inhibitors to sirolimus. The mechanisms responsible for proteinuria are far from being elucidated but possible hypothesis are apoptosis of podocytes, apoptosis of epithelial tubular cells inhibiting protein reabsorption, previous presence of proteinuria masked by the use of calcineurin inhibitors. Whatever the mechanism(s) the possible proteinuric effect, associated with drug-related hyperlipidemia, does not render sirolimus a very attractive alternative treatment for FSGS. As a matter of fact, some trials with sirolimus had to be interrupted because of severe side effects including rapid renal function deterioration, not always reversible after withdrawal of sirolimus, hyperlipidemia, or increasing proteinuria (Kamar et al., 2007).

In spite of these reservations, favorable results were reported by a single prospective, open-label uncontrolled trial conducted in 21 patients with idiopathic, steroid-resistant FSGS (Tumlin et al., 2006). After 6 months, sirolimus therapy (at doses not specified) was associated with complete remission in four (19%) patients and partial remissions in eight (38%). Among sirolimus-responsive patients, proteinuria decreased from a mean of 8.8 to 2.1g/24 h. In responsive patients, GFR was maintained throughout the study, whereas tended to decrease in non-responders. At present we remain concerned that in patients with FSGS the side effects of sirolimus may exceed its potential benefits, still not demonstrated, in a controlled trial, and do not recommend its use in FSGS. The drug is not approved for use in FSGS in the USA by the FDA or in Europe by the EMEA.

Rituximab

The anti-CD20 antibody rituximab has been used successfully as a rescue therapy in some patients with recurrent FSGS after renal transplantation. Anecdotal cases of patients with idiopathic FSGS who responded to rituximab have been reported. Relapse occurred with the reappearance of CD-19+ B– lymphocytes (a marker of CD-20+ B– lymphocytes) that had been eliminated by rituximab. The doses used varied between 375mg/m^2 per dose at weekly intervals for 4–6 weeks and a single dose of 1g repeated after 2 weeks. With the limited information available, no substantial adverse effects have been reported (Dötschet al., 2008), but over-immunosuppression could theoretically cause opportunistic infections to emerge. Although the preliminary results are promising, further studies with long-term follow-up for evaluation of both safety and efficacy are needed before using rituximab in FSGS. The drug is not approved for use in FSGS in the USA or by EMEA in Europe.

Apheresis and immunoabsorption

Plasmapheresis (plasma exchange) and *immunoabsorption* with protein A have been shown to be useful in reducing proteinuria in patients with post-transplant recurrence of FSGS, perhaps by removing a hypothetical circulating permeability factor. Some single-case reports pointed out good results with these techniques also in patients with primary FSGS and severe nephrotic syndrome refractory to treatment. There are no randomized clinical trials with such approaches in native FSGS.

Muso et al. (1994) treated with *LDL apheresis*, pravastatin, prednisone, and intravenous methylprednisolone eight adults with FSGS and steroid-resistant nephrotic syndrome. A partial remission of proteinuria to non-nephrotic levels was seen in five patients (but serum albumin remained under 3g/dL in one patient) while the three other patients remained nephrotic. These results are intriguing but were obtained in a small number of patients with short follow-up. Moreover one cannot exclude a beneficial role for the aggressive therapy with glucocorticoids. A few other single-case reports also found that LDL apheresis may obtain long-term remission in steroid-resistant patients. Waiting for further studies, this expensive procedure of unknown benefit and risk should be reserved, at present, for desperate cases in which the disorder and the accompanying nephrotic syndrome are truly life-threatening.

Pirfenidone

Pirfenidone is an orally available antifibrotic agent that has shown benefit in animal models of pulmonary and renal fibrosis and in clinical trials of pulmonary fibrosis, multiple sclerosis, and hepatic cirrhosis.

An open-label trial was performed to evaluate the safety and efficacy of pirfenidone in patients with idiopathic and postadaptive FSGS (Cho et al., 2007). Patients received angiotensin antagonist therapy if tolerated. Twenty-one patients were enrolled, and eighteen patients completed a median of 13 months of pirfenidone treatment. The monthly change in GFR improved from a median of -0.61 mL/min per 1.73m^2 during the baseline period to -0.45 mL/min per 1.73m^2 with pirfenidone therapy. This change represents a median of 25% improvement in the rate of decline. Pirfenidone had no effect on blood pressure or proteinuria. Adverse events attributed to therapy included dyspepsia, sedation, and photosensitive dermatitis. A larger trial with pirfenidone is now under way in the US.

Practical recommendations

Is focal glomerulosclerosis primary or secondary?

Before planning any treatment, the physician should always ascertain whether the FSGS is idiopathic in its nature or secondary to other diseases, conditions or drugs or conditions (see Table 6.2). This may prove difficult to establish in some particular instances (e.g., in the elderly, obese, hypertensive, or in patients with a congenitally single kidney, etc.). The secondary forms caused by maladaptive glomerular hemodynamic alterations may be distinguished by the absence of hypoalbuminemia, hypercholesterolemia, and edema in spite of nephrotic levels of proteinuria. Renal biopsy may provide some clues for differential diagnosis. Four histological features may allow a correct diagnosis of segmental glomerular lesions:

- The proportion of glomeruli affected (that is whether the lesions are focal or diffuse).
- The position of segmental lesions within glomeruli.
- The size of glomeruli.
- The ultrastructural features, notably the extent of foot-process effacement.

Table 6.7 Clinical and histological criteria used to differentiate idiopathic FSGS from secondary or maladaptive forms

Clinical features:	Hypoalbuminemia, hypercholesterolemia, and edema are generally present in patients with idiopathic FSGS along with nephrotic range proteinuria while they are often absent in patients with maladaptive FSGS in spite of nephrotic proteinuria.
Histological features:	In the idiopathic FSGS affected glomeruli are focally distributed while lesions are more diffuse in maladaptive FSGS. Initial sclerotic lesions are located at the tip of glomeruli in the idiopathic FSGS and in the hilar position in maladaptive forms. Mesangial proliferation may be seen in the idiopathic FSGS. In the maladaptive forms the glomeruli are larger.
	On electron microscopy there is a general effacement of foot processes in the idiopathic FSGS while <50% of glomeruli show effacement of foot processes in the maladaptive forms.

In the idiopathic, primary form of FSGS the sclerotic lesions are focally and randomly distributed, at least in the early stages of the disease. The presence of large glomeruli associated with sclerosing lesions confined to the hilus of the glomerular tuft lesions suggests hemodynamic or maladaptive changes, while the presence of Tip lesions recalls idiopathic FSGS or MCN. The presence of mesangial hypercellularity is more typical of the idiopathic form of FSGS. Very extensive presence of electron dense deposits in the mesangium or subendothelial areas should indicate another primary or systemic disease. The presence of <50% effacement of the foot-processes along the capillary surface should suggest a secondary rather than primary FSGS (Table 6.7).

HIV-associated and heroin-associated FSGS have a clear etiology; their histological findings are similar to those seen in idiopathic forms, but lesions are more severe, most often of the collapsing variety, and extensive tubulo-reticular structures may be found in endothelial cells. These forms progress to ESRD within a few months compared with the slower progression for idiopathic primary FSGS.

Which FSGS patients should be offered genetic testing?

There is agreement that genetic testing should be offered for the subjects with a familial form of FSGS, in order to identify the responsible gene. This will provide additional data on a genotype/phenotype correlation and might also be clinically informative in situations where living-related donor transplant is considered. Causal mutations in four genes *(NPHS1, NPHS2, WT1, LAMB2)* explain the majority (60%) of nephrotic syndrome that present in the first year of life. Thus, whenever a nephrotic syndrome develops in a very precocious age or in the presence of a strong family history suggesting an autosomal recessive or autosomal dominant inheritance pattern, a genetic screening should be performed before starting treatment.

In the absence of a positive family history, genetic testing still may be considered. Clinicians cannot establish on clinical grounds whether a given sporadic (non-familial) case of FSGS is or is not inherited, since in some (nuclear) families a recessive disease will be apparent in only one child. In sporadic patients, the role of genetic testing will depend on the frequency of the different forms of inherited FSGS and on the response to specific treatment, since most (although not all) inherited podocyte diseases do not respond to any therapy.

In a child ≥2 years or in an adult with nephrotic-range proteinuria and FSGS, genetic testing should not change the initial evaluation. However, it is now clear that a significant fraction (25%) of sporadic FSGS resistant to steroid treatment in children is due to *NPHS2* mutations. Thus, in a child with new-onset nephrotic syndrome that does respond to steroids, *NPHS2* testing is warranted. On the contrary, recessive *NPHS2* mutations are rare in adult white FSGS patients, and *NPHS2* mutation screening should not be recommended for FSGS adult population.

Mutations in other podocytopathy genes are much less likely to be a cause of FSGS, and it is hard to make the case for routine testing of any gene other than *NPHS2*.

Should non-nephrotic patients with FSGS be treated?

Patients with FSGS who have sustained non-nephrotic levels of proteinuria <2.0g/d usually do not progress to renal failure, are not exposed to the possible complications of the nephrotic syndrome, and are generally asymptomatic. Therefore 'specific' treatment is not strictly necessary for these patients. Control of blood pressure however should always be vigorous, preferably using angiotensin-converting enzyme inhibitors (ACEi), angiotensin receptor blockers (ARB), or both (see Chapter 1).

One of the most difficult areas of management of FSGS is for those patients who have persisting protein excretion rates between 2.0–3.5/d, do not have hypoalbuminemia, but have some mild-to-moderate decrease in renal function. These patients are often hypertensive and are good candidates for treatment with ACEi and/or ARB (see Chapter 1). Along with vigorous blood pressure control these agents have been shown to be able to decrease the level of proteinuria and slow the progression of renal insufficiency in patients with FSGS (Korbet, 2003), although randomized controlled trials specific for FSGS are lacking. These drugs are often given to patients with primary FSGS and appear to be of particular value for patients with FSGS secondary to conditions associated with hyperfiltration and/or reduced nephron mass and those patients with non-nephrotic primary FSGS. Statins are also recommended not only to lower lipid levels but also because they may have a protective role against cardiovascular disease and may even reduce proteinuria (Campese and Park, 2007). If proteinuria does not remit or fall below 2.0g/d with these measures and the overall clinical condition of the patient is favorable we feel justified a trial with glucocorticoids in a patient with sub-nephrotic proteinuria (2.0–3.5g/d) to obtain a full remission of proteinuria to <2.0g/d and hopefully slow the progression to renal failure.

Should nephrotic patients with FSGS be treated with 'specific' therapy?

An aggressive approach is justified in nephrotic patients with FSGS both because spontaneous complete remission of proteinuria is very rare and because patients with persistent nephrotic-range proteinuria usually progress to ESRD. On the contrary, if it is possible to induce complete or partial remission, the long term renal outcome is generally favorable. A further reason in favor of treatment is that nephrotic patients may be exposed to an increased risk of severe and even life-threatening complications, including intravascular thrombosis and cardiovascular disease. Moreover, nephrotic patients need several drugs to control edema, hyperlipidemia, electrolyte disorders, etc. Each of these drugs has a cost and potential side effects.

Treatment for nephrotic patients

Even if we lack randomized controlled trials showing the superiority of glucocorticoids over placebo in FSGS, a number of observational studies have shown that an initial short-term course with glucocorticoids, is generally safe and can obtain response in at least some patients (around 20–25%). Usually this first therapeutic approach consists of high-dose oral prednisone ($60mg/m^2/d$ for children; 1mg/kg/d for adults) for 2 months. For patients who respond the subsequent treatment may be similar to that of MCN, including the management of possible relapses (see Chapter 5). However, only a relatively few patients can be anticipated to respond to this initial treatment regimen (perhaps one in four to five treated patients).

It remains quite uncertain as to what is the best course for patients who do not respond to an initial short-term course of glucocorticoids. Until recently, many clinicians preferred to stop any form of 'specific' treatment and to provide only 'symptomatic' therapy, including angiotensin II inhibition (see Chapter 1) in order not to expose patients with little chances of responding to the possible iatrogenic morbidity of continued glucocorticoid or immunosuppressive therapy. In this regard, it must be pointed out that combined treatments with low-salt diet, diuretics, hypolipidemic drugs, ACEi or ARB, and anti-thrombotic agents may maintain some patients asymptomatic (including edema free), although their influence on progression to renal failure in primary FSGS specifically is still unproven. The attitude of nephrologists toward treatment of the patients with FSGS who do not display any response at all to short-term steroid treatment has changed after the demonstration that >50% of nephrotic patients with primary FSGS will respond to more prolonged steroid therapy or to other treatments. Thus, several different, but equally acceptable, therapeutic approaches may be suggested in patients who do not respond to a short-term course of glucocorticoids.

♦ Observational, non-randomized trials provided consistent evidence that patients with FSGS, who are resistant to an 8-week course with oral prednisone in high-dosage, may subsequently respond to a more prolonged steroid administration. Thus, according to the GRADE approach (Uhlig et al., 2006) it is possible to suggest that unless steroid toxicity develops after the first 8 weeks of intense high-dose steroid therapy, prednisone may be continued in tapering doses for another 8–16 weeks or longer, depending on response and side effects. About 50–60% of patients treated in this fashion can be expected to respond with a remission (complete or partial). However, some patients who tolerated a short-term course of glucocorticoids may develop steroid-related toxicity when treatment is prolonged (diabetes, obesity, Cushingoid appearance, infections, cataracts, bone complications, psychiatric reactions, etc.). Particularly delicate is the problem in children. In them, a prolonged administration of glucocorticoids can reduce the growth velocity and can be responsible for irreversible stature retardation. Moreover, a number of responders may develop frequent relapses or steroid dependency aggravating the problem further.

♦ A good therapeutical option for patients who do not respond to a short course of glucocorticoids is represented by calcineurin inhibitors. Observational and randomized controlled studies, showed that CsA, especially when associated with steroids, can induce complete or partial response of proteinuria in 50–60% of nephrotic patients with FSGS who were initially steroid unresponsive. These data provide a good quality of evidence and a rationale for recommending CsA, particularly in patients at risk of complications with glucocorticoids and in children, to allow to catch a normal growth rate, and to avoid the esthetic changes of steroids that may reduce the adherence to prescriptions. However, some guidelines must be carefully followed with the use of CsA (see Chapter 2). In particular, patients with sustained renal insufficiency (i.e., a GFR <60mL/min), arterial hypertension, diffuse glomerular sclerosis, and/or moderately advanced tubulointerstitial lesions at renal biopsy should be considered poor candidates for CsA therapy. CsA should be stopped in patients who do not respond within 6 months as they are unlikely to remit later (Cattran et al., 2007). In patients who respond with a partial or complete remission with CsA, the treatment may be gradually tapered off after 6–12 months in order to identify the minimal effective dosage. A few patients treated for 2 years or more may be able to maintain a stable remission after a progressive tapering of CsA to zero. Fewer studies with tacrolimus are available, but the impression is that the efficacy and the limits of tacrolimus are comparable to those of CsA.

♦ A further option, in steroid and/or CNI intolerant patients is represented by mycophenolate salts. MMF at a dose of 2g/d (or sodium mycophenolate at a dose of 1440mg/d) may be given for 6 months and continued at half doses for another 18–24 months. It should be pointed out, however, that the current evidence is insufficient to place much confidence that a good result will be obtained by this strategy, and the drug is not approved in the USA or the EC for its use in FSGS.

♦ An 8–12-week course with an alkylating agent may obtain the same rate of response than a short course of high-dose prednisone and may be therefore indicated as a primary treatment in patients who have contraindications to glucocorticoids. However, there is no evidence that cytotoxic drugs can obtain good results in patients with FSGS who do not respond to glucocorticoids and its use in steroid-resistant patients cannot be suggested.

In summary, we propose the following regimen for nephrotic patients with FSGS (Fig. 6.2). An initial course of 8 weeks with full-dose prednisone (60mg/m^2/d in children; 1mg/kg/d in adults) should be offered to all nephrotic patients who do not have specific contraindications to glucocorticoids. For responders who do not relapse, treatment should be stopped; for those patients who have frequent or infrequent relapses treatment should be the same as that used for steroid-sensitive relapsers with MCN (see Chapter 5). In case of poor response but good tolerance prednisone should be continued at tapering doses up to 4–6 months. A 12-week course with cyclophosphamide at a dose of 2mg/kg/d (with or without low-dose alternate day prednisone depending on the contraindications to steroids) can be proposed as a first treatment for patients with contraindications or intolerance to glucocorticoids. Alternatively,

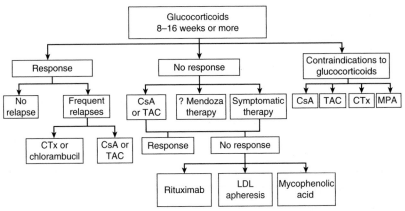

Fig. 6.2 Possible therapeutic options for a patient with primary FSGS and nephrotic syndrome. CsA: cyclosporine; TAC: tacrolimus; CTx: cyclophosphamide; MPA: mycophenolate mofetil or sodium mycophenolate.

cyclosporine may be given for 1–2 years. Mycophenolate salts may be offered to patients who have contraindications to glucocorticoids, cytotoxic drugs, or calcineurin inhibitors.

Whatever the therapeutic decision, it is mandatory that a nephrotic patient is followed carefully, so that the effectiveness and tolerance of the treatment can be checked on a regular basis. Clearly the therapeutic choice may be modified according to the clinical outcome or the development of side effects. A more aggressive approach from the outset may be tried in patients who develop severe, debilitating nephrotic syndrome or progressive renal failure. On the other hand, therapy may have to be stopped or modified in patients who do not respond or in those showing iatrogenic toxicity under the assigned treatment regimen.

What to do with patients with FSGS refractory to treatment?

There is little evidence that patients who do not respond to any of the previous treatments may benefit from further therapies, and the cumulative toxicity of treatment is a growing concern. In the case of no response, to the above described therapeutic regimens the physician may choose among *three* possible options for additional therapy according to the clinical status of the patient and his/her wishes and fears:

- Symptomatic therapy.
- Mendoza–Tune treatment.
- Oral cyclosporine (or tacrolimus) plus low-dose alternate day steroids (possibly combined with MMF).

Symptomatic therapy should be chosen in the case of a frail patient (often elderly or diabetic) particularly susceptible to the side effects of glucocorticoids or CsA. Mendoza treatment may be offered to those children who did not respond to glucocorticoids but showed a good tolerance to glucocorticoids. However, such a treatment is rarely used today because of the concern for its potential toxicity. CsA or tacrolimus may obtain some reduction of proteinuria even in patients refractory to glucocorticoids but should be used with caution in patients with reduced renal function. The choice between CsA and tacrolimus is mainly conditioned by the expected side effects and the tolerance of the individual patients for these effects. A few patients who did not respond to CsA were reported to respond to a switch to Tacrolimus—given however at relatively high dosage.

LDL apheresis, plasma exchange, immunoadsorption with column A, or rituximab have also been observed to be of benefit in sporadic case-reports. It is impossible to give recommendations on the basis of the scanty available data. Each treatment decision must be made on a case-by-case basis analyzing the potential (but largely unknown) benefits and the potential (and often known) risks. In taking these decisions we should always take into account the general clinical conditions of the patient and his/or her desires after an informed discussion of the benefits and risks. Written consent is often desirable when using approved drugs for off-label purposes

What to do in patients with FSGS and renal insufficiency?

Exceptional cases of improvement of renal function have been reported in patients with FSGS and advanced renal failure treated with plasmapheresis and low dose cyclophosphamide or with high-dose methylprednisolone pulses combined with oral cyclophosphamide. In general, however, there is not convincing evidence that any form of treatment is useful in patients who develop renal insufficiency despite treatment. Calcineurin inhibitors should not be used in these instances as they can further aggravate the kidney damage. Cytotoxic agents are generally ineffective and poorly tolerated by patients with reduced renal function. Glucocorticoids also should be used with caution. Mycophenolate salts may be better tolerated but there is no valuable information on their effectiveness in patients with deteriorating renal function due to progressive FSGS. Thus, in most cases we prefer not to insist with treatments which have little chances of efficacy and a high risk of iatrogenic toxicity; rather we maximize the symptomatic therapy with ACE-inhibitors, ARB, statins, antiplatelet agents. However, we suggest not to interrupt abruptly an immunosuppressive treatment, as this decision can accelerate the progression of renal failure in some cases. Therefore, it is better to reduce gradually the doses of the drugs used.

Transplantation

Recurrent FSGS

Patients with primary or idiopathic FSGS are at high risk of recurrence after renal transplantation. Approximately 20–40% of patients develop recurrence of FSGS in the first allograft and 90–100% have recurrence in the second allograft if a previous renal transplant failed because of FSGS recurrence. The risk of recurrence of FSGS in the renal allograft is higher in patients younger than 18 years, in recipients with good HLA matching (zero HLA mismatches), in patients with collapsing variant of FSGS, in patients with mesangial proliferative glomerulonephritis superimposed to FSGS, and in those who had a rapid progression to end stage renal disease (Table 6.8). Second grafts in those who have had recurrence in their first graft are generally accompanied by a further recurrence, but sporadic cases of success have also been reported. As mentioned earlier, the familial forms of FSGS associated with NPHS2 mutation seldom recur following transplantation, and even if a recurrence does develop it is generally mild and responsive to treatment. Also, patients with the sporadic variety of FSGS who also have homozygous or complex heterozygous podocin mutations have a low recurrence rate. In the other patients with sporadic FSGS, a more complex and likely multifactorial etiology accounts for the recurrence of FSGS. The results with living donation in FSGS are worse than in patients without FSGS, but better than those observed with cadaver renal transplantation. The risk of recurrence is higher in white than in non-white patients (Abbott et al., 2001).

Table 6.8 Factors that may influence the risk of post-transplant recurrence of FSGS

Risk factors for recurrence	Low risk of recurrence
Age under 18 years	Familial form
Good HLA match	Sporadic form with *NPHS2* mutation
Rapid progression to uremia	Slow progression to uremia
Positive circulating permeability factor (?)	Non nephrotic proteinuriain the original disease
Second transplant after loss of first transplant from recurrence	
White ancestry	
Superimposed mesangial proliferation at renal biopsy	

There are two clinical presentations of FSGS after transplantation; an *early recurrence* with massive proteinuria within hours to days after implantation of the new kidney and a *late* (more insidious) *recurrence* several months or years after transplantation. In patients with early recurrence, proteinuria, usually in a nephrotic range, may precede the development of histological lesions that develop in a median 10–18d after transplantation. Initial biopsies may show normal-appearing glomeruli by light microscopy but diffuse foot process effacement by electron microscopy (e.g., minimal change nephropathy). Segmental sclerosing lesions associated with endocapillary proliferation, foam cell accumulation may occur later and progress to glomerular sclerosis and interstitial fibrosis. Spontaneous remission of proteinuria is exceptional. Patients with early recurrence of FSGS have a high risk of graft failure. Late recurrence is rare and it is difficult to distinguish from *de novo* FSGS. The outcome is relentless but slower than in cases with early relapse.

The pathogenesis of recurrent FSGS is far from being established. The frequent occurrence of a rapid or even immediate relapse of proteinuria after transplantation suggests that at least some patients with FSGS have circulating factor(s) capable of altering glomerular permeability in normal grafts (Savin et al., 2003). However, despite an intensive research the presence and the nature of this factor are still speculative. Use of research bio-assays for this putative permeability factor and its utility in predicting recurrence has met with conflicting results. More recently the attention of the investigators focused on the inter-podocyte connection. The slit-diaphragm is structurally formed by extracellular proteins (such as nephrin, P-cadherin etc) anchored by a protein called podocin. It has been hypothesized that the permeability factors may induce redistribution and loss of nephrin as well as reduced expression of podocin. Cases of FSGS associated with mutation of *NPHS2* (encoding for podocin) have been reported both in familial and sporadic forms of FSGS. The risk of recurrence in patients with *NPHS2* (podocin) mutation is low but not zero, around 8%. However, caution should be recommended in transplanting these patients with *NPHS2* mutations with the kidney of their parents who are obligate carriers of *NPHS2* mutation, because it could increase the risk of recurrence (Vincenti and Ghiggeri, 2005). A role for costimulatory molecule B7-1 in podocytes as an inducible modifier of glomerular permselectivity has been suggested. B7-1 in podocytes was found in genetic, drug-induced, immune-mediated, and bacterial toxin-induced experimental kidney diseases with nephrotic syndrome. It is also possible that a subset of patients with FSGS may produce anti-actin, anti-ATP synthase, anti-nephrin autoantibodies that may co-operate in altering glomerular permeability.

The management of patients with recurrent FSGS and nephrotic syndrome is difficult and not well established (Table 6.9). An amelioration of proteinuria

Table 6.9 Treatment of recurrent FSGS after renal transplantation

Prevention:	Pre-transplant plasmapheresis (plasma exchange) may reduce the risk of recurrence
Treatment:	If proteinuria ≥2g/d, start with plasma exchanges (an exchange a day for 3d, then 2–3 exchanges per week for 2 weeks, followed by 1–2 exchange per week) or immunoadsorption with protein A (an exchange a day for 3 days, then 2–3 exchanges per week for 2 weeks, followed by 1–2 exchange per week)
	If no response one may try with rituximab ($375mg/m^2$ every week for 4 weeks)
	High-dose ACE-inhibitors or angiotensin-receptor blockers should be used as adjuvant therapy.

may be obtained in a few children with very high doses of CsA. The aim of such an approach is to compensate the lipid binding of CsA by elevated low density lipoprotein concentrations and the increase clearance of CsA seen in young children. However, the long-term efficacy and tolerance of such a therapy remains to be established.

The most commonly used therapeutic approach is represented by the use of plasmapheresis or immunoadsorption with protein A. The following patterns of response may be expected:

◆ Complete and sustained remission of proteinuria after a short course.

◆ Complete or partial remission with relapse of nephrotic proteinuria within weeks or months.

◆ Improvement of proteinuria with an early relapse after plasmapheresis is interrupted.

◆ No response.

However, it is impossible at present to predict which the response to plasmapheresis will be for the single patient. A protective role of prophylactic plasmapheresis before transplantation has also been reported (Gohh et al., 2005; Mahesh et al., 2008).

A long-term beneficial effect of rituximab, given weekly for 6 weeks, has been first reported in a child with a lymphoproliferative disorder and FSGS recurrence after transplantation by Pescovitz et al., (2006). Other single-case reports confirmed the benefit of rituximab, but the enthusiasm has been attenuated by the data of the group of Vincenti in San Francisco. No response at all was found after treatment with rituximab in four adults with recurrence of FSGS after kidney transplantation (Yabu et al., 2008).

In summary, a genetic evaluation is advisable before transplanting a patient with FSGS, since patients with mutation of a podocyte protein component have a low risk of recurrence. To prevent FSGS recurrence in the other patients we suggest preemptive plamapheresis whenever possible, and particularly in patients receiving the kidney from a living donor and in those who lost a previous transplant from recurrence. After transplantation, proteinuria may herald the development of FSGS even if early biopsy does not show glomerular abnormalities at light microscopy. Patients with FSGS due to the *NPHS2* mutation are at low risk of recurrence and thus would not need any preemptive management. Patients with post-transplant proteinuria >2g/d who have FSGS as their original disease should be treated as soon as possible with an intensive course of plasmapheresis (an exchange a day for 3d, then 2–3 exchanges per week for the first 2 weeks, followed by 1–2 exchanges per week using 5% albumin as the replacement fluid). It should be kept in mind that in some cases prolonged plasmapheresis, even for many months, is needed before seeing complete or partial remission of proteinuria. If a complete disappearance of proteinuria is obtained, plasmapheresis treatment may be stopped. A further course of plasmapheresis may be attempted in the case of relapse of nephrotic proteinuria. If proteinuria improves but remains over 2–3g/d, long-term plasma exchange therapy may be given at longer intervals. In one of our patients with recurrent nephrotic syndrome whenever plasmapheresis was interrupted, we continued plasmapheresis every 2–4 weeks for 7 years. We also recommend the administration of high-dose ACEi, ARB, and statins in order to exploit their anti-proteinuric and anti-lipemic effects. The role of rituximab should be better elucidated by further studies, but in the absence of contraindication a course with rituximab might be attempted if plasmapheresis is of no benefit. However the optimal doses and duration of treatment with rituximab have not been established. In the few available reports the schedules varied from $375mg/m^2$ every week for 4 weeks to 1g given 2 weeks apart, repeated at 6 months.

De novo FSGS

Cases of *de novo* FSGS after kidney transplantation are mainly sustained by the nephrotoxic calcineurin inhibitors. Studies of CsA in non-renal transplantation have clearly shown that CsA can induce FSGS. Some cases may occur also in patients with reduced renal mass due to a large discrepancy between the size of donor and recipient, or to polar resection needed to remove cysts, stones or tumors.

References

Abbate M, Zoja C, Rottoli D, Corna D, Tomasoni S, Remuzzi G (2002). Proximal tubular cells promote fibrogenesis by TGF-beta1-mediated induction of peritubular myofibroblasts. *Kidney International* **61**:2066–77.

Abbott KC, Sawyers ES, Oliver JD III, et al. (2001). Graft loss due to recurrent focal segmental glomerulosclerosis in renal transplant recipients in the United States. *American Journal of Kidney Diseases* 37:366–73.

Banfi G, Moriggi M, Sabadini E, Fellin G, D'Amico G, Ponticelli C (1991). The impact of prolonged immunosuppression on the outcome of idiopathic focal segmental glomerulosclerosis with nephrotic syndrome in adults. *Clinical Nephrology* 36:53–9.

Bazzi C, Petrini C, Rizza V et al. (2003). Fractional excretion of IgG predicts renal outcome and response to therapy in primary focal segmental glomerulosclerosis: a pilot study. *American Journal of Kidney Diseases* 41:328–35.

Bhimma R, Adhikari M, Asharam K, Connolly C (2006) Management of steroid-resistant focal segmental glomerulosclerosis in children using tacrolimus. *American Journal of Nephrology* 26:544–51.

Borges FF, Shiraichi L, da Silva MP, Nishimoto EI, Nogueira PC (2007). Is focal segmental glomerulosclerosis increasing in patients with nephrotic syndrome? *Pediatric Nephrology* 22:1309–13.

Boyer O, Moulder JK, Somers MJ (2007). Focal and segmental glomerular sclerosis in children: a longitudinal assessment. *Pediatric Nephrology* 22:1159–66.

Cade R, Mars D, Privette M et al. (1986). Effect of long-term administration of azathioprine in patients with minimal change glomerulonephritis and nephritic syndrome resistant to corticosteroids. *Archives of Internal Medicine* 146:737–41.

Cameron, J. S. (1992). The long-term outcome of glomerular diseases. In RN Schrier and CW Gottschalk (eds), *Diseases of the kidney*, 2nd edn, pp.1895–958. Little Brown, Boston, MA.

Campese VM, Park J (2007). HMG-CoA reductase inhibitors and renal function. *Clinical Journal of the American Society of Nephrology* 2:1100–3.

Cattran DC, Rao P (1998). Long-term outcome in children and adults with classic focal segmental glomerulosclerosis. *American Journal of Kidney Diseases* 32:72–9.

Cattran DC, Appel GB, Hebert LA, et al. (1999). A randomized trial of cyclosporine in patients with steroid-resistant focal segmental glomerulosclerosis. North America Nephrotic Syndrome Study Group. *Kidney International* 56:2220–6.

Cattran DC, Alexopoulos E, Heering P, et al. (2007). Cyclosporin in idiopathic glomerular disease associated with the nephrotic syndrome: Workshop recommendations. *Kidney International* 72:1429–47.

Cattran DC, Reich HN, Beanlands HJ, et al. (2008). The impact of sex in primary glomerulonephritis. *Nephrology Dialysis Transplantation* 23:2247–53.

Cho ME, Smith DC, Branton MH, Penzak SR, Kopp JB (2007). Pirfenidone slows renal function deterioration in patients with focal segmental glomerulosclerosis. *Clinical Journal of the American Society of Nephrology* 2:906–13.

Chun MJ, Korbet SM, Schwartz MM, Lewis EJ. (2004) Focal segmental glomerulosclerosis in nephrotic adults: presentation, prognosis, and response to therapy of the histologic variants. *Journal of the American Society Nephrology* 15:2169–77.

Crook ED, Habeeb D, Gowdy O, Nimmagadda S, Salem M. (2005) Effects of steroids in focal segmental glomerulosclerosis in a predominantly African-American population. *American Journal of Medical Science* 33:19–24.

D'Agati VD, Fogo AB, Bruijn JA, Jennette JC (2004). Pathologic classification of focal segmental glomerulosclerosis: a working proposal. *American Journal of Kidney Diseases* 43:368–82.

Deegens JK, Wetzels JF (2007). Fractional excretion of high- and low-molecular weight proteins and outcome in primary focal segmental glomerulosclerosis. *Clinical Nephrology* **68**:201–8.

Di Duca M, Oleggini R, Sanna-Cherchi S et al. (2006). Cis and trans regulatory elements in NPHS2 promoter: implications in proteinuria and progression of renal diseases. *Kidney International* **70**:1332–41.

Dixit M, Mansur A, Dixit N, Gilman J, Santarina L, Glicklich D (2002). The role of ACE gene polymorphism in rapidity of progression of focal segmental glomerulosclerosis. *Journal of Postgraduate Medicine* **48**:266–9.

Dötsch J, Müller-Wiefel DE, Kemper MJ (2008). Rituximab: is replacement of cyclophosphamide and calcineurin inhibitors in steroid-dependent nephrotic syndrome possible? *Pediatric Nephrology* **23**:3–7.

Dragovic D, Rosenstock JL, Wahl SJ, Panagopoulos G, DeVita MV, Michelis MF (2005). Increasing incidence of focal segmental glomerulosclerosis and an examination of demographic patterns. *Clinical Nephrology* **63**:1–7.

Frishberg Y, Becker-Cohen R, Halle D, et al (1998). Genetic polymorphisms of the renin-angiotensin system and the outcome of focal segmental glomerulosclerosis in children. *Kidney International* **54**:1843–9.

Gohh RY, Yango AF, Morrissey PE et al. (2005). Preemptive plasmapheresis and recurrence of FSGS in high-risk renal transplant recipients. *American Journal Transplantation* **5**:2907–12.

Grone EF, Grone H-J (2008). Does hyperlipidemia injure the kidney? *Nature Clinical Practice Nephrology* **4**:424–5.

Gulati S, Prasad N, Sharma RK, Kumar A, Gupta A, Baburaj VP (2008). Tacrolimus: a new therapy for steroid-resistant nephrotic syndrome in children. *Nephrology Dialysis Transplantation* **23**:910–3.

Habashy D, Hodson EM, Craig JC (2003). Interventions for steroid-resistant nephrotic syndrome: a systematic review. *Pediatric Nephrology* **18**:906–12.

Heering P, Braun N, Müllejans R, et al. (2004). Cyclosporine A and chlorambucil in the treatment of idiopathic focal segmental glomerulosclerosis. *American Journal of Kidney Diseases* **43**:10–8.

Hill GS (2008) Hypertensive nephrosclerosis. *Current Opinions in Nephrology and Hypertension* **17**:266–70.

Hinkes B, Wiggins RC, Gbadegesin R, et al. (2006) Positional cloning uncovers mutations in PLCE1 responsible for a nephrotic syndrome variant that may be reversible. *Nature Genetics* **38**:1397–405.

Hughson MD, Samuel T, Hoy WE, Bertram JF (2007). Glomerular volume and clinico-pathologic features related to disease severity in renal biopsies of African Americans and whites in the southeastern United States. *Archives Pathology Laboratory Medicine* **131**:1665–72.

Kamar N, Frimat L, Blancho G, Wolff P, Delahousse M, Rostaing L (2007). Evaluation of the efficacy and safety of a slow conversion from calcineurin inhibitor- to sirolimus-based therapies in maintenance renal-transplant patients presenting with moderate renal insufficiency. *Transplant International* **20**:128–34.

Kitiyakara C, Eggers P, Kopp JB (2004). Twenty-one-year trend in ESRD due to focal segmental glomerulosclerosis in the United States. *American Journal of Kidney Diseases* **44**:815–25.

Korbet SM (2003). Angiotensin antagonists and steroids in the treatment of focal segmental glomerulosclerosis. *Seminars in Nephrology* **23**:219–28.

Korbet SM, Schwartz MM., Lewis, EJ (1994). Primary focal segmental glomerulosclerosis. Clinical course and response to therapy. *American Journal of Kidney Diseases* **23**:773–83.

Kriz W, Le Hir M (2005). Patwhays to nephron loss starting from glomerular diseases – insights from animal models. *Kidney International* **67**:404 –19.

Mahesh S, Del Rio M, Feverstein D et al. (2008). Demographics and response to therapeutic plasma exchange in pediatric renal transplantation for focal glomerulosclerosis: a single center experience. *Ped Transplantation* **12**: 682–8.

Meyrier A (2005). Mechanisms of disease: focal segmental glomerulosclerosis. *Nature Clinical Practice Nephrology* **1**:44–54.

Meyrier A, Niaudet P (2005). Minimal change and focal. Segmental glomular sclerosis in A Davison, JS Cameron, JP Grunfeld, et al. (eds) *Oxford Textobook of Clinical Nephrology*, pp.439-67. Oxford University Press, Oxford.

Muso E, Yashiro M, Matsushima M, Yoshida H, Sawanishi K, Sasayama S (1994). Does LDL-apheresis in steroid-resistant nephrotic syndrome affect prognosis? *Nephrology, Dialysis and Transplantation* **9**:257–64.

Niaudet P (2004). Genetic forms of nephrotic syndrome. *Ped Neph* **19**: 1313–8.

Nayagam LS,Ganguli A, Rathi M, et al. (2008). Mycophenolate mofetil or standard therapy for membranous nephropathy and focal segmental glomerulosclerosis:a pilot study. *Nephrology Dialysis Transplantation* **23**:1926–30.

Onetti Muda A, Feriozzi S, Cinotti GA, Faraggiana, T (1994). Glomerular hypertrophy and chronic renal failure in focal segmental glomerulosclerosis. *American Journal of Kidney Diseases* **23**:237–41.

Pescovitz MD, Book BK, Sidner RA (2006). Resolution of recurrent focal segmental glomerulosclerosis proteinuria after rituximab treatment. *New England Journal Medicine* **354**:1961–63.

Plank C, Kalb V, Hinkes B et al. (2008). Cyclosporin A is superior to cyclophosphamide in children with steroid-resistant nephrotic syndrome-a randomized controlled multicentre trial by the Arbeitsgemeinschaft für Pädiatrische Nephrologie. *Pediatric Nephrology* **23**:1483–93.

Ponticelli C, Passerini P (1999). The place of cyclosporine in the management of primary nephrotic syndrome. *Biodrugs* **12**:327–41.

Ponticelli C, Passerini P (2003). Other immunosuppressive agents for focal segmental glomerulosclerosis. *Seminars in Nephrology* **23**:242–8.

Ponticelli C, Rizzoni G, Edefonti A et al. (1993) A randomized trial of cyclosporine in steroid resistant nephrotic syndrome. *Kidney International* **43**:1377–84.

Ponticelli C, Villa M, Banfi G, et al (1999). Can prolonged treatment improve the prognosis in adults with focal segmental glomerulosclerosis? *American Journal of Kidney Diseases* **34**:618–25.

Praga M, Morales E (2006). Obesity, proteinuria and progression of renal failure. *Current Opinion in Nephrology and Hypertension* **15**:481–6.

Savin VJ, Mc Carthy ET, Sharma M (2003). Permeability factors in focal segmental glomerulosclerosis. *Seminar in Nephrol* **23**: 147–60.

Schena PF, Cameron, JS (1988). Treatment of proteinuric idiopathic glomerulonephritis in adults: a retrospective study. *American Journal of Medicine* **85**:315–26.

Sepe V, Libetta C, Giuliano MG, Adamo G, Dal Canton A (2008). Mycophenolate mofetil in primary glomerulopathies. *Kidney International* **73**:154–62.

Stokes MB, Markowitz GS, Lin J, Valeri AM, D'Agati VD (2004). Glomerular tip lesion: a distinct entity within the minimal change disease/focal segmental glomerulosclerosis spectrum. *Kidney International* **65**:1690–702.

Swaminathan S, Leung N, Lager DJ et al. (2007). Changing incidence of glomerular disease in Olmsted County, Minnesota: a 30-year renal biopsy study. *Clinical Journal of the American Society Nephrology* **1**:483–7.

Tabel Y, Berdeli A, Mir S, Serdaroğlu E, Yilmaz E (2005). Effects of genetic polymorphisms of the renin-angiotensin system in children with nephrotic syndrome. *Journal of Renin Angiotensin Aldosterone System* **6**:138–44.

Tarshish P, Tobin JN, Bernstein J, Edelmann CM Jr (1996). Cyclophosphamide does not benefit patients with focal segmental glomerulosclerosis. A report of the International Study of Kidney Disease in Children. *Pediatric Nephrology* **10**:590–3.

Thomas DB, Franceschini N, Hogan SL et al. (2006). Clinical and pathologic characteristics of focal segmental glomerulosclerosis pathologic variants. *Kidney International* **69**:920–6.

Troyanov S, Wall CA, Miller JA, Scholey JW, Cattran DC; Toronto Glomerulonephritis Registry Group (2005). Focal and segmental glomerulosclerosis: definition and relevance of a partial remission. *Journal of the American Society Nephrology* **16**:1061–8.

Tumlin JA, Miller D, Near M, Selvaraj S, Hennigar R, Guasch A (2006). A prospective, open-label trial of sirolimus in the treatment of focal segmental glomerulosclerosis. *Clinical Journal of the American Society Nephrology* **1**:109–16.

Tune BM, Kirpekar R, Sibley RK, Reznik VM, Griswold WR, Mendoza SA (1995). Intravenous methylprednisolone and oral alkylating agent therapy of prednisone-resistant pediatric focal segmental glomerulosclerosis: a long-term follow-up. *Clinical Nephrology* **43**:84–8.

Uhlig K, MacLeod A, Craig J et al. (2006). Grading evidence and recommendations for clinical practice guidelines in nephrology. A position statement from Kidney Disease: Improving Global Outcomes (KDIGO). *Kidney International* **70**:2058–65.

Vincenti F, Ghiggeri M (2005). New insights into the pathogenesis and the therapy of recurrent focal glomerulosclerosis. *Amer J Transpl* **5**: 1179–84.

Waldo FB, Benfield MR, Kohaut EC (1992). Methylprednisolone treatment of patients with steroid-resistant nephrotic syndrome. *Pediatric Nephrology* **6**:503–7.

Winn MP (2008). 2007 Young Investigator Award: TRP'ing into a New Era for Glomerular Disease. *Journal of the American Society Nephrology* **19**:1071–75.

Yabu JM, Ho B, Scandling JD, Vincenti F (2008). Rituximab failed to improve nephrotic syndrome in renal transplant patients with recurrent focal segmental glomerulosclerosis. *American Journal Transplantation* **8**:222–7.

Chapter 7

Membranous nephropathy

Patrizia Passerini and Claudio Ponticelli

Introduction and overview

Definition

Membranous nephropathy (MN) is a glomerular disease which is characterized histologically by uniform thickening of the glomerular capillary due to the
presence of immunoglobulin-containing deposits on the outer or subepithelial
aspect of the glomerular basement membrane (GBM). It exists in idiopathic
(etiology unknown) or secondary (causally associated with another disorder)
forms. Differentiation of the idiopathic membranous nephropathy (IMN)
from secondary forms of MN may be difficult. It is a frequent cause of the
nephrotic syndrome in adults. It is also characterized by a tendency for spontaneous remission in some patients and by persistence of proteinuria and slow
progression to end-stage renal disease (ESRD) in others. Those patients with
severe and un-remitting nephrotic syndrome may also suffer from disabling
and even life-threatening extra-renal complications, such as thromboembolic
events.

Pathology

At light microscopy MN may show a spectrum of abnormalities of the GBM
caused by subepithelial deposits of immunoglobulins, presumed to be immune
complexes (see 'Pathogenesis'). These changes are diffuse, involving all glomeruli, and generalized or global, involving the whole glomerulus. Thus, a single
glomerulus in a renal biopsy specimen is sufficient to make a diagnosis with
precision. Usually in idiopathic cases there is little or no associated cellular
proliferation, although some mesangial hypercellularity may be detectable
using quantitative morphometry. Four pathologic stages of glomerular lesions
have been described by Ehrenreich and Churg (1968): stage 1 refers to the
presence of subepithelial deposits without any alteration in GBM morphology
or thickness which may be seen in the earliest stages detectable only on electron microscopy. At this stage the light microscopy (PAS and hematoxylin and
eosin stains) may be normal but the deposits may be seen with special stains

(Malory trichrome) (see Atlas plate 9); stage 2 is characterized by projections of basement membrane-like material ('spikes') that protrude from the external surface of the GBM in between the deposits. These abnormalities of GBM can also be seen at light microscopy with periodic acid-silver methenamine staining (Jones stain); in stage 3 the deposits are surrounded by basement membrane-like material ('domes') and incorporated into the GBM, which appears irregularly thickened (see Atlas plate 10); in stage 4 the deposits are becoming electron lucent and undergoing 'reabsorption.' They are reabsorbed into the GBM which may assume a 'bubbly' or 'Swiss-cheese' appearance and be quite remarkably and irregularly thickened. At all stages, the changes of GBM may also be associated with visceral epithelial cell foot effacement on electron microscopy.

By immunofluorescence examination there are granular subepithelial deposits of IgG (see Fig. 7.1) and C3 and in the idiopathic form the deposits contain predominantly IgG_4 subclass, lesser amounts of IgM or IgA and very rarely C1q. Fibrinogen stains are usually negative. In the more advanced phases progressive interstitial fibrosis and tubular changes are seen.

Generally, MN is a *diffuse and global* glomerular disease. However, cases of *segmental* IMN that show IgG deposits in a portion of the glomerulus have been reported in Japanese children. In segmental MN C1q deposits are more frequent than in classic IMN, and mesangial electron-dense deposits may be

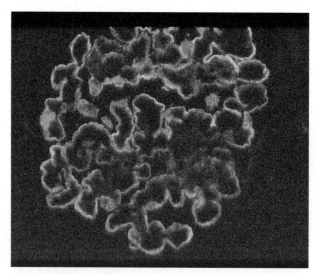

Fig. 7.1 MN immunofluorescence. Coalescent fine granular deposits of immunoreactants for IgG are globally and diffusely distributed along the capillary contours. (x 50)

seen in most cases. It is still unclear whether segmental MN should be considered a separate glomerular disease entity with child predominance distinctive from the typical idiopathic MN (Obana et al., 2006).

Atypical features, such as mesangial proliferation and/or a wide spectrum of different immunoglobulin and complement components deposits at immunofluorescence, suggest that the disease may be secondary to lupus, cancer, drug reaction, or infectious disease. The features which suggest a lupus related MN include: 'full-house' deposits of IgG, IgM, IgA, C3, and C1q by immunofluorescence, tubulo-reticular structures in endothelial cells, electron-dense deposits in mesangial or sub-endothelial areas, and prominent deposition of IgG_1 and IgG_2 (instead of IgG_4).

At immunofluorescence the intensity of glomerular deposits of IgG1 and IgG2 may be significantly stronger in patients with an underlying malignancy while IgG4 deposits prevail in patients with truly idiopathic MN (Ohtani et al., 2004). The number of inflammatory cells infiltrating the glomeruli has also been found to be significantly higher in patients with cancer-associated MN. The best cut-off value for distinguishing malignancy-related cases from controls was eight cells per glomerulus, with a specificity of 75% and a sensitivity of 92% (Lefaucheur et al., 2006).

Pathogenesis

MN is generally considered to be an immune complex-mediated disease. However, in the IMN circulating immune complexes are not commonly seen, and no study has yet shown that circulating immune complexes are the same as those deposited in the glomeruli. Rather, experimental studies have supported the hypothesis that in IMN there is an *in situ* formation of immune complexes as a consequence of a reaction between a circulating antibody and either an antigen planted in the subepithelial position or an intrinsic glomerular antigen in the same location.

As pointed out by Kerjaschki (2004), much of our current concepts about the pathogenesis of human MN derive from the Heymann models of experimental glomerulonephritis in rats. There are two models of Heymann nephritis. In the *active* model proteinuria and glomerular damage resembling that seen in human MN are induced by immunizing a rat with a suspension of Freund's adjuvant and an extract of crude brush border of proximal tubular cells. In the *passive* model, nephritis is caused by injecting antibodies prepared in rabbits or sheep against a rat kidney suspension into a normal rat. After years of intensive investigations the antigenic target has been eventually identified as a glycoprotein called *megalin*, because of its large size. Megalin is present in clathrin-coated pits located at the base of the microvilli in the proximal tubular brush border where it functions along with cubulin to assist in the reabsorption of filtered proteins. Megalin is also present in clathrin-coated pits along the base of the podocyte foot processes where it complexes with a specific protein, called receptor-associated-protein or RAP. RAP functions as the intracellular chaperon of megalin, assisting in the folding of megalin in the endoplasmic reticulum and its transport to the cell surface. In Heymann nephritis, circulating anti-megalin antibodies (IgG class) cross the GBM and bind to specific epitopes of megalin in the coated pits, forming *in situ* immune complexes that detach from the cell surface and attach covalently to the GBM (Fig. 7.2). The glomerular epithelial cells respond by increasing the rate of synthesis of megalin. Repeated cycles of this process lead to the accumulation of large aggregates of immune complexes in the same location, becoming visible to the electron microscope as an electron dense deposit in the subepithelial space, usually just beneath the slit-pore membrane. A cell-mediated response to the bound antibody may also occur. Nevertheless, anti-megalin

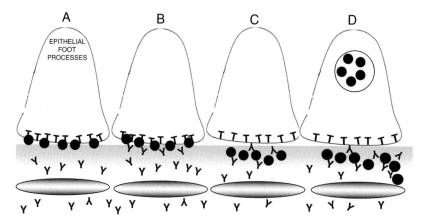

Fig. 7.2 Early events of the formation of an immune deposit in passive Heymann nephritis. A: circulating anti-megalin IgGs (Y) cross the GBM and bind to specific epitopes of megalin (●) located at the base of the epithelial foot processes. B: anti-megalin IgGs bind to megalin, forming *in situ* immunecomplexes. C: immunecomplexes are detached from the cell surface and attach covalently to the GBM as early as 15min after injection of the antibody. D: the immune deposits grow in size by repeated cycles of *in situ* immunecomplex formation and shedding into the lamina rara externa until it eventually encroaches on the area of the slit diaphragm. The glomerular epithelial cells respond by increasing the rate of synthesis of megalin which, like other membrane proteins, is assumed to be delivered via vesicles that eventually fuse with the cell membrane at the base of the foot processes. (T: clathrin coat; Y: anti-megalin IgG).

antibodies are unable per se to produce proteinuria, leading to the concept of a requirement for activation of local mediators of proteinuria, such as complement. Rarely a congenital form of MN may develop when a mother genetically deficient in neutral endopeptidase bears a child in which neutral endopeptidase is present. Transplacental transmission of anti-endopeptidase antibody formed in the mother produces MN in the child (Ronco and Debiec, 2006).

Couser and Nangaku (2006) have reviewed the paramount role of complement in triggering the lesions in MN. Experimental studies showed that C6-deficient rats do not develop proteinuria, despite the active formation of *in situ* immune complexes. Since the only known action of C6 is in the assembly of the late components of complement cascade C5b-9, also called membrane attack complex (MAC), this observation suggested that the membrane-lytic or membrane-altering properties of complement may contribute to glomerular damage. Further studies confirmed that proteinuria depends on insertion of complement proteins into podocyte cell membranes and activation of MAC. In turn, activated MAC, at sublytic levels, can trigger various intracellular events, including production of reactive oxygen species and proteases, and cytoskeletal changes. These result in degradation of GBM and redistribution of proteins that compose the slit diaphragm, eventually leading to the development of protein leakage into the Bowman's space. In addition C5b-9 attack leads to podocytopenia through apoptosis, lack of proliferation resulting from complement-induced DNA damage, and podocyte detachment. The extent of complement activation and glomerular injury is dependent, in part, on complement-regulatory proteins (such as factors H and I), which act at early or late steps within the complement cascade. Complement components in proteinuric urine also induce tubular epithelial cell injury and help to mediate progressive interstitial disease.

The presence of MAC within immune complexes has been documented in some human renal diseases, but in IMN stage 1 proteinuria is independent of the presence or absence of detectable C5b-9 in immune deposits. Proteinuria is rather correlated with the extent of tubular expression of adhesion molecules, such as alpha3beta1 integrin rather than tubular deposition of C5-C9. In deposits which are undergoing 'reabsortion,' one generally finds less C3 protein. Indeed the 'electron-density' of the deposits and the presence of C3 proteins may be a sign of 'active' formation of *in situ* immune deposits and an indirect feature of the 'activity' of the disease. Nonetheless, an important role of MAC in the pathogenesis of human IMN cannot be neglected as continuing urinary excretion of C5b-9 may correlate with poor clinical outcome. It has been suggested that measurements of urinary C5b-9 or podocyte excretion in the urine may be useful in the diagnosis of MN and may also be indicatory of disease activity and response to therapy.

In summary, we are still far from completely elucidating the pathogenesis of human IMN. However, there is broad agreement that the disease is probably triggered by circulating antibodies binding to an as yet poorly described protein target on podocyte membrane with consequent *in situ* formation of subepithelial immune deposits that produce glomerular injury by damaging and/ or activating podocytes through complement-dependent processes. It seems likely that the 'phenotype' of IMN may in fact be due to a very heterogeneous collection of putative antigenic targets. The strong association of IMN with deposits of IgG_4, which activates complement poorly if at all, remains unexplained. A search for the antigens involved in IMN in humans is continuing (Ronco and Debiec, 2006).

Etiology

Whereas megalin is the target antigen in Heymann nephritis it has not been found in human glomeruli or podocytes, nor has been detected in subepithelial immune deposits in patients with IMN. Taken into account the similarities between human and experimental MN, it is likely that in human MN circulating auto-antibodies cross the GBM and bind to an antigen on the podocyte foot processes. However, the identity of the human target antigen(s) remains unknown in the majority of cases, except for a rare form of antenatal MN, in which a neutral endopeptidase (NEP) represents the podocyte's cell membrane target antigen (Ronco and Debiec, 2006). Pathogenic antibodies directed against NEP originate in women who lack NEP epitopes because of truncating mutation. The mothers of the children were found to be homozygous deficient in a NEP and developed circulating allo-antibodies at the time of previous miscarriage. The anti-NEP antibodies produced by the pregnant woman were transferred across the placenta to her fetus, in which a severe form of MN developed prenatally.

In addition to NEP, other podocyte membrane proteins such as dipeptidyl peptidase IV and aminopeptidase A were shown to serve as target antigens for circulating antibodies in rabbits, rats and mice respectively. As both dipeptidyl peptidase IV and NEP are expressed on human podocyte it has been hypothesized that these two enzymatic antigens might play some role in the pathogenesis of human MN.

Although NEP has been identified as the target antigen in rare cases of MN in newborns, in the vast majority of human IMN the target antigen remains unknown. However, it is likely that there is not a 'universal' antigen in human MN and that several podocytes antigens might be probably involved.

A number of etiological factors have been recognized to be responsible of secondary MN (Table 7.1). The pathogenesis of these secondary forms has not

Table 7.1 Causes of secondary MN

Association with other diseases:	Autoimmune thyroiditis; bullous pemphigoid; Crohn's disease; dermatitis herpetiformis; diabetes mellitus; Guillain–Barré syndrome; hematopoietic stem cell transplantation; hemolytic uremic syndrome; mixed connective tissue disease; multiple sclerosis; myasthenia gravis; myelodysplasia; neoplasia (carcinoma; lymphoma, chronic lymphocytic leukemia); periaortic fibrosis; rheumatoid arthritis; psoriasis vulgaris; renal transplantation; renal vein thrombosis(?); sarcoidosis; sickle-cell disease; Sjögren's syndrome; systemic lupus erythematosus; temporal arteritis; thyroid disease
Exposure to drugs or toxic agents:	Captopril; clopidogrel; formaldheylde; heavy metals (mercury, gold); hydrocarbons; lithium; marijuana; non-steroidal anti-inflammatory drugs; penicillamine; probenecid; sulindac; trimetadione
Infections:	Enterococcal endocarditis; filariasis; hepatitis B or C; hydatid disease; leprosy; Quartan malaria; rectal abscess; schistosomiasis; Streptococcal infections; syphilis; tuberculosis

been clearly defined. *Helicobacter pylori* antigens, tumor antigens, and thyroglobulin have been detected in the subepithelial deposits, but there is no real proof that these antigens are pathogenic. MN is also frequently associated with HBV or HCV hepatitis, particularly in children and in patients from sub-Saharan Africa, Asia, and Eastern Europe. The presence of HCV antigen in the glomeruli has been demonstrated in a few patients but was not confirmed by other studies. The possibility that HCV trigger MN via an autoimmune mechanism cannot be ruled out. On the other hand, HCV infection is associated with a high prevalence of extra-hepatic immunological abnormalities, including synthesis of auto-antibodies, rheumatoid factor, and anti-smooth muscle antibodies, suggesting a possible link to the development of MN via an autoimmune mechanism.

The most frequent type of cancer associated with MN is lung carcinoma, followed by prostate, colon, kidney, breast, and stomach. Rare cases of MN associated with chronic lymphocytic leukemia or lymphoma have also been reported. In patients with MN secondary to carcinomas, the tumor may be an important source of antigens that can provoke the production of specific antibodies. However, the presence of tumor antigens and their corresponding antibodies in patients with paraneoplastic glomerulopathies does not necessarily mean that they are involved in the initial pathogenic process. In fact, these components can be passively deposited because of increased glomerular permeability to proteins as a result of the initial insult. Alternatively, it is possible that immune perturbations in cancer patients make them prone to developing immune-complex nephritis through the production of antibodies against tumor or self antigens.

Clinical presentation and features

IMN is considered to be one of the most common causes of nephrotic syndrome in adults, while it is rare in children. Secondary forms of MN only account for 20–25% of MN in adults whereas secondary forms account for >75% of cases of MN in children. Proteinuria is the hallmark of the disease. Usually proteinuria is non-selective and is often associated with microscopic (dysmorphic) hematuria. About 70–80% of patients referred to nephrologists because of IMN have a full-blown nephrotic syndrome at presentation, i.e., proteinuria ≥3.5g/d associated with hypoalbuminemia, hypercholesterolemia, and various degrees of edema. However, other patients may be asymptomatic and are discovered to be affected by the disease only at routine check-up visits or by incidental urinalyses. Renal dysfunction may be present at clinical onset in many cases, particularly if the diagnosis has been delayed. Few patients with severe nephrotic syndrome may develop thromboembolic complications at the onset of the disease, and these events may be the main reason for discovery of IMN.

The clinical presentation of IMN is similar in older and younger patients, although elderly patients more often present with a lower glomerular filtration rate (GFR), in part due to the physiological decline in GFR in advancing age. Arterial hypertension is seen more often in older patients.

In cases of secondary MN the clinical presentation is quite variable. Apart from the signs and symptoms of nephrotic syndrome when present, the clinical features may be dominated by the presence of an underlying disease, as in the case of malignancies, viral-associated liver diseases, systemic lupus erythematosus (SLE), etc. Secondary MN, especially associated with underlying malignancies, is more common in older patients and in children. More than 75% of MN in children is due to secondary causes (viral infections, drugs, auto-immune disease).

Around 10–20 % of patients with lupus nephritis may show a MN at renal biopsy. Rarely, SLE may present with proteinuria and abnormal urine sediment as the sole disease manifestation, antedating other clinical features and even immunological markers of the disease by years. These patients show an apparent idiopathic MN at presentation being the clinical or serological features of SLE absent. Atypical findings on renal biopsy may suggest the secondary nature of MN.

It is difficult to separate a MN secondary to malignancy from an IMN on the basis of renal histology alone (except perhaps the prominence of IgG_4 deposits in IMN). In approximately half of patients the neoplasia is recognized at the time of renal biopsy but in 40–50% of cases proteinuria may antedate by months or years the clinical signs and symptoms of an underlying carcinoma.

Thus, the evaluation of an adult (>50 years of age) with MN should include a diligent work-up (see 'Practical recommendations').

While the finding of diabetes is more common among patients with MN it is not well established that this association is of a causal nature. It may be fortuitous and related to a common genetically based predisposition. In patients with rheumatoid arthritis, MN may be triggered by the use of gold salts, non-steroidal anti-inflammatory drugs or penicillamine but in a number of cases no etiological agent may be found also suggesting a possible role for a common genetic background.

Younger patients with hepatitis B-associated MN and those with a smaller burden of subepithelial immune deposits may have spontaneous remission of proteinuria. Instead, spontaneous remission is rare in adults with MN due to hepatitis B viral infection and some of them may eventually progress to ESRD. MN may also be associated with malaria, tripanosomiasis, leprosy, or other infections particularly frequently in tropical areas. However, the true incidence of MN secondary to infection in tropical countries is unknown at the present.

The number of drugs potentially triggering a MN is continuously increasing. Proteinuria may appear rapidly after the drug is begun and usually disappears after its withdrawal. In other cases, MN may develop months or up to several years after treatment. In these patients the recovery of the disease after withdrawal of the offending drug may take a long time, roughly related to the length of the exposure to the drug. The exposure to substances such as solvents and hydrocarbons may also favor the development or progression of MN, but this remains as a highly controversial issue and the literature is not always consistent in demonstrating these association as having a causal nature.

Epidemiology

The current view is that IMN on a world-wide basis is largely prevailing over secondary MN. However, this estimate should be probably reassessed if one takes into account also the cases of MN in tropical areas. As a matter of fact, in those areas an indefinite number of cases of MN is associated with endemic infections, such as malaria, hepatitis B and C, or even tuberculosis. On the other hand, the increasing number and use of drugs that may cause MN will probably decrease the ratio idiopathic to secondary MN also in Western countries.

The association between MN and malignant neoplasia is well known. A recent review showed that 24 of 240 patients with MN (10%) had a malignancy at the time of renal biopsy or within a year thereafter. The incidence of cancer was significantly higher in patients with MN than in the general population, with a standardized incidence ratio of 9.8 in men and 12.3 in women. The frequency of malignancy increased with age, as it does in the general population, to as high as 20-25% after age 60 years (Lefaucher et al., 2006).

Until recently, IMN was considered to be the most frequent cause of idiopathic or primary nephrotic syndrome in adults. However, more recent reports have pointed out that focal segmental glomerular sclerosis (FSGS) is today the predominate cause of idiopathic nephrotic syndrome in Western countries (Braden et al., 2000). IMN accounts for about 22–33% of cases of nephrotic syndrome in adults, while it accounts for <5% of cases of nephrotic syndrome in children. Most textbooks still report that IMN has a peak incidence between 40–60 years (median about 55 years of age). Nevertheless the more liberal policy of renal biopsy in older patients has shown that the disease is more frequent than expected in the elderly. IMN is more frequent in men with a predominance of males over females, at 2 to 1 ratio (Hogan et al., 1995).

Natural history

A significant number of untreated patients with IMN may enter a partial or even a complete remission of proteinuria, which is more likely to occur in patients with sub-nephrotic proteinuria and in women (Laluck and Cattran 1999), while other patients maintain proteinuria fluctuating in a nephrotic range, and still others may slowly progress to ESRD over many years. However, it is difficult to assess the true percentage of patients with any of these possible outcomes in the absence of any treatment because most of the few relevant studies had too a short follow-up and included both nephrotic and non-nephrotic patients. The inclusion of non-nephrotic patients in natural outcome studies may lead to discrepant conclusions. For example, Schieppati et al. (1993) followed 100 Italian patients with MN and reported that 65% of those followed for at least 5 years developed a spontaneous remission of proteinuria. However, 37% of their patients did not have nephrotic syndrome at presentation (technically most of them were probably in 'partial remission') so that if one considers only nephrotic patients the probability of a true spontaneous remission should be probably halved to a value of about 30–35%. Moreover, many patients may show a relapse of nephrotic syndrome over time, so that only a part of those who entered remission may remain non-nephrotic in the long term. When patients with IMN are followed for a longer time without any specific therapy the results are much less optimistic. In a randomized study made in the same period as Schieppati et al. other Italian groups have shown that only 5% of untreated patients with IMN and nephrotic syndrome remained in complete remission and another 28% were in partial remission (33% in 'remission' in total) after 10 years of follow up (Ponticelli et al., 1995).

Besides other prognostic variables (see below), the probability of renal survival also depends on the length of follow-up. In systematic review including all studies reported up to 1994, Hogan et al. (1995) found that the renal survival averaged about around 50% at 14 years. Du Buf-Vereijken et al. (2005) also analyzed the reports published during the past 25 years. They excluded patients with a follow-up of <3 years and attributed a 100% renal survival rate to non-nephrotic patients. Overall, nearly 50% of the patients with IMN and nephrotic syndrome developed renal function deterioration and were probably destined to enter ESRD in the long term. Thus it is quite incorrect to assume that IMN is a benign disease, not requiring any specific therapy.

Apart from renal function deterioration, MN may also expose patients to the adverse clinical consequences of the nephrotic syndrome per se (see also Chapter 1). It is now generally agreed that persistently low levels of serum albumin (<2.5g/dL or 25g/L) represent a risk factor for survival and for fatal and non-fatal thromboembolic events. Most nephrotic patients also show hyperlipidemia and a highly pro-atherogenic lipid profile with hypercholesterolemia, hypertriglyceridemia, increase in LDL, IDL, and VLDL lipoproteins, while HDL levels are normal or reduced. An increase in lipoprotein (a) level further aggravates the atherosclerotic risk of nephrotic patients with IMN. Nephrotic syndrome is also associated with platelet activation, hypofibrinolysis, increased serum levels of procoagulant factors such as factor VIII, factor V, factor XIII, fibrinogen, plasminogen activator inhibitor, and decreased levels of anticoagulant factors, such as anti-thrombin III and vitamin B6 which are lost in the urine, having a low molecular weight. As a consequence, deep vein thrombosis and renal vein thrombosis are frequent in MN, and patients are at risk of developing a pulmonary embolism. Arterial thrombosis can also occur. The risk of thrombotic complications is particularly elevated in older patients and in those with a serum albumin level below 2.5g/dL. This heightened risk of thrombosis in MN with the nephrotic syndrome has led to suggest that prophylactic anticoagulation is indicated at least in some cases (Glassock, 2007).

Another important risk factor for cardiovascular events is renal dysfunction, which has been demonstrated to be a powerful independent predictor of fatal and non-fatal cardiovascular events in the general population and in patients who have already suffered from a myocardial infarction. In patients with chronic kidney disease the heightened risk of cardiovascular events becomes evident even with mild renal dysfunction, i.e., with creatinine levels as low as 1.4mg/dL or an estimated GFR around 60mL/min/1.73m^2. Mechanisms by which renal dysfunction increases the cardiovascular risk are not completely elucidated. However, it is likely that the association of renal dysfunction with traditional risk factors—such as arterial hypertension, glucose intolerance, abnormal lipoprotein profile, hyperuricemia—and non-traditional factors—such as anemia, oxidative stress, inflammation, hyperhomocysteinemia—may contribute to the development of cardiovascular complications in patients with elevated serum creatinine levels.

In summary, although IMN is often (erroneously in our view) considered as a 'benign' renal disease, the few studies examining the long-term outcome speak against this optimistic concept. On the other hand, it is likely that at present the long-term prognosis of the disease is improving since a prior nihilist attitude of not treating patients with MN has now changed. Today, most high-risk patients with IMN are receiving a regimen of specific treatment that may consistently alter the natural course of the disease and also receive the benefits of symptomatic treatment (see Chapter 1) based on statins, ACE-inhibitors, angiotensin-receptor blockers (ARB), diuretics, low-dose aspirin, and/or prophylactic anticoagulation. This more aggressive approach has considerably improved the outcome when compared to the recent past, so allowing the prevention of more severe complications of nephrotic syndrome and to improve the long-term prognosis of MN.

Prognostic factors (Table 7.2)

Age

Previously reported studies suggested a more favorable outcome of MN in children. However, a more recent review of the literature reported that nearly a quarter of children with nephrotic syndrome, whether untreated or treated with various immunosuppressive agents, developed chronic renal failure (Makker, 2003). Thrombotic complications are also quite frequent in children.

According to Deegens and Wetzels (2007) the prognosis of elderly patients with IMN is not very different from that of younger patients. However, older patients have higher than normal levels of serum creatinine at presentation and increased risk of developing renal insufficiency and vascular thrombosis than younger adults. Moreover elderly patients have a poorer tolerance than younger adults to treatments used in MN, and are more vulnerable to the consequences of the nephrotic syndrome.

Sex

There is general agreement that in IMN women fare better than men. This view has been substantiated by a large systematic review showing that female gender is associated with better probability of spontaneous remission and slower rate of progression (Cattran et al., 2008).

Table 7.2 Factors that may influence the prognosis of patients with IMN

Good	Prognosis	Bad
Children?	**Age**	Elderly
Female	**Sex**	Male
Asian subjects	**Ancestry (racial and ethnic origin)**	Caucasian patients?
Yes	**Any remission**	No
Absent	**Renal insufficiency**	Present
Non-nephrotic	**Proteinuria**	Profuse
Low urinary excretion of IgG, and β2 microglobulin	**?quality of proteinuria**	High urinary excretion of IgG, and β2 microglobulin
1–2	**?glomerular staging**	3–4 ?
Absent?	**Superimposed focal sclerosis**	Present?
±	**Tubulointerstitial changes**	++/+++
Low excretion	**Urinary C5b-9**	High excretion

Ancestry (racial and ethnic origin)

The disease seems to run a more favorable course in the Asian than in the Caucasian population. A large Japanese study involving 85 institutions and 949 patients with biopsy-proven IMN showed renal survival rates of 90.3% at 10 years and 81.1% at 15 years after diagnosis (Shiiki et al., 2004).

Proteinuria

The magnitude and the persistence of proteinuria impacts on the eventual outcome of MN. Cattran et al. (1997) elaborated a sophisticated prediction model for risk of progression in IMN, based on the severity of proteinuria over a 6-month observation, and validated the results on a large pool of Canadian, Italian, and Finnish patients. According to this model, a patient with normal serum creatinine and proteinuria <4g/d over 6 months has only 6% probability of progressing to chronic renal insufficiency at 52 months, while a patient with abnormal or deteriorating serum creatinine and/or proteinuria >8g/d over 6 months has 72% probability of entering renal insufficiency and patients with normal or nearly normal serum creatinine and variable amounts of proteinuria over 6 months have *intermediate* risks of progression.

The quality of proteinuria may also provide additional prognostic information. An elevation in the urinary excretion of IgG and alpha(1) microglobulin has been found to be associated significantly with the extent of tubulointerstitial damage and the likelihood of further progression (independently of the quantity of total protein excreted). A remission occurred in 100% in patients with IgG excretion <110mg/g urinary creatinine versus only 20% if the ratio was >110mg/g. Remission also occurred in 77% of patients with alpha (1) microglobulin excretion <33.5mg/g urinary creatinine versus 17% in patients with a higher ratio (Bazzi et al., 2001). Urinary excretion of beta2-microglobulin (Ubeta2m) and IgG (UIgG) were also found to be useful predictors of renal insufficiency in 52 patients with MN. At multivariate analysis Ubeta2m excretion >0.5mcg/min was the strongest independent predictor for the development of renal insufficiency. Sensitivity and specificity were 88 and 91%, respectively, for Ubeta2m, and both were 88% for UIgG >250mg/24h (Branten et al., 2005).

Remissions

In our experience, not only patients who entered a complete remission of proteinuria (<0.2g/d) but also those who attained a partial remission (defined as proteinuria <2g/d with normal serum creatinine) tend to maintain a stable renal function in the long term (Passerini et al., 1989). Similar results were also reported by Troyanov et al. (2004) who found that among 348 patients with IMN and nephrotic syndrome 136 (39%) had a partial remission. In the latter patients renal survival was 90% at 10 years and 70% at 15 years. The risk of relapse of nephrotic syndrome was high (47%) in the group with a partial remission but often reversible on further therapy.

Renal insufficiency

There is a general consensus that increased serum creatinine levels (>1.4mg/dL) at presentation presages the later development of ESRD. It should be pointed out, however, that in a number of cases with severe nephrotic syndrome renal insufficiency may be functional and reversible, being caused by a hypovolemia related to severe hypoalbuminemia, to excessive dosage of diuretics or to a complication of a drug-associated acute interstitial nephritis (often due to diuretics).

Glomerular lesions

There is no convincing evidence that the stage of glomerular lesions is consistently predictive of the future of progression (or remissions). Whether a superimposed FSGS is a discriminative parameter with independent prognostic value is still a matter of discussion. In a study on 53 patients with IMN, it was found that 22 patients with superimposed FSGS had a higher serum creatinine at time of biopsy, more severe interstitial fibrosis and higher glomerular stage of MN. The risk of renal failure was almost equally distributed between patients with and without FSGS. In Cox proportional hazard analysis, only the serum creatinine level at the time of biopsy was an independent predictor of subsequent renal failure—a not very surprising finding. It was concluded that FSGS is not an accurate prognostic marker in IMN (Heeringa et al., 2007). In the previously mentioned studies of Cattran et al. renal pathology could not be used to reliably predict either progression, remission, or response to treatment (Cattran et al., 1997; Troyanov et al., 2006).

Tubulo-interstitial lesions

A number of multivariate analyses reported that the factor more strongly associated to renal failure was the severity of tubulo-interstitial lesions (interstitial fibrosis and tubular atrophy). A large retrospective analysis (Troyanov et al., 2006) confirmed that a high degree of tubulo-interstitial lesions, vascular sclerosis, and FSGS taken together was associated with a reduced renal survival. However, these findings did not predict the outcome independently of the baseline clinical variables (e.g., serum creatinine level and proteinuria) nor did they correlate with the rate of decline in function or with baseline proteinuria. Furthermore, the severity of tubulo-interstitial and vascular lesions did not preclude a remission in proteinuria upon treatment. No pathological feature was able to reliably predict the presence or absence of a favorable response to therapy.

Urinary C5b-9

In Heymann nephritis, the subepithelial deposition of immune complexes activates the complement cascade leading to the formation of the terminal membrane attack complex C5b-9. The urinary excretion of C5b-9 might therefore reflect the activity of Heymann nephritis. Studies in humans would indicate that the urinary excretion of C5b-9 is related to the 'activity' of MN and associates with a poor outcome (Lehto et al., 1995). However, urine C5b-9 may be absent in about a third of patients with progression while the excretion may be high in about a fifth of patients with stable course. Moreover, the terminal complex of complement in the urine is not specific to MN but can be present also in lupus, diabetic nephropathy, and other primary glomerulonephritis.

HLA and tumor necrosis factor (TNF)

IMN has a strong association with the major histocompatibility complex HLA B8DR3 (17) DQ2 haplotype, but the influence of HLA on the outcome of the disease is still under evaluation. In 100 patients with IMN and 232 local controls, Thibaudin et al. (2007) reported that TNF-A2 and TNF-d2 alleles were strongly associated with occurrence/initiation of MN. However, there was not any significant and independent influence of these different genotypes on disease progression.

Specific treatment

Goals and objectives of treatment

The two primary goals of treatment in MN are:

- To avoid or minimize the adverse consequences of the nephrotic syndrome.
- To prevent the possible progression to renal failure.

There is still controversy among nephrologists on whether it is better to start therapy as early as possible, or to delay therapy until some 'marker' predictive of a likely poor outcome develops. This is essentially a 'risk stratification' maneuver in which only those 'destined' to have a poor outcome are treated initially, based on the presupposition that a delay in treatment will not adversely affect the responsiveness to therapy as compared to early treatment. This approach tends to neglect the adverse consequences of more prolonged exposure to the nephrotic state per se in those patients allocated to a 'delayed' treatment strategy. We will analyze in the following sections the arguments for an 'early start' versus a delayed treatment strategy in IMN with the nephrotic syndrome at presentation.

A number of drugs are now available for and have been evaluated in the treatment of IMN. Glucocorticoids in varying dosage and durations of treatment, alkylating agents chlorambucil and cyclophosphamide, and calcineurin inhibitors cyclosporine and tacrolimus, have received the greatest attention.

Glucocorticoids (Table 7.3)

In the past, oral administration of glucocorticoids has been a frequently recommended treatment approach in IMN. The results of retrospective uncontrolled studies have been inconsistent and controversial, mainly because the inclusion criteria, the doses of glucocorticoids, and the duration of treatment were extremely variable in the different studies.

Four prospective controlled trials of the use of glucocorticoids in nephrotic patients with IMN are available. Black et al. (1970) randomly assigned 19 patients with MN and nephrotic syndrome either to symptomatic therapy or

Table 7.3 Results with glucocorticoids in IMN

- Randomized trials did not show a benefit of glucocorticoids when given for short periods or for longer periods at moderate doses
- It is possible that a few patients may respond to a prolonged glucocorticoids treatments, but side effects are likely and it is difficult to recognize these potential 'responders'
- Asian patients seem to have a better rate of response than Caucasian patients

to oral prednisone, at a mean dose of 20–30mg/d for at least 6 months gradually tapered to 14mg/d at 1 year. After 2 years, 20% of the controls and 40% of the treated patients had daily proteinuria <1g, the difference being non-significant. Side effects were frequent and there were more cardiovascular deaths in the treated group. This study had two main defects: the power of the study to detect a difference was very low due to the small number of patients enrolled and the doses of prednisone were too small to obtain benefit but were high enough to produce side effects.

In a multicenter collaborative study in the USA (Collaborative Study of the Adult Nephrotic Syndrome, 1979), 72 nephrotic patients with biopsy-proven MN were randomized to symptomatic therapy or to alternate-day prednisone (mean dose 125mg every other day) for 2 months with an additional 2-month taper (4 months' total duration of therapy). During the study there were significantly more remissions of the nephrotic syndrome (proteinuria <2g/d) in the prednisone-treated patients than in untreated controls (22 vs. 11, p<0.05). However, relapses frequently occurred among the responders so that there were no differences in the frequency of complete remission at the end of a mean follow-up of 23 months, and this was also true at 4 years (RJ Glassock, personal communication). Of interest, the mean creatinine clearance declined much more steeply in controls (–10% per year) than in treated patients (–2% per year). Treatment was well tolerated with major side effects occurring in only two patients. This study has been criticized because the patients assigned to the control group appeared to have a worse outcome than that commonly observed. A total of ten of 38 (26%) of the untreated patients had a plasma creatinine >5mg/dL (440μmol/L), or died within 2 years of enrollment. This is much faster progression than usually observed in MN with severity comparable to the subjects enrolled in this study. On the other hand, the treatment was probably too short to obtain long-term remission.

The same therapeutic protocol was evaluated in another multicenter double-blind randomized trial organized by the Medical Research Council in the UK (Cameron et al., 1990). In that study, 107 adult nephrotic patients with biopsy-proven IMN were randomly allocated to prednisone, 125mg every other day for 8 weeks, or to placebo, followed by slow taper over 2 additional months. All patients had a potential follow-up of at least 3 years. No difference in the mean levels of proteinuria or serum creatinine could be seen between the two groups at 1, 2, or 3 years. The study had the advantages of a well designed, double-blind trial and an adequate number of enrolled patients. As with the previously mentioned American trial the main criticism concerns the short duration of administration of full-dose prednisone (2 months). As in the previous American trial, in the British study there was also a trend toward reduced proteinuria under prednisone treatment but many responders relapsed so that at 1 year there was no difference between the two groups.

In a Canadian study (Cattran et al., 1989), 158 patients with or without nephrotic syndrome were assigned to receive symptomatic therapy or prednisone at a dose of 45mg/m^2 on alternate days for 6 months No difference could be seen between the two groups at any time either in the mean urinary protein excretion or in the mean creatinine clearance during follow-up (up to 4 years). Therapy was usually well tolerated. The study was impeccable from a statistical point of view and, as the MRC study (Cameron, 1990), provided level 1 evidence *against* the use of glucocorticoids in IMN. However, the dosage of prednisone was probably too small to obtain therapeutic results. Moreover, the untreated controls had such a benign course that it would have been difficult to find any significant difference even if treatment was effective. This favorable outcome was partially due to the fact that non-nephrotic patients, who usually fare better than those with nephrotic syndrome, were included in the trial.

In summary, the available controlled trials have not shown a clear benefit of oral glucocorticoids (used in modest dosage over comparatively brief periods of time) over symptomatic therapy in IMN and this has been confirmed by a meta-analysis which did not find any difference either in the odds ratio of remission or in the 5-year renal survival between untreated patients and those treated with glucocorticoids (Hogan et al., 1995). These studies can be criticized as they employed oral prednisone either short term or at moderate doses, or both. One cannot exclude a better efficacy of glucocorticoids when given at high doses and for prolonged periods, but these approaches may result in severe side effects. In conclusion, the available data suggest that the concept of 'steroid-resistant' MN may be a misnomer. If a population of 'steroid-sensitive' patients with IMN does exist they are in a quite small minority (probably around 5–10% at the most), and cannot readily be distinguished from 'early' spontaneously remitting patients. It should be pointed out, however, that if glucocorticoids are of little benefit in Caucasian patients with MN, they may be effective in other ethnicities. In a large retrospective and uncontrolled Japanese study the renal survival rate in patients who had received a 4-week course of steroid therapy was significantly higher than in patients on supportive therapy alone (Shiiki et al., 2004). The results of this study are subject to a great deal of confounding (see Chapter 3).

Alkylating agents (Table 7.4)

Daily oral cyclophosphamide

In the past a few retrospective studies reported good results with the use of cyclophosphamide, generally given together with oral prednisone, while other

Table 7.4 Randomized controlled trials with daily oral alkylating agents versus symptomatic therapy in patients with MN and normal renal function

Authors	Patients (total)	Treatment	Results
Donadio (1974)	22	Oral cyclophosphamide for 1 year	No difference in reduction of proteinuria
Lagrue (1975)	41	Chlorambucil for 1 year vs. azathioprine for 1 year vs. placebo	Significantly more remissions in chlorambucil group but severe side effects
Tiller (1981)	54	Oral cyclophospha-mide+ warfarin/dipyri-damole for 3 years	Lower proteinuria; higher albuminemia; many serious side effects
Murphy (1992)	40	Oral cyclophosphamide for 6 months + warfa-rin/dipyridamole for 3 years	Greater reduction in proteinuria

investigators reported no benefit. The evaluation of these retrospective studies is difficult because of the different criteria of selection and the different durations of therapy. In some series cyclophosphamide was administered only to patients with a more ominous expected outcome, thus introducing a bias for comparison with untreated patients. In other studies, all patients with nephrotic syndrome were treated so that not even a historical control group was available for comparison.

Three randomized trials have been conducted with oral, daily cyclophosphamide in patients with normal renal function. Donadio et al. (1974) randomized 22 patients to be given either supportive therapy or oral daily cyclophosphamide monotherapy for 1 year at a mean dose of 1.8mg/kg/d. After a follow-up of 1 year, there was a trend to a greater decline of proteinuria in treated patients (mean reduction 4.7g per day in the treated subjects versus 2.6 g per day in the control subjects) but the difference was non-significant. The power of this study to detect a difference even if it was present was small.

Tiller et al. (1981) assigned 54 patients to symptomatic therapy or to oral daily cyclophosphamide plus warfarin and dipyridamole for 3 years. Therapy had to be discontinued in several patients because of side effects. Those who could complete the 3-year treatment showed significantly lower levels of proteinuria and higher levels of serum albumin than untreated controls. The mean levels of creatinine clearance did not differ in the two groups. The data on which this study was based were insufficient and the results were expressed only as mean values at the end of the follow-up. A possible criticism of the trial design is that a course of 3 years with daily oral cyclophosphamide and anticoagulants is disproportionately rich in side effects in comparison to its potential beneficial influence on proteinuria.

Murphy et al. (1992) randomized 40 patients either to symptomatic therapy alone or to daily oral cyclophosphamide for six months plus dipyridamole and warfarin for two years. In spite of the weak statistical power of the study, treated patients showed a significantly greater reduction of proteinuria and a larger number of complete and partial remissions when compared to controls.

Looking at these controlled trials it would seem that, with the exception of the study of Donadio et al, *daily* oral cyclophosphamide, given for prolonged periods can significantly reduce proteinuria or improve the chances of remission. The follow-ups were too short, however, to evaluate the effects of this immunosuppressive agent on renal function. The risks of daily prolonged therapy with oral cyclophosphamide cannot be discounted (see Chapter 2).

Finally, two controlled trials did not show any benefit with intravenous pulses of cyclophosphamide. Falk et al. (1992) found no difference in the risk of progression to ESRD between 13 patients with IMN and serum creatinine >2.0mg/dL randomized to receive alternate-day prednisone (2mg/kg/48h for 8 weeks) and thirteen patients assigned to intravenous methylprednisolone pulses plus oral prednisone plus intravenous cyclophosphamide for 6 months. In either arm of the trial four patients entered ESRD within 29 months. Reichert et al. (1994) reported that serum creatinine significantly increased in nine patients given monthly intravenous pulses of cyclophosphamide 750mg/m^2. Thus, there is no evidence for efficacy of intravenous pulse cyclophosphamide therapy, at least in moderately advanced MN.

Daily oral chlorambucil

Lagrue et al. (1975) randomly allocated 41 nephrotic patients with IMN to be given either chlorambucil for 1 year (sixteen patients), or azathioprine for 1 year (eleven patients), or symptomatic therapy (fourteen patients). After a mean follow-up of 2 years, nine chlorambucil-treated patients had complete remission of proteinuria and four had partial remission (total response rate = 81%). Of the azathioprine-treated patients, only one had a partial remission. Among the placebo patients two had complete and one had partial remission of proteinuria (total response rate = 23%). The design of this study and the randomization procedures used are not completely clear. In fact, not only patients with MN but also patients with other primary glomerulonephritis were apparently randomized. Moreover, at least some patients were given treatment for >12 months. The major criticism concerns the prolonged use of chlorambucil at a dose of 0.2mg/kg per day for 6 months plus 0.1mg/kg per day for another 6 months. The calculated cumulative dosage was not devoid of severe complications. Out of 37 patients with various types of glomerulone-phritis treated with chlorambucil for at least 1 year, *three* (8%) developed malignancy (skin cancer, gastric cancer, and acute leukemia respectively). This study, however, provided a rationale for further trials in which chlorambucil was used for shorter periods of time together with glucocorticoids in IMN.

Alternating glucocorticoids and cytotoxic drugs (cyclical therapy)

An Italian multicenter study (Ponticelli et al., 1995) assessed the efficacy of a treatment consisting of three cycles of a 2-month therapy. Each cycle began with 1g pulse of intravenous methylprednisolone repeated for 3 consecutive days followed by oral methylprednisolone (0.4mg/kg per day) for 1 month; then steroid was stopped and oral chlorambucil (0.2mg/kg per day) was given daily for 1 month. Eighty-one adult, nephrotic patients with biopsy-proven IMN were randomized to receive either supportive treatment or the combined therapy. The two groups were homogenous at randomization. Patients were followed for 10 years. The probability of surviving at 10 years without developing ESRD was significantly better in patients given cyclical methylprednisolone and chlorambucil than in controls (92% versus 60%). The probability of having a remission of the nephrotic syndrome as a first event (complete plus partial) was significantly higher in treated patients (83% versus 38%; p = 0.0038); it should be noted that about half of remissions occurred after the termination of treatment. The slope of the reciprocal of plasma creatinine with time, expressed in mg/dL, was significantly better after 10 years randomization from in treated patients (from 1.0 to 0.84) than in controls (from 1.0 to 0.51; p = 0.035). In the long term, one treated patient became obese and another developed diabetes. One control died of cardiac infarction. The main defect of this study is that it was unblinded (i.e., open label), and that it compared a combination of drugs to non-specific therapy (which did not include ACE inhibitors in all subjects, since the antiproteinuric effect of these agents was discovered after the trial was started).

Nevertheless, another randomized trial also provided level 1 evidence in favor of such a treatment. Jha et al. (2007) compared the effect of a 6-month course of alternating prednisolone and oral cyclophosphamide with supportive treatment in 93 adults with nephrotic syndrome caused by IMN. Patients were followed up for a median of 11 years. Data were analyzed on an intention-to-treat basis. Of the 47 patients who received the experimental protocol, 34 achieved remission (fifteen complete and nineteen partial) a total response rate of 72%, compared with sixteen (five complete, 11 partial), a total response rate of 35%, in the 46 controls (p<0.01). The 10-year dialysis-free survival was 89% and 65% for the experimental and control groups respectively, and the likelihood of survival without death, dialysis, and doubling of serum creatinine were

79% and 44%, both the differences being highly significant (p = 0.016 and p = 0.0006 respectively).

In another multicenter Italian trial (Ponticelli et al., 1992) the effects of combined treatment with methylprednisolone and chlorambucil were compared to those of methylprednisolone alone given at the same cumulative dosage as in the other arm (three pulses at months 1, 3, and 5 plus oral methylprednisolone 0.4mg/kg every other day for 6 months). The number of remissions, complete plus partial, was significantly higher at 1 year, 2 years, and 3 years for patients assigned to combined therapy. At 4 years there was still a 20% difference of remission in favor of the combined treatment (62% vs. 42%) but the difference was no longer significant. By the end of follow-up, averaging 54 months, the patients given the combined treatment were in remission longer than those given steroids alone (p = 0.008). The chances of remission were associated with the absence of mesangial sclerosis at initial biopsy, with the use of combined treatment, and with a plasma creatinine <88μmol/L (1.0mg/dL). One patient per group died. Four patients in the group treated with steroids and chlorambucil had severe side effects which completely reversed after treatment was stopped (infections in two cases, liver dysfunction, and gastric intolerance to chlorambucil). One patient treated with steroids alone stopped therapy because of pulmonary thrombosis. No other cases of vascular thrombosis were recorded. Since this study compared two potentially active treatments, the statistical power should have been stronger and the follow-up longer in order to better evaluate different outcomes with the two treatments. Thus, the 4-year outcomes shown by this study should be viewed as inconclusive rather than negative.

Ahmed et al. (1994) also compared the effects of a 6-month course of alternating prednisolone and cyclophosphamide with steroid alone. After a mean follow up of 46 ± 10 months, 33 of 36 patients who received the combined therapy achieved complete remission, and only one progressed to ESRD. In contrast, of the 35 patients assigned to steroids alone, fifteen achieved complete remission (p<0.001), three had a deterioration of renal function, and two other patients required dialysis.

In a third Italian trial a 6-month treatment cycle, alternating every other month methylprednisolone with oral chlorambucil, was compared with a 6-month treatment cycle alternating methylprednisolone with oral cylophosphamide in patients with biopsy-proven IMN and with a nephrotic syndrome (Ponticelli et al., 1998). Among 87 patients followed for at least 1 year, 36 of 44 (82%) assigned to methylprednisolone and chlorambucil entered complete or partial remission of the nephrotic syndrome, versus 40 of 43 (93%) assigned to methylprednisolone and cyclophosphamide. Of patients who attained remission of the nephrotic syndrome, eleven of 36 in the chlorambucil group (31%) and ten of 40 in the cyclophosphamide group (25%) had a relapse of the nephrotic syndrome between 6 and 30 months after completion of therapy. The reciprocal of plasma creatinine significantly improved in the cohort groups followed for 1 year for both treatment groups and remained unchanged when compared with basal values in the cohort groups followed for 2 and 3 years. Six patients in the chlorambucil group and two in the cyclophosphamide group did not complete the treatment because of side effects. One patient per group developed cancer, but were still alive at the last follow-up. As in the other two Italian trials, thrombotic events were very uncommon in both the treated and control subjects, much lower that had been reported in observational trials. The exact reason for the rarity of thrombo-embolic events in these trials is not known. Prophylactic anticoagulants were used only in patients with more severe nephrotic syndrome and no patient was studied for the occurrence of renal vein thrombosis prior to entry into the trial.

Taken all together, the results of trials using a cyclical treatment alternating steroids and an alkylating agent showed excellent renal survival and a high rate of remission even in the long-term (Table 7.5). A review of the three Italian trials showed that three patients among those who received chlorambucil (662 patient-years of follow-up) developed cancer, a ratio of 4.5/1,000 patient-years similar to the 4.3/1,000 patient-years observed in male Caucasian

Table 7.5 Results of randomized trials in patients with IMN and nephrotic syndrome treated with steroids (MP) alternated with an alkylating agent for 6 months (cyclical therapy). Data refer to patients who received therapy

Authors and treatment	Number of patients	Follow-up (years)	Renal survival at the last follow-up (including death)	Remission as a first event (complete + partial)
Ponticelli (1992): MP/chlorambucil	45	4	98%	62%
Ahmed (1994): MP/cyclophosphamide	36	4	100%	91%
Ponticelli (1995): MP/chlorambucil	42	10	92%	83%
Ponticelli (1998): MP/chlorambucil or MP/ cyclophosphamide	87	3	100%	87%
Jha (2007): MP/cyclophosphamide	47	11	89%	72%

Table 7.6 Results of treatment with glucocorticoids alternated with an alkylating agent in patients with IMN and renal insufficiency

Authors	Number of patients	Proteinuria g/24 h		Mean reduction	Plasma creatinine or creatinine clearance after treatment
		Before therapy	Last control		
Mathieson et al. (1988)	8	15.3	2.2	86%	81mL/min
Araque et al. (1993)	4	14	2.1	85%	1.3mg/dL
Warwick et al. (1994)	21	15	2.4	84%	–
Brunkhorst et al. (1994)	17	16.9	5.5	67%	1.7mg/dL
Branten et al. (1998)	15	9.1	7.6	16%	1.9mg/dL
Torres et al. (2000)	19	11.2	5.2	53%	2mg/dL

subjects examined in the same period of time (Ponticelli et al., 1998). Thus no oncogenic effect for chlorambucil could be found. However, longer periods of observation will be required to examine this point more critically.

Various schedules of combined treatments have also been used in patients with an already established renal insufficiency. This approach is often known as 'rescue therapy' or 'delayed intervention.' The response to a 6-month course with intravenous methylprednisolone and/or oral prednisone alternated with chlorambucil every other month was evaluated in 6 studies which considered 84 patients of MN with renal insufficiency (Table 7.6). Treatment obtained a mean reduction of proteinuria of 65% (from 16 to 86%) with an improvement or stabilization of renal function in all studies. Four studies considering 46 patients showed a benefit from cyclophosphamide associated with intravenous methylprednisolone and/or oral prednisone. Treatment achieved a mean reduction of proteinuria of 82% (from 80 to 86%) associated with an improvement or stabilization of renal function in all but one study. These studies would indicate that even a delayed treatment can still achieve good results. However, it should be noted that in most patients serum creatinine did not return to normal values. Moreover, the administration of glucocorticoids and cytotoxic agents to patients with renal insufficiency considerably increased the risk of side effects.

Synthetic adrenocorticotrophic hormone (ACTH)

Berg et al (1999) reported that synthetic ACTH administered intramuscularly twice per week for 1 year improved lipoprotein profile and obtained complete remission of proteinuria in three patients and partial remission in two of five patients with MN. In a further study, Berg and Arnadottir (2004) reported that all the fifteen patients treated with ACTH 0.75–1mg twice weekly for 9 months obtained remission of nephrotic syndrome as a first event. After a follow up of 18–30 months fourteen were still in remission. On the basis of these promising results a small randomized controlled trial was conducted in order to compare the 6-month regimen based on steroids alternated to an alkylating agent with intramuscular synthetic ACTH given at a dose of 1mg twice a week for 1 year (Ponticelli et al., 2006). In the first group, fifteen of sixteen patients entered complete or partial remission as a first event versus fourteen of sixteen in the second group. Median proteinuria decreased from 5.1g/d to 2.1g/d in the first group and from 6.0g/d to 0.3g/d in the ACTH group. No important side effects were seen in patients assigned to ACTH. However, in our experience, out of trial one patient had vertebral collapse and another one developed diabetes. Therefore, caution with such a therapy should be used, particularly in elderly patients. There is still little information on the risk of relapse after interruption of treatment and the long-term outcomes are not well understood. The mechanism responsible for the apparently beneficial effect of ACTH is unknown (see also Chapter 2). It is unlikely that it may depend on the enhanced secretion of endogenous glucocorticoids. A possible speculation is that by modifying apolipoprotein metabolism, ACTH might restore podocyte expression of apoliprotein J, which competes with the terminal components of complement, C5b-C9, for the same receptor in podocytes, namely megalin. Thus, ACTH therapy may be functionally equivalent to in situ down-modulation of complement-mediated podocyte injury.

Inhibitors of purine synthesis

Azathioprine

Goumenos et al., (2006) treated 33 patients with prednisolone (initially 60mg/d) and oral azathioprine (initially 2mg/kg/d) in gradually reducing doses for 26 months, whereas 17 'control' patients received no immunosuppressive drugs. The probabilities of doubling baseline serum creatinine, ESRD, persistent nephrotic syndrome, and remission rate were similar in treated and in untreated patients during the follow-up period, suggesting that azathioprine associated with glucocorticoids is of no benefit in patients with IMN. No adequately powered randomized controlled trials of azathioprine in IMN have ever been conducted.

Mycophenolate salts

Uncontrolled observational studies involving small numbers of patients reported the possibility of reducing proteinuria with mycophenolate mofetil (MMF) in nephrotic patients with IMN and normal renal function. The data, however, are scarce and conflicting. MMF was given orally at doses ranging between 0.5–2g per day for 3–7 months. Proteinuria decreased in many patients, but very few of them ever attained a complete remission. Mean serum creatinine remained stable. Side effects of MMF were infrequent and generally mild. In a small trial with short follow-up (mean 17 months) Nayagam et al. (2008) compared the efficacy of MMF with cyclical therapy in 21 neph-rotic adults with IMN, Of the eleven patients randomized to receive oral MMF (2g/d for 6 months) along with oral prednisolone at 0.5mg/kg/d for 2–3 months, seven (64%) entered complete or partial remission versus eight of ten (80%) assigned to cyclical treatment with steroids and cyclophosphamide for 6 months. On the other hand, another small controlled trial with 1 year of follow-up showed no difference in mean proteinuria or partial and complete remissions between nineteen patients given MMF alone (2g per day for 12 months) and 17 controls. Serious adverse effects were observed in four patients (20%) receiving MMF (Dussol et al., 2008).

MMF (usually with steroids) has also been used in patients with IMN and declining renal function as 'rescue' therapy. Branten et al. (2007) treated 32 patients with oral MMF, 1g twice daily, for 12 months and compared the results to those of 32 historical control patients treated with daily oral cyclo-phosphamide, 1.5mg/kg/d, for 12 months. Both groups also received intermit-tent intravenous methylprednisolone and alternate-day prednisone for 6 months. At 12 months, median serum creatinine levels fell from 1.8mg/dL (159μmol/L) to 1.4mg/dL (124μmol/L) in the MMF group and from 1.8mg/dL to 1.3mg/dL (115μmol/L) in the cyclophosphamide group. Proteinuria reduced from 8.4 to 1.4g/d in the MMF group and from 9.2 to 1.1g/d in the cyclophos-phamide group, respectively. Cumulative incidences of remission of proteinuria at 12 months were 66% in the MMF group versus 84% in the cyclophospha-mide group. Five patients (16%) in the MMF group versus none in the cyclo-phosphamide group did not respond to therapy (p = 0.05). Twelve patients (38%) experienced a relapse and nine patients (31%) were re-treated in the MMF group compared with four (13%) and two patients (6%) in the cyclo-phosphamide group, (p<0.01). At last follow up, patients treated with MMF were less likely to be in remission (44% versus 75%, p = 0.021).

Kidney function improved or stabilized in 28 patients and deteriorated in 4 in the MMF group, and improved or stabilized in 31 patients and deteriorated in 1 in the cyclophosphamide group. Side effects occurred in 24 patients (75%) in the MMF group and 22 patients (69%) in the cyclophosphamide group. Thus, a 12-month course of MMF decreased proteinuria and improved renal function in the majority of patients at least while therapy was being given, but did not appear as effective in achieving remission and preventing relapses. MMF was not better tolerated than cyclophosphamide.

In summary, the few small uncontrolled studies available seem to indicate a possible role for MMF in improving proteinuria, when associated with steroids; however, complete remissions are rare and relapses are frequent, the follow-ups are all short-term, and the optimal doses and length of treatment with MMF has not yet been established. A single small controlled trial of MMF monotherapy has shown disappointing results. On the basis of these data it seems premature to recommend the use of mycophenolate salts in the management of MN, except perhaps for those who are intolerant to other more established regimens and who still have full-blown nephrotic syndrome or as 'rescue' therapy in cyclophosphamide intolerant patients. Neither MMF nor sodium mycophenolate (Myfortic®) are approved for use in MN in the USA or by EMEA.

Mizoribine

In 34 patients with MN the slope of change in the proteinuria tended to be better in patients given mizoribine in addition to conventional treatment than in those given conventional treatment, but the difference was at borderline significance (Shibasaki et al., 2004).

Calcineurin inhibitors (Table 7.7)

Cyclosporine (CsA)

A number of uncontrolled studies reported a favorable anti-proteinuric effect of CsA in IMN. Taken together, the available retrospective data show that CsA may be effective in favoring the remission of nephrotic syndrome in 50–60% of patients (Cattran et al., 2007). The addition of small doses of prednisone may increase the probability of remission. Reduction of proteinuria usually occurs within 3–4 months of starting therapy. However, in a German study, fourteen of 41 patients given CsA obtained a complete remission and the median time for response was seven months (Fritsche et al., 1999). However, in spite of a high number of complete (50%) or partial remission (38%) obtained with an association of oral CsA, 3mg/kg/d and prednisone, 0.5mg/kg/d in sixteen patients with

Table 7.7 Randomized controlled trials with calcineurin inhibitors in patients with IMN

Authors	Number of patients	Treatment	Results
Cattran et al. (1995)	Seventeen with decline in GFR >8mL/min/year	CsA 3.5mg/kg/d for 6 months vs. placebo	Increase in GFR at 1 year 2.1 vs. 0.5mL/min (p <0.02)
Cattran et al. (2001)	51 with normal renal function	CsA 3.5mg/kg/d for 1 year vs. placebo	Response in 75% of CsA patients vs. 22% controls (p < 0.001) but relapse in 52% of responders
Praga et al. (2007)	25 with normal renal function	TAC 0.05mg/kg/d over 1 year with 6 months taper vs. symptomatic therapy	At 18 months 94% response in TAC group vs. 35% in controls (p<0.01) but relapse in 50% of responders.

CsA: cyclosporine; TAC: tacrolimus.

IMN a repeat renal biopsy performed after 18 months of treatment in ten patients with remission of NS showed that glomerular sclerosis, interstitial fibrosis, and vascular hyalinosis were deteriorated (Goumenos et al., 2004).

A single-blind randomized trial of Cattran et al., (2001) was conducted in 51 biopsy-proven IMN patients with nephrotic-range proteinuria 'resistant' to the effects of prednisone. Patients were randomly assigned to 26 weeks of oral CsA (averaging about 3.5mg/kg/d) plus low-dose prednisone (0.15mg/kg/d) or to placebo plus low-dose prednisone. All patients were followed for an average of 78 weeks (i.e., 52 weeks after the last dose of CsA). A partial or more rarely a complete remission of proteinuria occurred in 75% of treated patients versus 22% of the controls by 26 weeks. Relapse occurred in 52% of the CsA treated group with remissions and 40% of the placebo group by week 78. At the last follow-up, a doubling of baseline creatinine was seen in two patients in each group. No evidence of 'nephro-protection' for CsA could be identified in this study.

In another small randomized trial, Cattran et al. (1995) assigned seventeen patients with nephrotic syndrome and a decline in creatinine clearance of >8mL/min in a year either to placebo (eight patients) or to CsA, 3.5mg/kg per day (nine patients) for 12 months. Creatinine clearance declined by 2.0mL/min per month in the placebo group and by 0.73mL/min per month in the CsA group (p< 0.02). Twenty months after CsA was stopped, creatinine clearance remained stable in six of the eight patients. The ninth patient died of cardiac infarct.

In summary, both observational studies and small prospective randomized trials provide evidence that CsA may obtain remission of proteinuria in a number of nephrotic patients with IMN, although the rate of remission varies in different studies. However, little information is available on whether CsA therapy may be protective or harmful on renal function in the long-term. The risk of adverse events in patients with IMN is similar to that observed in patients with minimal change disease or FSGS (Cattran et al., 2007). The risk of nephrotoxicity is low if guidelines on CsA dosing and monitoring are followed (see Chapter 2). No head-to-head comparisons of CsA therapy with the standard cyclical alkylating agent-prednisone therapy regimen have been conducted to date.

Tacrolimus (TAC)

After sporadic cases of success with TAC in MN, two Spanish studies evaluated the role of this calcineurin-inhibitor in this disease. Ballarin et al. (2007) conducted a pilot study in 21 patients with IMN using initially low doses of oral steroids and TAC and adding MMF in nine patients with proteinuria >1g/d after 3 months. At the end of the treatment, eight patients (38.9%) entered complete remission and seven (33.3%) partial remission. At a mean time of 23.1 months after treatment was discontinued, eleven responders (73%) had relapsed. Praga et al. (2007) conducted a prospective randomized trial evaluating monotherapy with TAC in patients with biopsy-proven IMN. Twenty-five patients received TAC (0.05mg/kg/d) over 12 months with a 6-month taper, whereas 23 patients were in the control group. The probability of remission in the treatment group was 58% and 94% after 6 and 18 months but only 10% and 35%, respectively in the control group. No patient in the TAC group showed a relapse during the taper period, but nephrotic syndrome did eventually reappear in almost half of the patients who were in remission by the 18th month after TAC withdrawal.

In summary, TAC is a promising and perhaps useful therapeutic option for patients with IMN and preserved renal function who are intolerant of or choose not to receive CsA. The majority of patients will experience a remission with a significant reduction in the risk for deteriorating renal function but a high relapse rate can be expected when therapy is discontinued, just as with CsA. A role for 'triple therapy' with CsA (or TAC) plus MMF and steroids remains uncertain. It would likely be used only for the very uncommon patients who fail to respond to other better established forms of therapy.

Intravenous high-dose immunoglobulins

A completely different approach to the treatment of MN consists in an infusion of high-dose intravenous immunoglobulins (IVIgG). This has become a standard treatment for Kawasaki disease and idiopathic thrombocytopenic purpura, and has been used extensively in SLE and systemic vasculitis (see Chapter 2). Its method of action is unclear, although an important role may be played by the immunomodulating effect of anti-idiotype antibodies or of a sialylated Fc subfraction (see Chapter 2).

A few anecdotal uncontrolled reports suggested a possible benefit of IVIgG therapy in IMN. In a retrospective Japanese study (Yokoyama et al. 1999) 30 patients were given 1–3 courses of IVIgG (100–150mg/kg/d) for 6 consecutive days. Based on electron microscopic findings, the patients were divided into two subtypes, i.e., homogeneous type with synchronous electron-dense deposits, and heterogeneous type with various stages of dense deposits. For the homogeneous type, at 6 months post-treatment, IVIgG therapy had induced earlier remission (57%) as compared to treatments with glucocorticoids alone or together with cyclophosphamide (10%). However, there was no significant difference in the early therapeutic effect for the heterogeneous type or in the final outcome for all groups. No adverse effects were recorded during or after IVIgG therapy.

A number of questions remain unanswered regarding IVIgG therapy. It is unclear how long a patient should be treated before considering her/him as a non-responder and which is the optimal dosage. No information is available about the long-term outcome of these patients. Little information is available about the possible side effects of IVIgG therapy which may include respiratory distress and reduced renal function, mainly related to sucrose stabilized formulations. Finally, we do not know whether the potential response to treatment is influenced by the exact preparations of IVIgG, which may differ for each batch and for other features such as quantity and type of anti-idiotypic antibodies or IgA concentration.

Rituximab

As previously shown by the group of Remuzzi, the human-mouse chimeric anti-CD20 monoclonal antibody rituximab may reduce proteinuria in patients with IMN, but the response to treatment may vary from patient to patient. To identify which parameters may predict the response to rituximab, Ruggenenti et al. (2006) administered intravenous rituximab at a dose of 375mg/m^2 every week for 4 weeks to fourteen patients with IMN and proteinuria >3.5g/24h in spite of ACE inhibition for at least 6 months. Urinary protein excretion decreased in mean from 9.1 to 4.6g/24h in eight patients with tubulo-interstitial damage score <1.7, but did not change in six with a tubulo-interstitial damage score ≥1.7. Nine additional patients (seven untreated and two previously treated with rituximab) with IMN and a tubulo-interstitial score <1.7 were subsequently enrolled in a prospective study. Three-month proteinuria decreased in all patients from 8.9 to 4.9g/24h and serum albumin increased from 2.2 to 2.8mg/dL. In two patients proteinuria decreased to <3g/24h and in 4 additional patients to <1g/24h. Rituximab achieved circulating CD20 and CD19 lymphocyte depletion in all patients. The authors concluded that renal biopsy findings may help in predicting response to rituximab.

In another study, Fervenza et al. (2007) conducted an open-label uncontrolled pilot trial with rituximab in fifteen severely nephrotic patients with MN. Rituximab was given 2 weeks apart in doses of 1000mg and repeated again at 6 months in those patients who remained proteinuric but had recovered B-cell counts. The mean proteinuria was decreased from 9.8 ±.3.1g/24h to 6.0g/24h at 12 months, but the mean levels of the group remained in a nephrotic range. One patient was discovered to have a lung carcinoma 3 months after treatment and eventually died.In the 14 patients who completed follow-up, full remission was achieved in two and partial remission in six patients (total response rate = 57%). Of interest, the decline in proteinuria was greater after the 6th month. Minor side effects were frequent. Prospective identification of responsive patients was not possible.

Apart from the high cost of the treatment, these results do not generate a great deal of enthusiasm since in both the studies proteinuria significantly decreased but the mean values remained in a nephrotic range and complete remission was uncommon. Randomized trials with other therapeutic strategies have provided better results in nephrotic patients with IMN. No information is yet available on the long-term results, which will be particularly important for a disease which runs a long course and for a treatment that has marked and prolonged interference with the immune system. The doses and the duration of treatment are not well established. Treatment regimens geared to the level of circulating B-cells may reduce the overall dose (and thereby the cost) and allow for more prolonged therapy. Finally, there are contrasting results so far regarding about the possibility of predicting the response to rituximab by kidney biopsy. It seems appropriate to suggest that rituximab has not yet reached a point where it should be considered as standard therapy and long-term reports and randomized controlled trials are needed to formalize the indications for the use of rituximab in patients with IMN.

Practical recommendations

Before deciding whether, when, and how to treat a patient with MN, the clinician should always attempt to establish if the disease is primary or secondary in its aetiology; if the patient is oligo-symptomatic or symptomatically affected by a nephrotic syndrome; if his/her renal function is normal or deteriorating;

and should clearly consider the potential risks and benefits of the different possible treatments, particularly in the case of elderly or frail patients.

Is MN primary or secondary?

In some 10% of patients, depending upon age, MN is associated with malignancy, the percentage increasing significantly with age over 60 years (Lefaucheur et al., 2006). In approximately 40% of patients with cancer the neoplasia is recognized at the time of renal biopsy, but in 40–45% of cases proteinuria may antedate the initial manifestations of an underlying cancer by months or even years. Carcinomas of the lung, prostate, colon, rectum, kidney, breast, and stomach are the most frequent neoplasia but Hodgkin's disease, non-Hodgkin's lymphoma, and chronic lymphocytic leukemia may also be associated with MN. As pointed out earlier, it is difficult to differentiate the idiopathic from cancer-associated disease at renal biopsy. Extensive mesangial and/or subendothelial deposits, a high number of inflammatory cells infiltrating the glomerulus, and prominent IgG_1 and IgG_2 may suggest an underlying carcinoma. Still it is debated how extensive should be the investigation for detecting an 'occult' underlying cancer in a patient with MN. At least in the elderly patients and in heavy smokers, however, an extensive investigation is advisable, since some 20–25% of MN patients aged over 60 have an underlying malignancy (Glassock, 1992). Thus, especially in these patients, in addition to a thorough history and physical examination, a chest radiogram (preferably a CT because of its higher sensitivity in detecting small lung neoplasms), a colonoscopy (or at the very least a stool occult blood examination), a digital rectal exam of the prostate and a prostate specific antigen in men, a thorough breast examination and mammography in women, and renal ultrasonography (usually already done in connection with a renal biopsy) are suggested. A gastroscopy can also be done in selected patients, especially in the presence of upper gastrointestinal symptoms, early satiety, unexplained weight loss or iron-deficiency anemia. Moreover, patients should be closely followed as neoplasia may be undetectable on initial screening. The possibility that the surgical removal or successful chemotherapy of the cancer can result in a complete remission of MN is well established. In the study of Lefaucheur et al. (2006) there was a significant relationship between reduction of proteinuria and clinical remission of cancer. Treatment with steroids and chlorambucil may be indicated for patients with MN and low-grade non-Hodgkin's lymphoma. We have observed complete remission of both diseases in two patients with such an association.

In a number of patients MN can be secondary to drugs or toxic agents (see Table 7.1). Sometimes the drug exposure can be overlooked, leading to the 'misdiagnosis' of IMN. In MN due to drugs proteinuria usually remits after the removal of the offending agent. Although MN can develop in patients with rheumatoid arthritis who have never received any arthritis modulating therapy, it more often occurs, in this setting, after gold, non-steroidal anti-inflammatory drugs, or penicillamine and can be reversible after the drug has been stopped. Both topical as well as systemically administered agents have been associated with the occurrence of MN.

The infection most frequently associated with MN is hepatitis B virus (HBV). Many patients are asymptomatic but nearly all patients have hepatitis B surface antigenemia at the time of diagnosis. Hepatitis B-viral DNA and hepatitis Be antigen, indicating active viral replication are frequently found. An association between MN and HCV has also been reported. Therefore, patients with MN should be investigated for a possible association with both HBV and HCV infection. Liver disease may be very mild and consist only of 'transaminitis' in many cases. The use of glucocorticoids alone in hepatitis B/C viral-associated MN is contraindicated since it can reactivate viral replication. In a review of the literature Gan et al. (2005) reported that carriers of HBV with MN had an HBe antigen seroconversion along with improvement in nephrotic syndrome after lamivudine therapy. Reactivation of HBV after treatment discontinuation could be successfully treated again with lamivudine. Adefovir, dipivoxil, entecavir, and telbivudine may also be used when HBV develops resistance to lamivudine. Antiviral therapy with pegylate interferon-alpha-2 and ribavirin eradicate viral activity in a significant proportion of HCV-positive patients. Cases of complete remission have been reported in patients with MN secondary to HCV following therapy with interferon and ribavirin or even with ribavirin mono-therapy (Hu and Jaber 2005).

Should non-nephrotic patients with IMN be treated?

Almost all patients with sub-nephrotic proteinuria and IMN do not need 'specific' treatment and can be managed very effectively by conservative means (see also Chapter 1) with follow-up measurement of urine protein excretion and renal function. The risk of developing renal failure is minimal for these patients, unless they evolve into a full-blown nephrotic syndrome. Moreover, since non-nephrotic patients are nearly always asymptomatic and normo-albuminemic, they are not exposed to the potential harmful consequences of the nephrotic syndrome. Blood pressure should be kept ≤120/80mmHg. In some cases the administration of an ACE inhibitor or an ARB may obtain a further reduction and even the disappearance of proteinuria, in exceptional patients. Statins are also recommended in case of hyperlipemia resistant to dietary measures. Low-dose aspirin may be prescribed to prevent cardiovascular disease, although there is no clear-cut evidence that patients with non-nephrotic proteinuria and mild hypoalbuminemia have any increased risk of cardiovascular events after adjustment for other traditional risk factors (e.g., age, smoking, diabetes, hypertension). The risk of developing ESRD is minimal if any for patients who remain non-nephrotic over time. Nevertheless, it is mandatory that these patients are regularly followed, as a number of them may develop a full blown nephrotic syndrome sooner or later. The role of prophylactic anticoagulants is discussed in Chapter 1

Should nephrotic patients with IMN be treated and when?

A formal decision analysis showed that the difference in the expected quality-adjusted life expectancy for a 40-year-old man with IMN and nephrotic syndrome would be 7.2 years in favor of methylprednisolone/chlorambucil treatment in comparison with supportive therapy (Piccoli et al., 1994). Therefore, an effective specific treatment may be recommended in nephrotic patients with IMN, unless there are contraindications to the chosen drugs.

There is general agreement that a 'wait-and-see' policy is best for non-nephrotic patients; however, there are different attitudes for patients who present with nephrotic syndrome in IMN. At the two extremes, some clinicians are in favor of an early treatment at the time of presentation or shortly thereafter, independently from the age and sex of patients, while others prefer to treat the patient with symptomatic measures only (see Chapter 1), unless or until renal functional deterioration occurs or proteinuria is >10g/24h or a 'disabling' nephrotic syndrome develops. The partisans of the first choice argue that waiting to treat until renal insufficiency develops may be too late, since even a moderate increase of serum creatinine may reflect an underlying development of irreversible histological lesions that markedly reduce the chances of a beneficial response to treatment. Moreover, an early treatment can prevent, in responders, the potential complications of a severe and protracted nephrotic syndrome. Those who are against an early treatment argue that some 40–50% of patients, particularly if of female gender, would receive an unnecessary treatment since they will not develop ESRD or the ill-effects of a chronic nephrotic syndrome even after protracted follow-up (Table 7.8).

Unfortunately it is not easy to recognize at the time of initial presentation which patient will have an uncomplicated, favorable evolution and which patient is destined to develop renal failure, a thrombo-embolic event, or cardiovascular disease. Even the role of renal biopsy in deciding whether or not to treat is uncertain, as pointed out by the retrospective study from the Toronto Glomerulonephritis Study Group mentioned earlier (Troyanov et al., 2004).

Table 7.8 The pros and cons of an early initiation treatment in patients with IMN and nephrotic syndrome (NS)

	Pros	Cons
Elderly age	The response is similar to that of younger adults. The risk of extra-renal complications in patients with NS is higher than in younger adults	Increased risk of iatrogenic morbidity of glucocorticoids and cytotoxic agents. Elderly kidneys are more susceptible to renal toxicity of CNI
Female gender	The response to treatment is similar or even better in women than in men	The natural course of IMN is more favorable in women, thus it is better to wait and see
Nephrotic syndrome	The risk of complications and renal failure is higher in patients with NS than in those with asymptomatic proteinuria	A number of patients with NS may enter spontaneous remission and can avoid the potential toxicity of treatment.
Renal function	Even patients with reduced GFR may respond to treatment, therefore it is better to wait for treatment until GFR starts to decline.	Treatment may halt the progression and improve proteinuria even in patients with reduced GFR, but in most cases renal function does not improve. Thus it is better not to wait until GFR deteriorates before starting treatment.

In other words, any therapeutic decision entails either the risk of an unnecessary treatment of a 'benign' condition or of wrongful avoidance of effective therapy in a 'dangerous' disease. At the individual patient level this is a delicate balance affected by many imponderables.

A compromise could be an immediate treatment for adults with severe, symptomatic nephrotic syndrome (usually patients with proteinuria exceeding 10g/d, or with plasma albumin levels lower than 2g/dL), while postponing the treatment, of 6 months or so, in order to 'risk stratify' the relatively asymptomatic patients, depending on serial values of urinary protein excretion and creatinine clearance.

What is the initial treatment for nephrotic patients with IMN? (Table 7.9)

The results of randomized controlled trials show that three treatments offer advantages over symptomatic therapy, namely:

- ◆ Cyclical therapy with steroids and an alkylating agent.
- ◆ Calcineurin inhibitors (CNI)—either CsA or TAC.
- ◆ Synthetic ACTH.

Table 7.9 Treatments for IMN with NS. The quality of evidence and recommendations are based on the GRADE approach (Uhlig et al., 2006)

Glucocorticoids alternated with an alkylating agent:	The treatment can favor remission and protect renal function in the long term—high quality of evidence, confirmed by a number of RCT. Treatment may be recommended taking into account the potential side effects
Calcineurin inhibitors:	Both CsA and TAC favor remission—high quality of evidence provided by three RCT and several observational studies
	Serious limitations given by the little number of RCT and short-term follow-ups. Treatment may be suggested taking into account the high risk of relapses, the need of prolonged treatment, and the dose-dependent risk of nephrotoxicity
Synthetic ACTH:	May favor remission—evidence provided by a single RCT and an observational study but very serious limitations due to few, small-sized studies, and by the lack of information about the long-term outcome. Treatment may be suggested
Mycophenolate salts:	May favor remission—very low quality of evidence due to conflicting results of two small-sized RCT. Level of evidence limited by the little information about the optimal dosage, the usefulness of association with steroids, the duration of treatment and the results in the long-term. High risk of relapse after withdrawal of the drug. The consensus is based on the opinion of some experts
Rituximab:	May favor remission—low level of evidence. Only two observational studies and case-reports available. Evidence limited by the low number of complete remissions, the poor efficacy in patients with renal dysfunction, the lack of information about the long term, and by the high cost. The consensus is based on the opinion of some experts
IVIgG:	May favor remission—very low level of evidence. Only small-sized observational studies available. No information about the long term. Risk of acute renal failure with sucrose stabilized immunoglobulins. High cost. No consensus about this treatment
Glucocorticoids:	Neither effective in inducing remission nor in protecting from renal failure in Caucasian patients—high quality of evidence; negative results confirmed by RCT and meta-analyses. It is highly recommended not to use of glucocorticoids alone
	Possibly effective in inducing remission and protecting renal function in Asiatic patients—very low quality of evidence provided by observational studies

A 6-month course of *cyclical therapy* with methylprednisolone and an alkylating agents (either chlorambucil or cyclophosphamide) not only favors remission of the nephrotic syndrome, as shown by several randomized trials, but can also protect renal function in the long- term as shown by two trials with a follow-up of 10 years (Ponticelli et al., 1995; Jha et al., 2007). There is not evidence that a similar protective effect in the long-term may be obtained with ACTH or CNI, rather there is concern that a prolonged treatment with CNI may cause deterioration of renal function.

There is concern that alkylating agents administered in this fashion may cause serious side effects. This risk may be minimized following some guidelines (see Chapter 2). A matter of concern is represented by the risk of cancer. As extensively discussed in Chapter 2, this risk is mainly related to the cumulative dose of the cytotoxic drug. As reported above, the Italian trials showed that the incidence of cancer with 3 months of chlorambucil was comparable to that observed in the Caucasian general population. Alkylating agents can also cause irreversible azoospermia. This risk is more elevated with chlorambucil than with cyclophosphamide. Giving a cumulative dose of cyclophosphamide of 180mg/kg (i.e., 2mg/kg/d for 3 months) should keep the patient under the threshold of testicle toxicity, which is generally estimated to be around 200mg/kg. At any rate, young males should be encouraged to deposit their semen in a sperm bank before starting therapy. The ovary is more resistant to cytotoxic drugs but, to be on the safe side, fertile women should receive leuprolide therapy to induce gonadal arrest and decrease gonadal injury due to alkylating drugs. Alternatively, the cumulative dose of the alkylating agent may be decreased to protect gonadal function. Bone marrow toxicity may be prevented by monitoring blood cells every week during administration of the alkylating agent and by halving the dose if leukocytes are lower than 5000/cumm or withdrawing the drug if they are below 3000/cumm. Taking together the results of the three Italian trials, out of 174 patients only 9% of patients had to interrupt the cyclical treatment because of adverse events, which proved to be reversible after withdrawal of treatment (Passerini and Ponticelli, 2003). Other side effects occurred but were not severe enough to require interruption of treatment.

A higher incidence of side effects with this regimen may occur in patients with an already established renal insufficiency. It is well known that the bone marrow of patients with renal dysfunction is more vulnerable to the toxic effects of alkylating agents, and that these patients are more susceptible to infections. Therefore, it is highly recommended not to exceed daily doses of 0.1mg/kg when using chlorambucil and 1.5mg/kg when using cyclophosphamide in patients with a serum creatinine ≥ 2.0mg/dL or a creatinine clearance ≤ 60mL/min, also because these agents still showed to be effective at these doses (Brunkhorst et al. 1994; Reichert et al. 1994).

It is still unclear whether chlorambucil is better than cyclophosphamide or vice versa. Cyclophosphamide is an agent that is certainly more familiar to nephrologists and its long-term toxicity has already been well evaluated.

An Italian trial showed similar efficacy of the two drugs when given together with methylprednisolone, with less side effects in patients assigned to cyclophosphamide (Ponticelli et al., 1998). Intravenous cyclophosphamide appears to be ineffective in IMN (Falk et al., 1992) and cannot presently be recommended in any patient with IMN.

In summary, we find that cyclical therapy should be considered as the first therapeutic approach in those nephrotic patients with IMN who do not present contraindications to glucocorticoids or cytotoxic drugs. In case of poor response, intolerance, or contraindication to this regimen, an alternative option is represented by *calcineurin inhibitors*, with CsA being the best studied agent in this class. CsA may obtain a high initial rate of remission in patients with MN and nephrotic syndrome, in some circumstances comparable to the overall response rate seen with combined methylprednisolone and alkylating agents, but usually with inferior results for complete remissions. However, a prolonged administration and the association of CsA with moderate doses of glucocorticoids may improve the probability of complete remission. The main problem with CNI therapy is that in most responders proteinuria increases when the drug is stopped. The risk of relapse is particularly elevated when CNI are withdrawn abruptly and/or after short-term treatment. Moreover, in spite of clinical remission repeat biopsies may show histological progression of MN (Goumenos et al., 2004). To reduce the risk of relapse a Consensus Conference (Cattran et al., 2007) recommended continuing CsA for at least 3–4 months after complete remission is obtained. For patients with partial remission CsA should be continued at full doses for at least 1–2 years and then maintained at non-toxic serum levels indefinitely so long as serum creatinine concentration remains stable, if the patient has failed to respond to other treatments. TAC may induce a rate of remissions similar to CsA in nephrotic patients with MN. However, the risk of relapses is particularly elevated after treatments lasting 12 months (Ballarin et al., 2007; Praga et al., 2007). The recommendations for the use of TAC in MN are similar to those given for CsA. It should be pointed out that the experience thus far with TAC is considerably less than that of CsA in this setting. TAC should be avoided in obese patients with glucose intolerance and in patients with overt diabetes mellitus because of its diabetogenic effect. We suggest starting with doses not exceeding 4mg/kg/d for CsA and 0.1mg/kg/d for TAC. The time of response is unpredictable but if no change in proteinuria occurs after 6 months of treatment the chances of remission are low. In case of remission, most often partial, the initial doses may be gradually reduced in order to catch the minimal dose that may maintain proteinuria in an asymptomatic range. For maintenance treatment we suggest to keep trough blood levels between 50–100ng/mL for CsA and between 4–7ng/mL for TAC.

A further option is the administration of *synthetic ACTH* for 1 year. The reported results so far are impressive. However, the number of patients who received this treatment was too small and the follow-up was too short to recommend ACTH as a first-line treatment for IMN. The results should be substantiated by further trials. This regimen may be suggested for those patients who are reluctant to use cytotoxic drugs or a CNI for an indefinite period of time, and perhaps may be used also for patients who did not respond to other treatments. In this regard, it is of note that Berg et al. (2004) reported good results also in few patients who proved to be resistant to methylprednisolone and chlorambucil. Unfortunately this agent is not approved for treatment of IMN by FDA.

Other alternative treatments, with low level of evidence, have been used in IMN. The place of *MMF and sodium mycophenolate* in the therapy of IMN is still poorly defined. The results of small randomized trials are conflicting; it is interesting to note that the use of steroids favored a good rate of responses in one trial (Nayagam et al. 2008) while the administration of MMF as monotherapy resulted ineffective (Dussol et al., 2008). In a handful of patients resistant or intolerant to other treatments we have observed a good rate of remission when these agents were given together with moderate doses of prednisone or in alternate months with steroids. In order to prevent relapses which are frequent in responders (Branten et al., 2007) we are continuing treatment in responders for 2 or more years by halving the initial doses. Clearly, well designed randomized trials with adequate number of participants and follow-up are needed to better assess the effectiveness, dosage, duration of treatment, as well as the role of potential association with steroids for mycophenolate salts in IMN. At present, the quality of evidence for mycophenolate salts is very low and we do not recommend them for the initial therapy of IMN but limit their indication to cases who do not respond or have contraindications to other treatments.

Also low is the quality of evidence for *rituximab as initial therapy for IMN*. From an examination of the data reported by Ruggenenti et al. (2006) and Fervenza et al. (2007) it is unclear if rituximab may actually offer in IMN results better or at least comparable to those obtained with steroid-cytotoxic regimens or with CNI. No head- to- head comparisons of rituximab with these more standard approaches have yet been reported. Also disappointing is the fact that the chances of complete remission in males are minimal—if any— and that patients with tubulo-interstitial lesions do not apparently respond, although this point has not been confirmed by Fervenza et al. (2007). Hopefully, further studies will better clarify the initial effectiveness, relapse rate, requirement for repeated administrations and the long-term tolerance of rituximab in

IMN, although the high cost of this monoclonal antibody remains a major obstacle. Rituximab is not approved for use in IMN by the FDA or by EMEA

The results with high dose *IVIgG* are very preliminary and non-controlled. Generally the infusion is well tolerated but some risks of viral infections, allergic reactions and hyperviscosity exist and (sucrose-mediated) acute renal failure can rarely occur, particularly with sucrose-stabilized formulations (see Chapter 2). One of the major drawbacks of IVIgG treatment is represented by its very high cost.

Suggested treatment for nephrotic patients

On the basis of the available data and our own experience, we propose the following algorithm for nephrotic patients with IMN and normal renal function (see Fig. 7.3). According to the clinical conditions of the patient and his/her own conviction the physician can start with the regimen alternating methylprednisolone and an alkylating agent (probably oral cyclophosphamide preferred over chlorambucil) for 6 months. For patients who show remission and then relapse of nephrotic syndrome, a second course of treatment can be given, since the tolerance and probability of response to re-treatment are similar to those observed after the first course. In the case of refusal, intolerance, further relapses, or poor response to cyclical therapy either CsA or synthetic ACTH may be proposed. In case of response, CsA treatment should be prolonged for

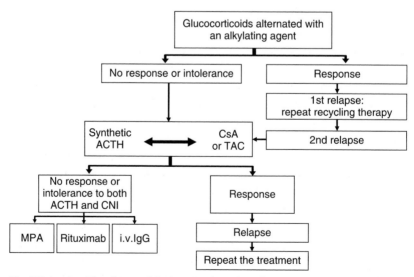

Fig. 7.3 An algorithm for possible therapeutic options for a patient with IMN and nephrotic syndrome.

1–2 years or even more at the minimal effective doses if the drug is well tolerated. Synthetic ACTH should be given at a dose of 1mg twice a week for 1 year. Mycophenolate salts, rituximab, or IVIgG may be tried in cases that have contraindications or intolerance to the other treatments.

In spite of the abundant evidence speaking against the utility of monotherapy with oral glucocorticoids, a number of patients with IMN are still given high-dose glucocorticoids for initial treatment, perhaps because of some lingering doubts that some patients may in fact be 'steroid-responsive.' It should be remembered that three out of four randomized controlled trials comparing glucocorticoids with symptomatic therapy showed non-superiority of steroid therapy versus symptomatic treatment, and 'steroid' responsive patients constituted only a minority. A meta-analysis of these studies (Hogan et al., 1995) concluded that there was no difference between treated and untreated patients in the probability of obtaining a remission at 3 years (odds ratio 0.97) or in the probability of renal survival at 5 years (80% in both groups). Although a few patients may 'respond' to initial monotherapy with oral glucocorticoids, they may have frequent relapses that require further courses of steroid treatment with the risk of developing iatrogenic morbidity. Therefore, *we do not recommend short (3–4 month) courses of daily oral steroid monotherapy for initial treatment of idiopathic MN* with the possible exception of Asian patients who seem to respond better than Caucasian subjects to steroid monotherapy.

What to do in patients with IMN and declining renal function?

Treatment of superimposed renal complications

Before deciding whether or not to treat patients with declining renal function, every effort should be made to recognize and appropriately handle any complication superimposed on the original disease. The three most frequent superimposed causes of deterioration of renal function in IMN are represented by acute drug-associated interstitial nephritis (most often due to diuretics), acute bilateral renal vein thrombosis, and extracapillary (crescentic) glomerulonephritis.

Acute hypersensitivity interstitial nephritis can be suspected by a rapidly progressive renal insufficiency associated with rash, fever, eosinophilia, and/or eosinophiluria in patients taking diuretic agents, antibiotics, allopurinol, or non-steroidal anti-inflammatory drugs. Renal biopsy is often necessary to confirm the diagnosis. Stopping the administration of the causal drug and an early course of high-dose oral prednisone (1mg/kg/d) can obtain the complete recovery of renal function in most of these instances.

Renal vein thrombosis (RVT) is frequent in patients with IMN (see Chapter 1), although the exact prevalence is a matter of controversy, ranging from 5% to over 50%. Unfortunately, the reasons underlying the development of RVT in IMN are still unknown. Clotting abnormalities, increased blood viscosity, and depletion of intravascular volume are probably the main factors involved in the pathogenesis of RVT. The same factors, however, can be present not only in IMN but in any other patient with nephrotic syndrome. The current opinion is that chronic RVT (unilateral or bilateral) has little influence on proteinuria or renal function but it can be responsible for pulmonary embolism. However, even if the deleterious role of chronic RVT on kidney function is still under discussion, there is clear evidence that an acute bilateral RVT can precipitate a sudden, often irreversible, deterioration of renal function. The diagnosis is suspected by the sudden onset of flank pain and macrohematuria and can be confirmed by an echocolor Doppler scan, renal venography, magnetic resonance or spiral computed tomography imaging. A prompt and correct diagnosis is of utmost importance in these symptomatic patients since early administration of fibrinolytic agents can obtain recovery of renal function in oligo-anuric patients.

The development of an *extracapillary (crescentic) glomerulonephritis* superimposed on IMN is an exceptional but well recognized possibility. Whenever the steady evolution of IMN is interrupted by a rapidly progressive course, such a complication should be considered. A sudden increase in dysmorphic erythrocytes and leukocytes in the urine sediment can signal the development of proliferative glomerular lesions in patients with a rapidly progressive course. The correct diagnosis can usually only be obtained by a renal biopsy. Either (or both) ANCA and anti-GBM auto-antibody pathogenetic mechanisms may be responsible for this occurrence in IMN. Treatment of these cases does not differ from that of rapidly progressive (crescentic) glomerulonephritis (see Chapter 10). The early institution of an aggressive therapy with intravenous high-dose methylprednisolone pulses and cytotoxic agents can often obtain recovery or substantial improvement of renal function.

Treatment of patients with steady progression and renal insufficiency

Patients with renal insufficiency and MN are more exposed to the risk of side effects caused by glucocorticoids, cytotoxic drugs, or CNI. Thus treatment should be limited to those cases having actual and reasonable chances of improving. Although there are neither controlled nor uncontrolled studies that attempt to correlate response to therapy with levels of serum creatinine or the histological picture, it appears from the available data that no patient with IMN has ever responded to therapy when his/her plasma creatinine exceeded 400μmol/L (4.5mg/dL) on a chronic progressive basis (see earlier sections for rapidly progressive or acute renal failure supervening in cases of MN).

Table 7.10 Indications for an aggressive treatment or no specific treatment in patients with IMN and declining renal function

	Treatment	No treatment
Plasma creatinine:	<400µmol/L	>400µmol/L
Ultrasonography:		
Size	Subnormal	Reduced
Hyperechogenicity	Moderate	Severe
Renal biopsy:		
Mesangial sclerosis	Moderate	Severe
Tubulointerstitial lesions	Moderate	Severe
Immune deposits	Fresh	Absent
Urine C5b-9:	Elevated	Low–absent

Patients with atrophic and hyper-echogenic kidneys at ultrasonography and/or those with very extensive glomerular sclerosis and severe chronic tubulo-interstitial changes at renal biopsy are also very unlikely to respond to any 'specific' treatment. Absence of C5b-C9 from urine may be a sign of 'inactive' disease. Therefore, patients with these characteristics should logically be excluded from attempts at 'rescue' treatment since such management is unlikely to obtain any sustained improvement but can cause considerable iatrogenic morbidity (Table 7.10).

Which treatment should be tried in patients with declining renal function who have not yet reached an irreversible stage? Even in 'responders' the effects of high-dose glucocorticoids (given orally or intravenously) seem to be transient and not sustainable. Good results have been reported with CsA (Cattran et al., 1995), but we discourage the use of CNI in patients with already established with severe interstitial fibrosis and/or with stable or declining values of estimated GFR <50–60mL/min. Most of the favorable results observed in patients with renal insufficiency have been obtained with the use of oral cyto-toxic agents either given alone or together with glucocorticoids. The best results were observed in patients treated with oral cyclophosphamide associated with glucocorticoids for at least 1 year or with a 6-month treatment alternating methylprednisolone and either cyclophosphamide or chlorambucil every other month (du Buf Vereijken et al., 2005). In contrast, two controlled trials did not find any particular benefit with intravenous pulses of cyclophosphamide (Falk et al., 1992; Reichert et al., 1994). The use of intravenous cyclophosphamide in patients with MN, with or without progressive renal function deterioration cannot be recommended.

On the basis of the available reports, we suggest the following options for patients with slowly progressive renal insufficiency. Patients showing a steady increase in plasma creatinine to >400µmol/l (4.5mg/dL) or those with a considerable reduction of kidney size at ultrasonography should be treated with symptomatic therapy alone (see Chapter 1). In the absence of contraindications, a renal biopsy should be carefully considered in patients with less marked renal insufficiency or in those with a sudden onset of a rapidly progressive course. If severe glomerular sclerosis and tubulo-interstitial changes are seen, any form of treatment is probably useless. If these lesions are not advanced and if fresh deposition of immune complexes (very electron dense deposits combined with strongly positive C3c deposition) is found, a specific treatment may be tried. Should the choice falls on a 6-month course of methylprednisolone and an alkylating agent, we recommend maintaining three courses of intravenous methylprednisolone pulses at doses of 0.5g each and reducing the doses of chlorambucil to 0.1mg/kg per day or cyclophosphamide to 1.5mg/kg per day (Table 7.11). As an alternative option, one may consider prolonged treatment (about 12 months) with low-dose prednisone (10–15mg per day or double doses every other day) and cyclophosphamide (1.0–1.5mg/kg/d). Whether occasional addition of methylprednisolone pulses may improve the response to the latter treatment is still unclear and remains untested. There is no information on the use of MMF, synthetic ACTH, IVIgG, or rituximab as 'rescue' treatments in patients with progressive IMN.

Table 7.11 Protocol based on methylprednisolone and alkylating agents in patients with renal insufficiency or old age

Months 1, 3, 5:	Three IV methylprednisolone pulses* (0.5g each) infused over at least 1h, every 48h
	Low serum potassium levels should be corrected and electrocardiogram should be checked before infusion
	Patients with pre-existing cardiac lesions should have continuous electrocardiographic monitoring
	Subcutaneous heparin should be given for 1 week to prevent thrombosis
	Glycemia should be returned to normal before giving a new pulse
	*After the three steroid pulses give oral prednisone 0.5mg/kg
Months 2, 4, 6:	Chlorambucil 0.1mg/kg per day *or*
	Cyclophosphamide 1.0–1.5mg/kg per day (MESNA or acetylcysteine to prevent bladder toxicity)

What treatment for elderly patients with IMN?

Older patients are particularly susceptible to the thrombotic and cardiovascular complications of the nephrotic syndrome. This might justify a therapeutic trial at least in the older patients with severe nephrotic syndrome and/or incipient renal failure. On the other hand, the choice of therapy is not easy since the available agents can have specific relative contraindications in many elderly patients. Glucocorticoids can aggravate arterial hypertension, arterial occlusive disease, glucose intolerance, cardiovascular disease, and other pathological conditions that may already be present. Alkylating agents carry an increased risk of leukopenia, bladder toxicity, and infections (both bacterial and viral) in the frail aged patient and are contraindicated, for their carcinogenic potential, in patients with a previous malignancy (see Chapter 2). Calcineurin inhibitors may worsen hypertension and may precipitate thrombotic complications or diabetes. Moreover, elderly subjects have often reduced levels of GFR and the 'aging' kidney is particularly vulnerable to the nephrotoxic effects of CNI. There is little experience with synthetic ACTH, but a prolonged treatment might cause osteoporosis, diabetes, and/or hypertension. Even symptomatic therapy should be prescribed with caution in the elderly since ACE-inhibitors, ARB, non-steroidal anti-inflammatory drugs, statins, and diuretics may precipitate a deterioration of renal function, which can be irreversible in some cases, especially if undiagnosed bilateral renal artery atheromas are present. No data are available with alternative therapies.

In summary, the decision on whether and how to treat an elderly patient should be based on the personal experience of the treating nephrologists and the clinical characteristics of the particular patient. A retrospective study reported a significant and persistent reduction of proteinuria (from a basal value of 6.8 ± 3.5 to 1.1 ± 0.4g/d at 5 years) in fifteen MN patients aged more than 65 years treated with cyclical methylprednisolone and chlorambucil for six months, while proteinuria remained stable in fourteen untreated patients. At 5 years serum creatinine remained stable in treated patients and doubled in untreated controls. However, 53% of patients given the combined treatment developed serious side effects and one patient died of sideroblastic anemia (Passerini et al., 1993). Thus, if a cyclical therapy is planned in elderly patients, we suggest to halve the doses of chlorambucil or cyclophosphamide and to halve the doses of methylprednisolone pulses to 0.5g (Table 7.11). If CsA is preferred, its use should be limited to patients with GFR >60mL/min/1.73 in view of its potential nephrotoxicity. We tend to keep the doses of CsA around 3mg/kg/d and the trough (Co) blood levels <150ng/mL. The role of mycophenolate salts is still to be investigated but is a reasonable option.

Transplantation

MN can develop in a transplanted kidney either as recurrence of the original disease or as a *de novo* form. About one-third of allograft MN is caused by recurrence and two-thirds by a *de novo* glomerulonephritis.

Recurrence of MN

The proportion of recurrence of MN is difficult to assess as the indications to graft biopsy are extremely variable among transplant centres. Moreover, a *de novo* form of MN may develop even in transplant recipients with an idiopathic MN as original disease with an indistinguishable histological pattern. The recurrence of MN is exceptional in children. In adults the rate of recurrence averages 30%, but it has been reported to be more elevated in single-centre series, which probably adopted a more aggressive policy for investigating the onset of proteinuria after renal transplantation.

No clinical or histological factor can predict the risk of recurrence. Nor could studies of HLA system find any significant difference between transplanted patients with or without recurrence. In Caucasian patients recurrence usually occurs within the 2nd and the 3rd year after transplantation while in Chinese patients MN occurs later, in a mean of 45 months after transplantation. Recurrence is not inhibited by the use of CNI, mTOR inhibitors, or biological reagents.

Histologically, the features of recurrent MN resemble those observed in cases of IMN although microscopic changes may be subtle initially and only granular GBM deposits at immunofluorescence play for the diagnosis. In an undefined number of cases the glomerular lesions are associated with vascular and tubulo-interstitial lesions caused by rejection, CNI toxicity, or infection.

Clinically, the recurrence of MN may be heralded by the appearance of proteinuria, which is often in a nephrotic range (>3.5g/d). However, the initial clinical manifestations of recurrence may be mild or absent (Dabade et al., 2008). The outcome may be as variable as in IMN but it is usually more severe in the recurrent form. Only rarely, proteinuria may spontaneously improve or even disappear. With the exception of these cases, the nephrotic syndrome is usually resistant to all forms of treatment and 60–65% of patients progress to ESRD, in a mean of 4 years after diagnosis of recurrence. This poor prognosis may be related to the fact that patients who arrived to transplantation were those with a more severe form of original MN. However, the very poor prognosis in these patients is not always attributable to the recurrent disease as many patients also showed histological evidence of chronic allograft rejection. There is not any convincing evidence that glucocorticoids, cytotoxic drugs, CNI, or purine synthesis inhibitors are of benefit in recurrent MN. Recently, some anecdotal cases of response to rituximab have been reported. The largest experience comes from the group of the Mayo Clinic in Rochester (Minnesota, USA). Fervenza et al. (personal communication) treated eight patients with recurrent MN and a mean proteinuria of 3.9 ± 5.3 (0.18 to 13.8) g/24h with rituximab (1g repeated after 1 week). After 1 year, four patients were in complete remission (50%) and graft function remained stable. No important side effects were encountered. These data are interesting and provocative and need confirmation. No information is available on the long-term outcome of treated patients. At any rate, independently from 'specific' treatments, in patients with recurrent MN a symptomatic treatment with diuretics, ACE-inhibitors, ARB, statins, and anticoagulants is recommended to attenuate the risk of complications related to the nephrotic syndrome (see Chapter 1).

De novo MN

De novo MN is one of the most common causes of nephrotic syndrome after renal allotransplantation. De novo MN usually occurs months or years after transplantation but rare cases may occur earlier, even within 3 months after engraftment. Contrary to primary MN, the recurrent form may develop not only in adults but also in children with similar frequency. It is particularly common in re-transplanted patients. These data may suggest that the etiology and the pathogenesis of de novo MN may be different from those of primary and recurrent MN. De novo MN is often associated with hepatitis B infection. Cases have also been described in HCV-positive patients. In some cases the HCV core protein was found in the glomeruli, suggesting that HCV infection may cause de novo MN through immune complex deposition.

The pathogenesis of de novo MN is unclear. The disease has been considered as an expression of chronic allograft rejection, since lesions of rejection may be associated with or may even antedate de novo MN. However, this hypothesis is challenged by the observation that de novo MN may also occur following transplantation between identical twins (Bansal et al., 1986). It is possible that MN is caused by an auto-immune or allo-immune response to unknown antigens of glomerular or tubular origin, with consequent in situ deposition of immune complexes in a subepithelial position.

The histopathological findings in some cases may either be similar to those of classical IMN, or may be more subtle, showing focal segmental variation in severity, often in conjunction with the features of chronic allograft nephropathy.

The prognosis as well as the risk factors that may predict a poor outcome are not well established. In a review the literature it was found that 42% of adults lost their allograft on average 3 years after the diagnosis. However, some investigators could not find differences in 5-year graft survival rate between the few patients with *de novo* MN and a large group of other renal transplant recipients. Discrepancies were also found in pediatric studies. Some investigators reported 60% children with *de novo* MN lost their graft on average 6 years after the diagnosis, while others did not find different outcomes between children with or without *de novo* MN (Ponticelli, 2007).

The *treatment* of 'idiopathic' *de novo* MN is elusive. There is no evidence that reinforcement of immunosuppressive treatment or introduction of new cytotoxic agents is of any benefit. However, in a few patients, remission of the nephrotic syndrome and stabilization of renal function were obtained by reinforcing the doses of oral prednisone. Antiviral therapy may be effective in cases associated with HBV infection.

References

Ahmed S, Rahman M, Alam MR, et al. (1994). Methylprednisolone plus chlorambucil as compared with prednisolone alone for the treatment of idiopathic membranous nephropathy-A preliminary study. *Bangladesh Renal Journal* 13:51–4.

Araque A, Mazuecos A, Andrés A, Sánchez R, Ortuño T, Praga M (1993). Tratamiento con esteroides y clorambucil de las glomerulonefritis membranosas idiopáticas con insuficiencia renal progresiva. *Nefrologia* 4:350–5.

Ballarin J, Poveda R, Ara J, et al. (2007). Treatment of idiopathic membranous nephropathy with the combination of steroids, tacrolimus and mycophenolate mofetil: results of a pilot study. *Nephrology Dialysis Transplantation* 22:3196–201.

Bansal VK, Koseny GA, Fresco R, et al. (1986). De novo membranous nephropathy following transplantation between conjoint twins. *Transplantation* 41:404–8.

Bazzi C, Petrini C, Rizza V, et al. (2001). Urinary excretion of IgG and alpha(1)-microglobulin predicts clinical course better than extent of proteinuria in membranous nephropathy. *American Journal of Kidney Diseases* 38:240–8.

Berg AL, Nilsson-Ehle P, Arnadottir, M (1999). Beneficial effects of ACTH on the serum lipoprotein profile and glomerular function in patients with membranous nephropathy. *Kidney International* 56:1534–43.

Berg AL, Arnadottir M (2004). ACTH-induced improvement in the nephrotic syndrome in patients with a variety of diagnoses. *Nephrology Dialysis Transplantation* 19:1305–7.

Black DAK, Rose G, Brewer DB (1970). Controlled trial of prednisone in adult patients with the nephrotic syndrome. *British Medical Journal* 3:421–6.

Braden GL, Mulhern JG, O'Shea MH, Nash SV, Ucci AA Jr, Germain MJ (2000). Changing incidence of glomerular diseases in adults. *American Journal of Kidney Diseases* 35:878–83.

Branten AJ, du Buf-Vereijken PW, Klasen IS, et al. (2005). Urinary excretion of beta2-microglobulin and IgG predict prognosis in idiopathic membranous nephropathy: a validation study. *Journal of the American Society of Nephrology* 16:169–74.

Branten AJ, du Buf-Vereijken PW, Vervloet M, Wetzels JF (2007). Mycophenolate mofetil in idiopathic membranous nephropathy: a clinical trial with comparison to a historic control group treated with cyclophosphamide. *American Journal of Kidney Diseases* **50**:248–56.

Brunkhorst R, Wrenger E, Koch KM (1994). Low-dose prednisolone/chlorambucil therapy in patients with severe membranous glomerulonephritis. *Clinical Investigation* **72**:277–82.

Cameron JS, Healy MJR, Adu D (1990). The Medical Research Council Trial of short-term high-dose alternate day prednisolone in idiopathic membranous nephropaty with nephrotic syndrome in adults. *Quarterly Journal of Medicine* **274**:133–56.

Cattran DC, Delmore T, Roscoe J, et al. (1989). A randomized controlled trial of prednisone in patients with idiopathic membranous nephropathy. *New England Journal of Medicine* **320**:8–13.

Cattran DC, Greenwood C, Ritchie S, et al. (1995). A controlled trial of cyclosporin in patients with progressive membranous nephropathy. *Kidney International* **47**:1130–5.

Cattran DC, Pei Y, Greenwood CM, Ponticelli C, Passerini P, Honkanen E (1997). Validation of a predictive model of idiopathic membranous nephropathy: its clinical and research implications. *Kidney International* **51**:901–7.

Cattran DC, Appel GB, Hebert LA, et al. (2001). North America Nephrotic Syndrome Study Group Cyclosporine in patients with steroid-resistant membranous nephropathy: a randomized trial. *Kidney International* **59**:1484–90.

Cattran DC, Alexopoulos E, Heering P, et al. (2007). Cyclosporin in idiopathic glomerular disease associated with the nephrotic syndrome: workshop recommendations. *Kidney International* **72**:1429–47.

Cattran DC, Reich HN, Beanlands HJ, et al. (2008). The impact of sex in primary Glomerulonephritis. *Nephrology Dialysis Transplantation* **23**:2247–53.

Collaborative Study of the Adult Nephrotic Syndrome (1979). A controlled study of short-term prednisone treatment in adults with membranous nephropathy. *New England Journal of Medicine* **301**:1301–6.

Couser WG, Nangaku M (2006). Cellular and molecular biology of membranous nephropathy. *Journal of Nephrology* **19**:699–705.

Dabade TS, Grande JP, Norby SM, Fervenza FC, Cosio FG (2008). Recurrent idiopathic membranous nephropathy after kidney transplantation: A surveillance biopsy study. *American Journal of Transplantation* **8**:1318–22.

Deegens JK, Wetzels JF (2007). Membranous nephropathy in the older adult: epidemiology, diagnosis and management. *Drugs Aging* **24**:717–32.

Donadio JV Jr, Holley KE, Anderson CF, Taylor WF (1974). Controlled trial of cyclophosphamide in idiopathic membranous nephropathy. *Kidney International* **6**:431–9.

Du Buf-Vereijken PWG, Branten AJW, Wetzels JFM (2005). Idiopathic membranous nephropathy: Outline and rationale of a treatment strategy. *American Journal of Kidney Diseases* **46**:1012–29.

Dussol B, Morange S, Burtey S, et al. (2008). Mycophenolate mofetil monotherapy in membranous nephropathy: a 1-year randomized controlled trial. *American Journal of Kidney Diseases* **52**:699–705.

Ehrenreich T, Churg J (1968). Pathology of membranous nephropathy. In SC Sommers (ed), Pathology Annual, pp. 145–86. Appleton-Century-Crofts, New York.

Falk RJ, Hogan SL, Muller KE, Jennette JC (1992). Treatment of progressive membranous glomerulopathy. A randomized trial comparing cyclophosphamide and corticosteroids with corticosteroids alone. The Glomerular Disease Collaborative Network. *Annals of Internal Medicine* **116**:438–45.

Fervenza FC, Cosio FG, Erickson SB, et al. (2007). Rituximab treatment of idiopathic membranous nephropathy. *Kidney International* **73**:117–25.

Fritsche L, Budde K, Farber L, et al. (1999). Treatment of membranous glomerulopathy with cyclosporin A: how much patience is required? *Nephrology Dialysis Transplantation* **14**:1036–8.

Gan SI, Devlin SM, Scott-Douglas NW, Burak KW (2005). Lamivudine for the treatment of membranous glomerulopathy secondary to chronic Hepatitis B infection. *Canadian Journal of Gastroenterology* **19**:625–9.

Glassock RJ (1992). Secondary membranous glomerulonephritis. *Nephrology, Dialysis and Transplantation* **7**(Suppl.1):64–7.

Glassock RJ (2007). Prophylactic anticoagulation in nephrotic syndrome: a clinical conundrum. *Journal of the American Society of Nephrology* **18**:2221–5.

Goumenos DS, Kalliakmani P, Tsakas S, Sotsiou F, Vlachojannis JG (2004). The remission of nephrotic syndrome with cyclosporin treatment does not attenuate the progression of idiopathic membranous nephropathy. *Clinical Nephrology* **61**:17–24.

Goumenos DS, Ahuja M, Davlouros P, El Nahas AM, Brown CB (2006). Prednisolone and azathioprine in membranous nephropathy: a 10-year follow-up study. *Clinical Nephrology* **65**:317–23.

Heeringa SF, Branten AJ, Deegens JK, Steenbergen E, Wetzels JF (2007). Focal segmental glomerulosclerosis is not a sufficient predictor of renal outcome in patients with membranous nephropathy. *Nephrology Dialysis Transplantation* **22**:2201–7.

Hogan SL, Muller KE, Jennette JC, Falk RJ (1995). A review of therapeutic studies of idiopathic membranous glomerulopathy. *American Journal of Kidney Diseases* **25**:862–75.

Hu SL, Jaber BL (2005). Ribavirin monotherapy for hepatitis C virus-associated membranous nephropathy. *Clinical Nephrology* **63**:41–5.

Jha V, Ganguli A, Saha TK, et al. (2007). A randomized, controlled trial of steroids and cyclophosphamide in adults with nephrotic syndrome caused by idiopathic membranous nephropathy. *Journal of the American Society of Nephrology* **18**:1899–904.

Kerjaschki D (2004). Pathomechanisms and molecular basis of membranous glomerulopathy. *Lancet* **364**:1194–6.

Lagrue G, Bernard D, Bariéty J, Druet P, Guenel J (1975). Traitement par le chlorambucil et l'azathioprine dans les glomérulonéphrites primitives: resultats d'une étude controlée. *Journal d'Urologie et Nephrologie* **81**:655–72.

Laluck BJ, Cattran DC (1999). Prognosis after a complete remission in adult patients with idiopathic membranous nephropathy. *American Journal of Kidney Diseases* **33**:1026–32.

Lefaucheur C, Stengel B, Nochy D, et al. (2006). Membranous nephropathy and cancer: Epidemiologic evidence and determinants of high-risk cancer association. *Kidney International* **70**:1510–7.

Lehto T, Honkanen E, Teppo AM, Meri S (1995). Urinary excretion of protectin (CD59), complement SC5b-9 and cytokines in membranous glomerulonephritis. *Kidney International* **47**:1403–11.

Makker SP (2003). Treatment of membranous nephropathy in children. Seminars in Nephrology **23**:379–85.

Mathieson PW, Turner AN, Maidment CG, Evans DJ, Rees AJ (1988). Prednisolone and chlorambucil treatment in idiopathic membranous nephropathy with deteriorating renal function. *Lancet* **2**:869–72.

Murphy BF, McDonald I, Fairley KF, Kincaid-Smith P (1992). Randomized controlled trial of cyclophosphamide, warfarin and dipyridamole in idiopathic membranous glomerulonephritis. *Clinical Nephrology* **37**:229–34.

Nayagam LS, Ganguli A, Rathi M, et al. (2008). Mycophenolate mofetil or standard therapy for membranous nephropathy and focal segmental glomerulosclerosis: a pilot study. *Nephrology Dialysis Transplantation* **23**:1926–30.

Obana M, Nakanishi K, Sako M, et al. (2006).Segmental membranous glomerulonephritis in children: comparison with global membranous glomerulonephritis. *Clinical Journal American Society Nephrology* **1**:723–9.

Ohtani H, Wakui H, Komatsuda A, et al. (2004). Distribution of glomerular IgG subclass deposits in malignancy-associated membranous nephropathy. *Nephrology Dialysis Transplantation* **19**:574–9.

Passerini P, Pasquali S, Cesana B, Zucchelli P, Ponticelli C (1989). Long-term outcome of patients with membranous nephropathy after complete remission of proteinuria. *Nephrology Dialysis Transplantation* **4**:525–9.

Passerini P, Como G, Viganò E, Melis P, Pozzi C, Altieri P, Ponticelli C (1993). Idiopathic membranous nephropathy in the elderly. *Nephrology Dialysis Transplantation* **8**:1321–5.

Passerini P, Ponticelli C (2003). Corticosteroids, cyclophosphamide, and chlorambucil therapy of membranous nephropathy. *Seminars Nephrology* **23**:355–61.

Piccoli A, Pillon L, Passerini P, Ponticelli C (1994). Therapy for idiopathic membranous nephropathy: Tailoring the choice by decision analysis. *Kidney International* **45**:1193–202.

Ponticelli C (2007). De novo renal diseases. In C. Ponticelli (ed) *Medical complications of Kidney Transplantation*, pp.187–204. Informa, London.

Ponticelli C, Altieri P, Scolari F, et al. (1998). A randomized study comparing methylpred-nisolone plus chlorambucil versus methylprednisolone plus cyclophosphamide in idio-pathic membranous nephropathy. *Journal of the American Society of Nephrology* **9**:444–50.

Ponticelli C, Passerini P, Salvadori M, et al. (2006). A randomized pilot trial comparing methylprednisolone plus a cytotoxic agent versus synthetic adrenocorticotropic hor-mone in idiopathic membranous nephropathy. *American Journal of Kidney Diseases* **47**:233–40.

Ponticelli C, Zucchelli P, Passerini P, Cesana B Italian Idiopathic membranous treatment study group. (1992). Methylprednisolone plus chlorambucil as compared with methyl-prednisolone alone for the treatment of idiopathic membranous nephropathy. *New England Journal of Medicine* **327**:599–603.

Ponticelli C, Zucchelli P, Passerini P, et al. (1995). A 10-year follow-up of a randomized study with methylprednisolone and chlorambucil in membranous nephropathy. *Kidney International* **48**:1600–4.

Praga M, Barrio V, Juárez GF, Luño J. Grupo Español de Estudio de la Nefropatía Membranosa. (2007). Tacrolimus monotherapy in membranous nephropathy: a randomized controlled trial. *Kidney International* **71**:924–30.

Reichert CJM, Koene KAP, Wetzels JFM, Huysmans FTM, Assman K (1994). Preserving renal function in patients with membranous nephropathy: daily oral chlorambucil compared with intermittent monthly pulses of cyclophosphamide. *Annals of Internal Medicine* **121**:328–33.

Ronco P, Debiec A (2006). New insights into the pathogenesis of membranous glomerulonephritis. *Current Opinions in Nephrology and Hypertension* **15**:258–63.

Ruggenenti P, Chiurchiu C, Abbate M, et al. (2006). Rituximab for idiopathic membranous nephropathy: who can benefit? *Clinical Journal of the American Society of Nephrology* **1**:738–48.

Schieppati A, Mosconi L, Perna A, et al. (1993). Prognosis of untreated patients with idiopathic membranous nephropathy. *New England Journal of Medicine* **329**:85–9.

Shibasaki T, Koyama A, Hishida A, et al. (2004). A randomized open-label comparative study of conventional therapy versus mizoribine onlay therapy in patients with steroid-resistant nephrotic syndrome (postmarketing survey). *Clinical Experimental Nephrology* **8**:117–26.

Shiiki H, Saito T, Nishitani Y, et al. (2004). Prognosis and risk factors for idiopathic membranous nephropathy with nephrotic syndrome in Japan. *Kidney International* **65**:1400–7.

Thibaudin D, Thibaudin L, Berthoux P, et al. (2007). TNFA2 and d2 alleles of the tumor necrosis factor alpha gene polymorphism are associated with onset/occurrence of idiopathic membranous nephropathy. *Kidney International* **71**:431–7.

Tiller DJ, Clarkson A, Mathew T, et al. (1981). A prospective randomized trial in the use of cyclophosphamide, dipyridamole and warfarin in membranous and mesangiocapillary glomerulonephritis. In W. Zurukzoglu, M. Papadimitriou, M. Pyrpasopoulos, et al. (eds), *Proceedings of the 8th International Congress of Nephrology*, pp. 345–54. University Studio and Karger, Thessaloniki.

Torres A, Dominguez-Gil B, Carreño A, et al. (2002). Conservative versus immunosuppressive treatment of patients with idiopathic membranous nephropathy. *Kidney International* **61**: 219–27.

Troyanov S, Wall CA, Miller JA, Scholey JW, Cattran DC. Toronto Glomerulonephritis Registry Group. (2004). Idiopathic membranous nephropathy: definition and relevance of a partial remission. *Kidney International* **66**:1199–205.

Troyanov S, Roasio L, Pandes M, Herzenberg AM, Cattran DC (2006). Renal pathology in idiopathic membranous nephropathy: a new perspective. *Kidney International* **69**:1641–8.

Uhlig K, Macleod A, Craig J, et al. (2006). Grading evidence and recommendations for clinical practice guidelines in nephrology. A position statement from Kidney Disease: Improving Global Outcomes (KDIGO). Kidney International **70**:2058-65.

Warwick GL, Geddes CG, Boulton-Jones JM (1994). Prednisolone and chlorambucil therapy for idiopathic membranous nephropathy with progressive renal failure. *Quarterly Journal of Medicine* **87**:223–9.

Yokoyama H, Goshima S, Wada T, et al. (1999). The short- and long-term outcomes of membranous nephropathy treated with intravenous immune globulin therapy. Kanazawa Study Group for Renal Diseases and Hypertension. *Nephrology Dialysis Transplantation* **14**:2379–86.

Chapter 8

Immunoglobulin A nephropathy

Richard J. Glassock and Grace Lee

Introduction and overview

The term *immunoglobulin A nephropathy* (IgA nephropathy or IgA N) refers to a primary glomerular disease characterized by the dominant or co-dominant, diffuse, and generalized mesangial deposition of IgA, often accompanied by deposition of IgG and the C3 component of complement in a similar distribution (Donadio and Grande, 2004; Barratt and Feehally, 2005; Tomino, 2007; Glassock, 2008; Lai, 2008). In the past, it has also been referred to as *Berger's disease*, to signify the senior author of the original publication describing the disorder that first appeared more than 4 decades ago in September of 1968 (Berger and Hinglais, 1968). IgA N is most likely the commonest primary glomerular disease in the developed world (D'Amico, 1987). The disease is characterized principally by episodic glomerular hematuria often with persistent proteinuria of a variable degree. It usually runs an indolent course, but may lead to end-stage renal disease (ESRD) in about 30–50% of cases after 25 years or more of follow-up.

Pathology

The light microscopic appearance of IgA N varies widely, but the most common findings are mesangial proliferation and expansion of the mesangial matrix (Donadio and Grande, 2004; Tumlin, 2004; Tomino, 2007,). These lesions are commonly focal and segmental (see Atlas plate 11) but may also be diffuse and generalized in distribution. As the lesion progresses areas of segmental or global glomerulosclerosis often ensue. The other lesions observed include diffuse crescentic glomerulonephritis (uncommon), membrano-proliferative glomerulonephritis (rare), and the minimal change lesion. It may co-exist with thin basement membrane nephropathy (see Chapter 11). Membranous nephropathy is very uncommon histologic pattern. A focal, necrotizing lesion ('capillaritis') may be seen and can signify the presence of a 'low-grade' renal-limited angiitis (D'Amico et al., 2001).

The glomerular IgA deposits (see Atlas plate 12) are often accompanied by IgG and/or IgM and C3, but the C1q component of complement is seldom found, indicating prominent involvement of the alternate or mannose binding lectin pathways for complement activation (Oortwijn et al., 2008). The J-chain is often found in the glomerular deposits of IgA, particularly after partial elution, indicating the polymeric nature of the deposits. The secretory component of IgA may also be present, but this is not very common (about 30%) (Oortwijn et al., 2008; Zhang et al., 2008).

The IgA deposits are principally composed of polymeric IgA_1 (Conley et al., 1980; Mestecky et al., 2008). The polymeric IgA_1 deposits very likely represent the deposition of immune complexes from the circulation composed of an under-galactosylated and over-sialylated form of IgA_1 and an IgA or IgG auto-antibody to the glycan or peptide region of the abnormal IgA_1 (see also 'Pathogenesis,' below).

Predominant IgA deposits in the glomeruli are also seen in a wide variety of other underlying diseases (also known as 'secondary' IgA nephropathy—see Table 8.1), including cirrhosis of the liver, various malignancies (lung cancer, mycosis fungoides), acute infections (staphylococcus, toxoplasmosis, human immunodeficiency virus), psoriasis, celiac disease (non-tropical sprue), and rheumatoid factor negative (sero-negative) spondyloarthropathies (Pouria and Barrattt, 2008). Deposits very similar to that described in subjects with clinical finding compatible with IgA N can also be found in otherwise normal individuals (revealed by autopsy following sudden accidental or suicidal death or by routine pre-implantation biopsies of donated kidneys in renal transplantation). The frequency of this finding varies from about 2–16%, depending on the study (Sinniah, 1983; Waldherr et al., 1989; Rosenberg et al., 1989, 1990; Curschellas et al., 1991; Varis et al., 1993; Suzuki et al., 2003; Glassock, 2008). IgA N is also closely related to a multi-system small vessel vasculitic disease known as Henoch–Schönlein (or anaphylactoid) purpura (HSP) (Philibert et al., 2002). IgA N may be considered to be a *mono-symptomatic or renal- limited form* of HSP and conversely HSP may be regarded as a multi-system form of IgA N. Intermediate forms having the renal-limited character of IgA N and the small vessel vasculitic features of HSP have been described (see 'capillaritis' above) (D'Amico, 2001). Very recently a uniform approach to the classification of the glomerular and tubulo-intestinal pathology of IgA N has been agreed upon (Roberts et al., 2008).

Pathogenesis

The pathogenesis of primary IgA N is now reasonably well understood (Barratt et al., 2007; Mestecky et al., 2008). A subset of B cells, including those in the palatine tonsils, bone marrow, and peripheral lymphoid tissue manufacture a form of IgA_1 that is deficient in galactose residues and has a surfeit of N-acetyl glucosamine (sialic acid) at several O-linked glycan side chains located in the 'hinge-region' of the molecule (Mestecky et al., 2008; Novak et al., 2008;

Table 8.1 A classification of disorders associated with glomerular IgA deposition (dominant or co-dominant)

Primary:
IgA nephropathy (Berger's disease)

Multisystem:
Henoch-Schönlein purpura

Secondary:
Celiac disease
Chronic liver disease (cirrhosis)
Crohn's disease
Cytomegalovirus
Dermatitis herpetiformis
Episcleritis
Familial immume thrombocytopenia
Galactosialadosis
Good pasture's disease
Hepatitis B infection
HIV infection
IgA monoclonal gammopathy
Leprosy
Mucin-secretin carcinoma
Multiple myeloma
Mycosis fungoides
Porto-systemic shunts
Post-staphyloccal acute nephritis
Psoriasis
Pulmonary hemosiderosis
Recurrent mastitis
Sero-negative spondylo-arthopathies
Sézary syndrome
Sicca syndrome
Small cell cancer of the lung
Thromboangiits obliterans
Toxoplasmosis
Vogt–Koyanagi–Harada syndrome

Suzuki et al., 2008). The cellular and molecular mechanisms underlying this glycosylation abnormality is not yet well understood. It may be due to an acquired imbalance of glycosylation/sialylation in a subset of B cells, perhaps driven by a perturbed local cytokine milieu (Mestecky et al., 2008; Suzuki et al., 2008). It might also be due to somatic or germ-line gene abnormalities of the main enzymes responsible for adding galactose or sialic acid to the glycan side chains (core β 1,3 galactosyltransferase or 1,6-sialyltrasferase or the molecular chaperone for these enzymes (COSM) (Beerman et al., 2007; Lai et al., 2007; Buck et al., 2008; Mestecky et al., 2008). The circulating IgA_1 of patients with IgA N has an increased concentration of these abnormally glycosylated molecules (which can be detected by abnormal binding to

Helix aspersa agglutinin) (Moldoveanu et al., 2007; Novak et al., 2008). This abnormality may provide a useful non-invasive diagnostic test for IgA N (Moldoveanu et al., 2007). An auto-antibody response (IgA or IgG class) to these abnormally glycosylated IgA $_1$ molecules results in the formation of immune complexes in the circulation, which can bind and localize to mesangial structures (predominantly via binding to the mesangial transferrin receptor) (Moura et al., 2008; Novak et al., 2008) and accumulate in the mesangium. The immune complexes also appear to be inefficiently cleared by the hepatic Kupfer cell mechanism. The deposition of aberrantly glycosylated IgA containing immune complexes provokes elaboration of various cytokines and growth factors and induces local activation of complement, via the alternative and mannose-binding lectin (MBL) pathways. IgA deposition alone may be insufficient to evoke a recognizable disease, as demonstrated by the high frequency (4–16%) of glomerular mesangial IgA deposits in otherwise normal healthy individuals (such as kidney transplant donors, and suicide/accident victims) (Sinniah, 1983; Rosenberg et al., 1989, 1990; Waldherr et al., 1989; Curschellas et al., 1991; Varis et al., 1993; Suzuki et al., 2003). Some additional event (a 'second hit') is required to bring the disease to its full clinical (and recognizable) form: such as, that a quantitative threshold for IgA deposition be exceeded; that characteristics of the IgA deposits (or the co-deposition of IgG) result in activation of mediators (such as the alternative complement pathway). Clearly something more than mere IgA deposition in the glomerular mesangium must be involved in determining the clinical expression of the disease. The study of subjects who undergo renal biopsy for the diagnosis of IgA nephropathy may underestimate the true nature of the disease, as expressed by glomerular mesangial deposits, both covert and overt.

Etiology

The precise etiology of the *primary* form of IgA nephropathy is unknown. It has been suggested that repeated exposure to a variety of environmental agents (bacterial, viruses) generates an over-stimulated B-cell population (in tonsils and bone marrow) which in turn secrete the abnormal IgA_1. It is also possible that environmental agents (e.g. *Staphylococcus aureus*) create a cytokine milieu within lymphoid tissue (including the tonsils) that favors the production of abnormal IgA_1. The mucosal immune system of patients with IgA N appears to be deficient in its protective response to ubiquitous neo-antigens in the environment, perhaps due to a fundamental defect in dendritic cells (antigen recognizing cells) (Eijgenraam et al., 2005, 2008). A condition closely resembling primary IgA N can be associated with staphylococcal infection (skin, viscera or wounds). This entity is called *IgA-predominant post-staphylo-coccal acute nephritis* (Nasr et al., 2003, 2007; Haas et al., 2008). There is little evidence to incriminate such staphylococcal infections in the overwhelming majority of patients with *primary* IgA N. From time to time reports have appeared identifying various antigens related to environmental agents (viruses, bacteria) in the glomerular mesangium of patients with otherwise typical IgA N (Hung et al., 1996; Ogura et al., 2000). These observations have been difficult to replicate (Park et al., 1994). Rarely, cytomegalovirus has been strongly implicated in the development of IgA N (Ortmanns et al., 1998) but this appears to be a rare event.

At the present time, the abnormally glycosylated *endogenous* IgA1 is believed to provide the dominant pathogenetic antigen in the primary form of IgA N. Thus, it appears that IgA N is an auto-immune disease involving pathogenic immune complex formation with an endogenous antigen (aberrantly glycosylated IgA_1 and a polyclonal auto-antibody (IgA or IgG class). A clear genetic influence is present in many cases of IgA N (Beerman et al., 2007; Gharavi et al., 2008). Familial clustering of cases of IgA N is seen, particularly in Europe (Italy) and the Southern United States (Kentucky, Tennessee, Alabama, Mississippi, and Louisiana) (Beerman et al., 2007). A familial tendency is seen in 10% to as many as 50% of cases, depending on the geographic region and case ascertainment. A genetic 'founder' effect as been suggested by genetic haplo-mapping. Several gene loci have been identified, particularly 6q22 (the IGAN1 locus) (Beerman et al., 2007). The precise relationship of these genetic loci to pathogenesis of sporadic or familial IgA N remains unknown, but is of intense interest. Genetic polymor-phisms may also influence susceptibility and /or progression of IgA N, but this has not been well worked out and some associations are hard to reproduce in all geographic sites and ancestry, perhaps because of the effect of population strati-fication. At the present time, it is not possible to *diagnose* IgA nephropathy by genetic testing alone nor does such testing offer much in the way of prognostica-tion. However, as methods improve, particularly whole genome scanning for single nucleotide polymorphisms (SNP) this may change dramatically.

However, it is clear that the aberrant IgA galactosylation abnormality under-lying idiopathic (primary) IgA N is inherited. As many as 25% of the (appar-ently healthy) blood relatives of subjects with proven IgA N and about 50% of the at-risk blood relatives of subjects with familial IgA N (assuming autosomal dominant inheritance) have abnormally elevated serum levels of the aber-rantly glycosylated IgA (Gharavi et al., 2008). Elevated serum levels of aber-rantly glycosylated IgA is not an acquired abnormality. Renal biopsies of the apparently normal subjects with elevated serum levels of aberrantly glycosylated IgA have not yet been performed but they might be presumed to contain IgA mesangial deposits.

Clinical presentation and diagnosis

Primary IgA nephropathy typically presents in older children and young or middle aged adults (Donadio and Grande, 2004; Tumlin et al., 2004; Lai, 2008). It is seldom seen in infancy or after the age of 80 years, at least in the idiopathic (primary) form. However, this observation may be due to the infrequency in which such patients at the extremes of age are subjected to renal biopsy. The peak age at diagnosis is somewhat older in males than in females (Briganti et al., 2001; Nasr and Walker, 2006). Males are more commonly affected than females, in a ratio of about 2 to 1, in most populations (Briganti et al., 2001). IgA N is much less often observed in African-American blacks but is particularly common in Caucasians, Asians, American Indians, Eskimos, and Hispanics. IgA N remains as the most common primary glomerular disease in young adult Caucasians in the USA (Nasr and Walker, 2006).

Recurrent episodes of macroscopic *dysmorphic (glomerular)* hematuria with or without proteinuria, often in association with upper respiratory infection (with or without tonsillitis), is a hallmark of the disorder, and the most common reason for its discovery. (Donadio and Grande, 2004). However, a substantial number of patients with IgA nephropathy do not have any history of recurrent bouts of macroscopic hematuria. Commonly about 50% of the erythrocytes in the urinary sediment are dysmorphic. In addition, asymptomatic microscopic hematuria with or without proteinuria can also be a presenting feature in those individuals whose disease is discovered upon screening testing of urine or when a urinalysis is performed for another indication. Persistent microscopic hematuria, without any episodes of macroscopic or gross hematuria at all, is more suggestive of thin basement membrane nephropathy or variants of *Alport syndrome* (see also Chapter 11). Loin pain— either unilateral or bilateral—and low-grade fever may also be present during these episodes. This may give rise to initial confusion with urinary tract infection or urolithiasis and prompt an erroneous referral to a urologist. Patients may (often unnecessarily) then undergo repeated urological investigations before the true diagnosis is established, because the presence of more than trivial proteinuria (1–2+ proteinuria on dipstick or >100mg/dL) or other urinary casts and dysmorphic erythrocytes (especially acanthocytes) are either not sought or their presence ignored. A frank nephrotic syndrome at presentation is relatively uncommon. Episodes of reversible acute renal failure in association with acute bacterial or viral upper respiratory infections and severe gross hematuria are not infrequent (Delclaux et al. 1993) but true rapidly progressive renal failure (with underlying extensive crescentic glomerulonephritis; see Chapter 10) is an uncommon event. This latter phenomenon is likely a manifestation of a severe form of renal limited vasculitis. Severe hypertension, even resembling malignant essential hypertension may occasionally be observed present (Clarkson et al., 1977). The diversity of clinical presentation of IgA nephropathy has recently been emphasized by Philibert and coworkers (Philibert, et al., 2008). The major differential diagnostic coinsiderations are: thin Basement membrane nephropathy (Chapter 11), membranoproliferative glomerulonephritis (Chapter 9), fibrillary glomerulonephritis (Chapter 11), resolving post-infectious glomerulonephritis (Chapter 4), and in familial cases both Alport syndrome (hereditary nephritis and deafness) and Fabry disease need to be considered as well. Henoch–Schönlein purpura can develop in a patient previously diagnosed as having primary IgA N.

Laboratory evaluation is of little help in establishing the diagnosis, but several abnormalities may provide clues. Serum IgA and IgA secretory-piece levels are elevated in about 50% of patients (Zhang et al., 2008). Serum IgA/C3 concentration ratios are elevated (greater than 4.0–4.5) but his has poor sensitivity despite reasonable specificity (Ishiguro, et al., 2002; Shen et al., 2007; Nakayama et al., 2008). Elevated IgA levels, presence of microalbuminuria or overt proteinuria, elevated blood pressure and increased IgA/C3 ratio≥3.0 has a reasonable ability to separate IgA N from other diseases causing hematuria, with a correct diagnosis rate of over 75% (Nakayama et al., 2008). Microalbuminuria in association with hematuria is a useful clue to underlying IgA N, at least in children (Assadi, 2005). This would likely be of less utility in adults and in obese subjects.

The most promising new tools for non-invasive diagnosis of IgA N are urinary proteomics and measurement of the serum levels of abnormally glycosylated IgA$_1$ (by the *Helix aspersa* assay) (Haubitz et al., 2005; Lai et al., 2007). IgA rheumatoid factor may be found in 80–85% of patients, and a variety of auto-antibodies to mesangial structural proteins may be present. These very likely are epi-phenomena. Serum complement levels (C3, C4, and C1q) are usually normal, but complement degradation products may be elevated in the serum, particularly during episodes of macroscopic hematuria (Janssen et al., 2000). CH50, C4, factor B, properdin and factor H and I levels are increased in IgA N (Onda et al., 2007). Interestingly C-reactive protein (CRP) levels, even with high-sensitivity methods, are not increased in IgA N (Baek et al., 2008). ANCA titers may be elevated in IgA N but tests using purified antigens

(MPO and PR3) are nearly always negative; thus, a positive ANCA in IgA N is usually a 'false positive' (Sinico et al., 1994). Biopsies of apparently normal skin on the volar surface of the forearm will show deposits of IgA in the dermal vessels in 30–70 per cent of patients (Hasbargen and Copley 1985).

Despite the advances in laboratory testing, at the present time a renal biopsy is still required for the definitive diagnosis of IgA N (Packham, 2007). Importantly, thin basement membrane nephropathy (see Chapter 11) cannot reliably be distinguished from IgA N on a clinical basis (Packham, 2007). However, patients presenting with persistent isolated microscopic (glomerular) hematuria and a positive family history of glomerular hematuria (autosomal dominant pattern) will more likely have thin basement membrane nephropathy than IgA N (Packham, 2007). Patients with isolated microscopic hematuria and a positive family history of hematuria (X-linked pattern) will more likely have Alport syndrome than IgA N. Hypocomplementemia is a feature of MPGN (persistent) (Chapter 9) or PSGN (Chapter 4) (transient), not IgA N.

Epidemiology

As stated above, asymptomatic, unrecognized (covert or 'lanthanic') deposition of IgA in the glomeruli (without any clinical abnormalities) is relatively common (averaging about 10%) in the general population (see above). Thus, it is not surprising that the frequency (incidence and prevalence) of IgA N in any given population is very intimately related to the indications for and the performance of renal biopsy. If the usual policy is to perform a renal biopsy in individuals with isolated hematuria (in the absence of any overt proteinuria) then the frequency of recognized IgA N in the population will be high, whereas if a more restrictive policy of renal biopsy is employed then the frequency of IgA N in the population will be lower. Due to the ancestral influences on the frequency of IgA N, populations with a high fraction of African-Americans will have a low frequency of IgA N. In Victoria, Australia, which has a relatively liberal renal biopsy policy (about 260 renal biopsies per million population per year in adults), the *incidence* of newly diagnosed IgA N is approximately 57 per million population per year in males and 30 per million population per year in females (total 87 per million population per year) (Briganti, et al., 2001). Lower values would be expected in the US and Europe, where the frequency of performing renal biopsies for a diagnosis of isolated hematuria tend to be lower. The prevalence of IgA N among adults undergoing renal biopsies of native kidneys for presumed primary glomerular disease is high, 25–50%, depending upon age and geographic region. IgA N remains as the most common primary renal disease encountered in *young* adults, at least in the *developed* world (Nair and Walker, 2006). A rise in the frequency of IgA N over time and a decline in the prevalence of membranoproliferative glomerulonephritis (see Chapter 9) has been suggested to be due to better hygiene and control of endemic infections (Johnson et al., 2003).

Differential diagnosis

The main conditions which need to be considered in a patient presenting with microscopic or macroscopic dysmorphic hematuria, with or without proteinuria, in the *absence* of a systemic disease are: IgA N, thin basement membrane nephropathy (TBMN) and variants of Alport syndrome (the type IV collagen disorders), membranoproliferative glomerulonephritis (MPGN), non-IgA mesangial proliferative glomerulonephritis, resolving acute post-infectious glomerulonephritis (AGN), fibrillary glomerulonephrits, and rarely crescentic glomerulonephritis (see relevant chapters for details). Persistence of low-grade microscopic dysmorphic hematuria in the absence of hypertension, proteinuria (including microalbuminuria), and normal renal function suggests TBMN, especially if there is a family history of hematuria with an autosomal dominant form of transmission. A persistently low C3 level is a clue for the presence of MPGN (type I or II). A history of a streptococcal or staphylococcal infection or a high anti-streptolysin O or anti-DNAase titer may suggest resolving AGN. Fibrillary glomerulonephrtis is almost always associated with a nephrotic syndrome; whereas, in IgA N nephrotic syndrome as a presenting feature in uncommon. A renal biopsy may be needed in most cases for accurate differentiation.

Natural history

Primary IgA N pursues a highly variable (and often unpredicatable) course (D'Amico, et al., 1993; Coppo and D'Amico, 2005; Berthoux et al., 2008). Most patients will experience multiple episodes of self-limited macroscopic hematuria, often occurring shortly (within 1–2 days) after an acute symptomatic viral or bacterial upper respiratory infection ('synpharyngitic' nephritis) (Clarkson et al., 1977). The majority of these patients will also display some degree of abnormal microscopic hematuria between episodes of gross hematuria. A minority will have only persistent microscopic hematuria, without any overt episodes of gross hematuria. The hematuria is dysmorphic in character (see Chapter 1), but not uncommonly only about 50% of the erythocytes in the urine specimen have the characteristic dysmorphism of glomerular hematuria. Proteinuria may be absent initially and slowly develop over many years. The presence of micro-albuminuria (excretion of albumin in the urine below the level usually detectable by qualitative testing (dipstick) but above normal) in conjunction with persistence of low- grade hematuria may predict the future evolution to a progressive disease (Nakayama et al., 2008). Occasionally, frank nephrotic syndrome is present initially and may undergo partial or complete remission in response to glucocorticoid therapy (see below). Spontaneous complete remissions and permanent disappearance of all abnormal findings are distinctly uncommon in adults (about 6%) but may be much more common in children (about 25–30%) (Schena 1990; Cameron 1993).

Progressive renal failure occurs in a substantial number of patients. Over 25 years of follow-up, about 30–50% of patients with IgA nephropathy will develop end-stage renal disease (ESRD) (Coppo and D'Amico, 2005; Berthoux et al., 2008). The average rate of development of ESRD is about 1.5% per year of follow-up. Some patients will experience a reduction in renal function and then stabilize at an abnormal level for many years (Fellin et al., 1988; D'Amico et al., 1993). Episodes of acute renal failure developing in association with macroscopic hematuria and upper respiratory infections is most often spontaneously reversible unless renal biopsy shows ESRD or very extensive (greater than 30–50%) diffuse crescentic involvement (Delclaux et al., 1993). A very prolonged course of macroscopic hematuria (>10 d) in association with acute renal failure in an older subject with IgA N may confer an adverse prognosis for compete recovery of renal function (Gutierrez et al., 2007). A rapidly progressive course to ESRD is distinctly unusual.

In those patients who develop progressive renal insufficiency the course to ESRD is usually slow but relentless in the absence of therapy. Arterial hypertension is common and may precede the development of progressive renal impairment by many years giving rise to a 'mis-diagnosis' of essential 'primary' hypertension. This seems to be particularly true in Caucasians and is much less true in African-American blacks. Elevated blood pressure is a significant contributor to the rate of progression towards ESRD (see Chapter 1).

Once impaired renal function is well established (e.g. an eGFR of about 30mL/min/1.73m^2 or less or a serum creatinine level above 2.0 to 3.0mg/dL, depending on age, ancestry, and gender) with chronic fibrotic and irreversible changes in the renal biopsy it becomes increasingly unlikely that any specific intervention will slow the rate of subsequent progression (other than control of blood pressure and the use of inhibitors of angiotensin II action). This stage of IgA N is often referred to as the 'point of no return' (D'Amico et al., 1993; Scholl et al., 1999; Komatsu et al., 2005).

Prognostic factors

Also see Table 8.2.

Table 8.2 Factors possibly indicating a poorer prognosis of IgA nephropathy

Clinical	Morphologic
◆ Impaired renal function at discovery (serum creatinine >1.4mg/dL)	◆ *Chronic tubulo-interstitial infiltrates/ fibrosis
◆ *Hypertension (uncontrolled or poorly controlled; >130/80mmHg)	◆ *Extensive crescents (>50%)
◆ *Magnitude, persistence and quality of proteinuria (>500mg/d total protein excretion; increased fractional excretion of IgG)	◆ *Advanced glomerulosclerosis
	◆ Arteriosclerosis and arteriolosclerosis (?hypertension related)
	◆ Extensive mesangial proliferation (some studies)
◆ Older age at diagnosis	◆ 'Capillaritis'
◆ Character of hematuria (macroscopic vs microscopic)	◆ Extensive peripheral capillary deposits of IgA
◆ HLA specificities (some studies)	◆ *Fibroblast specific protein-1 in interstitium
◆ *Low urinary EGF/MCP-1 ratio	◆ *'Tubulitis' (with GMP+ t-lymphocytes in tubules)
◆ Elevated IgA/C3 ratio (>3–4:1?)	◆ C3d deposits in mesangium and on tubular basement membrane
◆ Increased serum C4bp levels	◆ Reduced podocyte density
◆ Increased secretory IgA levels(?)	
◆ Angiotensin converting enzyme gene polymorphisms (DD genotype)	
◆ *Lack of use of inhibitors of the renin–angiotensin system	
◆ Metabolic syndrome (obesity/hyperuricemia/ hypertriglyceridemia)	
◆ Markers of inflammation (increased hs-CRP, low albumin, increased leucocytes)	
◆ Increased excretion of podocytes in urine	
◆ Exposure to volatile hydrocarbons (?)	

(* Most important)

Age

As stated previously, children have a higher likelihood of spontaneous clinical remission, providing they do not have established and persistent proteinuria or impaired renal function at the time of diagnosis. There is some clinical evidence that older age at presentation is associated with a worse prognosis (Cameron, 1993).

Gender

Gender-related differences in long-term outcome of IgA N have been inconsistently noted. Some studies have suggested a worse prognosis in males by univariate analysis (Cameron 1993; Hogg, 1995).

Ancestry

Black children appear to have a worse prognosis than Caucasian children (Hogg, 1995). However, ascertainment (lead-time) bias, may contribute to the differences observed.

Geographic site

Differences in long-term outcome have been reported according to the geographic site of diagnosis. Most, but not all, of these differences are probably due to differences in renal biopsy policy and the effects of an ascertainment (lead-time) bias (Geddes et al., 2003).

Renal function

In general, impaired renal function at discovery (e.g. an abnormally elevated serum creatinine concentration) is a poor prognostic sign unless it develops acutely in conjunction with macroscopic hematuria and acute upper respiratory infection (Cameron 1993; Delclaux et al., 1993). However, even mildly impaired renal function at the time of diagnosis does not guarantee a future progressive course (Fellin et al., 1988).

Hypertension

Established hypertension (blood pressure >140/90mmHg) generally reflects relatively advanced underlying disease and is often associated with a progressive course if untreated (Coppo and D'Amico, 2005). Management of hypertension is an important element in retardation of progression (see also Chapter 1). In the presence of proteinuria, the level at which 'hypertension' is diagnosed in a subject with IgA N should be lowered from ≥140/90mmHg to ≥130/80mmHg in adults.

Proteinuria

The presence of *persistent proteinuria*, over 500mg/d, has been repeatedly demonstrated to be associated with an adverse long-term prognosis, unless the renal biopsy shows only minimal change disease by light microscopy (Donadio and Grande, 2004; Coppo and D'Amico, 2005; Lv et al., 2008; Cattran et al., 2008). Persistence of >1.0g/d of proteinuria at presentation is an ominous finding (see below) (Coppo and D'Amico, 2005). The quality of proteinuria (e.g., increased fractional excretion of IgG) may indicate a worse prognosis, even at equivalent degrees of total daily urinary protein exertion (Bazzi and D'Amico, 2005). It is very clear from well-done retrospective studies in large cohorts of patients with IgA N that a partial remission of proteinuria to levels less than 1.0gm/d are associated with a dramatically better prognosis (Reich et al., 2007).

Hematuria

It has been reported that the *persistence of microscopic hematuria* carries a poor prognosis (Rauta et al., 2002), even in mild disease, but particularly when this is accompanied by overt proteinuria. Isolated persistent hematuria, in the absence of overt proteinuria, may have a favorable prognosis. However, as discussed in more detail below, this view may have to be altered as more studies show a deleterious effect for the combination of persistent micro-hematuria and micro-albuminuria on prognosis in IgA N (Shen et al., 2007). Persistent microscopic hematuria may be a sign of underlying 'capillaritis' (see above). On occasion, authors have associated episodes of *macroscopic hematuria* with progression to ESRD and a higher frequency of crescentic lesions. (Nicholls et al., 1984; Hogg et al., 1994), but others have shown the reverse (Ibels and Gyory, 1994; Rauta et al., 2002).

HLA antigens

Some but not all investigators have found an association between a poor prognosis and certain HLA specificities, most notably HLA Bw35 (Berthoux et al., 1988; Alamartine et al., 1991).

Genetically-based polymorphisms

Polymorphisms of the angiotensin-converting enzyme (ACE) gene have been associated with prognosis in IgA N. A deletion polymorphism in the ACE gene, the DD genotype, may be a risk factor for progression and predict therapeutic efficacy of ACE inhibitors in IgA nephropathy (Yoshida et al., 1995; Hunley et al., 1996) but this is not consistent across all populations

(Woo et al., 2004) The angiotensinogen-M235T polymorphism may predispose to progressive disease (Bantis et al., 2004). In epidemiologic cross-sectional studies many other single nucleotide polymorphisms (SNP) have been associated with susceptibility and/or prognosis of IgA N. These findings have been difficult to replicate and may have been due to systematic errors introduced by population stratification. At the present time, assessment of SNP in IgA N does not have any established role in determining prognosis. However, as methods improve for rapid and inexpensive genome-wide scanning for SNP, it remains possible, or even likely, that markers of susceptibility and/or progression may emerge that will have great value in both epidemiologic studies as well as in individual patients.

Familial disease

At one time, patients with a family history of IgA N were thought to have a worse prognosis. More recent studies have failed to demonstrate this effect (Izzi et al., 2006). The genetic loci currently identified as having an association with IgA N (such as the 622 locus or *IGAN1*) do not appear to have any prognostic significance.

Serum IgA and complement levels

Although commonly ($\approx 50\%$) elevated in patients with IgA N, the actual serum total or polymeric IgA levels have no prognostic utility (D'Amico 1992). The C3 level is almost always normal or slightly reduced. Some authors have suggested that an elevated IgA/C3 concentration ratio (>3 to 4 to 1) is a sign predicting a progressive disease, but this has not yet been confirmed in multiple populations (Ishiguro et al., 2002; Maeda et al., 2003 Komatsu et al., 2004; Nakayama et al., 2008). Elevated levels of C4bp may influence prognosis (Nakayama et al., 2008)

Urinary epidermal growth factor (EGF) to monocyte chemotactic peptide-1 (MCP-1) ratio (EGF/MCP1)

The group of Schena (Torres et al., 2008) has described the utility of measuring the urinary EGF/MCP-1 ratio at the time of renal biopsy in the determination of the prognosis of IgA N. In a prospective cohort study of 132 Italian patients with IgA N they found that this ratio was an independent predictor of outcome (measured as doubling of the serum creatinine from baseline and/or the development of ESRD). The factors studied in this multivariate analysis included sex, age, initial estimated creatinine clearance (by Cockcroft–Gault formula), urinary protein excretion, hypertension and histological grade (Lee classification). All patients were untreated, except for the use of ACEi or ARB (the use of which did not predict outcome). A *low* value for the EGF/MCP1 ratio (lowest tertile) was strongly associated with a progressive course. Over 60% of patients with the lowest tertile of the EGF/MCP-1 ratio developed progressive renal disease after 84 months of follow-up. None of the patients in the highest tertile had any manifestation of progressive disease. At a cutoff value of 23.2 (using concentrations of ECP and MCP-1 in ng/mg urinary creatinine) the sensitivity and specificity of the EGF/MCP1 ratio for the prediction for progression was 89% and 86% respectively. The actual levels of urinary protein excretion or blood pressure control *following* the diagnostic renal biopsy were not included in the multivariate model. There was also no adjustment for the red-cell excretion and the predictive power of the assay was not tested independently in another unselected cohort. Nevertheless, despite these caveats, the findings do suggest that measurement the EGF/MCP-1 ratio in urine at the time of renal biopsy may afford a more precise estimation of future likelihood of progression and thus have value in therapeutic decision making.

Obesity, hyperuricemia, hypertriglyceridemia

Obesity, elevated blood levels of uric acid and elevated triglyceride levels have been independently associated with a worse prognosis for IgA N (Syrjanen et al., 2000; Bonnet et al., 2001; Myllymaki et al., 2005; Nakayama et al., 2008). These are all components of the *'metabolic syndrome.'*

Inflammatory markers

Increased CRP, low serum albumin and increased leukocyte count may be markers of a poor prognosis; but these may simply reflect the state of underlying renal function (Kaartinen et al., 2008).

Exposure to volatile hydrocarbons (solvents)

Exposure to volatile hydrocarbons does not appear to be involved in the induction or susceptibility to IgA N. However, some studies have suggested that heavy and prolonged exposure to these substances may have a deleterious effect on prognosis and enhance progression to ESRD (Yaqoob et al., 1994; Jacob et al., 2007). These findings are based on case–control, and cohort studies. It may be prudent to advise individuals with established IgA N to avoid such exposures, whenever possible.

Other

Increased urinary excretion of podocytes may indicate a poor prognosis (Hara et al., 2007).

Renal biopsy morphology

Several morphologic findings in renal biopsy have been related to a poor prognosis, including the extent of *glomerulosclerosis, chronic tubulo-interstitial fibrosis, arteriosclerosis and arteriolosclerosis, and glomerular crescents* (Coppo and D'Amico, 2005). Podocyte injury and glomerular 'podocytopenia' has also been noted as a feature of severe and progressive injury to the glomerulus in IgA N (Lemley et al., 2002).

Several classifications and scoring systems for evaluating the character and the severity of these lesions have been developed and related to outcome in population studies (Radford et al., 1997, Cook, 2007). All of these show predictive power of the classification and scoring systems in determining the course of the disease to renal failure or ESRD. However, an *e*ffect of these morphologic findings, *entirely separate from and independent of the clinical variables of persistence of overt proteinuria, hypertension and reduced renal function,* has not been consistently observed (Cook, 2007). Thus, the actual contribution of the classification and scoring systems for renal biopsy findings to overall prognostication, over and above the application of simple clinical and laboratory findings at diagnosis or after short-term follow-up remains uncertain. At the present time these scoring systems are of greatest value in identifying, selecting, and stratifying patients for prospective controlled trials of therapeutic interventions. At the individual patient level they should be interpreted cautiously in the light of the associated clinical findings, particularly renal function and proteinuria, as a tool for prognostication. A large multi-institutional collaborative project is currently in progress to provide a definitive answer to this important gap in our knowledge concerning the independent prognostic value of renal biopsy (Feehally et al., 2007; Cook, 2007).

The extent and degree of IgA deposits as assessed by immunofluorescence microscopy do not uniformly predict the outcome, although some investigators have noted that very extensive peripheral capillary wall deposits of IgA are associated with a poorer outcome (D'Amico 1992). The presence of 'capillaritis' and associated segmental crescents may imply an 'active' vasculitic disease process and a poorer long-term prognosis (Ferrario et al., 1995 D'Amico et al., 2001). The coexistence of thin-basement membrane nephropathy is seen more commonly in females with a family history of renal disease, but is not accompanied by an improved prognosis (Berthoux et al., 1995). Superimposition of a lesion of FSGS may confer a worse long term prognosis, as does the presence of extensive and diffuse (>50%) crescents. Minimal change disease and nephrotic range proteinuria is associated with a favorable prognosis, so long as the patient is 'steroid-responsive (see below).

The application of newer techniques to the study of renal biopsy specimens, such as in situ hybridization, immuno-staining for specific molecules (such as fibroblast specific protein-1, cell surface markers for T-cells infiltrating the interstitium and/or tubules (tubulitis), and quantitative polymerase chain reaction assays on microdissected glomeruli) may yet prove to add great value to the more conventional approaches to estimating prognosis from renal biopsy (Nishitani et al., 2005; van Es et al., 2008). Extensive mesangial deposits of C4d (Espinosa et al., 2008) or peri- tubular deposits of C3d (Gherghiceanu et al., 2005) may also be a sign of progressive disease. Morphometric analysis of podocyte density may also be of value in prognostication (Lemley et al., 2002).

However, it must be remembered that renal biopsy is only a 'snapshot' of a disease at a single moment in time. Thus, the findings in a single biopsy sample will reflect the cumulative and lasting effects of past events and only by inference be viewed as a 'window' to the future, absent any intervention on the natural course of disease.

Formulas or indices to predict prognosis in individual patients

Several multi-variate analyses have been carried out in an attempt to refine the ability to reliably determine the prognosis in individual patients (Beukhof et al., 1986; D'Amico 1992, Bartosik et al., 2001; Rauta et al., 2002; Magsitroni et al., 2006; Wakai et al., 2006; Manno et al., 2007; Ballardie and Cowley, 2008, Lemley et al., 2008; Mackinnon et al., 2008). These studies have attempted to deduce 'scores', 'indices', or *formulae* which will allow prognosis to be determined from simple assessment of the additive effect of a variety of clinical and/or histological features present at the time of diagnosis or after a relatively short period of follow-up. While these analyses have been helpful in the determination of the factors that independently contribute to prognosis, the associations have been derived in *populations* of patients, usually examined retrospectively, and thus they have severe limitations when applied to *individual* patients. Because the course of IgA nephropathy can be very indolent with long periods of stable renal function punctuated by episodes of transient renal functional impairment, one should be cautious about prognosticating in individual patients using these methods, especially since they often give conflicting results when applied at the individual patient level. Nevertheless, groupings of prognostic indicators such as proteinuria, renal function, and renal histologic classifications have been quite useful for the selection of patients for studies of the influence of therapy on the course of disease and for the calculation of the expected frequency of selected end points in a placebo population (a critical part of determining sample size and power of a study (see Chapter 3) (Ballardie and Cowley, 2008). Some, but not all, of these formulas have been validated across populations and samples (MacKinnon et al., 2008).

The Wakai, et al. system of classification and scoring is a good recently published example of prognosis prediction and can serve as a prototype (Wakai et al., 2006). This scoring system estimates the 7-year risk of developing ESRD based on eight clinical and pathological variables examined retrospectively in 2269 patients with IgA N in Japan, with a cumulative total of 11,923 person years of follow-up. The variables examined were: gender, age, systolic blood pressure (<121mmHg to >158mmHg), proteinuria (qualitative), hematuria (rbc/hpf), serum total protein, histological grade (Japanese Society of Nephrology classification), and serum creatinine (<1.25mg/dL to >2.50mg/dL). Each variable was weighted with an assigned score value. The minimum score was −8 and the maximum score was +116. Scores between −8 and 22 were associated with a 1% or less risk of ESRD in 7 years; scores between 23 and 38 were associated with a 1–5% risk of developing ESRD in 7 years; scores between 39 and 52 were associated with a 5–20% risk of developing ESRD in 7 years; scores between 53 and 64 were associated with a 20–50% risk of developing ESRD in 7 years; scores between 65 and 80 were associated with a 50–75% risk of developing ESRD in 7 years; and scores above 80 were associated with a 75–100% risk of developing ESRD within 7 years. A sigmoid relationship between score and prognosis was observed. This risk stratification method may be useful, but it was determined by mail survey and included many patients who were treated, so it is not strictly a 'natural history' study.

It should also be re-emphasized that these systems for prognostication generally account for only about 50% of the variability in long-term outcome in IgA N, and some formulas *do not* include renal histologic abnormalities as such factors have not been *consistently* demonstrated to have an *independent* effect on prognosis, over and above simple clinical assessment (e.g. renal function, blood pressure, proteinuria, red cell excretion) (Bartosik et al., 2001). Importantly, the application of several different formulas, scoring systems, or indices to individual patients with similar or identical clinical characteristics do not always provide consistent and comparable results. Much improvement is needed in prognostic tools before they can be routinely applied to individual patients, beyond dividing patients into 'good,' 'moderate,' and 'poor' prognostic categories. It is hoped that in the future one may be able to determine with a high degree of precision the expected prognosis for all patients with IgA N, even at early stages of presentation, long before any impairment in renal function is evident (Lemley et al., 2008; Nakayama et al., 2008).

Specific treatment

No universal, evidence-based consensus has yet emerged on the specific treatment of IgA N, except in certain special circumstances. This is related, at least in part, to the lack of a full and complete understanding of the etiology and pathogenesis of the disease. Most current treatment strategies are empiric and 'non-specific' in that they are not targeted to a precise molecular or biological pathogenetic process. In addition, IgA N is such a clinically and pathologically heterogeneous disease that it is difficult to select a homogenous group of patients for a randomized prospective trial. This difficulty is compounded by the fact that none of the prognostic indicators identified can accurately predict outcome for an individual patient, thus making it difficult to identify patients who would most likely benefit from therapy, even though these indices are useful for stratification of subjects enrolled in randomized clinical trials. Finally, as the clinical course of IgA N is protracted and indolent, a large sample size and prolonged follow-up is necessary in order to yield meaningful results, using clinically relevant 'hard' end points such as death, dialysis, or transplantation.

Based on our current understanding of IgA N as an 'auto-immune,' immune-complex mediated disease, many of the therapeutic interventions have been directed at altering the abnormal immune response and its consequences including cellular proliferation, inflammation, and glomerulosclerosis (Table 8.3). The use of these therapeutic options in the following four clinical settings will be discussed:

- Isolated hematuria.
- Hematuria with proteinuria (normal or impaired renal function).
- Nephrotic syndrome.
- Acute renal failure or rapidly progressive glomerulonephritis.

Table 8.3 Specific agents/regimens that have been used to treat IgA nephropathy

Prevention or reduction of exogenous antigen entry:	Reduction of dietary antigens (gluten free diets; low-antigen diets)
	Removal of infective antigens (tonsillectomy, antimicrobials)
	Alteration of mucosal permeability (sodium cromoglycate, 5- amino salicylic acid, avoidance of alcohol)
Alteration of abnormal immune response or inflammations:	Reduction of serum IgA levels (phenytoin)
	Immunosuppression/Immunomodulation (glucocorticoids, cyclophosphamide, calcineurin inhibitors, azathioprine, MMF, high-dose IVIg)
	Dissolution of immune complexes (danazol)
	Anti-inflammation (glucocorticoids, fish oils, angiotensin inhibition)
Alteration of coagulation/thrombosis:	Inhibition of platelet aggregation (aspirin, dipyridamole, dilazep)
	Anti-coagulation (heparin, warfarin)
Other:	Anti-proteinuric agents (angiotensin converting enzyme inhibitors, angiotensin receptor blockers)

Isolated hematuria

Isolated hematuria is a relatively common mode of presentation for IgA N, especially when the disease is discovered a part of a 'screening' program or incidentally when a urinalysis is performed for some other indication. Various clinicopathological studies suggest that the outcome of IgA N is generally favorable in patients presenting with isolated episodes of gross or microscopic hematuria without any abnormal proteinuria or histological signs of indicating and active or severe disease process (see above) Hence, aggressive therapy is not usually recommended in this group of patients and there are no prospective randomized clinical trials in this area. However, recent studies have suggested that the prognosis may not be so benign in subjects with a biopsy proven lesion of IgA N who have in addition to hematuria, an increase in albumin exertion above the normal range but below that usually detected by qualitative tests (microalbuminuria) and those in whom the renal biopsy show early changes associated with future progression, including tubulo-interstitial inflammation ('tubulitis'), deposition of fibroblast specific protein-1 (FSP-1), T-cell markers or glomerular 'capillaritis' (see above). Perhaps, some of the patients with 'so-called' isolated hematuria demonstrating these 'poor prognosis' features early in the course of disease may become candidates for more aggressive specific therapy. However, it will be difficult to perform randomized controlled therapeutic trials with 'hard' end points (such as decline renal function or ESRD) because of the slow and indolent progression in these patients. If an *early* therapeutic intervention in patients presenting with isolated hematuria were found to be safe and effective, then there would be a radical change in the indications for performing renal biopsy in patients presenting with isolated hematuria. If blood pressure is elevated in subjects with IgA N and isolated hematuria it should be aggressively treated, preferably with angiotensin inhibition (see Chapter 1).

Hematuria with proteinuria (normal or impaired renal function)

This is a quite common mode of presentation for patients ultimately diagnosed as having IgA N. It may account for as many as 50–75% of such patients in some series. Most of the therapeutic trials have been conducted in this group of patients (see Table 8.4). Although it would be ideal to discuss treatment of patients with normal renal function separate from those with abnormal renal function, this is not possible as many of the clinical trials have included both categories of patients in the same trial. The level of proteinuria which was required for eligibility into a trial has varied, but most demanded persistent protein exertion above 1.0g/d, in order to enrich the trial for the expectation of events of distinctly impaired renal function and in order to assess the *surrogate*

Table 8.4 Effects of various therapies in patients with IgA nephropathy with haematuria and proteinuria

	IgA levels	IgAIC	Urine RBC	Urine protein	Histology	Renal function
Gluten-free diet	↓	↓	0	↓	↓	↓
Low-antigen diet	↓	↔	0	↓	↑	↔
Tonsillectomy	↓	↓	↓	↓	0	↔
Tetracycline	0	0	↓	↔	0	↔
Sodium cromoglycate	↓	↔	0	↓	0	↔
Phenytoin	↓	↓	↓	↔	↓	↓
Danazol	↔	0	↔	↓	0	↔
Corticosteroids	0	0	↓c	↓	↑*	↔**
Azathioprine	0	0	↔	↔	↑	↑
Cyclosporin A	↓	0	0	↓	0	↓
Intravenous immunoglobulin	↔	0	↓	↓	↑	↔
Antiplatelet agents	0	0	↔	↓	↔	↔
Urokinase	0	0	↓	↓	0	↑
Fish oil	0	0	↔	↔	0	↔, ↑
ACE inhibitors	0	0	0	↓	0	↔, ↑
Mycophenolate mofetil	0	0	↔	↓→	↓→	↔
Cyclophosphamate	0	0	↓	↓	↓→	↑

0 = not done; ↔ = not changed; ↑ = improved; ↓ = decreased; * = improved in children; ** = only in patients with preserved renal function; c = in children.
See text for references.

end point of a reduction in proteinuria consequent to treatment (see also discussion in Chapter 3). Unfortunately many trials did not require that all patients receive baseline treatment with ACEi or ARB, or both, as a condition of entry into the trial (see Chapter 1). Any imbalance in the arms of the study concerning treatment with these agents or in the degree of blood pressure control during follow-up could introduce a bias into the results.

Angiotensin-converting enzyme inhibitors (ACEi) and angiotensin receptor blockers (ARB)

ACE inhibitors and ARB, alone or in combination have shown beneficial effects on proteinuria and renal function in many experimental models of renal disease (reviewed in Chapter 1), in patients with diabetic nephropathy and in other chronic proteinuric nephropathies (GISEN, 1997; Ruggenenti et al., 1999, 2003). Apart from their ability to reduce glomerular capillary hypertension and thus provide protection against glomerular injury there is additional evidence that ACEi/ARB also have a direct effect on mesangial cell growth and proliferation, upon podocyte integrity and on inflammation and fibrosis. Inhibition of the renin--angiotensin system has pleiotropic effects, including hemodynamic, anti-inflammatory, anti-fibrotic, anti-proliferative, and anti-oxidant effects. Maximum effects on proteinuria are dose-related and are augmented by dietary sodium chloride restriction and/or diuretic-induced volume depletion (see also Chapter 1). The beneficial effects of these agents on the course of renal disease appear to be independent of the degree of blood pressure lowering, although some of the reported effects do appear to be directly due to lowering of systemic arterial (systolic) blood pressure.

ACEi and/or ARB have been used in many forms of non-diabetic glomerulopathies (GISEN, 1997) and many of these studies have included patients with IgA N. In these studies, ACEi/ARB inhibition significantly reduced proteinuria by 30–60% although the effect was variable and those that responded appeared to have higher pre-treatment proteinuria and were more likely to maintain stable renal function. Remuzzi and co-workers (Remuzzi et al., 1991) examined the effects of ACE inhibition on glomerular permselectivity in patients with proteinuria of above 1g/d and normal or moderately reduced renal function with creatinine clearances above 30 mL/min. Enalapril was given for a period of 1 month and there was a reduction in proteinuria and fractional albumin excretion during treatment which returned to baseline values when the enalapril was withdrawn. There was also a tendency for the glomerular filtration rate to decline during treatment although serum creatinine levels remained unchanged. The sieving coefficients of larger dextran molecules was reduced but there was no change in the sieving coefficients of the small dextran molecules.

In a landmark retrospective analysis of 115 patients with IgA nephropathy, Cattran and coworkers have shown better preservation of renal function among hypertensive patients receiving ACEi compared with other anti-hypertensive agents (Cattran et al., 1994).

In the first of several controlled trials in patients with IgA N (Rekola et al., 1991b) studied the effects of enalapril (an ACEi) in patients with a GFR above 40mL/min/1.73 m^2 and hypertension. Patients treated with β-blockers served as controls. Other medications were used when hypertension could not be controlled with monotherapy. After a mean follow-up of 1.7 years there was no deterioration in the GFR in the enalapril-treated group compared to the control group. There was also a decrease in proteinuria and increase in urine protein selectivity which did not reach statistical significance. Mean arterial blood pressures were not different between the two groups. However, no change in proteinuria was observed. Yoshida and colleagues have also added a new dimension to the analysis of the effectiveness of ACE inhibitors in IgA nephropathy (Yoshida et al., 1995). They found that the DD genotype of the ACE gene is found in 43% of Japanese patients with 'progressive' IgA nephropathy compared with only 7% of those with 'non-progressive' disease. Furthermore, proteinuria declined significantly only in patients with DD and not in ID or II genotypes when ACE inhibitors were employed. Similar findings have also been described in Caucasian populations (Hunley et al., 1996). Therefore the analysis of effectiveness of ACE inhibitors in IgA nephropathy probably should take into account ACE gene polymorphisms (Woo, et al., 2004).

The combination of an ACE1 with an ARB, both at maximal recommended dosage may be more effective than either drug given alone, in terms of reducing proteinuria, slowing the progression of renal disease and offering protection from ESRD. This finding was demonstrated in the COOPERATE study, which included a large number of subjects with IgA N (Nakao et al., 2003). Unfortunately, concerns have recently surfaced regarding the validity of the COOPERATE trial (Kunz et al., 2008a), so there remains much uncertainty regarding the overall efficacy and safety of combined ACEi and ARB therapy compared to monotherapy with maximum tolerated doses of an ACEi or an ARB. Nevertheless, a recent meta-analysis (excluding the COOPERATE trial results) supported the view that combinations of ACE inhibitors and ARB are more effective in reducing proteinuria than either drug used alone (Kunz et al., 2008). More multi-center controlled trials of combined therapy are needed to determine if this strategy is clearly more beneficial than monotherapy with either an ACE inhibitor or an ARB (in maximal tolerated dosage) in retarding progression of IgA N to ESRD (Fernandez-Juarez, et al., 2006).

Although relatively few controlled trials of monotherapy using an ACEi or an ARB have been carried out exclusively in those with IgA N and proteinuria (Praga et al., 2003; Coppo et al., 2007a), the bulk of evidence strongly indicates IgA N patients with proteinuria, above at least 1g/d and perhaps lower, benefit from therapies designed to inhibit the systemic and intra-renal effects of angiotensin II both in terms of reduction of proteinuria and slowing of the progression of renal disease. In this regard, it is possible to speculate a potential role for the new class of direct renin inhibitors, either given alone or in combination with an ACEi or an ARB.

Therapy of proteinuric subjects (>500mg/d) with an ACEi or ARB (or perhaps both if either one alone fails to reduce proteinuria to goal levels) is now considered the initial treatment of choice. It is possible that the response to ARB may be superior to ACEi, as the DD and ID genotypes of the ACE appear to respond less well to ACEi therapy. Because of this, some suggest that ARB is the preferred initial anti-angiotensin agents in IgA N (Woo, et al., 2008).

Other therapies (discussed below), such as steroids or cytotoxic agents should be reserved for those patients who exhibit unresponsiveness to ACEi or ARB, given in maximum tolerated doses or in combination of the two drugs, in terms of a decline in proteinuria of at least 30–40%% from baseline or who show progressive loss of renal function despite this therapy. Even a 'partial remission', a reduction of protein excretion to 1–2g/d is beneficial as measured by a delay in the progression of disease to ESRD (Reich et al., 2007). The goals of ACEi/ARB therapy should be to lower the protein excretion to the lowest possible value (preferably <500mg/d) without disabling or dangerous side effects. Sitting blood pressure levels should be maintained at between 115–130mmHg systolic and 70–80mmHg diastolic. The main issue is what to do with the patients who fail initial therapy with angiotensin inhibition (Locatelli et al., 2006 and 2006a). Whether angiotensin inhibition will also be effective in retarding progression of IgA N in milder cases is now being tested in the ACEARB trial (Pozzi et al., 2006). This addition of steroids to ACEi/ARB therapy on the *initial* approach may have added benefits, but this needs to be confirmed in a large trial (Lv et al., 2009).

Fish oils

Fish oil (menhaden oil, mackerel oil) is rich in ω3 fatty acids (eicosopentanoic and doxosohexanoic acid) and appears to exert its effects through limiting the production or action of inflammatory lipids and cytokines released during the inflammatory response (Donadio and Grande, 2004; van Ypersele de Strihou, et al., 1994).There is one uncontrolled trial (Cheng et al., 1990) and six controlled trials (Hamazaki et al., 1984; Bennett et al., 1989; Donadio et al., 1994; Petterson et al., 1994; Alexopoulos et al., 2004; Hogg et al., 2006a and 2006b) published using fish oil in IgA nephropathy. Cheng and co-workers (Cheng et al., 1990) used a dose of fish oil equivalent to 1.8g of eicosapentenoic acid and 1.2 g doxosahexanoic acid for a mean period of 43 weeks in 11 patients with advanced renal failure (mean serum creatinine levels of 319μmol/L (3.6mg/dL)) and observed that the renal function continued to deteriorate in all but two patients. It is probably unlikely that these patients would show a favorable response to any treatment in view of the advanced renal disease. Hamazaki and co-workers (Hamazaki et al., 1984) used a similar dose of fish oil for 1 year in a small trial in patients with mild renal impairment and found that the reciprocals of serum creatinine levels remained unchanged in the treatment group but deteriorated in the control group. Bennett and colleagues (Bennett et al., 1989) also used similar doses of fish oil for 2 years in a small trial in adults with mild renal impairment or active renal disease. They also could not show any benefit in either the creatinine clearance or degree of hematuria at the end of

2 years even when the patients with renal impairment were analysed separately. Petterson et al. (1994) conducted a 6-month controlled study using higher doses of fish oil (5.1g of ω-3-polyunsaturated fatty acids per day compared with about 3.0g in the earlier studies) in patients with IgA N and proteinuria exceeding 0.5g/d. Their results revealed a slight but significant *reduction* in creatinine clearances and glomerular filtration rate in the treatment group. There was also no change in the degree of proteinuria or hematuria.

The largest trial to date was reported from the Mayo Clinic by (Donadio et al., 1994) where 55 patients and 51 controls, who were stratified by serum creatinine levels, proteinuria, and blood pressure, received fish oil (Omacor®) for 2 years at doses similar to the studies of Hamazaki et al. (1984) and Bennett et al. (1989). The primary end point of a doubling of serum creatinine was observed in 6% of patients in the fish-oil group and 33% of patients in the control group. These findings were independent of the presence of renal impairment, degree of proteinuria, or presence of hypertension at baseline. There were no changes in bleeding times or lipid levels and no sustained effect on the magnitude of proteinuria. These encouraging results have to be tempered by the fact that the control group experienced a greater deterioration in renal function (7.1mL/min per year) than the controls in the study by Petterson (1.3mL/min per year) (Petterson et al., 1994) and another study by Rekola and co-workers (Rekola et al., 1991a) who examined the deterioration of renal function in IgA nephropathy using Cr^{51} EDTA clearance (3.6mL/min per year). The patients enrolled in the original Donadio et al. trial continued to show favorable results with more extended follow-up, so long as the patients continued to receive fish oil (Donadio and Grande, 2004). A more recent study of fish oils in IgA N was underpowered, but showed no beneficial effects on progression (Hogg et al., 2006a). Alexopoulos and coworkers in a small study also suggested that 'very low dose' fish oils (0.85g of EPA and 0.57g of DHA daily) also slowed the rate of progression of IgA N. If the latter study is correct, then there is no established 'dose-response' relationship for fish-oils. Some studies have suggested that dosage of fish oil should be should be on a weight basis (40mg/kg/d optimally) (Hogg et al., 2006) but this has not been consistently observed (Donadio et al., 2006).

A meta-analysis of all reported trials through 1996 suggested that the overall effects of fish oil were modest at best (Dillon, 1997). In addition, Fish oils may act synergistically with steroids or ACEi and/or ARB. The source of the fish oil (prescription grade versus over-the-counter diet supplements) might also be a factor in the effects. Side-effects are minimal, except for mild gastrointestinal distress, excess flatulence, and an unpleasant 'fishy' odor to the breath and perspiration. Easy bruising has been very minor and not of serious concern.

Fish oil therapy seems to have little effect on the magnitude of proteinuria in IgA N but its putative 'reno-protective' effect may be more evident in those with nephrotic-range proteinuria and those with more severe disease, as manifested by renal biopsy changes or impaired renal function (Donadio and Grande, 2004). In addition it is likely that fish-oils act synergistically with ACEi or ARB, so they should probably never be used alone to treat IgA N

Despite the caveats regarding overall effectiveness, fish oil therapy remains an attractive approach especially since it does not involve the risks associated with steroid and other immunosuppressive regimens. It may be especially useful in those with more 'severe' disease (including 'nephrotic-range' proteinuria) and a poorer prognosis. Whether it is effective in those with 'milder' disease and normal renal function remains uncertain. Because of the remarkable safety of fish-oil therapy, many nephrologists recommend it as a part of the routine therapy for IgA N, most often in combination with an ACEi or an ARB.

Glucocorticoids

As with other forms of glomerulonephritis, glucocorticoids (oral prednisone or prednisolone, intravenous methyl-prednisolone) have been used in the treatment of IgA nephropathy, in both uncontrolled and in randomized controlled trials.

In a small uncontrolled observational study of patients with IgA N and proteinuria of 2.0g/d or more Kobayashi and co-workers (Kobayashi et al., 1988) used an initial dose of prednisolone of 40mg/d and subsequently tapered the dosage to a maintenance level of 15mg/d given for a period of 1–3 years. Patients who had initially well-preserved renal function (creatinine clearances of 70mL/min or above) appeared to have stabilization of renal function with only one out of 15 patients developing renal failure after a follow-up of 74 months. Renal function, as measured by the serum creatinine level and creatinine clearance, continued to deteriorate at the same rate as before treatment in the group with creatinine clearances of <70mL/min. The complications from steroid therapy included one patient with avascular necrosis of the femoral head and another with a duodenal ulcer.

In another somewhat larger 'quasi-controlled' trial Kobayashi and co-workers (Kobayashi et al., 1989) studied 60 patients with IgA N and moderate proteinuria of 1–2g/d of which 18 were placed on a similar regimen of prednisolone as described above for a period of 2 years and who were compared to 42 'controls' treated with either indomethacin or dipyridamole. As with the previous study, patients with renal impairment (creatinine clearances <70mL/min) did poorly regardless of therapy. In patients with preserved renal function (creatinine clearance 70mL/min or above) and those with histological scores of 6 or less (by the scoring method of Pirani and Salinas-Madrigal (1968)) remained stable in both the treatment and control groups. However, in patients with well preserved renal function and histological scores of 7 or more, steroid therapy appeared to reduce proteinuria and slow the rapid deterioration of creatinine clearance. At the end of a follow-up of 79 months, 6 of 10 (60%) patients in the steroid group were stable compared to only one out of 20 (5%) in the control group. Complications included avascular necrosis of the femoral head in one patient. Another small controlled trial (Lai et al., 1986) failed to demonstrate any benefit of glucocorticoids.

In order to reduce the potential problem of steroid toxicity, Waldo and co-workers (Waldo et al., 1993) used an alternate-day prednisolone therapy given at a dose of 60mg/m^2 for a period of 2–4 years in children with IgA N and proteinuria of more than 1g/d (using historical controls). This study revealed that therapy normalized the urinalysis, preserved glomerular filtration rate, and resulted in a fall in the glomerular activity score in repeat renal biopsies. No steroid toxicity was observed in that there was no increase in the incidence of hypertension, cataracts, growth retardation, or bone disease. No random-ized controlled studies of long-term alternate day steroids in adults have been reported

More recently, in a large open-label randomized and controlled study of patients with IgA N and well preserved renal function (serum creatinine levels ≤1.5mg/dL; 132μmol/L) but with established proteinuria of 1–3g/d, Pozzi and colleagues (Pozzi et al., 2004) demonstrated a long-term benefit of gluco-corticoid therapy, in terms of a significant reduction in the surrogate end point of doubling of the serum creatinine concentration over time, using a regimen of steroid treatment compared to conservative treatment. Not all of the patients in this trial received treatment with ACEi or ARB, so the relevance of this approach to subjects with IgA N who fail to reduce proteinuria after aggressive treatment with ACEi or ARB is unknown (see Table 8.5 for a description of the 'Pozzi regimen'). Nevertheless, the benefit persisted over a long-term fol-low-up of at least 10 years and adverse effects were mild (Pozzi et al., 2004). From these studies it appears that patients with relatively well-preserved renal function, moderate proteinuria, and poor histological scores may benefit from steroid therapy. The role of such therapy in patients with more advanced degrees of renal insufficiency (Serum creatinine levels 1.5–2.5mg/dL) is debat-able, since no controlled studies have been performed in this group (Pozzi et al., 2002; Locatelli et al., 2003).

Table 8.5 A suggested regimen for glucocorticoid therapy in IgA nephropathy

Beginning of months 1, 3, and 5: 1.0g methylprednisolone intravenously for 3 consecutive days

Months 1–6: oral prednisone in doses of 0.5mg/kg every other day (at 8–9 a.m.)

Angiotensin converting enzyme inhibitors or angiotensin receptor blocker to maintain blood pressure <125/70mmHg

(Based on Pozzi et al., 2004)

Taken together, these relatively small studies of glucocorticoid therapy of IgA N demonstrate that such therapy can potentially offer meaningful benefits in surrogate end-points at a low risk of side effects. An older meta-analysis of trials (Schena et al., 1990) conducted in patients with IgA N and moderate to heavy proteinuria with or without the nephrotic syndrome, not including the one of Pozzi et al., also support the beneficial effect of steroid therapy on reduction of proteinuria in patients with proteinuria of more than 1–2g/d at the time treatment is initiated. Additional trials in which *all* patients are required to be treated for several months with ACEi and/or ARB prior to randomization to steroid or conservative (placebo) therapy still need to be done. The additive effect of steroid therapy over and above angiotensin inhibition therapy remains uncertain, but it must be pointed out that in the trial of Pozzi et al. using glucorticoids that the numbers of patients receiving ACEi or ARB were equal in both treatment and control arms.

Calcineurin inhibitors

The calcineurin inhibitors (cyclosporin A [CsA] and tacrolimus [TAC]) inhibit activation of both T and B lymphocytes and theoretically could have a beneficial therapeutic effect in IgA N. The cumulative experience with these drugs in IgA N is very limited and the results inconclusive. Lai and co-workers (Lai et al., 1988) conducted a small controlled trial comparing CsA (5mg/kg body weight/d for 12 weeks) to untreated placebo controls. All subjects had proteinuria of at least 1.5g/d and a creatinine clearance of >50mL/min. There was a significant reduction in proteinuria and increase in serum albumin as early as one week after the start of therapy. These effects were present even 12 months after discontinuation of treatment. There was also a significant *rise* in serum creatinine which returned to baseline level in all but one patient after cessation of treatment (presumably a manifestation of calcineurin toxicity). This study suggests a short course of CsA may be beneficial in patients with hypo-albuminemia and heavy proteinuria (because of the pronounced anti-proteinuric effects of CsA); however, nephrotoxicity severely limits the utility of this agent in the long-term management of the disorder unless it can be shown that CsA is effective at even lower doses(1–2mg/kg/d). Similar results would be expected with tacrolimus and these studies did not make any comparisons to patients treated with ACEi or ARB alone. It is likely that the effects of calcineurin inhibitors are no better than and perhaps inferior to ACEi/ARB therapy.

Mizoribine

Mizoribine is a purine synthesis inhibitor with similar effects to mycophenolate mofetil. Preliminary trials of mizoribine (carried out exclusively in Japan where the agent is approved for use) has shown efficacy, but only with short term- follow-up (Nagaoka et al., 2002; Kawasaki et al., 2004; Ikezumi et al., 2008). This agent may be of value in the treatment of patients who fail to benefit from steroids but further randomized controlled trials are needed to establish a role for this agent in IgA N.

Mycophenolate mofetil and mycophenolate sodium

Salts of mycophenolic acid (mycophenolate mofetil [MMF] and mycophenolate sodium [MPS]) have been use to treat IgA N. Only the former has been subjected to prospective randomized clinical trials and meta-analysis (Navaneethan et al., 2008). The results of the trials of MMF in IgA N have thus far been inconsistent or inconclusive. Two trials from China showed beneficial effects on proteinuria in short-tem follow up (Tang et al., 2005; Chen et al., 2002). Two trials in the USA showed no clear benefit for MMF, but both had low power to demonstrate efficacy and one enrolled patients with far-advanced disease (Hogg et al., 2004; Frisch et al., 2005). One well conducted randomized trial in Europe showed no benefit (Maes et al., 2004), despite a design that was very similar to the Chinese studies. It is possible that the divergent effects observed in these trials are consequent to some confounding variable, such a pharmacokinetics or pharmacodynamics of MMF which differ among the enrolled subjects (Yau et al., 2007). Further trials will be necessary to establish a role for MMF in the therapy of IgA N as the evidence for efficacy is presently contradictory.

Sequential cyclophosphamide–azathioprine

A small randomized controlled trial of low-dose (1.5mg/kg/d) oral daily cyclophosphamide for 3 months followed by long-term low dose azathioprine (also at 1.5mg/kg/d) (plus low-dose steroids) has been carried out by Ballardie and Roberts (2002). The patients were selected for randomization on the basis of progressive decline in renal function during a period of observation. All patients had a significant decline in renal function prior to randomization and the rate of decline would have predicted the early onset of ESRD. The use of the sequential cyclophosphamide/azathioprine regimen was associated with a marked protection from further decline in renal function and from ESRD. Not all of the patients randomized were treated with ACEi or ARB. No additional trials employing this sequential therapeutic strategy (similar to one used successfully in renal-limited vasculitis; see Chapter 10) have yet been reported to confirm these impressive results. Side effects have been minimal. Similar regimens have been reported to be successful in the treatment of severe crescentic glomerulonephritis associated with IgA N, but no controlled trials have been done (McIntyre et al., 2001) (see also Chapter 10).

Leflunomide

Small trials with short term follow-up have suggested beneficial effects of this agent in IgA N (Lou et al., 2006). A controlled comparative trial involving 60 patients with IgA N (30 treated with leflunomide and 30 treated with fosinopril [an ACEi]) has recently been reported (Lou et al., 2006). The composite complete remission rate (both groups combined) was 62% and there was no overall difference in the efficacy of leflunomide compared to fosinopril. Side effects were mild and equal in both groups. The long-term safety and benefits of this drug (approved for use in rheumatoid arthritis in the USA), including protection from the development of ESRD are not yet known and further trials are needed in order to establish a role for this drug in the treatment of IgA N.

Azathioprine

Azathioprine has been regarded as a weak and largely ineffective immunosuppressive agent for IgA N, despite its low risk for side effects and good long-term record of safety in renal allografts. However, the results of an extensive retrospective observational study conducted by Goumenos and colleagues at Sheffield Kidney Institute (UK) has stimulated a re-evaluation of this position (Goumenos et al., 1995). They studied 114 patients (adults and children) with IgA nephropathy; 66 were treated with long-term azathioprine (2mg/kg/d) plus low dose prednisolone and were compared with 48 patients not receiving either azathioprine or steroids. Both received vigorous conservative measures, including blood-pressure control, usually with agents other than ACEi or ARB. The clinical course in the treated patients was different from that in the 'untreated' patients only for those who presented with initial renal impairment (serum creatinine >110μmol/L, >1.25mg/dL). A 'non-progressive' course was seen in 80% of the treated group and in only 36% of the untreated group. No consistent effect on proteinuria was noted. Side effects occurred in 15% of treated patients, which were serious in 3%. Repeat renal biopsies showed stable lesions in patients with a 'non-progressive' course and deterioration in those with a 'progressive' course. Pretreatment biopsies showing mesangial proliferation, interstitial inflammation, and C3 and fibrin deposition (?possibly indicative of a 'capillaritis') predicted a beneficial response to therapy. Although this is an observational and retrospective study, the treated group had more factors indicating an unfavorable prognosis.

Very recently, the preliminary results of a randomized controlled trial comparing the Pozzi regimen of steroid therapy (see above) with and without added azathioprine has become available (Pozzi, 2007). No additional benefits of adding azathioprine were observed, and an increase in side effects were noted in those subjects assigned to the azathioprine arm of the study.

Thus, azathioprine, at least when given with steroids, is not considered to be effective and safe therapy for IgA N. Whether it will be more beneficial in children with severe disease (see below) in combination with other agents or in the 'subset' with continue glomerular inflammation or 'capillaritis' (manifested as persistence of hematuria, despite improvement in proteinuria following ACEi or ARB therapy) or as 'maintenance' therapy after short courses of oral daily cyclophosphamide (see sequential therapy, above) for more progressive disease remains uncertain.

Other combinations of immunomodulating agents

Yoshikawa and colleagues have conducted a series of controlled trials of a combination therapy approach, using prednisolone, azathioprine, heparin–warfarin, and dipyridamole, in children with 'severe' forms of IgA N associated with diffuse mesangial proliferation, including crescents in 16-21% of glomeruli (Yoshikawa et al., 1999, 2006). No studies of this combination approach have been carried out in adults. The comparison has been with the four-drug combination of prednisolone, azathioprine, heparin–warfarin, and dipyridamole to the two-drug combination of heparin–warfarin and dipyridamole (Yoshikawa et al., 1999), or the four-drug combination to prednisolone alone (Yoshikawa et al., 2006). In the study involving the four-drug comparison to the two-drug regimen of heparin and dipyridamole, the four-drug combination was superior in terms of reducing 'immune injury', proteinuria and hematuria, and glomerulosclerosis. No differences in renal function could be shown at 2 years of follow-up; most of the subjects had normal renal function at entry. In the study comparing the four-drug regimen to prednisolone alone, the primary end point of a complete remission of proteinuria ($<0.1g/m^2/d$) the group receiving the four-drug combination was 92% of patients randomized; while those assigned to the prednisolone-only arm of the study reached the primary end point in 74% of instances (p=0.0007 by log rank statistics). Glomerulosclerosis progressed only in the prednisolone only treated subjects. Adverse events were similar. These encouraging results have not yet been duplicated in adults with IgA N.

High-dose immunoglobulins

High-dose intravenous immunoglobulin therapy (see Chapter 2) have been effective in some forms of immune-mediated diseases (Hammarstromm et al., 1992) as there appears to be a deficiency in the IgG_1 subclass in proteinuric patients with IgA N and Henoch–Schönlein purpura (Rostoker et al., 1994). Rostoker and colleagues (Rostoker et al., 1995) studied the effects of high-dose intravenous immunoglobulin in a small uncontrolled study of patients with IgA N or Henoch-Schönlein purpura disease who had moderate to severe histological changes, proteinuria of >2g/d and a glomerular filtration rate >35mL/min. Intravenous immunoglobulins were given at a dose of 1g/kg body weight/d on 2 successive days each month for 3 months, followed by intramuscular immunoglobulins at a dose of 0.35mL/kg body weight twice each month for another 6 months. At the end of the study period there was a decrease in proteinuria, hematuria, and leukocyturia. The rate of decline in the glomerular filtration rate was reduced and repeat renal biopsies following therapy revealed a reduction in histological index of activity and a decrease in the staining intensity of glomerular IgA and C3 deposits. This may be a promising approach, especially in patients with a relatively rapid course of declining renal function, but randomized trials are necessary to fully evaluate the benefits and risks of this approach to treatment. Additional uncontrolled trials have in general supported these findings (Rasche et al., 2006). The recent discovery that an extremely potent anti-inflammatory fraction of heavily sialyted IgG can be isolated from polyclonal Ig preparations, may revolutionize the way we view this form of treatment (Kaveri et al., 2008) (see also Chapter 2).

Tonsillectomy

Surgical removal of the palatine tonsils has long-been advocated as a therapy for IgA N (particularly in some prefectures in Japan and in parts of France), usually combined with oral or pulse glucocorticoids (Bene et al., 1993; Hotta et al., 2001; Miyazaki et al., 2007; Suwabe et al., 2007; Komatsu et al., 2008). Unfortunately, this treatment strategy has never been subjected to a randomized clinical trial (although it is difficult to design one where tonsillectomy is believed to be universally indicated for 'chronic tonsillitis). However, such a trial is currently in progress in Japan. All of the observational and 'quasi-controlled' studies reported so far are biased by possible confounding or patient selection and most have used historical rather than concurrent case-controls. Komatsu and co-workers (Komatsu et al., 2008) recently reported on a trial where steroid 'pulse' therapy alone was compared to tonsillectomy plus 'pulse' steroids. This was not a randomized controlled trial. Nevertheless, the tonsillectomized patients (all of whom had 'chronic tonsillitis') did demonstrate a higher clinical remission rate at 24 months and had fewer proliferative lesions on re-renal biopsy. It could not be demonstrated that the treatment altered the progression to ESRD due to the short-term follow up.

This form of therapy is very popular in certain prefectures in Japan, but is seldom used for treatment of IgA N in the USA or in many other geographic areas. The rationale for this approach is that some of the circulating abnormally glycosylated IgA seen in and participating in the pathogenesis of the disease actually emanates from the tonsils (see 'Pathogenesis,' above). 'Chronic tonsillitis' and recurrent viral or bacterial pharyngitis is not uncommonly observed in patient with IgA N. An exacerbation of the clinical manifestations of disease can sometimes also be traced to an acute tonsillitis. Unfortunately, the results of tonsillectomy (usually accompanied by a course of oral prednisone or IV methyl-prednisolone), have been neither uniform nor consistent. Many of the observational studies describe a 'clinical remission' (disappearance of hematuria and proteinuria) in close conjunction with the treatment, and systematic reviews have shown an increase in the frequency of overall clinical improvement when tonsillectomy plus steroids is compared to steroids alone in uncontrolled studies. Long-term studies are generally lacking and when such observations were possible, clinical benefits were confined to diminution of proteinuria or hematuria (or both) with little demonstrated effect on 'hard' end points such as ESRD. Most subjects treated with tonsillectomy are children and generally this group is in an 'early' stage of disease and not infrequently displays 'spontaneous' remissions of clinical disease. It is noteworthy that in the controlled trial of Yoshikawa, et al., cited above (Yoshikawa et al., 2006), the complete remission rate for proteinuria in children with a 'severe' form of IgA N with steroid treatment alone is about 75%, very close to the frequency of 'clinical remission' claimed for treatment with tonsillectomy and steroids combined.

Spontaneous remissions of IgA N are common in the pediatric age group and very long-term observations of large numbers of patients would be required to show a difference in renal function and outcome consequent to tonsillectomy with adequate statistical power to show such an effect. Rarely, tonsillectomy may be associated with the development of macroscopic hematuria and acute renal failure. Tonsillectomy apparently does not prevent the recurrence of IgA N in the transplanted kidney. In sum, at present, tonsillectomy (with pulse steroids) is regarded as a promising but not established form of therapy for IgA N. Controlled trials are needed (the results of the Japanese trial is eagerly awaited).

Anti-platelet, anti-coagulant, and anti-thrombotic agents

The rationale for the use of anti-platelet and anti-coagulant therapy in IgA N has been based on the findings that platelets play a role in the pathogenesis of glomerular disease, and also that micro-thrombotic lesions within the glomerulus may contribute to the progression of renal disease (Cameron, 1984). Dipyridamole and warfarin have been used in the treatment of other forms of glomerulonephritis and there are only two controlled trials using the 'triple therapy' of cyclophosphamide, dipyridamole, and warfarin in patients with IgA N (Woo et al., 1987a; Walker et al., 1990).

Woo et al. (1987) conducted a small controlled trial in patients with IgA N and normal renal function comparing cyclophosphamide (1.5mg/kg body weight/d) for 6 months, dipyridamole (300mg/d) and low-dose warfarin (to maintain a thrombotest between 30–50%) for 3 years to a group of untreated control patients. At the end of this period the serum creatinine levels and creatinine clearances remained unchanged in the treated group but deteriorated in the control group while proteinuria was reduced in the treatment group but remained unchanged in the control group. Follow-up renal biopsies revealed a significant *increase* in the degree of glomerulosclerosis and the total histological score in the control group (Woo et al., 1987a). While there was also an increase in the degree of glomerulosclerosis in the treatment group, this did not reach statistical significance. In an extension study some patients elected to continue on dipyridamole and warfarin while the others did not (Woo et al., 1991). Both groups continued on follow-up and after 5 years the patients who chose to continue therapy had a small rise in serum creatinine levels. Those who discontinued treatment experienced a significant elevation in serum creatinine levels. Both groups experienced a significant fall in creatinine clearance. There were no patients with ESRD in the treatment group and six with ESRD in the non-treatment group. This was not a controlled trial, as the results are biased by the fact that the more compliant patients would choose to stay on therapy and therefore tend to have better outcomes, the results are still worth noting as it gives an indication that this form of therapy might be effective over the long term in this slowly progressive disease.

Walker and coworkers (Walker, et al., 1990) performed a similar study in patients with IgA N who had one or more of the following criteria: significant hematuria (>200,000 RBC/mL); proteinuria of >1g/d; an elevated serum creatinine level of >120μmol/L (1.36mg/dL) but <200μmol/L (2.27mg/dL); or a renal biopsy showing >10% crescents. 'Triple therapy' consisting of oral cyclophosphamide (1–2mg/kg/d) for 6 months, and dipyridamole (400mg/d) and warfarin (at anticoagulant doses) was compared to no therapy and the follow-up was 2 years. At the end of the trial, there was an increase in serum creatinine levels in both groups, and an apparent, although not significant, fall in a hematuria in the control group. Proteinuria was reduced in the treatment group and remained unchanged in the control group. Therefore, the results of this trial were not as encouraging as those in the trial of Woo et al. (1987). The differences in the results could be related to differences in doses of warfarin and the duration of the two trials. Both studies, however, revealed a reduction of proteinuria with treatment.

In order to avoid the serious drawbacks of long-term cyclophosphamide therapy, Lee and colleagues (Lee et al., 1989) used a combination of dipyridamole and low-dose warfarin, without cyclophosphamide, for 3 years in a small, controlled study of patients with renal impairment who had serum creatinine levels between 1.6mg/dL (140μmol/L) and 3.0mg/dL (265μmol/L). At 10 months of follow-up serum creatinine levels significantly increased in the control group but remained unchanged in the treatment group. At 3 years of follow-up, the findings were similar and four patients from the control group and one from the treatment group were in end-stage renal failure (Lee et al., 1997).

Another controlled trial examined the effects of combination therapy using diypridamole and aspirin in patients with slightly elevated serum creatinine levels was reported by Chan et al. (1987) who found that after 33 months there was no difference in serum creatinine levels, creatinine clearances, or proteinuria between the treatment and control group. Combinations of azathioprine, steroids, heparin, and anti-thrombotic agents have been shown to be beneficial in children with severe IgA N in a small controlled trials (see 'Combined therapies,' above). A meta-analysis of this treatment of IgA N with anti-platelet agents, including the use of dilazep, an anti-platelet drug approved in Japan but not in the USA, showed relatively minor benefits in IgA N (Taji et al., 2006).

The overall long-term benefits (and risks) of anti-platelet and anti-coagulant therapy in IgA N remain unclear at present although the therapy generally reduces proteinuria modestly over the short term. The long-term use of cyclophosphamide, in conjunction with these agents, also does not appear to be justifiable in this group of patients (Chan et al., 1987), due to the risk of side-effects with long-term treatment with this cytotoxic agent. Shorter term use of daily oral cyclophosphamide (sequentially with oral Azathioprine) and steroids (but without anti-platelet or anti-thrombotic agents) in patients with overtly progressive disease is discussed above (see 'Sequential therapy').

Urokinase

Several investigators have used urokinase, a fibrinolytic agent, in IgA N because of the finding of fibrinogen in the glomerulus of many IgA nephropathy patients (Miura et al., 1985; Miura 1987), particularly in those with segmental crescents and 'capillartiis'. Miura et al. (1989) reported a controlled trial using urokinase given at a dose of 48,000 to 60,000IU for periods of 2 weeks in 27 patients, and continued at once a week in another 14 patients for a period of between 2-47 months. There were 16 controls on anti-platelet agents. All patients had improved serum creatinine levels and proteinuria during the study period but these changes were not sustained and after 65 months of follow-up there was no significant difference in the serum creatinine levels between urokinase-treated and control patients. It is therefore difficult to draw any conclusions regarding the benefits of urokinase therapy and this approach is not currently recommended.

Anti-microbials

There is only one brief report of a controlled trial using *tetracycline* for 1 year in patients with IgA N (Kincaid-Smith and Nicholls 1983). This small trial showed that although there was a significant reduction in the magnitude of hematuria, the serum creatinine and proteinuria remained unchanged. There have also been numerous anecdotal reports of the use of antibiotics in children with IgA N where they were found not to change the rate of gross hematuria.

Sodium cromoglycate and 5-aminosalicylic acid

Both sodium cromoglycate, an anti-allergic agent, and 5-aminosalicylic acid alter mucosal permeability to food antigens. Two trials have been performed in IgA N using these agents, one controlled (Sato et al., 1990) and using either sodium cromoglycate (1200mg/d for 4 months) or 5-aminosalicyclic acid and another uncontrolled study by. Bazzi and co-workers (Bazzi et al. 1992) in which patients with serum creatinine levels <2mg/dl and proteinuria of >1.5g/d received either sodium cromoglycate (400mg/d for 6 months or 5-aminosali-cyclic acid 2.4 g/d for 6 months). Apart from a reduction in serum IgA levels in the sodium cromoglycate-treated group no changes were noted in serum creatinine levels, degree of proteinuria, or circulating IgA immune complex levels.

Phenytoin

Phenytoin sodium, an anticonvulsant agent with pleotropic properties, has been shown to consistently reduce serum total IgA levels (Aarli and Tunder 1975; Seager et al., 1975) and to depress cellular immunity (Aarli, 1980) thus justifying the trial of its use in patients with IgA N. Two controlled trials have been reported (Clarkson et al., 1980; Egido et al., 1984b). Clarkson and co-workers (Clarkson et al., 1980) administered phenytoin sodium at a dose of 5–6mg/kg body weight/d to achieve therapeutic anticonvulsant levels in patients with IgA N with proteinuria and normal renal function for a period of 2 years while Egido et al. (1984b) gave similar doses (phenytoin 300mg/d) to patients with IgA N and normal renal function to moderate renal failure (creatinine up to 3.0mg/dL) for a mean period of 17 months. Phenytoin reduced serum IgA levels in 54% to 74% of treated patients the episodes of macro-hematuria, but it did not appear to have a beneficial effect on the outcome of the disease, at least over relatively short periods of follow-up.

Danazol

Danazol, a heterocyclic anabolic steroid, increases serum complement levels in patients with complement deficiency such as hereditary angioneurotic edema (Gelfand et al., 1976) and may thus assist in solubilizing IgA glomerular deposits. In an observational study, Tomino and co-workers (Tomino et al., 1984) administered danazol at a dose of 200mg/d to patients with IgA N (with serum creatinine between 0.8mg/dL and 2.7mg/dL) for 4–10 months and observed a reduction in proteinuria in patients with mild renal histology. There was no change in serum creatinine, degree of hematuria, and serum IgA levels. These interesting findings have not yet been substantiated by further clinical trials.

Restricted diets

Increased levels of IgA antibodies to a variety of alimentary antigens, most frequently anti-gliadin IgA (Fornasieri et al., 1987; Rodriguez-Soriano et al., 1988; Rostoker et al., 1988) have been described in patients with IgA N and a few studies have also demonstrated that food antigens participate in the formation of IgA immune complexes (Fornasieri et al., 1988; Sancho et al., 1988). Only two uncontrolled trials have been performed to study the effects of a reduction in dietary antigens. Coppo and co-workers (Coppo et al., 1990) used a *gluten-free* diet in adults with serum creatinine ranging from 0.5–2.7mg/dL, for a period of 6 months to 4 years. There was a reduction in proteinuria and microscopic hematuria after six months on the gluten-free diet. However, serum creatinine levels continued to rise suggesting that although some immunological abnormalities were corrected, the diet did not favorably alter the clinical course. A short anecdotal report by Ferri et al. (1992) showed that an *oligo-antigenic diet* could reduce proteinuria, but there were no changes in renal function. Follow-up of patients upon return to 'normal' diet was lacking.

It appears from these limited trials that dietary restrictions (gluten) do not offer much benefit apart from a reduction in proteinuria, but larger-scale trials and longer follow-up are probably warranted. It is noteworthy that patients with proven gluten- sensitive enteropathy (with anti-gliadin antibody positivity and an abnormal small intestinal biopsy) do have an increased incidence of IgA glomerular deposits and in such patients a gluten- free diet may be beneficial.

Oral calcitriol

A single small trial reported beneficial effects on proteinuria of oral calcitriol (0.5mcg twice weekly) in IgA nephropathy (Szeto et al., 2008). No controlled trials have yet been conducted.

Nephrotic syndrome associated with minimal glomerular lesions

The nephrotic syndrome is a rather uncommon presentation of IgA N with a frequency ranging from 0–13%. Although nephrotic-range proteinuria has been associated with a poor prognosis (see above) (Katz et al., 1983; Neelakantappa et al., 1988) there have been reports of a subset of patients (frequently Chinese) who respond to steroid therapy or who have spontaneous remission of the nephrotic syndrome. Virtually all the reported cases of *steroid-responsive nephrotic syndrome* in adults and children with IgA nephropathy have only minimal glomerular changes on renal biopsy. In such cases, the nephrotic syndrome runs a course similar to *idiopathic* minimal change nephropathy (see also Chapter 5) with relapses that usually remain steroid responsive. It is uncertain, at present, if this entity constitutes two separate diseases; that is, IgA N and minimal change nephropathy, occurring at the same time by chance alone, whether it is a variant of IgA nephropathy, or whether it is actually minimal change disease with IgA deposits (Southwest Pediatric Nephrology Study Group 1985). Two studies (Cheng et al., 1989; Fukushi et al., 1989) report the disappearance of the IgA deposits in four patients following steroid therapy, with one concluding that this was more likely the result of a variant of minimal change nephropathy (Fukushi et al., 1989) and the other suggesting that it is a distinct clinical syndrome (Cheng et al., 1989). Despite the confusion in classifying this entity, there is general agreement that this group of patients should be treated with steroids as they have a favorable prognosis.

Lai et al. (1989) conducted a small controlled trial of nephrotic patients with IgA N of prednisolone or prednisone at a dose of 40–60mg/d with subsequent tapering of the dose after 8 weeks and a total treatment period of 4 months. The controls received no treatment. Patients with varying severity of histology on renal biopsy were enrolled in the trial and after a mean follow-up of 38 months there was no significant difference in the serum creatinine levels and creatinine clearances between the two groups. Moreover, 40% of patients on steroid therapy developed complications. However, despite the *overall* lack of benefit of steroid therapy in IgA N with nephrotic syndrome, there was excellent remission rate of 80% of patients with mild histological changes only. This study confirms the observation that patients with IgA N, mild renal histology and the nephrotic syndrome clearly benefit from steroid therapy. Relapses in these patients usually respond again to steroids although cyclophosphamide at a dose of 1.5–2.0mg/kg body weight for about 8–12 weeks (Southwest Pediatric Nephrology Study Group 1985) may be required in the frequent relapsing patient.

Acute and/or rapidly progressive renal failure

Acute or rapidly progressive renal failure are uncommon presentations in IgA N, occurring in about 10% or less of patients of which 20–25% might require temporary dialysis. Acute renal failure occurs: i) in association with the development of *diffuse and extensive crescentic glomerulonephritis;* or ii) following an episode of *gross hematuria* in which the renal biopsy reveals minor glomerular changes (including occasional segmental crescents involving <25% of glomeruli) but marked *acute tubular necrosis, interstitial nephritis* and marked red cell casts in the tubule lumina (Delclaux et al., 1993; Fogazzi et al., 1995). A separate discussion of these two clinical forms are needed.

With extensive crescentic glomerulonephritis

Crescentic glomerulonephritis is seen in 5% or less of patients with IgA N in series that report such cases (Rocatello et al., 1995). Some large series, however, have not reported the presence of crescentic glomerulonephritis at all (Abuelo et al., 1984). The histological finding of a crescentic glomerulonephritis, where 30–50% or more of the glomeruli are involved with cirumferential crescent formation, is frequently associated with the clinical presentation of a rapidly progressive glomerulonephritis (Chapter 10). This, however, is not always the case in IgA N as there are patients with 'crescentic glomerulonephritis' on biopsy who have relatively benign presentations with reversible acute renal failure and/or stable renal function (Delclaux et al.,1993; Fogazzi et al., 1995).

Not surprisingly, there have been no controlled therapeutic studies as the condition of rapidly progressive glomerulonephritis is uncommon in IgA N. Anecdotal reports have described the use of various therapeutic regimens which include steroids, cytotoxic agents, anticoagulants, and plasmapheresis

(Rocatello et al., 1995). Most of the regimens use a combination of glucocorti-coid—either oral prednisolone or intravenous methylprednisolone pulses—and cytotoxic agents such as cyclophosphamide and/or azathioprine. The combination of prednisolone and cytotoxic agents does not appear to be uni-formly effective in controlling progression of the disease (Hene et al., 1982; Lai et al., 1987; Itami et al., 1989), but anecdotal reports of success has been claimed (see also Chapter 10).

Plasmapheresis added to a regular dose of steroids and cytotoxic agents has been shown to stabilize renal function during treatment but a variable course was observed following cessation of therapy with some reporting a deteriora-tion of function several months later (Coppo et al., 1985). The reports of Lai and others have noted a more sustained effect (Lai et al., 1987; Boobes et al., 1990; Rocatello et al., 1995). Intravenous methlyprednisolone 'pulse' therapy has been thought to be beneficial according to the observational study of Habib and co-workers (Habib et al., 1994) who reported that in a group of 38 patients who had crescent formation in 50% or more of glomeruli, nephrotic syndrome, or both, all nine (100%) who remained untreated progressed to end-stage renal failure, whereas seven out of 17 (41%) who were treated with combination therapies including oral steroids immunosuppressive agents, anticoagulants, and non-steroidal anti-inflammatory agents progressed to end-stage renal fail-ure while none of the 12 (0%) who were given methylprednisolone alone were in end-stage renal failure. However, this observation has not always been repro-ducible as others have found no benefit with the use of methylprednisolone pulse therapy alone (Coppo et al., 1985; Itami et al., 1989).

Without extensive crescentic glomerulonephritis

Some patients with acute renal failure have been noted to exhibit minor glom-erular abnormalities and/or scattered segmental glomerular crescents (<30% of glomeruli involved) accompanied by acute tubulo-interstitial lesions on renal biopsy (Kincaid-Smith et al., 1983; Delclaux et al., 1993; Fogazzi et al., 1995). These patients typically present with an episode of macro-hematuria, sometimes associated with flank pain, shortly following an acute upper respiratory illness. The episodes of acute renal failure may be recurrent in individual patients. Rarely, these episodes may follow surgical tonsillectomy, especially in the face of an active or chronic tonsillitis. The episodes of acute renal failure are thought to occur as a result of extensive glomerular bleeding, leading to tubular damage due to the local production of toxic hemoglobin degradation products and/or toxic oxygen radicals (Fogazzi et al., 1995) within the tubular lumina. Temporary dialysis therapy is required in some patients during the period of acute renal failure but nearly all patients eventually recover renal function.

Practical recommendations

Isolated hematuria

Because of an intrinsically favorable prognosis, in the absence of progression to overt proteinuria, this group of patients requires no specific therapy. Observation with angiotensin II inhibition for hypertension is indicated.

Persistent proteinuria and hematuria (with or without reduced renal function)

A consensus on the treatment of patients with IgA nephropathy who present with hematuria and significant (but often non-nephrotic) proteinuria (e.g., >0.5–3.0g/d) with or without mild renal impairment has emerged in the past few years. Table 8.4 provides a summary of the effects of various therapies in this group of patients and Fig. 8.1 provides a suggested algorithm for *initial* management. A trial of ACEi and or ARB is recommended in all patients. The dose of ACEi or ARB should be gradually increased to maximum recommended

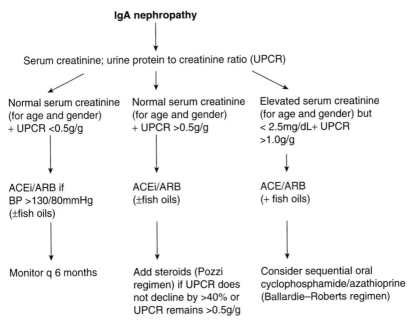

ACEi: angiotensin converting enzyme inhibitor; ARB: angiotensin II receptor blocker; UPCR: urine protein to creatinine on spot first morning voided urine

Fig. 8.1 A suggested algorithm for initial treatment of IgA nephropathy based on urine protein excretion and serum creatinine (without minimal change lesions, extensive crescents or advanced glomerulosclerosis/interstitial fibrosis on renal biopsy). See text for additional details.

dosage using proteinuria as the guidepost of an effect, with a goal of reducing proteinuria to 500mg/d or less in the absence of symptoms related to low blood pressure (<110mmHg systolic) or orthostatic hypotension. The additional of a low-salt diet and/or diuretics potentiates the anti-proteinuric actions of these agents. Blood pressure should be maintained at 120–130mmHg systolic and 70–80mmHg diastolic. If goal proteinuria cannot be met with the use of one agent alone, then treatment with both agents (an ACEi and an ARB) should be considered, Even a partial reduction of proteinuria to levels higher than 500mg/d (1–2g/d) can be of benefit in slowing the pace of progression of renal disease.

If a substantial reduction in proteinuria cannot be achieved by monotherapy with ACEi or ARB therapy in maximum tolerated dosage or by a combination of an ACEi and an ARB (or if disabling side-effects ensue limiting this treatment approach), then adjunctive therapy can be considered. There is no reason not to use fish oils (preferably prescription forms) in doses of 40mg/kg/d usually in two divided doses, concomitantly with the ACEi/ARB regimens, but the true added value of this treatment approach is not well known. Side effects are usually mild. Anti-platelet agents (such as dilazep or dipyridamaole) can also be given but the overall safety and efficacy of this 'add-on' is not well known, especially in the face of concomitant fish-oil and ACEi/ARB therapy. Monotherapy with anti-platelet agents, alone or in combination with anti-coagulants, cannot be recommended at this time.

The choice of adjunctive therapy for patients who do not respond to the above regimens must be individualized. Evidence from controlled trials suggests that a course of steroids using the *'Pozzi' regimen* (described above) will reduce proteinuria and slow the rate of progression of renal disease. The level of renal function at the time such treatment is started may influence the response, and patients with serum creatinine concentrations ≤1.5mg/dL (132μmol/L, creatinine clearance >70mL/min) without moderate-to-marked tubulo-interstitial fibrosis on renal biopsy appear to respond better than those with more advanced chronic disease, but exception to this general rule do exist (Mitsuiki et al., 2007). Thus, the decision to use steroids for therapy should be made before significant progression of disease has occurred. The addition of oral azathioprine alone to the steroid regimen is of no proven benefit and may even be harmful. We remain uncertain about the possible role of immunosuppressive agents (such as azathioprine or MMF) in the small subset of patients with persistence of hematuria and red-cell casts who have evidence of 'capillaritis' in renal biopsies. These patients may represent examples of a 'smoldering' renal-limited small vessel vasculitis and might be considered candidates for a more aggressive immunomodulating approach, although proof of efficacy and safety for this is lacking.

If the serum creatinine concentration is >2.5mg/dL (220µmol/L; estimated GFR <30mL/min/1.73m^2—'the point-of-no-return') and advanced tubulo-interstitial chronic lesions are present in the renal biopsy, further treatment is generally futile, except that ACEi/ARB should be continued with intensified monitoring of serum potassium concentration in order to retard the rate of progression to ESRD.

Adult patients who exhibit features of progression with a loss of estimated GFR >5–7mL/min/year (in the absence of rapidly progressive glomerulone-phritis with extensive glomerular crescent involvement, see below) should be considered candidates for a low-dose sequential oral daily cyclophosphamide/oral azathioprine regimen, such as originally described by Ballardie and Roberts (see above) (Ballardie and Roberts, 2002). Children with severe proliferative (and crescentic) IgA N could be considered for treatment using the four-drug combination regimen described by Yoshikawa, et al. (see above) (Yoshikawa et al., 2006).

The therapeutic roles of other adjunctive agents, such as mycophenolate mofetil [MMF] or enteric coated mycophenolate sodium [MPS]), sirolimus, cyclosporin, tacrolimus, IVIg, and leflunomide are not well established and cannot be generally recommended. No trials with rituximab (a chimeric anti-CD20 monoclonal antibody agent) have yet been reported in IgA N. While MMF as therapeutic option for IgA N has been studied in randomized and controlled trials (conducted in China, Europe, and the USA) the results are inconsistent and contradictory. The effects of MMF appear to be better in Asians than in Caucasians, but this has not been formally evaluated in a prospective fashion. High-dose IVIg has been claimed to have a benefit in IgA N, but this is based on small uncontrolled trials only. There is no consistent body of evidence that calcineurin inhibitors on sirolimus may be indicated for long-term use in IgA N.

Tonsillectomy, usually performed in conjunction with short-term oral or 'pulse' steroids, seems to have an effect to promote 'clinical remission', particularly in children. However, no randomized, controlled long-term trials have yet been conducted and the available observational studies do not support the view that this therapy has any material and consistent effect on long-term outcome (Rasche et al., 1999), even though episodes of hematuria may decrease in frequency and urinary protein excretion may diminish contemporaneously with this treatment. Thus, at the present time, tonsillectomy (with or without pulse steroid therapy) cannot be generally recommended for the treatment of IgA N. Other therapies, such as danazol, phenytoin, urokinase, sodium cromoglycate, or chronic broad-spectrum antimicrobials have no significant lasting effect on the course of IgA N and are not recommended. High dose immunoglobulin therapy may eventually be found to be effective (especially with the identification of an 'anti-inflammatory IgG'), but at present the limited observational studies are only suggestive of a beneficial long-term effect in severe and progressive diseases (Rasche et al., 2006).

Nephrotic syndrome with minimal glomerular changes

Treatment of the nephrotic syndrome associated with minimal glomerular histological changes in IgA N should follow the lines of treatment in patients with idiopathic nephrotic syndrome and MCN as pointed our in Chapter 4. Patients can be given a course of prednisone at an initial dose of 40–60mg/d (60mg/m^2 in children) for a total treatment period of 3–4 months. Relapses usually respond to steroids although cyclophosphamide at a dose of 1.5–2.0mg/kg body weight for 8–12 weeks may be required in the frequent relapser. Treatment of patients with the *nephrotic syndrome* and IgA N who have more severe changes on renal histology is more difficult to define as there has only been one controlled study (Lai et al., 1989) which showed that a short course of prednisolone did not confer any benefits on this group of patients. As discussed above, other controlled trials have shown benefits when steroids are given to patients with IgA N exhibiting lower levels of proteinuria (see above). Consistent with other recommendation in other settings, patients with the nephrotic syndrome and IgA deposits in glomeruli, should be offered ACEi/ARB therapy, although the benefit of this approach in those with underlying minimal change nephropathy who are also very steroid-sensitive is not well understood.

Acute or rapidly progressive glomerulonephritis

With extensive crescents

Because of the conflicting findings in small uncontrolled trials using different regimens, it is difficult to provide any 'evidence-based' recommended therapy in patients with rapidly progressive IgA N associated with extensive glomerular crescents (>30–50% glomerular crescents), but aggressive therapy, including IV methylprednisolone pulses and even plasma exchange might be justified because of the uniformly dismal outcome in untreated patients. Thus, until more definitive data are available, patients with rapidly progressive IgA N associated with very extensive glomerular crescents should be treated in the standard fashion, as other forms of crescentic glomerulonephritis (see Chapter 10), with prednisolone at an initial dose of 1mg/kg body weight/d and oral cyclophosphamide at a dose of 2mg/kg body weight/d. A methylpred-nisolone pulse of 500mg to 1g/d for 3 days can be given prior to initiation of the oral prednisolone. There is no standard regimen for plasma exchange and, if required, the plasma exchanges can be tailored according to the clinical progress of the patient

Without extensive crescents

No definitive treatment, apart from supportive therapy (including dialysis), is recommended for this group of patients, who often have a picture like acute tubular necrosis with mild crescentic involvement (<30% of glomeruli affected by segmental crescents), because of the marked tendency for 'spontaneous' recovery. It should be emphasized that a renal biopsy is often needed to separate these two differing forms if IgA N with rapid loss of renal function, even though the patient may already carry a diagnosis of IgA N from a prior diagnostic renal biopsy.

Advanced chronic kidney disease

Patients with IgA N who present with or who advance to chronic kidney disease (Stage 4) with eGFR of <30mL/min/1.73m^2 and serum creatinine concentrations >2.0–3.0mg/dL and who show very chronic tubulo-interstitial changes and advanced glomerulosclerosis are not very likely to benefit from any of the 'specific' treatment modalities listed above. This stage is often called the *'point-of-no-return'* (D'Amico et al., 1993; Lai et al., 2002; Coppo and D'Amico, 2006). At this period, management of hypertension should be aggressive with a goal for systolic blood pressures of 120–130/70–80mmHg, using inhibitors of angiotensin II action as preferred agents.

Summary of practical recommendations

Patients with *isolated hematuria* and normal renal function without significant proteinuria (<500mg/d) do not warrant an initial aggressive therapeutic approach as their prognosis is generally excellent. However, a subset of this category will be destined to evolve over time into progressive disease. The magnitude of proteinuria, including microalbuminuria and selected morphological findings (such as tubulitis and T-cell infiltation), might 'predict' such an evolution, but in the absence of randomized controlled trials of therapy enrolling patients at this 'early' stage of disease a conservative, symptomatic approach is recommended (see Chapter 1). Similarly, patients with advanced *chronic renal failure* (serum creatinine ≥2.5mg/dL [220μmol/L]; eGFR <30mL/min/1.73m^2), *the 'point-of-no-return'*, should be treated conservatively with general measures to retard the further progression of disease, including ACEi/ ARB with rigorous control of systemic arterial blood pressure to <130/80mmHg (see Chapter 1).

The dilemma in treatment is found in the much larger subset of patients with hematuria and significant proteinuria (>0.5g/d) with normal to mildly impaired renal function (GFR >50mL/min) often accompanied by hypertension and chronic glomerular and tubulo-interstitial lesions on biopsy (see Barratt and Feehally, 2006; Ballardie, 2007; Floege and Eitner, 2008 for reviews) A regimen of ACEi and/or ARB should be tried as initial therapy in all cases (unless contraindications exist), monitoring the blood pressure and urinary protein excretion. The goal of this therapy is to reduce the proteinuria to the lowest possible value (preferably to <500mg/d) without disabling side effects. A trial of at least 3–6 months in duration is in order before moving on to other adjunctive regimens. Fish oils may be used in combination with the ACEi/ARB regimen. A steroid-based regimen (Pozzi regimen) or a potentially more toxic oral low-dose cyclophosphamide/azathioprine sequential regimen (Ballardie and Roberts regimen) can be used for patients who do not attain goals of ACEi/ARB therapy, depending on the level of renal function and its rate of progression.

There are only two circumstances in which steroid therapy is definitely indicated in the *initial* therapy of IgA nephropathy: i) in the *nephrotic syndrome with mild glomerular changes on histology*—frequent relapses of the nephrotic syndrome can be treated with a short course of cyclophosphamide; ii) *rapidly progressive glomerulonephritis* with extensive crescents where intravenous methyl-prednisolone is used in combination with a cytotoxic agent and/or plasmapheresis.

The long-term therapy with orally administered cytotoxic agents (combined with steroids) is uncertain in those patients with IgA N who have persistent dysmorphic hematuria (sometimes with red-cell casts), despite a reduction of proteinuria to <500mg/d, or a partial remission from higher levels of proteinuria. This finding may reflect ongoing glomerular injury from a smoldering 'capillaritis' due to ongoing activity of the underlying auto-immune process.

Transplantation

Glomerular IgA deposition occurs in between 10–60% of renal allografts in patients who have undergone renal transplantation for progressive IgA N (Cameron, 1994; Floege, 2004; Ivanyi, 2008), According to Ponticelli and co-workers (Ponticelli et al., 2001, 2004), a recurrence of IgA deposits was found in 23% of patients at a median of 4 years post-transplantation, but this may not be a true reflection of the 'recurrence rate' since only patients with micro-hematuria and/or proteinuria underwent a transplant kidney biopsy. A recurrence of IgA deposition develops in both living related, living unrelated and deceased (cadaveric) donor organ recipients, probably at roughly equal frequency. Some studies however have shown a slightly increased risk for recurrence if living related donors are used (Wang et al., 2001), but this is not a consistent finding. Very probably these deposits represent recurrence of the original disease, rather than *de novo* IgA N, however, the risk of finding such deposits in subsequent renal biopsies of the transplanted kidney is enhanced if the donor had (clinically unrecognizable) glomerular deposits of IgA *prior* to implantation of the kidney (Moriyama et al., 2005). Early rejection episodes may also be increased when patients receive kidneys from donors with mesangial IgA deposits (Ji et al., 2004). Rarely, the IgA deposits are transferred from a donor not recognized to have IgA nephropathy (Sanfillipo et al., 1986). The prevalence of *recurrent* deposits of IgA in recipients with IgA N as their original disease depends on the duration of the post-transplant period, but by 2–5 years post-transplant about 20–40% or more of renal allograft biopsies reveal IgA deposits (Hartung et al., 1995).

The eventual risk of recurrence of IgA deposition may approach 100% for very long post-transplant graft survival (10–20 years). Fortunately such recurrences of IgA deposition have only a modest and inconsistent effect on graft survival. The deleterious effect of recurrent IgA deposition may be offset by a somewhat better graft outcome (in the first 10 years), in terms of freedom from acute or chronic allograft rejection in recipients with IgA N, particularly when the donor and recipient are well–matched (zero-mismatches) (McDonald and Russ, 2006). While recurrences of IgA N in renal allografts may be more frequent in subjects receiving well matched (zero mismatched) donor kidneys, the long-term graft survival is not materially affected, probably because of the off-setting effects of the recurrence and the better matching of donor and recipient (McDonald and Russ, 2006). The consequences of using zero-mismatched kidneys in patients with IgA N has not be thoroughly studied and has not been confirmed. Graft loss due to recurrence was as low as 3% in a series of 101 patients from Malaysia (Ng et al., 2007). Also, in a very large series of patients from Hong Kong, only 3 of 75 patients (4%) had graft loss due to recurrence after a mean follow-up of about 8 years (Choy et al., 2003). Longer term follow-up (>12 years) shows a suggestion of greater graft loss due to recurrence compared to non-IgA N recipients (Choy et al., 2003).

Hartung and associates (Hartung et al., 1995) found about a 15% lower cumulative graft survival rate at 5 years post-transplant for recipients with recurrence of IgA N compared to those without recurrence. However, Ponticelli and coworkers (Ponticelli, et al., 2001) found that the slope of the reciprocal of serum creatinine concentration was not different for up to 10 years post-transplantation for patients with and without biopsy proven recurrence. Overall, patients with IgA nephropathy may enjoy somewhat favored graft survival compared with other glomerulopathies, perhaps due to IgA 'blocking' antibodies (Lim et al., 1991), but other studies have not shown that overall graft survival differ between IgA N and Non-IgA N transplant recipients.

The combination of dysmorphic hematuria and low-grade proteinuria may signify recurrent disease. Rarely, crescentic glomerulonephritis may be a manifestation of recurrent disease. This is seen more often in patients who present with HSP, than with IgA N.

No conventional pre-transplant clinical or serologic characteristics, other than a positive intra-operative renal biopsy of the donor kidney showing pre-existing IgA deposits or the existence of aggressive crescentic disease in the recipient (Moriyama et al., 2005; Mousson et al., 2007),are predictive of the risk for recurrence (Coppo et al., 1995, 2007a). Polymorphisms of IL-10 and/or TNF alpha may be associated with protection from recurrence of IgA N (Coppo et al., 2007).Very recently Berthoux and co-workers (Berthoux et al., 2008b) have suggested that renal allograft recipients who receive anti-thymocyte globulin (ATG) therapy for prevention of allograft rejection have a lower risk of recurrence of IgA N. This observation has not yet been independently confirmed. Patients receiving MMF for post-transplant maintenance immunosuppression do not have a lower risk of recurrence (Chandrakantan et al., 2005). The effect of steroid-avoidance protocols for maintenance immunosuppression in renal allografts is not yet known, but theoretically these protocols might increase the risk of recurrent disease.

In sum, IgA N should not be regarded as a 'contra-indication' for renal transplantation, but prospective recipients should be informed regarding the likelihood of a recurrence. An intra-operative renal biopsy is recommended to see if the donor has clinically unrecognized IgA deposits.

Ordinarily, no specific therapy is needed for mild-moderate recurrent disease. No data are available on the safety or efficacy of fish oil, low-antigen diets, IVIg, cytotoxic agents or rituximab for recurrent disease. The protocol used for suppression of transplant rejection does not appear to have any consistent influence on the likelihood of a recurrence (Chandrakantan et al., 2005). ACEi/ARB should be prescribed if hypertension and/or proteinuria are present. Recurrent crescentic glomerulonephritis, which is quite rare, should be treated as the *de novo* disease is treated with steroids, cytotoxic agents, and plasma exchange (see Chapter 10).

References

Aarli JA (1980). Effects of phenytoin on the immune system. In *Phenytoin-induced teratology and gingival pathology*, (ed. Hassell, Johnston, and Dudley, pp. 25–34. Raven Press New York.

Aarli JA, Tunder A (1975). Effects of anti-epileptic drugs on serum and salivary IgA. *Scand J Immunol* **4**:391–403.

Abuelo JG, Esparza AR, Matarese RA, et al. (1984). Crescenteric IgA nephropathy. *Medicine* **63**:396–406.

Alexopoulos E, et al. (2004). Treatment of severe IgA nephropathy with omega-3 fatty acids: the effect of a 'very-low-dose' regimen. *Renal Failure* **26**:453–9.

Almartine E, Sabatier J, Guerin C, et al. (1991). Prognostic factors in mesangial IgA glomerulonephritis: an extensive study with invariable and multivariable analysis. *Am J Kidney Dis* **18**:1–19.

Assadi FJ. (2005). Value of urinary excretion of microalbumin in predicting glomerular lesions in children with isolated microscopic hematuria. *Pediatr Nephrol* **20**:1131–5.

Baek JE, et al. (2008). Serum high-sensitivity C-reactive protein is not increased in patients with IgA nephropathy. *Nephron Clin Pract* **108**:c35–c40.

Ballardie FW (2007). Quantitative appraisal of treatment options for IgA nephropathy. *J Am Soc Nephrol* **18**:2806–2809.

Ballardie F, Roberts TS. (2002). Controlled prospective trial of prednisolone and cytotoxics in progressive IgA nephropathy. *J Am Soc Nephrol* **13**:142–8.

Ballardie FW, Cowley RD. (2008). Prognostic indices and therapy in IgA nephropathy: toward a solution. *Kidney Int* **73**:249–251.

Baldree LA, Wyatt RJ, Julian B, et al. (1993). Immunoglobulin A–fibronectin aggregate levels in children and adults with immunoglobulin A nephropathy. *Am J Kidney Dis* **22**:1–4.

Bantis C, et al. (2004). Influence of genetic polymorphisms of the renin–angiotensin system on IgA nephropathy. *Am J Nephrol* **24**:258–67.

Barratt J, Feehally J (2005). IgA nephropathy. *J Am Soc Nephrol* **16**:2088–97.

Barratt J, Feehally J (2006). Treatment of IgA nephropathy. *Kidney Int* **69**:1934–8.

Barratt J, et al. (2007). Immunopathogenesis of IgAN. *Semin Immunopathol* **29**:427–43.

Bartosik LP, et al. (2001). Predicting progression in IgA Nephropathy. *Am J Kidney Dis* **38**:728–35.

Bazzi G, Sinico RA, Petrini G, et al. (1992). Low doses of drugs able to alter intestinal mucosal permeability to food antigens (5-amino-salicylic acid and sodium cromogly-cate) do not reduce proteinuria in patients with IgA nephropathy: a preliminary non-controlled trial. *Nephron* **61**:192–5.

Bazzi G, D'Amico G (2005). Qualitative aspects of proteinuria predict progression and response to therapy better than its quantity. *NephSAP* **4**:111–16.

Beerman I, et al. (2007). The genetics of IgA nephropathy. *Nat Clin Pract Nephrol* **3**: 325–38.

Bene MC (1994). Tonsils in IgA nephropathy. *Contr Nephrol* **104**:153–61.

Bene MG, Hurault de Ligny B, Kessler M, et al. (1991). Confirmation of tonsillar abnor-malities in IgA nephropathy: a multicenter study. *Nephron* **58**:425–8.

Bene MG, Hurault de Ligny B, Kessler M, et al. (1993). Tonsils in IgA nephropathy. In *IgA nephropathy: the 25th year*. (ed. M. C. Bene, G. C. Faure, and M. Kessler), Vol. **104**, pp. 153–61. Karger, Basel.

Bennett WM, Walker RG, and Kincaid-Smith P (1989). Treatment of IgA nephropathy with eicosapentaenoic acid (EPA): a two-year prospective trial. *Clin Nephrol* **31**: 128–31.

Berger J, Hinglais N (1968). Les depots intercapillaries d'IgA–IgG. *J Urol Nephrol* (Paris), **74**:694–700.

Berthoux F, Alamartine F, Pommier G, et al. (1988). HLA and IgA-nephritis revisited 10 years later. HLA-B35 antigen as a prognostic factor. *New Eng J Med* **319**:1609–10.

Berthoux F, Laurent B, Koller J-M, et al. (1995). Primary IgA glomerulonephritis with thin glomerular basement membrane: a peculiar pathological marker versus thin membrane nephropathy association. In *IgA nephropathy: pathogenesis and treatment*, (ed. A., Clarkson and A. Woodroffe), vol. III, pp.1–7. Karger, Basel.

Berthoux FC, et al. (2008a). Natural history of primary IgA nephropathy. *Semin Nephrol* **28**:4–9.

Berthoux F, et al. (2008b). Antithymocyte globulin (ATG) induction therapy and disease recurrence in renal transplant recipients wtih primary IgA nephropathy. *Transplantation* **85**:1505–7.

Beukhof J, Kardaun O, Schaafsma W, et al. (1986). Towards individual prognosis of IgA nephropathy. *Kidney Int* **29**:549–56.

Bonnet F, et al. (2001). Excessive body weight as a new indépendant risk factor for clinical and pathological progression in primary IgA nephritis. *Am J Kidney Dis* **37**: 720–27.

Boobes Y, Baz M, Jaber DK, et al. (1990). Early start of intensive therapy in malignant form of IgA nephropathy. *Nephron* **54**:351–3.

Briganti EM, et al. (2001). The incidence of biopsy-proven glomerulonephritis in Australia. *Nephrol Dial Transplant* **16**:1364–7.

Buck KS, et al. (2008). B-cell O-galactosyltransferase activity and expression of O-glycosylation genes in bone marrow in IgA nephropathy. *Kidney Int* **73**:1128–36.

Cameron JS (1984). Platelets in glomerular disease. *Ann Rev Med* **35**:175–80.

Cameron JS (1993). The long-term outcome of glomerular disease. In *Disease of the Kidney*, (5th edn), (ed. R. Schrier and G Gottskalk), pp.1914–16. Little Brown, Boston.

Cameron JS (1994). Recurrent renal diseases after renal transplantation. *Curr Opin Nephrol Hypertens* 3:602–7.

Cattran D, Greenwood G, Ritchie S (1994). Long-term benefit of angiotensin converting enzyme inhibitor therapy in patients with severe immunoglobulin A nephropathy: a comparison to patients receiving treatment with other antihypertensive agents and to patients receiving no therapy. *Am J Kidney Dis* **23**:247–54.

Cattran D, et al. (2008). The impact of sex in primary glomerulonephritis. *Nephrol Dial Transplant* **23**:2247–53.

Chan MK, Kwan SYL, Chan KW (1987). Controlled trial of antiplatelet agents in mesangial IgA glomerulonephritis. *Am J Kidney Dis* **9**:417–21.

Chen X, et al. (2002). A randomized trial of mycophenolate mofetil treatment in severe IgA nephropathy. *Zhonghua Yi Xue Za Zhi* **82**:796–801.

Chandrakantan A, et al. (2005). Recurrent IgA nephropathy after renal transplantation despite immunosuppressive regimens with mycophenolate mofetil. *Nephrol Dial Transplant* **20**:1214–31.

Cheng IKP, Chan KW, Chan MK (1989). Mesangial IgA nephropathy with steroid-responsive nephrotic syndrome: disappearance of mesangial IgA deposits following steroid-induced remission. *Am J Kidney Dis* **14**:361–4.

Cheng, IKP, Chan PG K, Chan MK (1990). The effects of fish-oil dietary supplement on the progression of mesangial IgA glomerulonephritis. *Nephrol Dial Transplant* **5**:241–6.

Choy BY, et al. (2003). Renal transplantation in patients with primary immunoglobulin A nephropathy. *Nephrol Dial Transplant* **18**:2399–2404.

Clarkson AR, Seymour AE, Thompson AJ, et al. (1977). IgA nephropathy: a syndrome of uniform morphology, diverse clinical features and uncertain prognosis. *Clin Nephrol* **8**:458–71.

Clarkson AR, Seymour AE, Woodroffe AJ, et al. (1980). Controlled trial of phenytoin therapy in IgA nephropathy. *Clin. Nephrol* **13**:215–18.

Conley ME, Cooper MD, Michael AF (1980). Selective deposition of immunoglobulin A, in immunoglobulin A nephropathy, anaphylactoid purpura nephritis, and septuric lupus erythematosus. *J Clin Invest* **66**:1342–9.

Cook HT (2007). Interpretation of renal biopsies in IgA nephropathy. *Contr Nephrol* **157**: 44–9.

Coppo R, Basolo B, Giachino O, et al. (1985). Plasmapheresis in a patient with rapidly progressive idiopathic IgA nephropathy: removal of IgA-containing circulating immune complexes and clinical recovery. *Nephron* **40**:488–90.

Coppo R, Rocatello D, Amore A, et al. (1990). Effects of a gluten-free diet on primary IgA nephropathy. *Clin Nephrol* **33**:72–86.

Coppo R, Amore A, Curina P, et al. (1995). Characteristics of IgA and macromolecular IgA in sera from IgA nephropathy transplanted patients with and without IgAN recurrence. In *IgA nephropathy: pathogenesis and treatment*, (ed. A., Clarkson and A. Woodroff), Vol. **III**, pp. 85–92. Karger, Basel.

Coppo R, D'Amico G (2005). Factors predicting progression of IgA nephropathy. *J Nephrol* **18**:503–12.

Coppo R, et al. (2007a). Serological and genetic factors in early recurrence of IgA nephropathy after renal transplantation. *Clin Transplant* **21**:728–37.

Coppo R, et al. (2007b). IgACE: a placebo controlled, randomized trial of angiotensin-converting enzyme inhibition in children and young adults with IgA nephropathy and moderate proteinuria. *J Am Soc Neprhol* **18**:1880–8.

Curschellas E, et al. (1991). Morphologic findings in 'zero-hour' biopsies of reanl transplants. *Clin Nephrol* **36**:215–22.

D'Amico G (1987). The commonest glomerulonephritis in the world: IgA nephropathy *Quart J Med* **245**:709–27.

D'Amico G (1992). Influence of clinical and histologic features on actuarial renal survival in adult patients with idiopathic IgA nephropathy, membranous nephropathy, and membranoproliferative glomerulonephritis. Survey of the recent literature. *Am J Kidney Dis* **20**:315–23.

D'Amico G, et al. (1993). Typical and atypical natural history of IgA nephropathy in adult patients. *Contr Nephrol* **104**:6–13.

D'Amico G, et al. (2001). Idiopathic IgA nephropathy with segmental necrotizing lesions of the capillary wall. *Kidney Int* **59**:682–92.

Delclaux C, Jacquot C, Callard P, et al. (1993). Acute reversible renal failure with macroscopic hematuria in IgA nephropathy. *Nephrol Dial Transplant* **8**:195–9.

Dillon JJ (1997). Fish oil therapy for IgA nephropathy: efficacy and interstudy variability. *J Am Soc Nephrol* **8**:1739–44.

Donadio JV, Grande JP (2002). IgA nephropathy. *N Engl J Med* **347**:738–48

Donadio JV, Grande JP (2004). The role of fish oil/omega-3 fatty acids in the treatment of IgA nephropathy. *Semin Nephrol* **24**:225–43.

Donadio JV, Bergstrahl EJ, Offord KP, et al. (1994). A controlled trial of fish oil in IgA nephropathy. *New Eng J Med* **331**:1194–9.

Donadio JV, et al. (2006). Is body size a biomarker for optimizing dosing of omega-3 polyunsaturated fatty acids in the treatment of patients with IgA nephropathy? *Clin J Am Soc Nephrol* **1**:933–99.

Egido J, Blasco R, Lozano J, et al. (1984a) Immunological abnormalities in the tonsils of patients with IgA nephropathy: inversion in the ratio of IgA: IgG bearing lymphocytes and increased polymeric IgA synthesis. *Clin Exp Immunol* **57**:101–6.

Egido J, Rivera F, Sancho J, et al. (1984b) Phenytoin in IgA nephropathy: a long-term controlled trial. *Nephron* **38**:30–9.

Eijgenraam JW, et al. (2005). Dendritic cells of IgA nephropathy patients have an impaired capacity to induce IgA production in naive B cells. *Kidney Int* **68**:1604–12.

Eijgenraam JW, et al. (2008). Immuno-histological analysis of dendritic cells in nasal biopsies of IgA nephropathy patients. *Nephrol Dial Transplant* **23**:612–20.

Emancipator SN (1990). Immunoregulatory factors in the pathogenesis of IgA nephropathy. *Kidney Int* **38**:1216–29.

Espinosa M, et al. (2008). Mesangial cell C4d deposition: a new prognostic factor in IgA nephropathy. *Nephrol Dial Transplant* Oct 8 [Epub ahead of print].

Feehally J, Baratt J, Coppo R, et al. (2007). International IgA nephropathy network clinico-pathological classification of IgA nephropathy. *Control Nephrol* **157**:13–8.

Fellin G, et al. (1988). Renal function in IgA nephropathy with established renal failure. *Nephrol Dial Transplant* **3**:17–23.

Fernandez-Juarez G, et al. (2006). Dual blockade of the renin-angiotensin system in the progression of renal disease: the need for more clinical trials. *J Am Soc Nephrol* **17** (Suppl. 3):s250–4.

Ferrario F, et al. (1995). Capillaritis in IgA nephropathy. *Control Nephrol* **111**:8–12.

Ferri C, Puccini R, Paleologo G, et al. (1992). IgA nephropathy: preliminary results of low-antigen-content diet treatment. *Arch Int Med* **152**:249.

Floege J (2004). Recurrent IgA nephroapthy after renal transplantation. *Semin Nephrol* **24**:287–91.

Floege J, Eitner F. (2008). Immune modulating therapy for IgA nephropathy: rationale and evidence. *Semin Nephrol* **28**:38–47.

Fogazzi G, Imbasciati E, Moroni G, et al. (1995). Reversible acute renal failure from gross hematuria due to glomerulonephritis, not only in IgA nephropathy and not associated with intratubular obstruction. *Nephrol Dial Transplant* **10**:624–9.

Fornasieri A, Sinico RA, Maldifassi P, et al. (1987). IgA-antigliadin antibodies in mesangial IgA nephropathy (Berger's disease). *Br Med J* **295**:78–80.

Fornasieri A, Sinico RA, Maldifassi P, et al. (1988). Food antigens, IgA immune complexes and IgA mesangial nephropathy. *Nephrol Dial Transplant* 3:738–43.

Frisch G, et al. (2005). Mycophenolate mofetil (MMF) vs placebo in patients with moderately advanced IgA nephropathy: a double blind randomized controlled trial. *Nephrol Dial Transplant* **21**:39–45.

Fukushi K, Yamabe H, Ozawa K, et al. (1989). Disappearance of glomerular IgA deposits in steroid-responsive nephrotic syndrome. *Nephron* **51**:553–4.

Geddes CC, et al. (2003). A tricontinental view of IgA nephropathy. *Nephrol Dial Transplant.* **18**:1541–8.

Gelfand JA, Sherins RJ, Ailing DW, et al. (1976). Treatment of hereditary angioneurotic edema with danazol. Reversal of clinical and biochemical abnormalities. *New Eng J Med* **295**:1444–8.

Gharavi AG, et al. (2008). Aberrant IgA1 glycosylation is inherited in familial and sporadic IgA nephropathy. *J Am Soc Nephrol* **19**:1008–14.

Gherghiceanu M, et al. (2005). The predictive value of peritubular C3d deposition in IgA glomerulonephritis. *J Cell Mol Med* **9**:143–52.

GISEN (Gruppo Italiano di Studii Epidemiolgici in Nefologia. (1997). Randomized placebo controlled trial of the effect of ramipril on decline in glomerular filtration rate and risk of terminal renal failure in proteinuric, non-diabetic nephropathy. *Lancet* **349**:1857–63.

Glassock RJ (2008). Future prospects for IgA nephropathy. In KN Lai (ed), *Advances in IgA Nephropathy.*

Goumenos D, Ahuja M, Shortland J, and Brown C. (1995). Can immuno-suppressive drugs slow the progression of IgA nephropathy. *Nephrol Dial Transplant* **10**:1173–81.

Gutierrez E, et al. (2007). Factors that determine an incomplete recovery of renal function in macrohematuria-induced acute renal failure in IgA nephropathy. *Clin J Am Soc Nephrol* **2**:51–7.

Haas M, et al. (2008). IgA-dominant posttinfectious glomerulonephritis: a report of 13 cases with common ultrastructural features. *Hum Pathol* **39**:1309–16.

Habib R, Niaudet P, and Levy M. (1994). Schönlein-Henoch purpura nephritis and IgA nephropathy. In Tisher C and Bremner BM (eds.), *Renal pathology: with clinical and pathological correlations,* (2nd edn), pp. 472–523. Lippincott, Philadelphia.

Hamazaki T, Tateno S, and Shishido S. (1984). Eicosapentaenoic acid and IgA nephropathy. *Lancet* **i**:1017–18.

Hammarstromm L, Lundkvist I, Petterson A, et al. (1992). The use of IVIG in immunological disorders other than cytopenias. In PL Yap (ed), *Clinical applications of intravenous immunoglobulin therapy,* pp.117–37. Churchill Livingstone, Edinburgh.

Hara M, et al. (2007). Cumulative excretion of urinary podocytes reflects disease progression in IgA nephropathy and Schonlein–Henoch purpura. *Clin J Am Soc Nephrol* **2**:231–8.

Hartung R, Livingston B, Excell L, et al. (1995). Recurrence of IgA deposits/disease in grafts. In Clarkson A and Woodroffe A (eds.), *IgA nephropathy: pathogenesis and treatment,* Vol. III, pp. 13–17. Karger, Basel.

Hasbargen J. and Copley J (1985). Utility of skin biopsy in the diagnosis of IgA nephropathy. *Am J Kidney Dis* **6**:100–6.

Haubitz M, et al. (2005). Urine protein patterns can serve as diagnostic tools in patients with IgA nephropathy. *Kidney Int* **67**:2313–20.

Hene RJ, Valentijin RM, Kater L (1982). Plasmapheresis in nephropathy of Henoch–Schönlein purpura and primary IgA nephropathy. *Kidney Int* **22**:409 (Abstract).

Hogg RJ (1995). Prognostic indicators and treatment of childhood IgA nephropathy. *Contrib Nephrol* **111**:194–9.

Hogg RJ, et al. (2004). A randomized controlled trial of mycophenolate mofetil in patients with IgA nephropathy. *BMC Nephrol* **5**:3.

Hogg RJ, et al. (2006a). Efficacy of omega-3 fatty acid in children and adults with IgA nephropathy is dosage and size-dependent. *Clin J Am Soc Nephrol* **1**:1167–72.

Hogg RJ, et al. (2006b). Clinical trial to evalaute omega-3 fatty acids and alternate day prednisone in patients wtih IgA nephropathy: report from the Southwest Pediatric Nephrology Study Group. *Clin J Am Soc Nephrol* **1**:467–74.

Hotta O, et al. (2001). Tonsillectomy and steroid pulse therapy significantly impact on clinical remission in patients with IgA nephropathy. *Am J Kidney Dis* **38**:736–43.

Hung KY, et al. (1996). Adult primary IgA nephropathy and common viral infections. *J Infect* **32**:227–30.

Hunley TE, Julian BA, Phillips JA 3rd, et al. (1996). Angiostensin converting enzyme gene polymorphism: potential silencer motif and impact on progression in IgA nephropathy. *Kidney Int* **49**:571–7.

Ibels LS and Gyory AZ (1994). IgA nephropathy: analysis of the natural history, important factors in the progression of renal disease, and a review of the literature. *Medicine (Baltimore)* **73**:79–102.

Iino Y, Ambe K, Kato Y, et al. (1993). Chronic tonsillitis and IgA nephropathy. *Acta Otolaryngol* **508**(Suppl.): 29–35.

Ikezumi Y, et al. (2008). Use of Mizoribine as a rescue drug for steroid-resistant pediatric IgA nephropathy. *Pediatr Nephrol* **23**:645–50.

Ishiguro C, et al. (2002). Serum IgA/C3 ratio may predict diagnosis and prognosis grading in patients with IgA nephropathy. *Nephron* **91**:755–8.

Itami N, Akutsu V, Kusonoki Y, et al. (1989). Does methylprednisolone pulse therapy deteriorate the course of rapidly progressive IgA nephropathy? *Am J Dis Child* **143**:441–2 (Letter).

Ivanyi B (2008). A primer on recurrent and de novo glomerulonephritis in renal allografts. *Nat Clin Pract Nephrol* **4**:446–57.

Izzi C, et al. (2006). IgA nephropathy: the presence of familial disease does not confer an increased risk for progression. *Am J Kidney Dis* **47**:761–69.

Jacob S, et al. (2007). Effect of organic solvent exposure on chronic kidney disease progression: the GN-PROGRESS Cohort study. *J Am Soc Nephrol* **18**:274–81.

Janssen U, et al. (2000). Activation of the acute phase response and complement C3 in patients with IgA nephropathy. *Am J Kidney Dis* **35**:21–8.

Ji S, et al. (2004). The fate of glomerular mesangial deposition in the donated kidney after allograft transplantation. *Clin Transplant* **18**:536–40.

Johnson RJ, et al. (2003). Hypothesis: dysregulation of immunologic balance resulting from hygiene and socioeconomic factors may influence the epidemiology and causes of glomerulonephritis world wide. *Am J Kidney Dis* **42**:575–81.

Julian BA, Barker C (1993). Alternate-day prednisone therapy in IgA nephropathy. *Control Nephrol* **104**:198–206.

Julian BA, Barker CV, Woodford SY (1993). Alternate-day prednisone treatment in patients with IgA nephropathy. *J Am Soc Nephrol* **4**:681 (Abstract).

Kaartinen K, et al. (2008). Inflammatory markers and the progression of IgA glomerulonephritis. *Nephrol Dial Transplant* **23**:1285–90.

Katz A, Walker JF, and Landy PJ (1983). IgA nephritis with nephrotic range proteinuria. *Clin Nephrol* **20**:67–71.

Kaveri SV, et al. (2008). The anti-inflammatory IgG. *N Engl J Med* **17**:307–9.

Kawasaki Y, et al. (2004) Efficacy of multidrug therapy combined with mizoribine in children with diffuse IgA nephropathy in comparison with multidrug therapy without mizoribine and methylprednisolone pulse therapy. *Am J Nephrol* **24**:576–81.

Kincaid-Smith P, Bennett W. M, Dowling J. P, et al. (1983). Acute renal failure and tubular necrosis associated with hematuria due to glomerulonephritis. *Clin Nephrol* **19**:206–10.

Kincaid-Smith P, Nicholls K (1983). Mesangial IgA nephropathy. *Am J Kidney Dis* **3**:90–102.

Kobayashi Y, Fujii K, Hiki Y, et al. (1988). Steroid therapy in IgA nephropathy: a retrospective study in heavy proteinuric cases. *Nephron*, **48**:12–17.

Kobayashi Y, Hiki Y, Fujii K, et al. (1989). Moderately proteinuric IgA nephropathy: prognostic prediction of individual clinical courses and steroid therapy in progressive cases. *Nephron* **53**:250–6.

Kohaut E, Waldo F (1989). IgA nephropathy in black children. *Pediatr Nephrol* **3**:C135.

Komatsu H, et al. (2004). Relationship between serum IgA/C3 ratio and the progression of IgA nephropathy. *Intern Med* **43**:1023–8.

Komatsu H, et al. (2005). 'Point of no return' (PNR) in progressive IgA nephropathy; significance of blood pressure and proteinuria management up to PNR. *J Nephrol* **18**:690–5.

Komatsu H, et al. (2008). Effect of tonsillectomy plus steroid pulse therapy on clinical remission of IgA nephropathy: A controlled study. *Clin J Am Soc Nephrol* **3**:1301–7.

Kunz R, et al. (2008). The COOPERATE trial. A letter of concern. *Lancet* **371**:1575–6.

Kunz R, et al. (2008a). Meta-analysis: effect of monotherapy and combination therapy with inhibitors of the renin-angiotensin system on proteinuria in renal dissease. *Ann Intern Med* **148**:30–48.

Lai KN, Lai FM, Ho C, et al. (1986). Corticosteroid therapy in IgA nephropathy: a long-term controlled trial. *Clin Nephrol* **26**:174–80.

Lai KN, Lai FM, Leung ACT, et al. (1987). Plasma exchange in patients with rapidly progressive idiopathic IgA nephropathy: a report of two cases and review of literature. *Am J Kidney Dis* **10**:66–70.

Lai KN, Lai FM, Vallance-Owen J (1988). A short-term controlled trial of cyclosporin A in IgA nephropathy. *Trans Proceedings* **20**(Suppl. 4):297–303.

Lai KN, Lai FM, Ho CP, et al. (1989). Corticosteroid therapy in IgA nephropathy with nephrotic syndrome: a long-term controlled trial. *Clin Nephrol* **26**:174–80.

Lai FM, et al. (2002). Primary IgA nephropathy with low histologic grade and disease progression: is there a 'point of no return'? *Am J Kidney Dis* **39**:401–6.

Lai KK, et al. (2007). Serum levels of galactose-deficient IgA in children with IgA nephropathy and Henoch–Schonlein purpuraa. *Pediatr Nephrol* **22**:2067–72.

Lai KN (ed) (2008). *Advances in IgA Nephropathy.*

Lee GSL, Woo KT, Lim CH (1989). Controlled trial of dipyridamole and low dose warfarin in patients with IgA nephritis with renal impairment. *Clin Nephrol* **31**:276.

Lee GSL, Choong HL, Chiang GCS, et al. (1997). Three year randomized controlled trial of dipyridamole and low-dose warfarin in patients with IgA nephropathy and renal impairment. *Nephrology* **3**:117–21.

Lemley KV, et al. (2002). Podocytopenia and disease severity in IgA nephropathy. *Kidney Int* **61**:1475–85.

Lemley KV, et al. (2008). Prediction of early progression in recently diagnosed IgA nephropathy. *Nephrol Dial Transplant* **23**:213–22.

Li GS, et al. (2007). Variants of the ST6GALNAC2 promoter influences transcriptional activity and contribute to genetic susceptibility to IgA nephropathy. *Hum Mutat* **28**:950–7.

Lim E, Chia D, Terasaki P (1991). Studies of sera from IgA nephropathy patients to explain high kidney graft survival. *Hum Immunol* **32**:81–6.

Locatelli F, et al. (2003). Advanced IgA nephropathy: to treat or not to treat ? *Nephron Clin Pract* **93**:c119–21.

Locatelli F, et al. (2006). IgA glomerulonephritis: beyond angiotensin-converting enzyme inhibitors. *Nat Clin Pract Nephrol* **2**:24–31.

Locatelli F, et al. (2006a). IgA nephritis. ACE inhibitors, steroids, both or neither. *Nephrol Dial Transplant* **21**:3357–61.

Lou T, et al. (2006). Randomized controlled trial of leflunomide in the treatemnt of Immunoglobulin A nephropathy. *Nephrology (Carlton)* **11**:113–16.

Lozano L, Garcia-Horo R, Egido J, et al. (1985). Tonsillectomy decreases the synthesis of polymeric IgA by lymphocytes and clinical activity in patients with IgA nephropathy. *Proc Eur Dial Transplant Assoc* **22**:800–4.

Lv J, Zhang H, Chen Y, et al. (2009). Combination therapy of prednisone and ACE inhibitor versus ACE inhibitor therapy alone in patients with IgA nephropathy: a randomized controlled trial. *Am J Kidney Dis* **53**:26–32.

Lv J, Zhang H, Zhou Y, et al. (2008). Natural history of immunoglobulin A nephropathy and predictive factors of prognosis: a long-term follow-up of 204 cases in China. *Nephrology* (Carlton) **13**:242–6.

McDonald SP, Russ GR (2006). Recurrence of IgA nephropathy among renal allograft recipients from living donors is greater among those with zero HLA mismatches. *Transplantation* **27**:759–62.

McIntyre CW, et al. (2001). Steroid and cyclophosphamide therapy for IgA nephropathy associated with crescentic change: an effective treatment. *Clin Nephrol* **56**:193–8.

MacKinnon B, et al. (2008). Validation of the Toronto formula to predict progression of IgA nephropathy. *Nephron Clin Pract* **109**:c148–53.

Maeda A, et al. (2003). Significance of serum IgA levels and serum IgA/C3 ratio in diagnostic analysis of patients with IgA nephropathy. *J Clin Lab Anal* **17**:73–6.

Maes BD, et al. (2004). Mycophenolate Mofetil in IgA nephropathy: results of a 3-year prospective placebo-controlled randomized study. *Kidney Int* **65**:1842–9.

Magsitroni R, et al. (2006). A validated model of disease progression in IgA nephropathy. *J Nephrol* **19**: 32–40.

Manno C, et al. (2007). A novel simple histological classification for renal survival in IgA nephropathy: a retrospective study. *Am J Kidney Dis* **49**:763–5.

Mestecky J, et al. (2008). Role of aberrant glycosylation of IgA1 in the pathogenesis of IgA nephropathy. *Kidney Blood Pres Res* **31**: 29–37.

Mitsuiki K, et al. (2007). Histologically advanced IgA nephropathy treated successfully with prednisone and cyclophosphamide. *Clin Exp Nephrol* **11**:297–303.

Miura M (1987). Intraglomerular coagulation and fibrinolysis in patients with IgA nephropathy. *Jap J Nephrol* **29**:1189–97.

Miura M, Tomino Y, Tagume M (1985). Immunofluorescent studies of alpha$_2$-plasmin inhibitor in glomeruli from patients with IgA nephropathy. *Clin Exp Immunol* **62**:380–6.

Miura M, Endoh M, Nomoto Y, et al. (1989). Long-term effect of urokinase therapy in IgA nephropathy. *Clin Nephrol* **32**:209–16.

Miyazaki M, Hotta O, Komatsuda A, et al. (2007). A multicenter prospective cohort study of tonsillectomy and steroid therapy in Japanese patients with IgA nephropathy: a 5-year report. *Control Nephrol* **157**:94–8.

Moldoveanu Z, et al. (2007). Patients with IgA nephropathy have increased serum galactose-deficient IgA1 levels. *Kidney Int* **71**:1148–54.

Moriyama T, et al. (2005). Latent IgA deposition from donor kidney is the major risk factor for recurrent IgA nephropathy in renal transplantation. *Clin Transplant* **19**(Suppl. 14): 41–8.

Moura IC, et al. (2008). The glomerular response to IgA deposition in IgA nephropathy. *Semin Nephrol* **28**:88–95.

Mousson C, et al. (2007). Recurrence of IgA nephropathy with cresccnts in kidney transplants. *Transplant Proc* **39**:2595–6.

Myllymaki J, et al. (2005). Uric acid correlates with the severity of histopathological findings in IgA nephropathy. *Nephrol Dial Transplant* **20**:89–95.

Nagaoka R, et al. (2002). Mizoribine treatment for IgA nephropathy. *Pediatr Int* **44**:217–23.

Nair R, Walker PD (2006). Is IgA nephropathy the commonest primary glomerulopathy among young adults in the USA? *Kidney Int* **69**:1455–8.

Nakao M, et al. (2003). Combination treatment of angiotensin II receptor blocker and angiotensin converting enzyme inhibitor in non-diabetic renal disease (COOPERATE): a randomized controlled trial. *Lancet* **361**:117–24.

Nakayama K, et al. (2008). Prediction of diagnosis of immunoglobulin A nephropathy prior to renal biopsy and correlation with urinary sediment findings and prognostic grading. *J Clin Lab Anal* **22**:114–19.

Nasr SH, et al. (2007). Acute post-staphyloccal glomerulonephritis superimposed on diabetic glomerulosclerosis. *Kidney Int* **71**:1317–21.

Nasr SH, et al. (2003). IgA-dominant acute post-staphylocoocal glomerulonephritis complicating diabetic nephropathy. *Hum Pathol* **34**:1235–41.

Navaneethan SD, et al. (2008) Meta-analysis of mycophenolate mofetil in IgA nephropathy. *Nephrology (Carlton)* **13**:90.

Neelakantappa K, Gallo RG, and Baldwin DS. (1988). Proteinuria in IgA nephropathy. *Kidney Int* **33**:716–21.

Ng YS, et al. (2007). Long-term outcome of renal allografts in patients with immuno-globulin A nephropathy. *Med J Malaysia* **62**:109–13.

Nicholls K, et al. (1984). The clinical cause of mesangial IgA associated nephropathy in adults. *Quart J Med* **210**:227–36.

Nishitani Y, et al. (2005). Fibroblast specific protein-1 is a specific prognostic marker for renal survival in patients with IgAN. *Kidney Int* **68**:1078–85.

Novak J, et al. (2008). IgA glycosylation and IgA immune complexes in the pathogenesis of IgA nephropathy. *Semin Nephrol* **28**:78–87.

Ogura Y, et al. (2000) Hemophilus influenza antigen and antibody in children with IgA nephropathy and Henoch–Schonlein purpura. *Am J Kidney Dis* **36**:47–52.

Onda K, et al. (2007). Hypercomplementemia in adult patients with IgA nephropathy. *J Clin Lab Anal* **211**:77–84.

Oortwijn BD, et al. (2008). The role of secretory IgA and complement in IgA nephropathy. *Semin Nephrol* **28**:58–65.

Ortmanns A, et al. (1998). Remission of IgA nephropathy following treatment of cytomeg-alovirus with ganciclovir. *Clin Nephrol* **49**:379–84.

Packham DK (2007). Thin basement membrane nephropathy and IgA glomerulonephritis: can they be distinguished without a renal biopsy? *Nephrology (Carlton)* **12**:481–6.

Park JS, et al. (1994). Cytomegalovirus is not specifically associated with immunoglobulin A nephropathy. *J Am Soc Nephrol* **4**:1623–6.

Petterson EE, Rekola S, Berglund L, et al. (1994). Treatment of IgA nephropathy with omega-3-polyunsaturated fatty acids; a prospective, double-blind, randomised study. *Clin Nephrol* **41**:183–90.

Philibert D, et al. (2008) Clinicopathologic correlations in IgA nephropathy. *Semin Nephrol* **28**:10–17.

Pillebout E, et al. (2002). Henoch-Schönlein purpura in adults: outcome and prognostic factors. *J Am Soc Nephrol* **13**:1271–8.

Pirani CL, Salinas-Madrigal L (1968). Evaluation of percutaneous renal biopsy. *Pathol Ann* **3**:249–96.

Ponticelli C, et al. (2001). Kidney transplantation in patients with IgA mesangial glomeru-lonephritis. *Kidney Int* **60**:1948–54.

Ponticelli C, et al. (2004). Kidney transplantation in patients wtih IgA mesangial glomeru-lonephritis. *Pediatr Transplant* **8**:334–8.

Pouria S, Barratt J. (2008). Secondary IgA nephropathy. *Semin Nephrol* **28**:27–37.

Pozzi C, et al. (2002). Can immunosuppression therapy be useful in IgA nephropathy when the « point of no return » has already been exceeded ? *Nephron* **92**:699–701.

Pozzi C, et al. (2004). Corticosteroid effectiveness in IgA nephropathy: long term results of a controlled randomized clinical trial. *J Am Soc Nephrol* **15**:157–62.

Pozzi C, et al. (2006). ACE inhibitors and angiotensin II receptor blockers in IgA nephro-pathy with mild proteinruia: the ACEARB study. *J Nephrol* **19**:508–15.

Pozzi C (2007). Treatment of IgA nephropathy with chronic renal failure. *G Ital Nefrol* **25**(Supplement 44):83–7.

Praga M, Gutierrez-Millet V, Navas JJ, et al. (1985). Acute worsening of renal function during episodes of macroscopic hematuria in IgA nephropathy. *Kidney Int* **28**:69–74.

Praga M, et al. (2003). Treatment of IgA nephropathy with ACE inhibitors: a randomized and controlled trial. *J Am Soc Nephrol* **14**:1578–83.

Radford MG, et al. (1997). Predicting Renal Outcome in IgA Nephropathy. *J Am Soc Nephrol* **8**:199–207.

Rasche FM, et al. (1999). Tonsillectomy does not prevent a progressive course in IgA nephropathy. *Clin Nephrol* **51**:147–52.

Rasche FM, et al. (2006). High-dose intravenous immunoglobulin pulse therapy in patients with progressive immunoglobulin A nephropathy: a long term follow-up. *Clin Exp Immunol* **146**:47–53.

Rauta V, Finne P, Fagerudd J, et al. (2002). Factors associated with progression of IgA nephropathy are related to renal function - a model; for estimating risk of progression in mild disease. *Clin Nephrol* **58**:85–94.

Reich HN, et al. (2007). Remission of proteinuria improves prognosis in IgA nephropathy. *J Am Soc Nephrol* **18**:3177–83.

Rekola S, Bergstrand A, Bucht H (1991a). Deterioration in GFR in IgA nephropathy as measured by ^{51}Cr-EDTA clearance. *Kidney Int* **40**:1050–4.

Rekola S, Bergstrand, A, Bucht H (1991b). Deterioration rate in hypertensive IgA nephropathy: comparison of a converting enzyme inhibitor and β-blocking agents. *Nephron* **59**:57–60.

Remuzzi A, Peritcucci E, Rùggenenti P, et al. (1991). Angiotensin converting enzyme inhibition improves glomerular size-selectivity in IgA nephropathy. *Kidney Int* **39**:1267–73.

Roberts ISD. A new approach to classification: the clinician - pathologist collaborative project. *American Society of Nephrology Annual Meeting.* Philadelphia 2008.

Rocatello D, Ferro M, Coppo R, et al. (1995). Treatment of rapidly progressive IgA nephropathy. In A Clarkson, A Woodroffe (eds), *IgA nephropathy: pathogenesis and treatment*, vol. 111, pp. 177–83. Karger, Basel.

Rodriguez-Soriano J, Arrieta A, Vallo A, et al. (1988). IgA antigliadin antibodies in children with IgA mesangial glomerulonephritis. *Lancet* **i**:1109–10 (Letter).

Rosenberg H, et al. (1989). A morphologic study of 103 kidneys donated for reanl transplantation. *Rev Med Chil* **117**:1344–50.

Rosenberg H, et al. (1990) Morphological findings in 70 kidneys of living donors for renal transplants. *Pathol Res Pract* **186**:619–24.

Rostoker G, Laurent J, Andre C, et al. (1988). High levels of IgA antigliadin antibodies in patients who have IgA mesangial glomerulonephritis but no coeliac disease. *Lancet* **i**: 356–7.

Rostoker G, Pech M. A, Del Prato S, et al. (1989). Serum IgG subclasses and IgM imbalances in adult IgA mesangial glomerulonephritis and idiopathic Henoch–Schönlein purpura. *Clin Exp Immunol* **75**:30–4.

Rostoker G, Desvaux-Belghiti D, Pilatte Y, et al. (1994). High-dose immunoglobulin therapy for severe IgA nephropathy and Henoch–Schönlein purpura. *Ann Intern Med* **120**:476–84.

Rootoker G, Desvaux-Belghiti D, Pilatte Y, et al. (1995). Immunomodulation with low-dose immunoglobulins for moderate IgA nephropathy and Henoch-Schönlein purpura. Preliminary results of a prospective uncontrolled trial. *Nephron* **69**:327–34.

Ruggenenti P, et al. (1999). In chronic nephropathies prolonged ACE inhibition can induce remission: dynamics of time-dependent change inGFR. Investigations of the GISEN Group. *J Am Soc Nephrol* **10**:997–1006.

Ruggenenti P, et al. (2003). Retarding progression of chronic renal disease: the neglected issue of residual proteinuria. *Kidney Int* **63**:2254–61.

Sancho J, Egido J, Rivera F, et al. (1988). Immune complexes in IgA nephropathy: presence of antibodies against diet antigens and delayed clearance of specific polymeric IgA immune complexes. *Clin Exp Immunol* **73**:295–301.

Sanfillipo F, Crocker P, Bollinger R (1986). Fate of four cadaveric donor allografts with mesangial IgA deposits. *Transplantation* **42**:511–15.

Sato M, Takayama K, Kojima H, et al. (1990). Sodium cromoglycate therapy in IgA nephropathy: a preliminary short-term trial. *Am J Kidney Dis* **15**:141–6.

Schena F. R, Montenegro M, Scivittaro V (1990). Meta-analysis of randomised controlled trials in patients with IgA nephropathy (Berger's disease). *Nephrol. Dial. Transplant* **5** (Suppl. 1):47–52.

Scholl U, et al. (1999). The 'point of no return'and the rate of progression in the natural history of IgA nephritis. *Clin Nephrol* **52**:285–92.

Seager J, Wilson J, Jamieson DL, et al. (1975). IgA deficiency, epilepsy and phenytoin treatment. *Lancet* **ii**:632–5.

Shen P, et al. (2007). Useful indicators for performing a renal biopsy in adult patients with isolated microscopic hematuria. *Int J Clin Pract* **61**:789–94.

Shigematsu H, Kobayashi Y, Tateno S, Tsukada M. (1980). Ultrastructure of acute glomerular injury in IgA nephritis. *Arch Pathol Lab Med* **104**:303–7.

Sinico RA, et al. (1994). Lack of IgA neutrophil cytoplasmic antibodies in Henoch–Schönlein purpura and IgA nephropathy. *Clin Immunol Immunopathol* **73**:19–26.

Sinniah (1983). Occurrence of mesangial IgA and IgM deposition in a control necropsy population. *J Clin Pathol* **36**:276–9.

Southwest Pediatric Nephrology Study Group (1985). Association of IgA nephropathy with steroid-responsive nephrotic syndrome. *Am J Kidney Dis* **5**:157–64.

Sugiyama N, Shimizu J, Nakamura M, et al. (1993). Clinicopathological study of effectiveness of tonsillectomy in IgA nephropathy accompanied by chronic tonsillitis. *Acta Otolaryngol* **508**(Suppl.): 43–8.

Suwabe T, Ubara Y, Sogawa Y, et al. (2007). Tonsillectomy and corticosteroid therapy with concomitant methylprednisolone pulse therapy for IgA nephropathy. *Control Nephrol* **157**:99–103.

Suzuki K, et al. (2003). Incidence of latent mesangial IgA deposition in renal allograft donors in Japan. *Kidney Int* **63**:2286–94.

Suzuki H, et al. (2008). IgA1-secreting cells lines from patients with IgA nephropathy produce aberrantly glycosylated IgA1. *J Clin Invest* **118**:629–39.

Syrjanen J, et al. (2000). Hypertriglyceridemia and hyperuricemia are the risk factors fro progression of IgA nephropathy. *Nephrol Dial Transplant* **15**:34–42.

Szeto CC, et al. (2008). Oral calcitriol for the treatment of persistent proteinuria in immunoglobulin A nephropathy: an uncontrolled trial. *Am J Kidney Dis* **51**:724–31.

Taji Y, et al. (2006). Meta-analysis of anti-platelet therapy for IgA nephropathy. *Clin Exp Nephrol* **10**:268–73.

Tang S, et al. (2005). Mycophenolate mofetil alleviates proteinuria in IgA nephropathy. *Kidney Int* **68**:802–12.

Tamura S, Masuda Y, Inokuchi I, et al. (1993). Effect of and indication for tonsillectomy in IgA nephropathy. *Acta Otolaryngol* **508**(Suppl.):23–8.

Tomino Y, Sakai H, Miura M, et al. (1984). Effect of danazol on solubilization of immune deposits in patients with IgA nephropathy. *Am J Kidney Dis* **4**:135–40.

Tomino Y (ed) (2007). IgA nephropathy today. *Control Nephrol* **157**:1–255.

Torres DD, et al. (2008). The ratio of epidermal growth factor to monocyte chemotactic peptide-1 in the urine predicts renal prognosis in IgA nephropathy. *Kidney Int* **73**: 327–33.

Tumlin JA, Henniger RA (2004). Clinical presentation, natural history and treatment of crescentic Proliferative IgA nephropathy. *Semin Nephrol* **24**:256–68.

Tumlin JA, et al. (2004). Idiopathic IgA nephropathy: Pathogenesis. Histopathology and Therapeutic Options. *Clin J Am Soc Nephrol* **2**:1054–11.

van Es LA (1992). Pathogenesis of IgA nephropathy. *Kidney Internat* **41**:1720–9.

van Es LA, et al. (2008). GMP-17-positive T-lymphocytes in renal tubules predict progression in the early stages of IgA nephropathy. *Kidney Int.* **73**:1426–38.

van Ypersele de Strihou C (1994). Fish oil for IgA nephropathy? *New Eng J Med* **331**:1227–9.

Varis J, et al. (1993). Immunoglobulin and complement deposition in glomeruli of 776 subjects who had committed suicide or met with a violent death. *J Clin Pathol* **46**: 215–22.

Wakai K, et al. (2006). A scoring system to predict renal outcomes in IgA nephropatht: from a nationwide prospective study. *Nephrol Dial Transplant.* **21**:2800–8.

Waldo B, Wyatt RJ, Kelly DR, *et al.* (1993). Treatment of IgA nephropathy in children: efficacy of alternate-day prednisolone. *Pediat Nephrol* **7**: 529–32.

Waldherr R, et al. (1989). Frequency of mesangial IgA deposits in a non-selected autopsy series. *Nephrol Dial Transplant* **4**:943–46.

Walker RG, Yu SH, Owen JE, et al. (1990). The treatment of mesangial IgA nephropathy with cyclophosphamide, dipyridamole and warfarin: a two year prospective trial. *Clin. Nephrol* **34**:103–7.

Wang AY, et al. (2001). Recurrent IgA nephropathy in renal transplant allografts. *Am J Kidney Dis* **38**:588–96.

Woo KT, Chiang GSC, Lim CH (1987a). Follow-up renal biopsies in IgA nephritic patients on triple therapy. *Clin. Nephrol* **28**:304–5.

Woo KT, Lee GSL, Lau YK, et al. (1991). Effects of triple therapy in IgA nephritis: a follow-up study 5 years later. *Clin Nephrol* **36**:60–6.

Woo KT, Edmondson RPS, Yap HK et al. (1987). Effects of triple therapy on the progression of mesangial proliferative glomerulonephritis. *Clin Nephrol* **27**:56–64.

Woo KT, et al. (2004). Polymorphisms of renin –angiotensin system genes in IgA nephropathy. *Nephrology (Carlton)* **9**:304–9.

Woo KT, Lau YK, Chan CM, et al. (2008). Angiotensin-converting enzyme inhibitor versus angiotensin 2 receptor antagonist therapy and the influence of angiotensin-converting enzyme gene polymorphism in IgA nephritis. *Ann Acad Med Singapore* **37**: 372–6.

Yaqoob M, et al. (1994). Relationship between hydrocarbon exposure and nephropatholgy in primary glomerulonephritis. *Nephrol Dial Transplant* **9**:1575–9.

Yau WP, Vathsala A, Lou HX, et al. (2007). Is a standard fixed dose of mycophenolate mofetil ideal for all patients? *Nephrol Dial Transplant* **22**: 3638–45.

Yoshida H, Mitarai T, Kawamura T, et al. (1995). Role of deletion polymorphisms of the angiotensin converting enzyme gene in the progression and therapeutic responsiveness of IgA nephropathy. *J Clin Invest* **86**:2162–9.

Yoshikawa N, et al. (1999). A controlled trial of combined therapy for newly diagnosed severe childhood IgA nephropathy. *J Am Soc Nephrol* **10**:101–9.

Yoshikawa N, et al. (2006). Steroid treatment for severe childhood IgA nephropathyhy: a randomized, controlled trial. *Clin J Am Soc Nephrol* **1**:511–17.

Zatz R, Dunn B R, Meyer T W, et al. (1986). Prevention of diabetic nephropathy by pharmacological amelioration of glomerular capillary hypertension. *J Clin Invest* **77**:1925–30.

Zhang JJ, et al. (2008). The level of secretory IgA of patients with IgA nephropathy is elevated and associated with pathological phenotypes. *Nephrol Dial Transplant* **23**:207–12.

Chapter 9

Membranoproliferative glomerulonephritis

Richard J. Glassock

Introduction and overview

Definition

Membranoproliferative glomerulonephritis (MPGN, also known as mesangiocapillary glomerulonephritis) is a designation given to a very heterogeneous collection of disorders that manifest by light microscopy both mesangial hyper-cellularity and proliferation accompanied by broadening of the peripheral capillary loops (Holley and Donadio, 1994; Glassock et al., 1995; Strife and West, 2001; Glassock, 2008) due to reduplication of the glomerular capillary basement membrane (known as 'double-contour'). In many instances, these broadened capillary loops also display prominent interposition of cells between the layers of the basement membrane and/or subendothelial or intra-membranous electron-dense deposits that may be accompanied by fragmentation or distortion of the basement membrane itself. The disorders encompassed by this definition also frequently display persistent reduction in serum complement levels (West et al., 1965).

Pathology

Both primary (idiopathic) and secondary forms of the pattern of MPGN by light microscopy are recognized; the latter frequently associated with autoimmune disease (e.g., systemic lupus erythematosis, SLE), chronic infections (e.g. viral hepatitis B and C), chronic thrombotic microangiopathy (TTP/HUS), complement regulatory factor deficiencies (factor H and I) and various monoclonal immunoglobulin deposition diseases (MIDD) (see Table 9.1 for full descriptions). Immunofluorescence and electron microscopy are particularly useful in separating the various underlying causes of MPGN (Holley and Donadio 1994; Rennke and Renounce 1995; Glassock et al., 1995; Glassock, 2008)). Chronic hepatitis viral C infection may result in MPGN associated with mixed (IgG/IgM) cryoglobulinemia. (Johnson et al. 1994a).

Table 9.1 Classification of disorders which may be associated with an MPGN pattern by light microscopy*

Primary (idiopathic)	Secondary
Type I MPGN (with subendothelial electron dense deposits- hepatitis C virus infection excluded) **Type II MPGN** (dense deposit disease) **Type III MPGN** (with deposits and fragmentation of basal lamina-also known as the Strife and Adams variant) **Type IV MPGN** (with subendothelial and subepithelial electron dense deposits—also known as the Burkholder variant)	**Infections** *(usually with type I MPGN pattern):* Hepatitis C virus infection (with or without cryoglobulinemia); hepatitis B virus infection (rare) Chronic bacterial, fungal, helminthic or parasitic infections ('shunt nephritis,' indwelling catheters, visceral abscesses, mycoplasma, malaria, schistosomiasis, filariasis, histoplasmosis, coccidiodomycosis, etc.) **Autoimmune diseases** *(usually with type I or IV MPGN pattern):* Lupus nephritis (class IV; diffuse proliferative) Mixed connective disease **Heredo-familial disorders** Factor H antibody Complement deficiency/dysregulation disorders (often with type II MPGN pattern) Factor H (or CR-1 or I) deficiency (congenital or acquired, with or without partial lipodystrophy—Dunnegan–Koeberling syndrome) C2 or C4 deficiency (often with a lupus-like syndrome) **Monoclonal immunoglobulin deposition disorders** *(with type I or II MPGN pattern- some with deposits with an organized substructure-glomerulonephritis with organized monoclonal immunoglobulin deposits):* Light chain deposition disease (kappa-chain nephropathy (may mimic primary type II MPGN) Heavy chain deposition disease (with hypocomplementemia) Monoclonal IgG deposition disease Type I (monoclonal) cryoglobulinemia Crystal cryoglobulinemia **Chronic thrombotic microangiopathies** *(TMA) (no electron dense deposits)* Atypical hemolytic uremia syndrome (with or without factor H deficiency) Drug-induced chronic TMA Radiation nephritis Transplant glomerulopathy

(Continued)

Table 9.1 (continued) Classification of disorders which may be associated with an MPGN pattern by light microscopy*

Primary (idiopathic)	Secondary
	Other disorders:
	Sickle cell disease
	Sjogren syndrome (?hepatitis C viral infection)
	Sarcoidosis
	Cyanotic congenital heart disease (?chronic infection)
	Malignant neoplasm (lung, lymphoma— without monoclonal immunoglobulin deposition disease)
	Antitrypsin deficiency
	Castleman's disease
	Buckley syndrome
	Kartagener syndrome (?chronic infection)

*Adapted with permission from Glassock RJ (2008). Membranoprolfierative glomerulonephritis. In D Molony and J Craig (eds), *Evidence-Based Nephrology.* Wiley Blackwall

Among the *primary* forms of MPGN, unassociated with any known underlying cause and largely confined to the kidneys, *four* morphologic subtypes are described (Holley and Donadio 1994; Glassock, Cohen and Adler, 1995; Glassock, 2008):

- *Type I MPGN*, (see Atlas plate 13) accounting for approximately 80% of cases, is characterized by electron-dense subendothelial deposits (see Atlas plate 14) which contain immunoglobulins and complement (C3) by immunofluorescence (Holley and Donadio, 1994; Glassock, 2008).

- *Type II MPGN*, which accounts for 15–20% of cases and is also known as dense deposit disease (DDD), is characterized by intramembranous electron-dense deposits (see Atlas plate 15) and is sometimes associated with partial lipodystrophy, retinal degeneration, and factor H (or I) deficiency (Appel, et al., 2005). The intramembranous dense deposits are negative by immunofluorescence but the surrounding basal lamina contains C3 and nodular deposits of C3 are found in the mesangium. This subtype is often classified as a separate disease entity, since it may lack the feature of MPGN by light microscopy (Walker, 2007; Walker, et al., 2007). It also may be 'mimicked' by light-chain deposition disease when the monoclonal light chain deposits are amorphous and/or intra-membranous and when 'false-negative' stains for monoclonal light chain deposition is noted by immunofluorescence.

- *Type III MPGN*, originally described by Strife and co-workers (Strife et al., 1975), accounts for <5% of cases and is often associated with extensive fragmentation of the basal lamina.

- *Type IV MPGN* is also considered by some to be a part of the morphologic spectrum of MPGN. This variant (also known as mixed membranous and proliferative glomerulonephritis), first described by Burkholder (Burkholder et al., 1970) accounts for much less than 5% of cases and is associated with both subendothelial and subepithelial deposits which are positive for immunoglobulins by immunofluorescence. These lesions have a strong resemblance to those found in lupus nephritis but serological studies for SLE are negative or inconclusive.

Any of the morphological variants of MPGN can be complicated by the development of segmental or diffuse crescentic glomerulonephritis, which greatly worsens the prognosis (see below and Chapter 10).

The *most important* step in assessing MPGN diagnosed by light microscopic pattern is to exclude the secondary disorders that can produce this morphological pattern of disease, particularly chronic infections such as hepatitis C viral infection (with or without associated cryoimmunoglobulinemia), Complement regulatory protein deficiencies (factor H/I), auto-immune disease (lupus nephritis), MIDD (such as light or heavy chain deposition disease or immunotactoid nephropathy and a chronic form of thrombotic microangiopathy (atypical hemolytic-uremia syndrome) (Glassock, 2008).

Pathogenesis

The pathogenesis of MPGN is diverse (Glassock, 2008). Deposition or *in situ* formation of immune complexes is believed to play a role in MPGN type I—with the antigen usually derived from an infectious agent or an autochthonous neoplastic or other proliferating endogenous cell (such as in SLE). The pathogenesis of MPGN type II is uncertain but may be due to inherited or acquired dysregulation of complement activation, particularly of the alternative pathway (Appel et al., 2005). MPGN type II is strongly associated with deficiencies of factor H (or I) and also with an auto-antibody to the C 3 convertase enzyme (C3Bb) of the alternative pathway. This autoantibody is known as C3 nephritic factor (C3Nef) (Smith et al., 2007; Walker, 2007).

Etiology

As already stated, the primary forms of MPGN must be clearly separated from the secondary forms (See Table 9.1), Ordinarily this can be easily accomplished by a careful examination of the renal biopsy specimen with light, immunofluorescence, and electron microscopy supplemented with serological studies, including anti-ds DNA autoantibody, serum complement (C3, C4m and C'H50), serum and urine immuno-fixation for monoclonal immunoglobulin-related proteins, Hepatitis B and C antibody and viral genome assays, a search for signs of thrombotic microangiopathies (hemolytic anemia with schistocytosis, thrombocytopenia) and (if appropriate) measurement of the functional activity and protein content of factor H and I. The presence of C3Nef in the circulation may herald an underlying primary form of MPGN type II (Glassock, 2008).

Clinical presentation

Despite this morphologic heterogeneity, the clinical expression of the various primary (as well as secondary) forms of MPGN is similar with a prominent tendency for the development of macroscopic or microscopic hematuria, heavy proteinuria (including nephrotic syndrome), and progressive impairment of renal function. Hypertension, which is sometimes severe, is also a common finding. In general, the morphological findings will direct the diagnostic evaluation (see 'Etiology').

Primary MPGN is a diagnosis of exclusion and no patient should be so labeled or considered for treatment until all reasonable efforts to identify a potential secondary cause have been carried out (Glassock, 2008). Omission of this step may lead to incorrect choices of therapy and thereby poor long- or short-term outcomes. Failure to recognize an underlying disease may adversely affect prognosis.

MPGN may present at any age although it most commonly involves children, adolescents, and young adults (Donadio and Holley 1982). MPGN type I characteristically affects a somewhat younger age population compared to MPGN type II. Males are slightly more commonly affected than females although in many series the male:female ratio is unity. The typical features leading to a diagnosis include the relatively abrupt onset of hematuria, heavy proteinuria, edema, and hypertension. This acute nephritic/nephrotic presentation can also be seen in post-streptococcal glomerulonephritis, lupus nephritis, vasculitis, cryoimmunoglobulinemia, and several other glomerulopathies (including fibrillary or immunotactoid glomerulonephritis).

It is important to re-emphasize that occult chronic infection with hepatitis C virus (HCV), with or without features of liver injury, commonly underlies MPGN type I. As many as 80% (or even more in some parts of the world where HCV infection is endemic) of patients with a light microscopic finding of MPGN type I can be shown to be chronically infected with HCV (Johnson et al., 1994a). About 50–60% of such patients will also have cryoglobulinemia (Kamar et al., 2008), but one-third of patients with HCV-associated MPGN (type I or III) have *no evidence* of cryoglobulinemia or multisystem involvement. Thus, all patients with MPGN type I or III should be screened for HCV antibody and/or HCV RNA by polymerase chain reaction. Identification of HCV infection has important therapeutic implications (see below).

A feature which often leads to the suspicion of MPGN is the concomitant presence of persistent hypocomplementemia; decreased serum levels of the C3 and/or C4 components of complement (West et al., 1965; Varade et al., 1990). A brief episode of decreased C3 level lasting 8 weeks or less is more typical of post-streptococcal glomerulonephritis, whereas the hypocomplementemia associated with MPGN is generally long-lasting. C3 is often decreased to a greater extent than C4 (Varade et al., 1990) in idiopathic (primary) MPGN and that associated with SLE; whereas the reverse is true in cryoglobulinemia-associated glomerulonephritis, including the glomerular disease accompanying chronic HCV infection (Johnson et al., 1994a). In MPGN type I, C1q levels may also be low, suggesting classical complement pathway activation. On the other hand, in MPGN type II MPGN, C1q is most often normal suggesting alternative complement pathway activation (Varade et al., 1990). C3 nephritic factor (C3Nef), which is an autoantibody to the alternative pathway convertase (C3Bb), is present predominantly in type II MPGN, where it acts to stabilize the alternate pathway convertase and to protect it from natural inhibitors (Daha et al. 1978; Berger and Daha 2007).

MPGN type II (DDD) has additional distinctive features such as partial lipodystrophy (Dunnigan–Koeberling disease) and the development of retinal degeneration (which may uncommonly cause blindness) (Appel, 2005). The retinal changes are recognized by the presence of extensive'drusen' by indirect retinoscopy.

Despite these clinical-serologic correlations a renal biopsy with immunofluorescence and electron microscopy is required for appropriate subcategorization of MPGN. Such subtyping may be important since underlying pathology has important diagnostic, prognostic, and therapeutic implications. The clinical course varies among the subtypes.

Epidemiology

Overall, primary MPGN appears to be decreasing in frequency in developed countries but remains as a relatively common finding in patients presenting with the nephrotic syndrome in the developing countries of Asia and Africa (Barbiano di Belgiojoso et al., 1985; Simon et al., 2004; Asinobi et al., 1999). MPGN type I in South Africa is not related to HCV infection (Madala, et al., 2003). In series emanating from developed countries the prevalence of MPGN among subjects undergoing renal biopsies for evaluation of nephrotic syndrome is usually <5% overall with a higher prevalence in children and young adults than in older adults. Some investigators have suggested that the changing epidemiology of MPGN is related to the control of infectious disease (through improved hygienic measures and use of anti-microbials—also known as the'hygiene hypothesis' (Johnson, et al., 2003).

Natural history

In adults, the actuarial renal survival at 10 years for MPGN type I is between 54–64% (Table 9.2) (D'Amico 1992). The prognosis for MPGN type II and type III disease may be somewhat worse (Cameron et al., 1983; Southwest Pediatric Nephrology Study Group 1985; Glassock, 2008), perhaps because of a greater prevalence of superimposed crescentic glomerular disease. Studies in children undergoing various therapies also have suggested a 10-year actuarial renal survival of about 50–60% (Habib et al., 1973; Cameron et al., 1983; Donadio and Offord, 1989; Glassock, 2008), so the overall prognosis for adults and children with MPGN is similar. Donadio (Donadio et al., 1984) found that the average decline in GFR was 20mL/min/year in a group of adults with severe MPGN receiving a placebo, almost 50% had developed ESRD by 33 months after entry into the trial. These subjects had a long history of disease before being entered into the trial so these ominous prognostic features from placebo-treated patients with MPGN are unduly pessimistic. Spontaneous complete clinical remissions of MPGN are quite uncommon, although they have been reported. Several clinical and morphological features affect the likelihood of developing end-stage renal failure, as will be discussed below (Cameron 1993; Glassock, 2008) (see also Table 9.3).

Prognostic factors

Age/sex

Neither the age at presentation nor gender has any consistent effect on long-term prognosis. A few studies have suggested a better prognosis for children

Table 9.2 Renal survival in MPGN type I*

Study	Year	N	Renal survival at 10 years
Cameron	1983	69	62%
Valles-Prats	1985	72	54%
Schmitt	1990	220	64%
Gruppo Italiano Di Immunopatholgica Renale	1990	259	60%
Overall		620	61%

*Reproduced from D'Amico G (1992). Influence of clinical and histological features on actuarial renal survival in adult patients with idiopathic IgA nephropathy, membranous nephropathy and membran-oproliferative glomerulonephritis. Survey of the recent literature. *American Journal of Kidney Disease* **20**:315–23. With permission of Elsevier

Table 9.3 Factors indicating a poor prognosis in MPGS type I

Clinical:	Older age at presentation (not consistently observed)
	Persistent nephrotic-range proteinuria (3.5g/d)
	Impaired renal function at discovery
	Persistent poorly controlled hypertension (systolic>diastolic)
	Positive viral serology (MPGN secondary to chronic hepatitis C viral infection)
Pathological:	Extensive crescents (>50% glomerular involvement)
	Superimposed segmental glomerulosclerosis
	Advanced tubulointerstitial fibrosis
	Arteriolo-nephrosclerosis (hypertension-related)

(Cameron et al., 1983; Yanagihara et al., 2005; Glassock, 2008), but this is not a consistent finding.

Proteinuria

The magnitude of proteinuria and its persistence has a significant effect on prognosis (D'Amico, 1992) as is true for all primary glomerular diseases. Cameron and his colleagues have found a 10-year renal survival rate of only 40% in patients with MPGN type I presenting with nephrotic syndrome whereas the 10-year survival rate was 85% in those presenting with non-nephrotic proteinuria (Cameron et al., 1983). Similar findings have been noted by some but not all studies. It is generally agreed that the greater the proteinuria the worse the long-term prognosis. In subjects with the nephrotic syndrome the 50% actuarial survival will be reached somewhere between 5–9 years after discovery, depending on how well the blood pressure is controlled.

Impaired renal function at presentation

An elevated serum creatinine and/or reduced creatinine clearance (or estimated GFR) at discovery is often, but not invariably, associated with a poor long-term outcome both in adults and in children (Valles-Prats et al., 1985; Gruppo Italiano di Immunopathologia Renale 1990; D'Amico 1992; Cansick et al., 2004; Glassock, 2008). The Italian study concluded that reduced GFR at presentation was an independent risk factor for eventual development of end-stage renal disease (ESRD). Fluctuations in the level of renal function, representing exacerbations of disease due to superimposed infection, may punctuate the course of the disease.

Complement levels

The pattern of complement levels (C3, C4) has little impact on prognosis in MPGN type I or II (Varade et al 1990; Ohi and Tanuma 1991). The levels may fluctuate and show no clear-cut relationship to the clinical activity of the disease. Persistently low C3 levels are more commonly observed in MPGN type II than in type I (Glassock, 2008).

Viral serology

As noted previously, chronic infection with HCV and, to a much lesser extent, HBV may be associated with clinical features which closely resemble primary (idiopathic) MPGN type I (Adler et al., 1995; Kamar et al., 2008). While long-term studies have not been conducted, the prognosis for these patients may be worse because of a high prevalence of impaired renal function at discovery and a very high frequency of nephrotic syndrome at presentation (Johnson et al., 1994a), but they may respond to anti-viral therapy such as interferon and ribaviran for HCV and lamuvidine adefovir, or other new antiviral agents (dipivoxil, entecavir, elbivudine) for HBV.

Hypertension

As is commonly noted in many glomerular disease, the presence of hyper-tension (usually now defined for proteinuric subjects as >130/80mm/Hg) is usually a feature indicating a worse prognosis. This has been confirmed as an independent risk factor by multivariant analysis (D'Amico 1992; Vikse et al., 2002).

Morphologic features

Only the presence of superimposed extensive crescents and/or chronic tubu-lointerstitial lesions have consistently been shown to affect prognosis adversely (Schmitt et al., 1990; D'Amico 1992; Vikse et al., 2002; Glassock, 2008). The severity of mesangial cellular interposition and/or hypercellularity are not particularly helpful in prognostication. Arteriolar damage, perhaps reflecting the severity of hypertension, can indicate a poor outcome. The somewhat worse prognosis of MPGN type II seen in some studies could be explained by a greater tendency for superimposition of crescents in this variant (Habib et al., 1973). Segmental glomerulosclerosis and/or nodular lesions have shown an adverse affect on renal survival in some studies (D'Amico 1992).

Specific treatment

At present there is no proven effective treatment for primary MPGN in any of its variations (Glassock, 2008). However, several regimens have been suggested to be efficacious in small, relatively short-term controlled trials, often using surrogate end points (such as improvement in proteinuria), or in larger and longer term observational, uncontrolled trials. In nearly all the therapeutic tri-als reported to date the analysis of the effect of treatment is confounded by morphologic and pathogenetic heterogeneity of the subjects with MPGN enrolled in the treatment trials. Additionally, many uncontrolled trials have used historical controls as the basis for comparison. Such analyses are biased since treatment groups must survive from clinical onset to the initiation of treatment whereas control patients have no such constraints. By intention-to-treat analysis from the onset or discovery of disease, many of the claims of efficacy cannot be supported (Donadio and Offord, 1989).

Glucocorticoids

Long-term but uncontrolled studies of children with predominantly type I MPGN conducted at the University of Cincinnati Children's Hospital have suggested that *high-dose, alternate-day prednisone* therapy preserves renal function, reduces glomerular inflammation, and increases renal survival (McAdams et al., 1975; McEnery et al., 1980, 1985; McEnery 1990). Alternate-day prednisone is usually begun at 2–2.5mg/kg or 60mg/m^2 (maximum dose 80mg) every other day (with appropriate careful and initial observation for exacerbation of hypertension) and subsequently slowly reduced to 1–1.5 mg/kg every other day at 2 years and 0.2–1.0mg/kg every other day at 4 years. Repeat biopsies in patients so treated have shown resolution of hypercellularity and 'improved' glomerular architecture. In the absence of an untreated cohort of patients with similar characteristics at onset it is not possible to definitively conclude that glucocorticoid therapy itself is responsible for the observed changes.

In 1990, McEnery updated the cumulative University of Cincinnati Children's Hospital uncontrolled experience with a high-dose, alternate-day prednisone regimen in MPGN (McEnery, 1990). Seventy-one pediatric patients with primary MPGN seen at this center have been treated *exclusively* with the alternate-day prednisone regimen described above. Of the patients treated with this regimen since 1957, 43% have been type I MPGN, 22% type II MPGN, and 34% type III MPGN. The average duration of disease prior to treatment was 1.5 years and the average total duration of treatment was 7.7 years. Overall, nineteen of 71 treated patients (27%) developed ESRD and the actuarial renal survival in this group at 10 and 20 years from the *start of therapy* was 75% and 59% respectively. Survival at 10 and 20 years from the *time of diagnosis* was 82% and 56% respectively. The development of ESRD was not greater in patients treated for 1 or more years (averaging 3.5 years) after the diagnosis or discovery of disease compared to patients treated early in the course of disease (average 0.3 years following discovery). While an 82% 10-year renal survival rate from disease discovery is substantially greater than the expected 50–60% 10-year renal survival rate mentioned earlier, the absence of contemporaneous controls makes it difficult to ascribe the better outcome to glucocorticoid therapy alone (Glassock, 2008). Other improvements in management, particularly better control of hypertension or the use of angiotensin II inhibiting agents (Guo et al., 2008), could have also affected the outcome in comparison to historical controls. Nevertheless, repeat renal biopsies in treated patients showed improvement in inflammation (McAdams et al., 1975) and patients with normal or near-normal renal function 15 or more years after the onset (more accurately discovery) of disease continued to enjoy stable renal function, although with discontinuation of glucocorticoid therapy exacerbations and relapses have been observed. Therefore, McEnery and colleagues continue to recommend careful observation of patients with MPGN treated with alternate-day glucocorticoids following tapering and discontinuance of this therapy (McEnery, 1990).

Only one prospective, randomized, placebo-controlled trial of alternate-day glucocorticoids in MPGN has been reported. The full-length report of the International study of kidney disease in children trial appeared in 1992 (Tarshish et al., 1992), approximately 12 years following the closure of the study to entry of new patients and 10 years after the initial abstract appeared recording the preliminary results of the trial. All patients admitted to the trial were children with primary MPGN (53% MPGN type I). Eligibility included a creatinine clearance $\geq 70mL/min/ 1.73 m^2$ and persistent proteinuria $>40mg/h/m^2$. A total of 80 patients were randomized to receive either prednisone $40mg/m^2$ every other day or a placebo (lactose). The average duration of treatment was 41 months, with the onset of renal failure the most common reason for termination of treatment. Forty-two patients had MPGN type I, fourteen MPGN type II, and seventeen had MPGN type III/IV. Seven patients had unclassified MPGN. Treatment failure was defined as a *30% increase* in serum creatinine concentration from baseline and this event occurred in *33%* of patients with MPGN type I or type III allocated to prednisone treatment compared with *58%* in the placebo group ($p = 0.05$). Kaplan–Meier analysis indicated that 61% of treated patients and 12% of placebo patients had stable renal function over the first 10 years of follow-up ($p = 0.07$). Repeat renal biopsy showed no important differences between treated and placebo patients. There was no difference in outcome relative to whether treatment was instituted early (<1 year) after diagnosis or discovery compared with late treatment (>1 year). It is noteworthy that the duration of disease prior to entry was only 8.9 ± 1.3 months in the prednisone-treated group and 18.1 ± 3.9 months in the placebo group ($p <0.05$). A stable course was noted more often in patients whose red cell excretion rate fell and whose urinary protein excretion decreased during the observation periods.

Side effects were encountered, particularly worsening of hypertension. Aggravation of hypertension led to discontinuance of prednisone in five of 47 treated patients and in two of 33 placebo patients. The conclusion offered by the authors was that 'long-term treatment with prednisone appears to improve the outcome of children with MPGN.' The differences in outcome were of marginal statistical significance and the power to detect substantial differences was small (0.35). In terms of stability of renal function the differences between treated and placebo patients were not observed until after 90 months of observation when only eleven prednisone and seven placebo patients were under observation. Thus, the strength of the data supporting the conclusions is weak and when interpreted strictly the study is at best inconclusive.

Mota-Hernadez et al. (1985) conducted a small trial of alternate day steroids in children with an up to 5-year follow-up. Only one of nine (11%) subjects in the steroid treated group developed ESRD whereas four of nine (44%) in the placebo group went on to develop ESRD.

Most of the studies of steroids in MPGN have indicated that types II and III MPGN are 'resistant' to such therapy as would be expected from presumed pathogenesis (Braun et al., 1999) Data on the use of oral alternate-day prednisone in adults is scarce and largely anecdotal—no controlled trials of alternate day steroids have yet been reported in adults.

Ford et al. (1992) carried out a small uncontrolled trial of oral and/or intravenous glucocorticoids in nineteen children with MPGN I utilizing regimens which were 'tailored to the severity of disease based on creatinine clearance and proteinuria' (treatment was generally instituted within 1 year of the diagnosis of disease. The most intensive regimens included intravenous methylprednisone (30mg/kg/d for three doses) and oral prednisolone (2mg/kg/d, up to 60mg/d). This regimen was utilized for patients with creatinine clearances <50mL/min and any level of proteinuria. The least intensive regimen was 20mg of prednisone every other day. This regimen was used for patients with a creatinine clearance >80mL/min and proteinuria <40mg/h/m^2. Those with disease severity between these two extremes received oral glucocorticoids either daily or every other day in doses of 2mg/kg. Therapy was subsequently tapered slowly according to clinical course. Other immunosuppressive agents were not used. Hypertension was controlled 'medically' and 90% of patients received an angiotensin-converting enzyme inhibitor. Follow-up averaged 6.5 years with total duration of therapy of 38 ± 3 months. Repeat renal biopsies were performed after about 3 years of treatment and showed reduced inflammatory activity in the great majority of patients. Interestingly, progressive glomerulosclerosis was seen only in those patients treated with *daily* as opposed to *every other day* glucocorticoid regimens. Eight of nineteen (42%) treated patients entered a complete remission with normal urinalyses. The average creatinine clearance for the entire group rose from 78 ± 7 to 126 ± 5mL/min over the course of treatment and follow-up. No patient developed ESRD. Significant side effects were observed in the treated patients, which included seizures, hypertension, growth retardation, osteoporosis, and obesity. This experience, although uncontrolled, suggests that early and very aggressive intravenous glucocorticoid therapy, based on the severity of illness at presentation, may afford benefit in children with MPGN type I. Nevertheless, it is possible that the good outcomes observed in this trial were also a function of better control of hypertension and the use of angiotensin-converting enzyme inhibitors. It is also worth re-emphasizing that progressive glomerulosclerosis was associated with the use of *daily* glucocorticoid regimens. Other limited studies of prednisone therapy conducted in children have suggested that the initiation of therapy early in the course of disease, before the establishment of chronic irreversible lesions, may be important in determining the final outcome of treatment (Warady et al., 1985; Yanagihara et al., 2005; Bahat et al., 2007; Glassock, 2008).

Very limited trials of glucocorticoids have been conducted (none controlled) in adults with MPGN but they have generally reached conclusions similar to those in children. In extensive reviews of data from several trials using an intention-to-treat analysis, Donadio and Offord at the Mayo Clinic and a meta-analysis by Schena and colleagues have concluded that the available information does not support a beneficial effect of glucocorticoids in adults (Donadio and Offord 1989; Schena et al., 1999), since in many studies treatment was started years after onset of disease. A role for very intensive therapies with high-dose intravenous pulses of glucocorticoids (with or without concomitant cytotoxic agents) has been suggested by small observational trials with limited follow-up (Emre et al., 1995; Bahat et al., 2007).

Alkylating agents

Prior to 1980, numerous anecdotes had appeared regarding the use of adjunctive cytotoxic (alkylating) immunosuppressive agents in MPGN (see Kincaid-Smith 1972; Chapman et al., 1980; Glassock, 2008). These reports were generally unimpressive and mostly demonstrated unfavorable results. As a consequence, the use of these agents in MPGN has, until recently, not been recommended and no prospective trials of this category of therapeutic modalities have been conducted, except in combination with warfarin or heparin and dipyridamole (see below). These latter trials also concluded that cytotoxic therapy was ineffective in MPGN (Chapman et al., 1980; Tiller et al., 1981; Cattran et al., 1985).

A few studies, largely of an uncontrolled nature, have suggested that more aggressive regimens combining intravenous 'pulse' intravenous methylprednisolone with oral cyclophosphamide initially followed by short-term maintenance therapy with alternate-day prednisone and oral cyclophosphamide may be beneficial. Faedda and colleagues (Faedda et al., 1994) studied nineteen patients, ages 9–65 years, with a variety of types of MPGN. Fifteen of nineteen (79%) patients treated with this aggressive glucocorticoid and cytotoxic regimen experienced complete remission while three additional patients (15%) experienced partial remissions. Relapses occurred in six of the eighteen responders and overall four patients progressed to ESRD. After an average follow-up of 7.4 ± 0.8 years, the renal survival rate was 79%. Because of the lack of contemporaneous controls, it is not possible to conclude that the favorable outcome was a result of treatment, although a complete remission rate of 79% is higher than one would have predicted from historical 'controls.' However, it should be pointed out that a renal survival rate of approximately 80% following 7.5 years of follow-up is not greatly different from that found in other trials which utilized glucocorticoids alone in children. A controlled randomized study is needed to confirm these encouraging results from observational trials (Glassock, 2008).

Inhibitors of purine synthesis

Azathioprine and mycophenolate mofetil

No controlled trials of azathioprine (AZA) or mycophenolate mofetil (MMF) or its parent compound mycophenolate sodium have been reported to date. Numerous anecdotes and small short term observational trials have been reported. usually in combination with steroids (Choi et al., 2002; Bayazit et al., 2004; Jones et al., 2004; Glassock, 2008);. Short-term results have included a diminution of urinary protein excretion and stabilization of renal function. The long-term benefits and risks of azathioprine and/or MMF in MPGN are unknown.

Calcineurin inhibitors

Cyclosporine A and Tacrolimus

Limited uncontrolled trials and case-reports of cyclosporine A (CsA), usually in doses of 4–6mg/kg/d and tacrolimus (0.1–0.15mg/kg/d) accompanied by low doses of oral prednisolone have demonstrated a modest decline in proteinuria (Lagrue et al., 1982; Erbay et al., 1988; Cattran, 1991; Glassock, 1994; Matsumoto et al., 1995; Kiyomasu et al., 2002) or more rarely complete remission (Haddad et al., 2007). However, because of the potential for nephrotoxicity with a drug- and dose-related decline in GFR and aggravation of hypertension, these agents are not currently widely used or recommended (Radhakrishnan and Halevy 2000; Glassock, 2008). Buckley's syndrome associated with MPGN might be helped by CsA (Lagrue et al., 1982).

Plasma exchange/infusion

Intensive plasma exchange with immunosuppression may be of benefit for the occasional patient with superimposed extensive crescentic glomerulone-phritis and the syndrome of rapidly progressive glomerulonephritis (see also Chapter 10) (D'Apice and Kincaid-Smith 1979; Montoliu et al., 1982; McGinley et al., 1985; Morton and Bannister 1993; Kurtz and Schlueter, 2002). Plasma infusion might conceivably be of benefit in Type II MPGN associated with Factor H deficiency (Licht et al., 2005).

Interferon-α/Ribavirfan

High-dose recombinant human interferon-α (3 million units subcutaneously, twice weekly for 6–12 months) will reduce the load of infectious virions, reduce proteinuria, and perhaps improve or stabilize renal function in HCV-associated MPGN (Johnson et al. 1994a,b). Unfortunately relapses are very common when treatment is stopped. Side-effects are common. Treatment of HCV-associated MPGN with steroids and cytotoxic agents may be hazardous. Combination of interferon-α and ribaviran may be more effective but requires further trials (Lai et al., 1993; Bruchfeld et al., 2003). Better results may be expected with the use of pegylated interferon associated with ribavirin.

Anticoagulant and antithrombotics

As already mentioned, early uncontrolled trials suggested that anticoagulants (heparin or warfarin), frequently combined with glucocorticoids and cyto-toxic agents, had beneficial effects in MPGN, but prospective trials generally failed to support this view and this therapeutic approach fell out of favor (Tiller et al., 1981; Cattran et al., 1985). Combinations of aspirin (975mg/d) and dipy-ridamole (325mg/d) were initially shown to significantly delay or slow the rate of deterioration of GFR (as measured by radioisotopic methods) in a prospec-tive, randomized trial conducted by Donadio and co-workers in 1984 (Donadio et al., 1984). This study examined the impact of this therapeutic regimen over the first 4 years following therapy, not from the time of the original recogni-tion of disease. In this trial, platelet survival time was improved but there was no change in proteinuria, urinalysis, hematuria, or complement profile. Mild-to-moderate bleeding complications required discontinuance of active drug combinations in 15% of patients. In addition, combinations of warfarin and dipyridamole were also demonstrated as having beneficial effects on renal function in another prospective, cross-over design study, but the frequency and severity of complications related to bleeding limited the utility of this approach, and it is not currently recommended (Zimmerman et al., 1983).

In 1994, a further non-blinded prospective controlled trial of aspirin and dipyridamole therapy was reported from the Collaborative Glomerulone-phritis Therapy Study Group (Zauner et al., 1994). Eighteen adult patients (fifteen with type I MPGN and three with type II MPGN) were randomly assigned to receive to aspirin 500mg/d plus dipyridamole 75mg/d or symptomatic therapy only for 36 months. Both treated and control patients had impaired renal function and proteinuria of a similar extent (serum creatinine 1.8mg/d and proteinuria 7–8g/d. During the post-randomization period, proteinuria fell in both groups, but to a greater extent in the aspirin–dipyridamole-treated patients. A partial remission of nephrotic-range proteinuria occurred in seven of ten of the aspirin–dipyridamole group versus only two of eight in the control group. Serum creatinine values did not change in either group. The post-randomization observation period may have been too brief to detect any effect of reduced proteinuria on the course of renal function. Combinations of cyclophosphamide, dipyridamole, and anticoagulants in MPGN have yielded disappointing results, but many of these were underpowered to show a beneficial effect (Cattran, 1985; Harmankaya et al., 2001).

Taken together, the data suggest that aspirin combined with dipyridamole, even in relatively low doses, may have a beneficial effect on the course of MPGN; however, as stressed by Donadio and Offord (1989) one should be cautious not to overinterpret the results of these studies since they followed the course of disease *from introduction of therapy*, not from the *onset of diagnosis of disease*. Due to the relatively brief periods of follow-up, conclusive statements on the long-term impact of this therapy on the natural history of disease remains uncertain.

Non-steroidal anti-inflammatory drugs

Non-steroidal anti-inflammatory drugs (NSAID), particularly indomethacin, have been used for several decades (predominantly in Europe) in the treatment of MPGN, mostly in uncontrolled trials and sometimes in combination with cytotoxic agents (Michielsen et al., 1973; Vanrenterghem et al., 1975). Mild-to-moderate reduction in proteinuria has been observed, particularly in salt-depleted patients. Stabilization of renal function, after an initial decline, has also been noted. These effects rapidly dissipate with discontinuance of the agent. Complications, particularly of a gastrointestinal nature, are common and this form of therapy is seldom used outside selected centers in Europe. Controlled trials are lacking (Glassock, 2008).

Practical recommendations

As discussed previously, one should always carry out a thorough investigation of possible secondary causes before initiating any therapy for MPGN. This would include a careful search for chronic infections (particularly endocarditis, visceral abscesses, and viral hepatitis C or B), cryoglobulinemia, autoimmune disease (particularly SLE), complement regulatory deficiencies (particularly factor H), thrombotic microangiopathies and various forms of plasma cell dyscrasia or immunoglobulin-deposition diseases. Light chain disease can mimic MPGN type II and requires careful consideration when the clinical and morphologic features are atypical for MPGN type II. Specific therapy of these disorders with antimicrobials, interferon-α, pegylated interferon, ribaviran, lamivudine and other anti-HBV agents, plasma exchange/plasma infusion, rituximab, or chemotherapy (melphalan, thalidomide, or bortezomib) may be indicated. Electron microscopy is particularly helpful to characterize the lesions and to exclude any of the non-amyloid (Congo-red negative) fibrillary glomerulopathies. Having obtained sufficient data to reliably exclude secondary causes of MPGN, one may then proceed to a consideration of optimal therapeutic approaches to primary MPGN according to the morphological classification.

Patients with *primary MPGN type I or type III/IV* disease could be offered one of the four approaches (Table 9.4) described next (see also reviews by Levin, 1999 and Glassock, 2008):

- *Long-term alternate-day oral glucocorticoids (prednisone or prednisolone)*: this approach is preferred in children with relatively well preserved renal function and nephrotic-range proteinuria; very little evidence of efficacy in adults is available. Blood pressure must be carefully monitored and aggressively treated, preferably with agents affecting the rennin–angiotensin–aldosterone system, to values <130/80mmHg. The child and parent should be made aware of potential long-term complications.

- *Combinations of aspirin and dipyridamole*: this approach may be preferred in adults, especially those with modest impairment of GFR accompanied by heavy proteinuria. The risk of bleeding should be explained. This therapy has a very limited potential for any long-term beneficial effects but has a low likelihood of inducing adverse events. It is not likely to reduce the development of ESRD.

- *Combinations of high-dose intravenous glucocorticoids and oral cyclophosphamide (or MMF)*: this form of combination therapy could be offered to those patients with an aggressive course, especially those in whom the disease has been complicated by superimposed crescentic disease (see also Chapter 10). The addition of a course of plasma exchange (daily or every other day for 7 sessions) to a regimen of steroids and cytotoxic agents may also be helpful in this group, but this has not yet been proven.

- *Conservative therapy*: a program of watchful waiting is recommended for any patient with normal GFR and non-nephrotic proteinuria. Blood pressure should be vigorously treated, preferably with angiotensin-converting enzyme inhibitors (ACEi) or angiotensin receptor blockers (ARB). If proteinuria is >3.5g/d or the urinary protein to creatinine ratio >3gm/gm (in an adult), ACEi/ARB may be tried for an anti-proteinuric effect even if hypertension is absent. The goal of such treatment is to reduce the proteinuria to the maximum extent possible without disabling symptoms. A small controlled trial in MPGN has generally confirmed the benefits for such an approach (Giri et al., 2002). The benefits of ACEi/ARB are usually seen only when there is a distinct lowering of proteinuria (by at least 25% from baseline). Patients with advanced renal insufficiency and marked chronic tubulointerstitial damage should be managed conservatively.

At present there does not appear to be any good justification for the use of calcineurin inhibitors (CsA or tacrolimus), oral anticoagulants or NSAID in type I or III MPGN except as a part of a randomized clinical trial (Glassock, 2008).

The therapy for *type II MPGN* is very problematical. Immunosuppressive therapy, of any kind, is not likely to be of benefit and may be harmful, therefore it cannot be recommended. According to the Hixton Retreat on Dense Deposit Disease (Smith et al., 2007), if C3Nef is present then a trial of plasma exchange/ infusion therapy is indicated. If a factor H deficiency is present due to a factor H gene mutation then plasma infusion therapy is indicated. If a factor H deficiency is due to an inhibiting auto-antibody then rituximab and plasma exchange could be tried. The use of eculizumab (a monoclonal antibody to C5) requires further evaluation in the therapy of type II MPGN. Finding an effective and non-toxic therapy for type II MPGN is a very important goal because of the high recurrence rate and graft loss with renal transplantation (see next section).

Recurrence in renal transplants

All forms of MPGN have been noted to recur in renal allografts (Glassock, 2008; Ivanyi 2008). The recurrence rate is about 67–100% in MPGN type II whereas only 20–33% of patients with MPGN type I will manifest a clinical recurrence (Curtis et al., 1979; Briganti, et al., 2002; Braun et al., 2005; Ivanyi, 2008). The recurrence rate is related more to the severity of the underlying disease, particularly the presence of superimposed crescentic glomerulone-phritis, than to the type of MPGN (Little et al., 2006). There are no clinical features prior to transplantation, other than superimposed extensive crescen-tic disease, which will reliably predict the risk of recurrence of MPGN in a renal allograft. Fortunately, in many, but not all patients without superim-posed crescentic disease, the recurrence of disease does not lead to graft loss (Ivanyi, 2008); however, graft loss due to recurrence is overall relatively common in MPGN and is particularly likely with MPGN type II where graft loss due to recurrence is reported to be 34–66% (Ivanyi, 2008), largely due to the higher prevalence of superimposed crescentic disease (Little et al., 2006). Treatment of recurrent disease is generally unsatisfactory, but a few anecdotal reports have claimed success for aggressive treatment with oral cyclophosph-amide, plasma exchange, and/or high-dose MMF and intravenous steroids, but the true benefits of these approaches have not yet been tested in a con-trolled trial (Lien and Scott, 2000; Kurtz and Schlueter, 2002; Wu et al., 2004; Glassock, 2008). If a factor H deficiency is the cause of type II MPGN, plasma exchange/infusion may be used in the pre- and post-transplant management to try to avoid a recurrence.

References

Adler S, Cohen A, Glassock R (1995). Secondary glomerular disease. In B Brenner (ed), *The Kidney*, 5th edn, pp.1543–55. WB Saunders, Philadelphia, PA.

Appel GB, Cook HT, Hageman G, et al. (2005) Membranoproliferative glomerulonephritis type II (dense deposit disease): an update. *J Am Soc Nephrol* **16**:1392–1403.

Asinobi AO, Gbadegesin RA, Adeyemo AA, et al. (1999). The predominance of membranoproliferative glomerulonephritis in childhood nephrotic syndrome in Ibadan, Nigeria. *West Afr J Med* **18**:203–6.

Bahat E, Akkaya BK, Akman S, et al. (2007). Comparison of pulse and oral steroid in childhood membranoproliferative glomerulonephritis. *J Nephrol* **20**:234–45.

Barbiano di Belgiojoso G, Baroni M, Pagliari B, et al. (1985). Is membranoproliferative glomerulonephritis really decreasing? *Nephrol* **40**:380–4.

Bayazit AK, Noyan A, Cengiz N, et al. (2004). Mycophenolate mofetil in children with multi-drug resistant nephrotic syndrome. *Clin Nephrol* **61**:25–29.

Berger SP, Daha MR (2007). Complement in glomerular injury. *Semin Immunopath* **29**:375–84

Briganti EM et al. (2002). Risk of renal allograft loss from recurrent glomerulonephritis. *N Engl J Med* **347**:103–9.

Braun MC, Stablein DM, Hamiwka LA, et al. (2005). Recurrence of membranoproliferative glomerulonephritis type II in renal allografts: The North American Pediatric Renal Transplant Cooperative Study experience. *J Am Soc Nephrol* **16**:2225–33.

Braun MC, West CD, Strife CF (1999). Difference between membranoproliferative glomerulonephritis type I and III in long-term response to an alternate-day prednisone regimen. *Am J Kidney Dis* **34**:1022–32.

Bruchfeld A, Lindahl K, Ståhle L, et al. (2003). Interferon and ribavirin treatment in patients with hepatitis C-associated renal disease and renal insufficiency. *Nephrol Dial Transpl* **18**:1573–80.

Burkholder P, Marchand H, and Krueger R (1970). Mixed membranous and proliferative glomerulonephritis. A correlative light, immunofluorescence and electron microscopic study. *Lab Invest* **23**:450–7.

Cameron JS (1993). The long-term outlook of glomerular diseases. In R Schrier and C Gottschalk (eds), *Diseases of the kidney*, 5th edn, pp.1919–24. Little Brown, Boston, MA.

Cameron J, Turner D, Heaton J, et al. (1983). Idiopathic mesangiocapillary glomerulonephritis. Comparison of type I and II in children and adults and long-term prognosis. *Am J Med7* **4**:175–92.

Cansick JC, Lennon R, Cummins CL, et al. (2004). Prognosis, treatment and outcome of childhood mesangiocapillary (membranoproliferative) glomerulonephritis. *Nephrol Dail Transpl* **19**:2769–7.

Cattran D (1991). Current status of cyclosporin A in the treatment of membranous, IgA and membranoproliferative glomerulonephritis. *Clin Nephrol* **35**(Suppl. 1): 543–7.

Cattran DC, Cardella C, Roscoe J, et al. (1985). Results of a controlled drug trial in membranoproliferative glomerulonephritis. *Kidney Int* **27**:436–41.

Chapman S, Cameron J, Chantler C, et al. (1980). Treatment of mesangiocapillary glomerulonephritis in children with combined immunosuppression and anticoagulation. *Arch Dis Child* **55**:446–57.

Choi MJ, Eustace JA, Giminez LF, et al. (2002). Mycophenolate mofetil treatment for primary glomerular diseases. *Kidney Int* **61**:10981114.

Curtis J, Wyatt R, Bhathena D, et al. (1979). Renal transplantation for patients with type I and type II membranoproliferative glomerulonephritis: serial complement and nephritic factor measurement and the problem of recurrence of disease. *Am J Med* **66**:216–23.

D'Amico G (1992). Influence of clinical and histological features on actuarial renal survival in adult patients with idiopathic IgA nephropathy, membranous nephropathy and membranoproliferative glomerulonephritis. Survey of the recent literature. *Am J Kidney Dis* **20**:315–23.

D'Apice AJF, Kincaid-Smith G (1979). Plasma exchange in the treatment of glomerulonephritis. In P Kincaid-Smith, AJF D'Apice, R Atkins (eds), *Progress in glomerulonephritis*, pp.371–84. John Wiley, New York, NY.

Daha M, Austen K, Fearon D (1978). Heterogenicity, polypeptide chain composition and antigenic reactivity of C3 nephritic factor. *Z Immunol* **120**:1389–93.

Donadio JV, Holley KE (1982). Membranoproliferative glomerulonephritis. *Semin Nephrol* **2**:214–19.

Donadio J, Offord K (1989). Reassessment of treatment results in membranoproliferative glomerulonephritis, with emphasis on life-table analysis. *Am J Kidney Dis* **6**:445–51.

Donadio J, Anderson C, Mitchell J, et al. (1984). Membranoproliferative glomerulonephritis, a clinical trial of platelet inhibitor therapy. *New Engl J Med* **310**:1421–6.

Emre S, Sirin A, Alpay H, et al. (1995). Pulse methylprednisolone therapy in children with membranoproliferative glomerulonephritis. *Acta Paediatr Jpn* **37**:626–9.

Erbay B, Karatan O, Duman N, et al. (1988). The effect of cyclosporine in idiopathic nephrotic syndrome resistant to immunosuppressive therapy. *Transplant Proc* **20**(Suppl. 4):292.

Faedda R, Satta A, Tanda F, et al. (1994). Immunosuppressive treatment of membranoproliferative glomerulonephritis. *Nephron* **67**:59–65.

Ford P, Briscoe D, Shanley P, Lum G (1992). Childhood membranoproliferative glomerulonephritis type I. Limited steroid therapy. *Kidney Int* **41**:1606–12.

Giri S, Mahajan SK, Sen R, et al. (2002). Effects of angiotensin converting enzyme inhibitors on renal function in patients with membranoproliferative glomerulonephritis with mild to moderate renal insufficiency. *J Assoc Physicians India* **50**:1245–9.

Glassock R (1994). The role of cyclosporine in glomerular disease. *Cleveland Clin J Med* **61**:363–9.

Glassock RJ (2008). Membranoprolfieratvei glomerulonephritis. In D Molony and J Craig (eds), *Evidence-Based Nephrology*. In Press.

Glassock R, Cohen A, Adler S (1995). Primary glomerular disease. In B Brenner (ed), *The Kidney*, 5th edn, pp.1458–66. WB Saunders, Philadelphia, PA.

Gruppo Italiano di immunopathologica renale (1990). Le glomerulonefrite membranoproliferativo. *Giorn Ital Nephrol* **7**:67–102.

Guo S, Kowalewska J, Wietecha TA, et al. (2008). Renin-angiotensin system blockade is renoprotective in immune complex-mediated glomerulonephritis. *J Am Soc Nephrol* **19**:1168–76.

Habib R, Kleinknecht C, Gubler M-C, et al. (1973). Idiopathic membranoproliferative glomerulonephritis in children. Report of 105 cases. *Clin Nephrol* **1**:194–214.

Habib R, Gubler M-C, Loriat C (1975). Dense deposit disease: a variant of membranoproliferative glomerulonephritis. *Kidney Int* **7**:204–10.

Haddad M, Lau K, Butani L (2007). Remission of membranoproliferative glomerulonephritis type I with the use of tacrolimus. *Pediatr Nephrol* **22**:1787–91.

Harmankaya O, Basturk T, Ozturk Y, Karabiber N, Obek A (2001). Effect of acetylsalicylic acid and dipyridamole in primary membranoproliferative glomerulonephritis type I. *Int Urol Nephrol* **33**:583–7.

Holley K, Donadio J (1994). Membranoproliferative glomerulonephritis. In C Tisher, B Brenner (eds), *Renal Pathology, with clinical and functional correlations*, 2nd edn, pp. 294–349. Lippincott, Philadelphia, PA.

Ivanyi B (2008). A primer on recurrent and de-novo glomerulonephritis in renal allografts. *Nat Clin Pract Nephrol* **4**:446–57.

Johnson RJ, Gretch D, Couser W, et al. (1994a). Hepatitis C virus associated glomerulonephritis. Effect of interferon therapy. *Kidney Internat* **46**:1701–4.

Johnson RJ, Gretch D, Yamabe H. et al. (1994b). Interferon α in the treatment of membranoproliferative glomerulonephritis associated with hepatitis C virus infection: do we have enough data or are we still in the learning stage? *J Nephrol* **1**:336–9.

Johnson RJ, Hurtado A, Merszei J, et al. (2003). Hypothesis: dysregulation of immunologic balance resulting from hygiene and socio-economic factors may influence the epidemiology and cause of glomerulonephritis worldwide. *Am J Kidney Dis* **42**:575–81.

Jones G, Juszczak M, Kingdon E, et al. (2004). Treatment of idiopathic membranoproliferative glomerulonephritis with mycophenolate mofetil and steroids. *Nephrol Dial Transplant* **19**:3160–4.

Kamar N, Izopet J, Alric L, et al. (2008). Hepatitis C virus-related kidney disease: an overview. *Clin Nephrol* **69**:149–60.

Kincaid-Smith P (1972). The treatment of chronic mesangiocapillary glomerulonephritis with impaired renal function. *Med J Aust* **2**:587–92.

Kiyomasu T, Shibata M, Kurosu H, et al. (2002). Cyclosporin A treatment for membranoproliferative glomerulonephritis type II. *Nephron* **91**:509–11.

Kurtz KA, Schlueter AJ (2002). Management of membranoproliferative glomerulonephritis type II with plasmapheresis. *J Cin Apher* **17**:135–7.

Lagrue G, Laurent J, Dubertret L, et al. (1982). Buckley's syndrome and membranoproliferative glomerulonephritis. *Nephron* **31**:279–83.

Lai M, Pang P, Kao J, et al. (1993). Combination therapy of α interferon and ribavirin in patients with clinical hepatitis C: an interim repeat. *Hepatology* **18**:933A (Abstract).

Levin A (1999). Management of membranoproliferative glomerulonephritis: Evidence-based recommendations. *Kidney Int* (Suppl. 70):s41–6.

Licht C, Weyersberg A, Heinen S, et al. (2005). Successful plasma therapy for atypical hemolytic uremia syndrome caused by Factor H deficiency owing to a novel mutation in the complement cofactor protein domain 15. *Am J Kidney Dis* **45**:415–21.

Lien YH, Scott K (2000). Long-term cyclophosphamide treatment for recurrent type I membranoproliferative glomerulonephritis after transplantation. *Am J Kidney Dis* **35**:539–43.

Little MA, Dupont P, Campbell E, et al. (2006). Severity of primary MPGN, rather than MPGN type determines renal survival and post-transplantation recurrence risk. *Kidney Int* **69**:504–11.

Madala ND, Naicker S, Singh B, et al. (2003). The pathogenesis of membranoproliferative glomerulonephritis in KwaZulu-Natal, South Africa is unrelated to hepatitis C virus infection. *Clin Nephrol* **60**:69–73.

Matsumoto H, Shibasaki T, Ohno I, et al. (1995). Effect of cyclosporin monotherapy on proteinuria in patients with membranoproliferative glomerulonephritis. *Nippon Jinzo Gakkai Shi* **37**:258–62.

McAdams A, McEnery P, West C (1975). Mesangiocapillary glomerulonephritis: changes in glomerular morphology with long-term alternate-day prednisone therapy. *J Pediatr* **86**:23–30.

McEnery P (1990). Membranoproliferative glomerulonephritis: the Cincinnati experience—cumulative renal survival 1957–1989. *J Pediatr* **116**:5109–14.

McEnery P, McAdams A, West C (1980). Membranoproliferative glomerulonephritis: improved survival with alternate-day prednisone therapy. *Clin Nephrol* **13**:117–24.

McEnery P, McAdams A, West C (1985). The effect of prednisone in a high-dose, alternate-day regimen on the natural history of idiopathic membranoproliferative glomerulonephritis. *Medicine* (Baltimore) **6**:401–18.

McGinley E, Watkins R, McLay A, et al. (1985). Plasma exchange in the treatment of mesangiocapillary glomerulonephritis. *Nephron* **40**:385–90.

Michielsen P, Van Damme B, Dotremont G, et al. (1973). Indomethacin treatment of membranoproliferative and lobular glomerulonephritis. In P Kincaid-Smith, T Mathew, E Becker (eds), *Glomerulonephritis*, pp.611–20. John Wiley, New York, NY.

Montoliu J, Bergada E, Arrizabalaga P, et al. (1982). Acute renal failure in dense-deposit disease: recovery after plasmapheresis. *Br Med J* **384**:940–3.

Morton MR, Bannister K (1993). Renal failure due to mesangiocapillary glomerulonephritis in pregnancy—use of plasma exchange therapy. *Clin Nephrol* **40**:74–8.

Mota-Hernandez F, Gordillo-Paniagua G, Munoz-Arizpe R, et al. (1985). Prednisone versus placebo in membranoproliferative glomerulonephritis: long-term clinicopathologic correlation. *Int J Pediatr Nephrol* **6**:25–8.

Ohi H, Tanuma N (1991). Does nephritic factor relate to disease activity in hypocomplementuric membranoproliferative glomerulonephritis? *Nephron* **62**:116–17.

Radhakrishnan J, Halevy D (2000). Cyclosporin treatment of glomerular diseases. *Expert Opin Invest Drugs* **9**:1053–63.

Rennke H, Renounce H (1995). Secondary membranoproliferative glomerulonephritis (nephrology forum). *Kidney Int* **47**:643–56.

Schena FP (1999). Primary glomerulonephritides with nephrotic syndrome. Limitations of therapy in adult patients. *J Nephrol* **12**(Suppl.2):si25–130.

Schmitt H, Bohle H, Reinke T, et al. (1990). Long-term prognosis of membranoproliferative glomerulonephritis type I. Significance of clinical and morphological parameters. *Nephrol* **55**:242–50.

Simon P, Ramee MP, Boulahrouz R, et al. (2004). Epidemiologic data of primary glomerular diseases in Western France. *Kidney Int* **66**:905–8.

Smith RJH, Alexander J, Barlow PN, et al. (2007). New approaches to the treatment of Dense Deposit Disease. *J Am Soc Nephrol* **18**:2447–56.

Southwest Pediatric Nephrology Study Group (1985). Dense deposit disease in children. Prognostic value of clinical pathologic observations. *Am J Kidney Dis* **6**: 161–71.

Strife CF, West CD (2001). Membranoproliferatvie glomerulonephrits. In S Massry, R Glassock (eds), *Textbook of Nephrology*, 4th edn, pp.713–16. Lippincott, Williams and Wilkins, Philadelphia, PA.

Strife CF, McEnery P, McAdams J, et al. (1975). A third ultrastructural variant of membranoproliferative glomerulonephritis. *Kidney Int* **8**:454–9.

Tarshish P, Bernstein J, Tobin T, et al. (1992). Treatment of mesangiocapillary glomerulonephritis with alternate-day prednisone. A report of the International study of kidney disease in children. *Pediatr Nephrol* **6**:123–30.

Tiller D, Clarkson A, Mathew T (1981). A prospective randomized trial of the use of cyclophosphamide, dipyridamole and warfarin in membranous and membranoproliferative glomerulonephritis. In *Proceedings of the 8th International Congress on Nephrology*, pp.345–51. Karger, Basel.

Valles-Prats M, Espinel GE, Alloza J, et al. (1985). Glomerulonephritis mesangiocapillar idiopathica. Estudio de 72 cases. *Nephrologia* **5**:17–23.

Vanrenterghem Y, Roels L, Verberckmoes R, et al. (1975). Treatment of chronic glomeru-lonephritis with a combination of indomethacin and cyclophosphamide. *Clin. Nephrol* **4**, 218–22.

Varade W, Forrestal J, West C (1990). Patterns of complement activation in idiopathic membranoproliferative glomerulonephritis; types I, II, III. *Am J Kidney Dis* **16**:196–206.

Vikse BE, Bostad L, Aasarød K, et al. (2002). Prognostic factors in mesangioproliferative glomerulonephritis.*Nephrol Dial Transpl* **17**:1603–13.

Walker PD (2007). Dense deposit disease: new insights. *Curr Opin Nephrol Hypertens* **16**:204–12.

Walker PD, Ferrario F, Joh K, et al. (2007). Dense deposit disease is not a membranoprolif-erative glomerulonephritis. *Mod Pathol* **20**:605–16.

Warady B, Guggenheim S, Sedman A, et al. (1985). Prednisone therapy of membranopro-liferative glomerulonephritis in children. *J Pediatry* **107**:702–7.

West CD, McAdams J, McConville J, et al. (1965). Hypocomplementemic and normocom-plementemic persistent (chronic) glomerulonephritis: clinical and pathological characteristics. *J Pediatr* **23**:459–67.

Wu J, Jaar BG, Briggs WA, et al. (2004). High-dose mycophenolate mofetil in the treatment of post-transplant glomerular disease in the allograft: a case series. Nephron Clin Pract **98**:c61–6.

Yanagihara T, Hayakawa M, Yoshida J, et al. (2005). Long-term follow-up of diffuse mem-branoproliferative glomerulonephritis type I. *Pediatr Nephrol* **20**:585–90

Zauner I, Bohler J, Braun N, et al. (1994). Effect of aspirin and dipyridamole on proteinu-ria in idiopathic membranoproliferative glomerulonephritis: a multicenter prospective clinical trial. *Neph Dial Transp* **9**:619–22.

Zimmerman SW, Moorthy A, Dreher W, et al. (1983). Prospective trial of warfarin and dipyridamole in patients with membranoproliferative glomerulonephritis. *Am J Med* **75**:920–9.

Chapter 10

Crescentic glomerulonephritis

Patrick Nachman and Richard J. Glassock

Introduction and overview

Definition

The term *crescentic glomerulonephritis* (CrGN) refers to a diverse collection of disorders of widely different etiology and pathogenesis having in common the development of extensive proliferation of cells within Bowman's space (Couser, 1988; Glassock et al., 1995; Nachman et al., 1998; Pusey and Rees, 1998; Morgan et al., 2006; Lionaki, et al., 2007). The resulting accumulation of cells gives rise to a '*crescent*' enveloping the glomerular tuft itself. Polymerization of fibrinogen in Bowman's space due to passage of fibrinogen through gaps in the capillary wall, the elaboration of procoagulant factors by infiltrating monocytes and impaired fibrinolysis all contribute to the pathogenesis of the crescent (Couser, 1988, Glassock et al., 1995). Usually >50% of glomeruli are involved with crescentic lesions. Such patients also frequently manifest rapid and progressive deterioration of renal function leading to the clinical syndrome of *rapidly progressive glomerulonephritis*. Early and aggressive treatment can often delay or prevent the development of end-stage renal disease (ESRD). See Table 10.1 for an etiologic and pathogenetic classification of CrGN.

Pathology

The fundamental morphologic lesion of CrGN is the accumulation of cells in Bowman's space (see Atlas plate 16), believed to be derived from both proliferating and de-differentiated visceral and parietal epithelial cells (Ferrario and Rastaldi, 1998; Ng et al., 1999; Bariety et al., 2003, 2005; Thorner et al., 2008). Ruptures in the integrity of the capillary wall (gaps or focal discontinuities) are common if not universal (Bonsib, 1985). Similar gaps may appear in Bowman's capsule leading to the invasion of Bowman's space by T-cells, macrophages, and myofibroblasts from the adjacent interstitium (Ng et al., 1999). Proliferating podocytes and parietal cells of Bowman's capsule as well as macrophages and infiltration by lymphocytes contribute to the cellularity of the crescent.

Table 10.1 A classification of crescentic glomerulonephritis* according to serology (anti-glomerular basement membrane [GBM] antibody and anti-neutrophil cytoplasmic antibody [ANCA])

Anti-glomerular basement membrane antibody mediated disease (Anti-GBM antibody positive, ANCA negative):	Primary (renal-limited) crescentic glomerulonephritis without pulmonary hemorrhage*
	Goodpastures's disease (with pulmonary hemorrhage)
	Superimposed on another primary glomerular disease (e.g. membranous nephropathy)
	Secondary to drugs, neoplasia, viruses, renal trauma, environmental exposure (?hydrocarbons)
	De-novo in the transplant renal allograft in a patient with X-linked Alport syndrome
Immune complex mediated disease (anti-GBM antibody negative, ANCA negative or positive):	Primary (renal-limited) glomerular disease with crescents*
	Superimposed on another primary glomerular disease (e.g., IgA nephropathy)*
	Multisystem disease (SLE, HCV cryoglobulinemia, HSP)
	Secondary to infections, neoplasia, drugs, other
Pauci-immune necrotizing and crescentic glomerulonephritis (ANCA positive, anti-GBM antibody negative)- also known as ANCA-associated crescentic glomerulonephritis:	Primary (renal-limited) glomerular disease with crescents or renal-limited microscopic polyangiitis*
	Multisystem disease (systemic microscopic polyangiitis, Wegener's granulomatosis)
	Drug-induced (penicillamine, propylthiouracil, allopurinol, hydralazine, etc.)
	Viral- or environmental exposure-related (Parvovirus B19?; silica)
Dual-antibody disease (anti-GBM antibody positive and ANCA positive):	Primary (renal-limited) disease*
Idiopathic pauci-immune necrotizing and crescentic glomerulonephritis (Anti-GBM antibody negative and ANCA negative):	Primary (renal-limited) disease*

* Forms of crescentic glomerulonephritis that are discussed in this chapter. SLE: systemic lupus erythematosus; HCV: hepatitis C virus; HSP= Henoch–Schönlein purpura.

(Lan et al., 1997; Ng et al., 1999; Bariety et al., 2003; Thorner et al., 2008). The crescents may be accompanied by glomerular capillary lesions, most often segmental, necrotizing glomerulonephritis or exudative and proliferative glomerulonephritis. The former is likely a manifestation of a microscopic form of polyangiitis. Early in the course of CrGN the cellular proliferation in the crescent dominates, but later fibrosis ensues leading to glomerular obsolescence.

Crescents evolve from cellular, to fibrocellular, to fibrous lesions (Wiggins, 1998). This process may often develop quite rapidly, in a matter of weeks or months, or can develop over a more prolonged period. Various degrees of interstitial inflammation, particularly in a peri-glomerular location may be seen. Vasculitis is uncommon, but can be seen under certain circumstances (see later sections).

The underlying pathogenetic mechanisms responsible for the CrGN determines the features observed by light, immunofluorescence (see Atlas plate 17) and electron microscopy. For example, in anti-glomerular basement membrane (anti-GBM) antibody-mediated CrGN, the glomerular tufts are compressed by a proliferating crescent, gaps are common, IgG is deposited in a linear and continuous fashion along the inner aspect of the capillary wall, and no electron-dense deposits are seen (Turner and Rees, 1998). In immune-complex mediated CrGN, there is often cellular proliferation within the glomerular tufts, gaps are less common, granular deposits of IgG/IgM or IgA decorate the capillary loops and/or mesangium and electron- dense deposits are seen in the capillary walls and mesangium. In the anti-neutrophil cytoplasmic autoantibody (ANCA) associated CrGN, a necrotizing lesion is often seen in the glomerular tufts, crescents are exuberant and cellular, gaps are common, and only scanty deposits of IgG ('pauci-immune') are seen and no electron-dense deposits are observed (Nachman, et al., 1998). In the latter case an extra-glomerular 'angiitis' may be observed. Regardless of the underlying pathogenetic mechanism, extensive deposits of partially or fully polymerized fibrin are interspersed between the proliferating cells. Bridges between the basement membrane and Bowman's capsule appear early and the entry of Bowman's space to the proximal tubule is often occluded with cells and a fibrin clot (Le Hir, et al., 2001). These lesions may in part account for the rapid decline in glomerular filtration rate observed in CrGN. The extent of glomerular involvement may vary considerably from case to case, in part due to 'sampling error.' Most cases exhibiting a progressive decline in GFR will have >50% of the glomeruli involved with crescents and patients with oliguric renal failure may have 100% of the glomeruli in the biopsy sample involved with crescents. At the individual glomerular level, crescents can be segmental or circumferential, the latter having more ominous prognostic implications. Segmental crescents can resolve, leaving a focal scar or adhesion, but circumferential crescents frequently lead to total glomerular obsolescence, which may be followed by complete glomerular 'reabsorption,' leaving behind 'aglomerular' atrophic tubules (Kriz and Le Hir, 2005).

Pathogenesis

The pathogenetic mechanisms found to underlie CrGN are quite heterogeneous (see also Table10.1.) (Pusey and Rees, 1998) About 10–15% of cases will be due to the deposition of an autoantibody to epitopes on the alpha 3 chain of type IV collagen located in the globular NC-1 domain (the Goodpasture antigen) expressed uniformly along the inner aspect of the GBM (Kalluri et al., 1975; Turner and Rees, 1998; Borza et al., 2003). The glomerular injury is due to local (not systemic) complement activation and polymorphonuclear leukocyte activation. Such patients frequently have high levels of circulating anti-GBM antibody but normal serum complement levels. Although direct injury of the glomerular capillary wall, involving complement activation and polymorphonuclear leukocytes is believed to be the main mechanism for the glomerular disease, it is very clear that T cells may also be independently operative in the pathogenesis of the disease (Huang et al., 1994; Kitching et al., 1999; Salama et al., 2003).

In another 15–20% of cases immune complexes are involved. This mechanism is due to the formation of immune complexes in the circulation and their subsequent deposition in glomerular capillary tufts or to the in situ formation of immune complex within the glomerular capillaries (Cameron, 1998; Holdsworth, et al., 1998). The antigens involved in such immune complexes are quite diverse and range from replicating exogenous antigens (bacteria, viruses) to autologous antigens(nuclear antigens, tumor antigens). The immunoglobulin may be IgG, IgM, and/or IgA. Local as well as systemic complement activation may be a prominent feature of the disorder depending on the nature of the antigen-antibody systems involved. Immune complex-mediated CGN can also arise as a complication of another primary glomerular disease (such as membranous nephropathy, MPGN type I, or IgA nephropathy (see Chapters 7, 8, and 9). It may also complicate MPGN type II (see Chapter 9).

In about 50–75% of cases, an ANCA mechanism is involved (Morgan et al., 2006). ANCA are directed to either myeloperoxidase (anti-MPO) or to proteinase-3 (PR-3) or rarely both (as measured by ELISA and purified antigens). The anti-MPO-ANCA commonly gives a perinuclear or p-ANCA pattern on indirect immunofluorescence using alcohol-fixed, buffy-coat human leukocytes, whereas the anti-PR-3 ANCA most commonly give a cytoplasmic or c-ANCA pattern on similarly prepared leukocyte substrates. The precise mechanism by which ANCA arise is still debated, but it appears that these autoantibodies can activate neutrophils and cause them to injure capillary walls in the glomeruli and in blood vessels elsewhere (Jennette and Falk, 2008). Complement (C) activation is not a necessary feature, and the injury is directly mediated by cells rather than by antibody deposits in the glomerular capillaries; however, C activation via the alternative pathway can participate in glomerular injury associated with ANCA in some circumstances (Xiao et al., 2007).

In a small number (about 5–15%) of cases of CrGN, both anti-GBM and ANCA mechanisms coexist and, in an equally small number of cases (<10%), no anti-GBM immune complexes or ANCA mechanism can be identified (Rutgers et al., 2005; Lionaki et al., 2007). It is entirely possible, even likely, that antibody-independent, T-cell mediated processes are involved in some or even most forms of CrGN (Tipping and Holdsworth, 2005).

Regardless of the fundamental immunopathological mechanisms, the crescent forms and evolves by proliferation of visceral and parietal epithelial cells, polymerization of fibrin (from fibrinogen escaping into Bowman's space through the 'gaps'), infiltration with monocytes, macrophages and T cells, and invasion by myofibroblastic cells from the interstitium. These processes are driven by local accumulation of chemical mediators such as interleukin-1 (IL-1), tumor necrosis factor (TNF-alpha), macrophage chemotactic protein-1 (MCP-1), macrophage inflammatory factor (MIF), membrane prothrombinase, and transforming growth factor (TGF)-beta production (Khan et al., 2005). An important role may be played by transcription factors T-bet and Jun D. T-bet is a transcription factor that is essential for T helper (Th)1 lineage commitment and optimal IFN-gamma production by CD4(+) T cells. Phoon and coworkers (Phoon et al., 2008) showed that T-bet directs Th1 responses that induce renal injury in experimental CrGN. Behmoaras and co-workers (Behmoaras et al., 2008) recently demonstrated that the activator protein-1 (AP-1) transcription factor JunD, a major determinant of macrophage activity, is strongly associated with CrGN susceptibility. Eventually the TGF-beta stimulated myofibroblasts from the interstitium differentiate into fibroblasts secreting collagens I, III, and IV leading to the organization and fibrosis of the crescent (Wiggins, 1998).

Etiology

Not surprisingly, the etiology of CrGN is very diverse and in many cases entirely unknown, even though its pathogenesis can be accurately described in most instances (>90%) (de Lind van Wijngaarden et al., 2008). Secondary forms of CrGN occur in infectious disease (post-streptococcal GN—see Chapter 4) (Cameron, 1998), viral disease, such as hepatitis B or C), malignant neoplasia (such as lung cancer), drug exposure, autoimmune disease (such as SLE), or in association with multisystem diseases such as Goodpasture's disease (anti-GBM disease with nephritis and pulmonary hemorrhage), systemic granulomatous angiitis (Wegener's granulomatosis), microscopic polyangiitis, Henoch–Schönlein purpura and Churg-Strauss allergic granulomatosis. These secondary forms of CrGN are not the primary focus of this volume, but rather it will deal primarily with those forms of CrGN that are *not* accompanied by systemic features, other than those resulting from loss of renal function and in which the etiology is unknown (no drug exposure, silica exposure infectious agent, neoplasia, or systemic autoimmune disease is present). These are the so-called 'renal-limited' forms of CrGN—although extra-renal involvement may in fact be present, it is too subtle to be recognized easily by clinical means. Thus, from an etiological standpoint this chapter will deal with anti-GBM mediated disease, without pulmonary involvement (no alveolar hemorrhage), immune complex disease arising *de novo* without systemic features, and the renal-limited form of ANCA-associated CrGN (also called pauci-immune necrotizing and crescentic glomerulonephritis- P-ICGN). A background of heavy exposure to silica may be ascertained in patients with ANCA-associated CrGN (Hogan et al., 2007), and several hypothesis have been put forward to possibly explain the cause of ANCA-associated CrGN (de Lind van Wijngaarden et al., 2008; Yang et al., 2008). Viral infections (HIV, influenza, hantavirus), neoplasia (lymphoma, lung carcinoma, multiple myeloma), exposure to vola-tile hydrocarbons or renal trauma (extra-corporeal shock wave lithotripsy) might be etiological factors in some cases of anti-GBM antibody CrGN (Ma, et al., 1978; Stevenson et al., 1995; Billheden et al., 1997; Maes et al., 1999; Xenocostas et al., 1999; Borza et al., 2005; Weschler, et al., 2008).

Clinical presentation and features

In addition to a rapid progressive decline in renal function, other clinical features of glomerulonephritis are usually present, including dysmorphic hematuria, erythrocyte casts, and glomerular proteinuria (Glassock et al., 1995). Nephrotic syndrome is relatively uncommon, perhaps because of the rapid loss of glomerular filtration. Hypertension is quite variable and may be entirely absent (Glassock et al., 1995). The onset of CrGN is usually rather abrupt with overt symptoms and signs suggesting glomerulonephritis such as gross hematuria and edema (Glassock et al., 1995). In the absence of specific treatment, the disorder rapidly culminates in features of renal failure (weak-ness, nausea, vomiting, and easy fatigability). Nevertheless, insidious develop-ment of renal failure over several months may also occur. An antecedent 'viral-like' illness is not uncommon and mild arthralgias, myalgias, and low-grade fever may occasionally be seen, especially in immune complex and ANCA-associated CrGN. *By definition* (see 'Etiology'), evidence of multisystem, extrarenal involvement is lacking in *primary CGN,* but vascular congestion resulting from greatly impaired glomerular filtration rate and fluid retention may cause pulmonary edema and even mild hemoptysis. Frank pulmonary hemorrhage should not occur in primary disease and, if present, suggests a multisystem disorder such as Goodpasture's disease, pulmonary angiitis

(Wegener's granulomatosis, microscopic polyangiitis), systemic lupus erythematosus, Henoch–Schönlein purpura, or cryoimmunoglobulinemia. Concomitant cutaneous leukocytoclastic vasculitis ('palpable purpura') suggests Henoch–Schönlein purpura, lupus nephritis, or microscopic polyangiitis (Jennette et al., 1994). Upper and lower airway involvement (otitis, sinusitis, tracheitis, bronchitis) suggests Wegener's granulomatosis. Mononeuritis multiplex suggests polyangiitis, especially that associated with chronic viral hepatitis (hepatitis B viral infection). Purpura, splenomegaly, and liver abnormalities suggest chronic hepatitis C virus-associated cryoimmunoglobulinemia (Johnson et al., 1994). Patients with anti-PR3 auto-antibody associated CrGN (including Wegener's granulomatosis) may be at increased risk for venous thrombo-embolism due to concomitant antibody to plasminogen (preventing normal fibrinolysis) (Bautz et al., in press) (see also Chapter 1).

Overall, both males and females are affected in nearly equal proportions (Glassock et al., 1995). Anti-GBM antibody-mediated CrGN is seen most frequently in young males and in older females (Turner and Rees, 1998). Immune complex and ANCA-associated CrGN are seen in all ages but are much more common in older individuals, especially ANCA-associated CrGN (Jennette and Falk, 1990). The combination of ANCA and anti-GBM mediated CrGN is seen more commonly in older females. Secondary forms of CrGN also may have strong age and sex associations; for example, lupus nephritis as seen in young females, cryoimmunoglobulinemia in older females, and hepatitis B- and hepatitis C viral infection associated vasculitis and cryoglobulinemia in younger males, especially intravenous drug abusers (Johnson et al., 1994).

Renal function, as assessed by serum creatinine or estimated GFR, is often impaired at discovery or shortly thereafter in CrGN. It then rapidly worsens over several weeks or months. Oliguric acute renal failure may be the presenting feature in patients with very severe, fulminating disease with very extensive crescentic involvement of glomerular. A more indolent course is seen uncommonly. Urinalyses are almost always abnormal with dysmorphic hematuria (often with numerous acanthocytes and erythrocyte casts) and modest proteinuria. Very heavy proteinuria and early development of hypoalbuminemia is distinctly uncommon. Blood pressure is normal or only modestly elevated in the majority of patients; elevated blood pressure is more likely to occur in immune complex-mediated CrGN, especially with glomerular infiltration with monocytes, as might be associated with cryoglobulinemia or in MPGN type I (see Chapter 9). Very severe or malignant hypertension should make one suspicious of polyarteritis nodosa, renal arterial occlusive disease, atheroembolic renal disease, scleroderma, hemolytic uremic syndrome, or malignant hypertension with fibrinoid necrosis of renal arterioles (Glassock et al., 1995).

Laboratory features, especially serology, are *crucial* for the identification of the underlying pathogenetic mechanism which will then guide therapy and assist in prognostication (see below and Table10.2). Anti-GBM mediated CrGN is characterized by circulating anti-GBM antibodies (best measured by a commercially available ELISA assay using recombinant COLIVA3NCI antigen) (Turner and Rees, 1998; Borza et al., 2003). About 95% of patients will be positive if specimens are taken early in the course of disease before treatment is begun. False-positive assays are very uncommon. The titer of the anti-GBM antibody is only weakly correlated with the severity of the renal disease. Most of the anti-GBM antibody is IgG but rarely it may be IgA (Border et al., 1979). About 20–30% of patients with anti-GBM antibody also may develop concomitant ANCA, so all patients with CrGN must be assessed for both anti-GBM and ANCA regardless of their clinical presentation (see below) (Rutgers et al., 2005). C3 and C4 levels are normal and cryoimmunoglobulins are absent in anti-GBM-mediated disease.

In immune-complex mediated CrGN, the serological finding varies according to the underlying disease. ASLOT may be increased and C3 decreased in post-streptococcal disease (see also Chapter 4). Serum C3 and or C4 may also be abnormally low (for example in SLE or in cryoglobulinemia with chronic hepatitis C viral infection or in monoclonal immunoglobulin deposition diseases).

In ANCA- associated CGN, the ANCA levels measured by indirect immunofluorescence (IIF) and antigen-specific ELISA assays are increased, most often anti-PR3-ANCA and anti-MPO in renal-limited disease. The sensitivity and specificity for these assays are best when they are used together (Hagen et al., 1998). In renal-limited ANCA-associated CrGN (PI-NCGN) the sensitivity and specificity are around 85–90% and 95% respectively, but since these assays are not standardized, one must know the characteristics of the individual laboratory performing the test in order to interpret its diagnostic

Table 10.2 Factors affecting the prognosis of crescentic glomerulonephritis

Clinical	Pathology
◆ Age at onset of disease	◆ Extent of crescentic involvement (% normal glomeruli)
◆ Infectious/drug etiology	
◆ Renal function at discovery (oliguria, dialysis dependency)	◆ Nature of the crescent (cellular, fibro-cellular, fibrous)
◆ Serology (ANCA, anti-GBM, dual antibody)	◆ Extent of glomerulosclerosis
	◆ Chronic tubulointerstitial lesions
◆ Genetics (HLA)	◆ Disruption of Bowman's capsule

value. Highly sensitive tests for ANCA have been developed, but are not yet commercially available (Hellmich et al., 2007).

Up to one-third of patients with anti-GBM disease also have circulating ANCA (Savage and Lockwood, 1990; Hellmark et al., 1997; Kalluri et al., 1997; Rutgers et al., 2005). Both anti-MPO specific P-ANCA and anti-PR3 specific C-ANCA can occur in patients with anti-GBM disease. Interestingly, no differences in the antigenic specificity of anti-GBM antibodies were detected between sera with or without concurrent expression of ANCA (Hellmark et al., 1997). Coexistence of ANCA in patients with anti-GBM antibodies is associated with small vessel vasculitis in organs in addition to lung and kidney (Levy et al., 2004). In experimental models, antibodies to myeloperoxidase (MPO) aggravate experimental anti-GBM disease (Heeringa et al., 1996).

Epidemiology

Primary forms of CrGN are relatively uncommon. The multisystem forms are seen much more frequently. Anti-GBM antibody nephritis is seen world-wide but is rather rare (Turner and Rees, 1998) with an incidence rate of 0.5–1.0 new cases diagnosed per million population per year. It is much more common in Caucasians and Asians than in black populations. It may be more common in the spring and summer months. It may even occur in mini-epidemics or clusters of cases, suggesting a viral etiology. The occurrence of anti-GBM disease with respect to age and gender is bimodal. Two peaks are seen—one in the second and third decades mostly in males and another is the sixth to seventh decade, predominantly in women. The disease is very rare in children younger than 10 years of age and is not seen over the age of 70 years.

ANCA-associated CrGN is much more common with an annual incidence rate of around 5–20 newly diagnosed cases per million population, depending on the region. There is a marked predilection to affect older individuals (over age 50 years), both males and females (Gaskin and Pusey, 1998). Caucasians, Hispanics, and Asians are most commonly affected and the disorder is relatively uncommon in black populations. There may be differences in frequency between regions, such as Southern and Northern Europe. No seasonal differences in occurrence of ANCA-associated CrGN have been consistently noted.

Natural history

Data concerning the natural history of CrGN in the pretreatment eras are quite limited and do not separate the various pathogenetic subcategories listed above. It is generally believed that glomerulonephritis with extensive circumferential crescents (>50% glomerular involvement) seldom undergoes spontaneous remission and that survival with endogenous renal function in the absence of specific treatment for more than 6–12 months is uncommon (Cameron, 1977). Lesser degrees of crescentic involvement (e.g., <30% glomerular involvement), especially when superimposed on another glomerular disease (e.g. IgA nephropathy, post-streptococcal glomerulonephritis) (see also Chapters 4 and 8), may spontaneously regress and, even if renal function is initially impaired, recovery to baseline is the rule rather than the exception. Patients with moderate crescentic involvement (30–50% of glomeruli) may have a more indolent course, but if untreated, will still probably experience the eventual onset of ESRD. When biopsy samples contain relatively few glomeruli (<10), it may be difficult to estimate the true extent of glomerular involvement with crescents (Glassock et al., 1995) due to sampling error considerations. Prognostication based on the degree of crescentic involvement should be made with great caution if the numbers of glomeruli in the biopsy specimen are limited.

Thus, nearly every patient with CrGN and extensive glomerular involvement (defined here as >50% glomerular crescents) and probably also those with a percentage of crescents between 30 and 50% should be considered as candidates for aggressive therapy (see 'Specific treatment') unless treatment is contraindicated by excessive risks or unless clinical and morphologic parameters strongly suggest an unfavorable outcome even with aggressive treatment (see 'Specific treatment'). Assessing futility of treatment based on clinical and morphological findings at discovery of CrGN is possible, but there is always some residual uncertainty. The factors that can be used to assess the prognosis for outcome (freedom from ESRD, death, relapse of disease after initial induction therapy) are outlined as follows (see also Table 10.2).

Prognostic factors

Treatment timeliness

As will be discussed later, the *single* most important factor affecting prognosis is the speed with which treatment is instituted following recognition and categorization of disease. A delay in treatment can allow the disease-related damage to glomeruli to become irreversible (Little and Pusey, 2004).

Age and gender

Overall, the age and gender of patients may influence prognosis, largely because of the age-associated difference and the prevalence of the underlying subtypes of CrGN, the predilection for subtypes to affect certain genders, and the rising risk of complications in older patients (Cameron, 1977; Glassock et al., 1995). The prognosis for older patients with combined ANCA-associated CrGN and anti-GBM disease appears particularly grim (Bonsib et al., 1993). Children with crescentic glomerulonephritis secondary to a well-recognized streptococcal illness or exposure to drugs (such as anti-thyroid medications) may have a favorable prognosis, particularly with mild crescentic involvement (Cameron, 1977). Nevertheless, age alone is not a powerful determinant of prognosis Even in children the outcome of the disease is mainly related to timely diagnosis and treatment (Dewan et al., 2008).

Proteinuria

The magnitude of proteinuria at discovery has no particular prognostic significance in CrGN. Following treatment, persistent proteinuria or the emergence of nephrotic-range proteinuria may indicate a poor long-term outcome. This may be a manifestation of 'oligonephronia' resulting from irreversible damage to a large population of nephrons with maladaptive functional and morphologic changes (e.g., focal and segmental glomerulosclerosis) in the residual hyper-functioning nephrons (see also Chapter 1).

Renal function

Severe acute onset of oligo-anuric renal failure is usually a reflection of very extensive crescentic involvement or an associated tubulointerstitial lesion (e.g., acute tubule necrosis or acute tubulointerstitial nephritis) and usually confers a worse prognosis (Cameron, 1977). Patients with anti-GBM antibody mediated CrGN treated *before* the onset of dialysis dependency (e.g., a serum creatinine ≤ 6.8mg/dL or 600µm/L) have an improved prognosis (see below) (Glassock, 1995; Levy et al., 2001). Patients with ANCA-associated CGN may sustain and maintain substantial improvement in renal function even if treatment is delayed to dialysis dependency, depending on the treatment regimen used (see below) (Falk et al., 1990; Hauer et al., 2002; Hogan et al., 2005; Mukhtyar et al., 2008; Pagnoux et al., 2008). Although serum creatinine levels at the time of presentation and the initiation of therapy are important predictors of renal outcome (survival free of dialysis), there is no absolute level of serum creatinine above which treatment is deemed futile (Hogan et al., 2005).

Renal morphology and pathogenetic subtype

In general, the extent of crescentic involvement of the glomeruli (usually assessed by counting the percentage of normal glomeruli in the biopsy specimen) relates to prognosis (and response to treatment) (Cameron, 1977). A focal lesion characterized by a few glomeruli (<30%) involved with segmental crescents (<50% of individual glomerular involvement) generally has a more favorable prognosis and spontaneous resolution is not uncommon. Renal functional impairment in these circumstances may be the consequence of associated tubulointerstitial lesions (e.g., acute tubule necrosis, tubulointerstitial nephritis).

Such lesions are seen more frequently in IgA nephropathy and post-strepto-coccal glomerulonephritis. On the other hand, diffuse (100%) glomerular involvement with circumferential crescents has an unfavorable prognosis, especially if the crescents are fibrocellular and if significant glomerular capillary collapse and segmental sclerosis is present (Glassock et al., 1995). The combination of circumferential fibrocellular glomerular crescents involving 100% of the glomeruli and oligo-anuria is particularly ominous.

Diffuse and global glomerulosclerosis and chronic tubulointerstitial lesions (atrophy and fibrosis) also confer a poor prognosis (Neild et al., 1983). Disruption of Bowman's capsule, which allows for invasion of the crescent with interstitium-derived myofibroblasts, also indicates a poor outcome (Ferrario et al., 1994).

The pathogenetic subtype of the lesion is a somewhat less important determinant of prognosis (see 'Serology'), especially if treatment is instituted early in the course of disease. Nevertheless, very extensive crescentic involvement in anti-GBM antibody-mediated disease may indicate a very poor outcome (Cameron, 1977; Glassock et al., 1995). A very high titer of circulating anti-GBM antibodies, 100% crescentic involvement and oligo-anuria with dialysis-dependence indicates a very poor prognosis, even with aggressive therapy (see 'Specific treatment') in anti-GBM antibody mediated disease (Levy et al., 2001). Patients with ANCA-associated CrGN may also have a poor prognosis when extensive glomerular involvement (<2% normal glomeruli) is accompanied by severe interstitial fibrosis, but with aggressive therapy some of these patients may recover useful renal function even if they have required dialysis therapy for treatment of rapidly progressive renal failure (See 'Specific treatment') (de Lind van Wijngaarden et al., 2006, 2007). Patients with combined ANCA and anti-GBM associated CrGN behave more like severe anti-GBM antibody- only disease than severe ANCA-only associated disease (Levy et al., 2004). Extensive endocapillary proliferation with subepithelial 'humps' unaccompanied by glomerulosclerosis or tubulointerstitial atrophy and fibrosis may be associated with a more favorable outcome, especially with a background of an acute infectious disease (Cameron, 1977; Neild et al., 1983). Extensive necrotizing lesions of the glomerular capillary tuft, as is seen commonly in P-INCGN, may also be associated with the persistence of proteinuria and impaired renal function even with initially successful treatment. The late emergence of heavy proteinuria, hypertension, and progressive renal failure is a common sequela of very severe initial disease (Leaker and Neild, 1991). As indicated above, this latter process may be non-immunologically mediated and related to hemodynamic adaptations occurring in surviving nephrons (see also Chapter 1). Therapy designed to modify these adaptations (e.g., angiotensin-converting enzyme inhibitors) may have a salutary effect on long-term prognosis (Leaker and Neild, 1991) (see also Chapter 1).

Serology

The pre-therapy titer of autoantibodies (e.g., anti-GBM, ANCA) correlates rather poorly with disease severity and renal outcome, at least in those patients with renal-limited disease. Overall, high initial levels of anti-GBM antibodies are more associated with a poor outcome than high levels of ANCA (Jennette and Falk, 1991; Herody et al., 1993; Lionaki et al., 2007). In a large series, however, the titer of anti-GBM antibodies neither correlated with the fraction of crescentic glomeruli nor with serum creatinine (Fischer and Lager, 2007).Thus, initial serologic studies in anti-GBM antibody mediated disease are primarily useful for diagnosis rather than prognosis. A possible exception may be represented by patients with both anti-GBM antibodies and anti-MPO ANCA who may have worse renal survival than patients with anti-MPO ANCA only, at least in some series (Levy et al., 2004; Rutgers et al 2005).

Whether serial serologic monitoring of ANCA (anti-MPO and/or antiPR-3) or anti-GBM antibody titers following successful induction therapy may have value in predicting subsequent relapses is also disputed. Relapses of anti-GBM antibody disease after successful therapy are quite uncommon (<5%) and monitoring of antibody levels after initial therapy is not needed, unless a clinical recurrence is evident. The available data relating relapse to serology in ANCA-associated CrGN is more extensive for C-ANCA/PR3-ANCA than for P-ANCA/MPO-ANCA. The literature on the subject also lacks homogeneity on the testing methodology and the definition of significant changes in titers. However, a substantial (4-fold or greater) rise in ANCA titer after reaching an nadir post-therapy may herald a clinical relapse (Han et al., 2003), but the positive predictive value of such a change in titer for a relapse is only about 60–80% (Cohen Tervaert et al., 1990; Davenport et al., 1995; de'Oliviera et al., 1995) and the timing of a relapse may be delayed by several months. Relapse is well known to be far more common in anti-PR3-positive patients (>50%) compared to anti-MPO-positive patients (about 10–15%), so monitoring is likely to be of greater value in the patient with anti-PR-3-positive disease. Some studies have suggested that patients with Wegener's granulomatosis (who are often positive for anti-PR-3 antibodies) may benefit from a prophylactic approach of reinstituting therapy when ANCA reappears or titer increases (Cohen Tervaert et al., 1990). However, in an analysis of serially obtained PR3-ANCA titers as part of the large randomized and controlled trial of etanercept in Wegener's granulomatosis, increases in ANCA titers were not associated with relapse (Finkelman et al., 2007). At this point in time, there is little evidence to support the notion that serial ANCA testing (especially in anti-MPO positive patients) can be used effectively and safely to predict future relapses and guide 'preemptive' increases in the intensity of (or reinsttution of) immunosuppression. Nevertheless, some patients may exhibit a consistent and recurring pattern of a rising ANCA titers preceding each clinical relapse of disease (this is mostly found in anti-PR3 positive patients). Such patients might become candidates for a prophylactic approach to therapy with immunosuppressive agents (including cyclophosphamide, intravenous immunoglobulin [IVIg], Rituximab, and/or MMF) (see 'Specific treatment').

Genetics

There is both a genetically determined predisposition to anti-GBM and ANCA associated CrGN as well as an influence of underlying genetic makeup on prognosis. Certain alleles at the HLA chromosome (chromosome 6), e.g. HLA DR-2 and/or B-7 may determine the severity of disease and its outcome (Rees et al., 1984; Fisher et al.,1987; Borgmann and Haubnitz, 2004; Tsuchiya et al., 2006; Heckmann et al., 2008). At the present time these genetic influences on susceptibility, severity, and prognosis are mainly of research interest and they do not have any role in therapeutic decision making. An alpha-1-antitrypsin deficiency may rarely be encountered.

Specific treatment

See also Table 10.3

Table 10.3 Initial therapy of crescentic glomerulonephritis based on pathogenetic category (see Table 10.1) and dialysis-dependency* (see text for details)

Category	Dialysis-independent	Dialysis-dependent
Anti-GBM	Oral or IV glucocorticoids Oral cyclophosphamide Plasmapheresis	Conservative[a]
Immune complex	Oral or IV glucocorticoids Oral or IV cyclophosphamide	Oral or IV glucocorticoids Oral or IV cyclophosphamide[b]
ANCA-associated	Oral or IV glucocorticoids Oral or IV cyclophosphamide	Oral or IV glucocorticoids Oral or IV cyclophosphamide[b] Plasmapheresis[c]
Dual antibody	Same as for Anti-GBM	Same as for ANCA
Idiopathic	Same as for ANCA	Same as for ANCA

*Dialysis-dependency defined as requiring dialysis for treatment of renal failure for >1 week.
[a]Some patients may receive therapy as for dialysis independent patients if acute onset of renal failure and very cellular (non-fibrotic) crescents present;
[b]Reduced dosage of cyclophosphamide may be required.
[c]Plasmapheresis should be used for acute renal failure even if dialysis required for treatment.

Treatment of ANCA positive, anti-GBM negative disease (ANCA associated small vessel vasculitis—ANCA-SVV)

Data on the treatment of ANCA positive pauci-immune necrotizing and crescentic glomerulonephritis is derived from the literature of ANCA-associated small vessel vasculitis including Wegener's granulomatosis and microscopic polyangiitis (Little and Pusey, 2004). There is scant data directly derived specifically from patients with renal-limited CrGN. The *induction treatment* of ANCA-associated glomerulonephritis (with or without systemic vasculitis) rests primarily on the use of *methylprednisolone, high-dose glucocorticoids, and cyclophosphamide.*

Initiation of therapy with *pulse methylprednisolone* (7mg/kg per day for 3d) is used to curb the active inflammation as soon as possible (Bolton, 1995; Little and Pusey, 2004). This is followed by prednisone at a daily dosage of 1mg/kg per day (not to exceed 80mg/d for the first month of therapy). Prednisone is then tapered over the second month to alternate-day dosing and subsequently decreased by 10mg per day every week until they are eventually discontinued by the end of the fourth to fifth month. The rate of decrease in glucocorticoid dosing should be tailored based on an assessment of each patient's disease activity.

The beneficial role of *cyclophosphamide* in the treatment of acute ANCA-associated small-vessel vasculitis is evidenced by the substantial improvement in the rate of remission (from 56% to 85%) and a 3-fold decrease in the risk of relapse is associated with the use of this drug (Nachman et al., 1996). Cyclophosphamide may be administered as a daily oral regimen or as monthly intravenous pulses. When the intravenous route is used, it is usually started at a dose of $0.5g/m^2$ of body surface area, which is subsequently increased to a maximum dose of $1g/m^2$. This dose is adjusted to maintain the 2-week leukocyte nadir at more than $3000/mm^3$. When the daily oral regimen is used, cyclophosphamide is given at 1.5–2mg/kg/d, adjusting the dose to maintain the leukocyte count above $3000/mm^3$ throughout therapy. Cyclophosphamide is traditionally continued for a total of 6–12 months, depending on the patient's response to treatment. The optimal form of cyclophosphamide therapy (daily oral vs. intravenous pulse) is a subject of continued investigation. In general, the intravenous regimen allows for a ~2-fold smaller cumulative dose of cyclophosphamide than the oral regimen and is associated with a significant decrease in the rate of clinically significant neutropenia and other complications. The regimen of daily oral cyclophosphamide is purported to be associated with a decreased risk of relapse (Guillevin et al., 1997). However, when analyzed in a meta-analysis of three randomized controlled trials, the rate of relapse associated with pulse cyclophosphamide was not statistically higher than with a daily oral regimen; but attained a statistically higher rate of remission, and lower rates of leucopenia and infections (de Groot et al., 2001). The final outcomes of patients (death or ESRD) were no different between the two dosing regimen.

If the patient has reached a complete remission after 3 months of treatment with cyclophosphamide, an alternative approach consists of switching from cyclophosphamide to oral azathioprine. Oral *azathioprine* (1–3mg/kg/d) is then continued for 12–18 months. This regimen offers the advantage of limiting the use of cyclophosphamide and results in similar rates of remission and relapse as the cyclophosphamide-only-based therapy in a large randomized and controlled study (Jayne et al., 2003). It is noteworthy that patients whose PR3-ANCA titers remain positive at the time of the switch have about a 2-fold increased risk of subsequent relapse when compared to patients whose ANCA titers have reverted to negative (Sanders et al., 2006).

The addition of *plasmapheresis* to conventional induction therapy with glucocorticoids and cyclophosphamide is currently indicated for patients presenting with either advanced renal failure or with diffuse alveolar hemorrhage. The addition of plasmapheresis is indicated for the treatment of patients presenting with severe renal dysfunction (serum creatinine >500mol/L, or 5.8mg/dL). In a large, multicenter controlled trial (Jayne et al., 2007), 137 patients with a new diagnosis of ANCA-vasculitis confirmed by renal biopsy were randomly assigned to either seven treatments (sessions) of plasmapheresis (n = 70), or 3000mg of intravenous methylprednisolone (n = 67). Both groups received standard therapy with oral cyclophosphamide and oral prednisone followed by azathioprine for maintenance therapy. Plasmapheresis consisted of seven treatment sessions within 14d of study entry with a volume of 60mL/kg on each occasion; the replacement was with 5% albumin. Fresh frozen plasma at the end of the procedure was used in patients who were at risk of hemorrhage (or may be used in subjects who have recently (<72 hours) undergone a percutaneous renal biopsy). Compared to pulse methylprednisolone, plasmapheresis was associated with a significant increase in renal recovery at 3 months (69% of patients who received plasmapheresis vs. 49% of patients in the intravenous methylprednisolone group), and of dialysis-free survival at 12 months. The hazard ratio for ESRD over 12 months for the plasmapheresis versus methylprednisolone groups was 0.47 (95% CI 0.24–0.91, $P = 0.03$). Importantly, a subgroup analysis of the 69 patients who presented with dialysis-dependent acute renal failure at the beginning of this trial (de Lind van Wijngaarden RA et al., 2007) revealed that the point at which the chance of dying from therapy with plasmapheresis exceeds that of the chance of recovery was reached only in patients with severe tubular atrophy and <2% of glomeruli remaining normal. This analysis suggests that there is essentially no histological determinant that would render a trial of therapy futile in the management of patients with ANCA-vasculitis presenting with advanced renal failure. Among patients who require hemodialysis, those who do recover sufficient renal function nearly always do so within the first 3 months of treatment (Nachman et al., 1996; de Lind van Wijngaarden et al., 2007). In a retrospective analysis of outcomes of 46 patients receiving maintenance immunosuppression while requiring chronic dialysis, no patient died of active vasculitis (Weidanz et al., 2007). Rather, the major cause of death was infection, and the vast majority of non-fatal infections occurred in patients receiving immunosuppression. Importantly, the relapse rate post-dialysis was significantly less than pre-dialysis (RR 0.4, 95% CI 0.15–0.98, $P = 0.044$). This study suggests that the risk of fatal and non-fatal infection is higher than the risk of relapse or death from active disease. Considering that most patients who will recover renal function after suffering acute renal failure from P-INCGN do so in the first 3 months after initiation of dialysis (Nachman et al., 1996; de Lind van Wijngaarden et al., 2007), a rational approach would be to discontinue immunosuppressive therapy in all patients who do not have clinical evidence for active disease and who have not recovered renal function by that point.

The addition of plasmapheresis is also strongly indicated for patients with alveolar hemorrhage. Diffuse alveolar hemorrhage is associated with an elevated risk of death. Based on several uncontrolled case series, early and aggressive institution of plasmapheresis appears associated with a substantially diminished mortality rate from massive pulmonary hemorrhage (Klemmer et al., 2003). Plasmapheresis is typically performed daily until the pulmonary hemorrhage ceases and then every-other day for a total of 7–10 treatments. Plasma is replaced with a solution of 5% albumin, but 2 units of fresh-frozen plasma are administered at the end of the treatment to replace clotting factors and minimize the risk of persistent or renewed bleeding.

Whether the addition of plasmapheresis to conventional therapy is beneficial for patients without pulmonary hemorrhage or without severe renal involvement (such as dialysis dependent acute renal failure) is not supported by the currently available data. A large, multicenter, randomized controlled trial addressing this issue is in preparation.

The use of *methotrexate* in lieu of cyclophosphamide has been advocated for patients suffering from mild ANCA small-vessel vasculitis without significant renal impairment (Sneller et al., 1995). In a randomized controlled trial of induction therapy among patients with 'early' ANCA- vasculitis comparing weekly methotrexate to daily oral cyclophosphamide, the rate of remission at 6 months was comparable among the two treatment groups (De et al., 2005).

However, the onset of remission in methotrexate-treated patients with relatively extensive disease or pulmonary involvement was delayed. Methotrexate was also associated with a significantly higher rate of relapse than cyclophosphamide (69.5% vs. 46.5%), and 45% of relapses occurred while patients were receiving methotrexate. Importantly, methotrexate is relatively contraindicated for patients with renal impairment. The dose of methotrexate must be reduced in patients with a creatinine clearance <80mL/min, and its use is contraindicated when creatinine clearances are <10mL/min. Overall, the role of methotrexate in ANCA-vasculitis appears to be limited to a select group of patients with mild extra-renal and extra-pulmonary disease. It is not appropriate for patients with P-INCGN and renal failure.

Over the last decade, there has been a great deal of interest in using *mycophenolate mofetil* (MMF) in lieu of cyclophosphamide in ANCA vasculitis as in other autoimmune diseases. Several small uncontrolled case series have appeared that suggest some benefit of MMF in the treatment of patients with active vasculitis and glomerulonephritis (Joy et al., 2005). MMF has not been evaluated in the treatment of patients with moderate or severe renal impairment. Two recent reports on the potential role of MMF have recently been published. In an uncontrolled case series, the effect of MMF and oral prednisolone was analyzed retrospectively in a cohort of 32 consecutive patients who could not receive cyclophosphamide (because of prior insufficient response, prior complications, unacceptable cumulative dose, cancer, or patient refusal) (Stassen et al., 2007), complete remission was obtained in 78% and partial remission in 19% of patients. However, relapses occurred in 61% of patients who achieved a remission, with a median relapse-free survival of 16 months. Importantly, 90% of relapses occurred while the patients were still receiving MMF.

In another small randomized and controlled study from China, induction therapy with MMF (1.5–2.0g/d) was compared to monthly pulse cyclophosphamide (0.75–1.0gm/m^2 body surface area) (Hu et al., 2008) in a total of 35 patients (28 with MPO-ANCA, and two with PR3-ANCA) with mild-to-moderate disease (serum creatinine <500μm/L, and without pulmonary hemorrhage or CNS involvement). All patients received intravenous methylprednisolone pulse therapy (0.5g, once daily × 3), followed by oral prednisone. While the intention-to-treat analysis suggested a better response to MMF than cyclophosphamide, this apparent superiority dissipated upon exclusion of the 23% of patients assigned to the cyclophosphamide group who were lost to follow up. Nevertheless, the results of these two studies do add to the body of literature suggesting a beneficial response to MMF in the therapy of patients with mild-to-moderate ANCA-vasculitis. Whether treatment with MMF is superior or equivalent to, or better tolerated than cyclophosphamide will await a large, randomized controlled trial. Such trials are currently underway in Europe (clinicaltrials.gov identifiers NCT00103792 and NCT00414128).

Management of therapy-resistant disease

Several agents have been evaluated as adjunctive therapy for patients with disease resistant to conventional therapy with glucocorticoids and cyclophosphamide.

Adjunctive therapy with *IVIg* (single course of a total of 2gm/kg) was evaluated in a randomized controlled trial in patients with persistently active ANCA vasculitis despite conventional therapy. Patients treated with IVIg experienced a more rapid decline in disease activity (as measured by a 50% reduction in BVAS) and C-reactive protein at 1 and 3 months, but there was no significant difference between the two groups after 3 months with respect to disease activity or frequency of relapse (Jayne et al., 2000).

Rituximab, a chimeric monoclonal antibody directed against the CD20 antigen effectively depletes B lymphocytes, but not plasma cells. Several small, uncontrolled case series suggest a role for rituximab for the management of ANCA vasculitis that is resistant to, or relapsing after standard therapy (Eriksson, 2005; Keogh et al., 2005; Stasi et al., 2006). In these reports, the use of rituximab (375mg/m2 IV weekly × 4, or 500mg IV weekly × 4 fixed doses) in conjunction with corticosteroids resulted in remission in the majority of patients, and was generally well tolerated. In contrast, other case series reported limited efficacy of rituximab in patients with severe, refractory Wegener's granulomatosis (Aries et al., 2005). The role of rituximab as induction therapy in ANCA-vasculitis awaits the results of an ongoing large randomized controlled trial comparing it to cyclophosphamide (clinicaltrials.gov identifier: NCT00104299).

Alemtuzumab (Campath-1H®) is a humanized monoclonal IgG1 antibody directed against the CD52 antigen expressed on the surface of peripheral blood lymphocytes, monocytes, and macrophages (Kirk et al., 2003). Treatment with alemtuzumab leads to complement-mediated lysis, antibody-dependent cellular cytotoxicity, and induction of apoptosis of target cells and results in depletion of T cells and B cells (Isaacs et al., 1996). Alemtuzumab has been used to treat a select group of 71 patients with refractory or multiply relapsing ANCA vasculitis (63 patients with Wegener's granulomatosis and eight with microscopic polyangiitis) (Jayne, 2002). These patients received at least one course of 134mg intravenous alemtuzumab over 5d. Clinical remission on no immunosuppression was achieved in 65% of patients. Unfortunately, this treatment regimen was associated with high rates of serious infection and death (mortality rate of 0.09 per patient-year), and 60% experienced a relapse with a median relapse-free survival of 9.2 months. Alemtuzumab has also been associated (paradoxically) with the development of anti-GBM antibody nephritis (Clatworthy et al., 2008).

Tumor necrosis factor (TNF)-α is thought to play an important role in the pathogenesis of ANCA vasculitis based on *in vitro* and *in vivo* data (Lamprecht et al., 2007). The chimeric monoclonal antibody directed against TNF-α, *infliximab*, was evaluated in a small, open-label, uncontrolled case series of patients where infliximab was used in conjunction with corticosteroids, and either cyclophosphamide or other immunosuppressive agents. In the largest of these studies, which included 32 patients with acute or resistantdisease, infliximab was associated with a remission rate of 88% and a relapse rate of 20% (Booth et al., 2004). These promising results are mitigated, however, by an elevated rate of serious infectious complications. In addiction, the use of TNF inhibitors has paradoxically been associated with an increased risk of developing an auto-immune disease resembling systemic lupus erythematosus

Calcineurin inhibitors (cyclosporin) have been used successfully in ANCA-associated Cr GN, but a high relapse rate is to be expected (Allen et al., 1993)

Relapsing disease

Relapsing ANCA-associated vasculitis responds to immunosuppression with glucocorticoids and cytotoxic agents with a similar response rate as the initial disease (Nachman et al., 1996). The decision regarding the repeated use of cyclophosphamide should be based on the severity of the relapse taking into account the cumulative dose previously received by the patient over the course of the disease. Patients with a history of relapsing disease pose a particular challenge because they are particularly subject to the cumulative toxic effects of cytotoxic agents and glucocorticoids. This has been the impetus to find alternatives to cyclophosphamide, especially for patients with mild-to-moderate disease. In addition to the agents described for induction therapy, the use of 6 monthly pulses of IVIg (0.5g/kg/d ×4 d) was evaluated for the treatment of relapse occurring while on glucocorticoids and/or immunosuppressants (cyclophosphamide, azathioprine, methotrexate, or MMF) (Martinez et al., 2008). IVIg was added to the same immunosuppressant regime the patient was receiving. All patients (n = 22) initially responded to IVIg therapy. Complete or partial remission occurred in 83% or patients at 6 months and in 63% of patients by month 9. IVIg was well tolerated with mild transient side effects, although one patient suffered a rapid deterioration of the underlying kidney disease. In patients with renal dysfunction, it is preferable to use a sucrose-free formulation of IVIg in order to minimize the risk of osmotic agent induced acute renal failure (Dickenmann et al., 2008).

Maintenance therapy and prevention of relapses

Several agents have been evaluated for maintenance immunosuppressive therapy with a goal to prevent future relapses. In evaluating studies of prevention of relapse, important considerations should be kept in mind:

◆ The risk of relapse is not uniform among all patients with ANCA vasculitis. Depending on the number of risk factors, the incidence of relapse may vary from 26% over a median of 62 months, to 47% over a median of 39 months (Hogan et al., 2005).

◆ The efficacy of a drug in preventing relapse can only be assessed if compared to a placebo or active comparator. Therefore, in order to convincingly demonstrate efficacy in preventing relapse, a study should target a population at high risk for relapse, followed for a sufficiently long period of time, and include a control group treated with placebo or an active comparator. Unfortunately, most published reports on the subject have been open-label, uncontrolled cohort studies with a small number of patients followed over a relatively short period of time. The only placebo-controlled study evaluated benefit of cotrimoxazole in the prevention of relapses in patients with Wegener's granulomatosis. In this study, cotrimoxazole was effective in preventing relapses involving the nose and upper respiratory tract, but no benefit was seen in disease affecting the kidneys or other organ systems (Guillevin et al., 1999).

The best documented therapeutic option in ANCA vasculitis remains inferred from the large randomized controlled trial of *azathioprine* versus cyclophosphamide for the maintenance of remission (Jayne et al., 2003). Although not specifically designed to demonstrate the ability of azathioprine to prevent relapses (compared to a placebo for example), that study established that substituting cyclophosphamide for azathioprine after 3 to 6 months versus 12 months resulted in similar rates of relapse (Jayne et al., 2003).

The efficacy and safety of the TNF receptor–Fc fusion protein *etanercept* in the maintenance of remission among patients with Wegener's granulomatosis was evaluated in a randomized controlled trial. In that study, etanercept or placebo were added to a traditional regimen of daily oral cyclophosphamide or methotrexate and corticosteroids. The use of etanercept failed to affect the rate or the severity of relapses, and was associated with a higher rate of solid tumors (Stone, 2003).

One prospective, multicenter, randomized controlled trial compared the use of *methotrexate to leflunomide* in 54 patients with the diagnosis of generalized Wegener's granulomatosis (Metzler et al., 2007). All patients received induction therapy with prednisone and oral cyclophosphamide (2mg/kg/d) for 6 months.

In the methotrexate group, patients were then started on 7.5mg/week orally, and then titrated upward to 15mg/week by week 5, and 20mg/week after week 8. Leflunomide was started with a loading dose of 100mg/d orally for the first 3d, followed by 20mg/d for up to 4 weeks and continued at 30mg/d thereafter. This study was terminated early because of a significantly higher rate of major and minor relapse in the methotrexate group compared with the leflunomide group. Significant adverse events occurred in the leflunomide group, including hypertension, persistent leukopenia, and peripheral neuropathy in one patient. It appears from this study that methotrexate is inferior to leflunomide in preventing relapse of Wegener's granulomatosis. Whether a lower dose of leflunomide would be equally as effective but associated with fewer side effects remains to be determined.

Whether MMF is effective in preventing relapses has only been evaluated in small uncontrolled cohort studies. Thus, in a retrospective analysis of 29 patients who received MMF for maintenance therapy, fourteen (48.3%) patients relapsed with a mean time to relapse of 14.1 ± 13.9 months (Koukoulaki and Jayne, 2006). Because of the absence of a control group, it is not possible to assess whether MMF effectively prevented relapses from occurring in some patients or decreased their severity. The efficacy of MMF in preventing relapses is currently being compared to that of azathioprine in a randomized trial (IMPROVE) by the European Vasculitis Study Group.

ANCA negative and anti-GBM negative pauci-immune necrotizing/crescentic glomerulonephritis or ANCA negative small vessel vasculitis

About 5–10% of patients with P-INCGN may present with a persistently negative ANCA and anti-GBM antibody tests. Likewise, a small number of patient may present with signs and symptoms that are characteristic of microscopic polyangiitis or Wegener's granulomatosis (with pulmonary nodules which on biopsy reveal non-caseating granulomata), and yet have consistently negative ANCA tests both by indirect immunofluorescence microscopy and by antigen-specific ELISA. These patients are typically treated according to the same guidelines as for patients who are ANCA-positive. The number of these patients is small, and no specific studies or outcome measures have been published specifically for this group of patients. A therapeutic dilemma occurs when such patients present with advanced renal failure or diffuse pulmonary hemorrhage, i.e., with indication for plasmapheresis. Here again, there is unfortunately no data to support or refute the use of plasmapheresis. Because of the severity of these presentations and the narrow window of opportunity to intervene successfully, we have erred on the side of providing plasmapheresis in these circumstances. It is conceivable that these patients have autoantibodies to either other antigens or to epitopes of PR3 or MPO that are not readily detected by the currently available tests (Hellmich et al., 2007). It is noteworthy that such patients were indeed included in the controlled trial of plasmapheresis vs. methylprednisolone (Jayne et al., 2007).

ANCA negative and anti-GBM negative immune complex mediated crescentic glomerulonephritis

As already described, ANCA and anti-GBM negative immune complex crescentic glomerulonephritis may be secondary to infections, malignancy, or autoimmune diseases such as SLE, and IgA nephropathy. Truly 'idiopathic' immune complex glomerulonephritis is very uncommon. Therefore, prior to commencing immunomodulating, anti-inflammatory therapy, patients should undergo a thorough screen for occult malignancy or infection. As noted previously, drug associated CrGN is usually anti-MPO ANCA positive and the lesions are typically P-INCGN. A careful clinical and serologic investigation for subtle signs of systemic autoimmune disease should also be undertaken. There is no direct information on the treatment of idiopathic immune complex crescentic glomerulonephritis. The treatment of such patients is therefore mirrored on that of ANCA-positive patients or patients with lupus nephritis using pulse *intravenous methylprednisolone* followed by *oral glucocorticoids* and IV or oral cyclophosphamide for patients with severe renal impairment and diffuse crescents (>50% of glomeruli). Patients with milder form of disease may conceivably receive therapy with oral glucocorticoids and MMF (1–1.5g twice daily).

ANCA negative, and anti-GBM positive disease (anti-GBM disease)

The standard treatment for anti-GBM disease consists of oral *glucocorticoids*, *cyclophosphamide*, and intensive *plasmapheresis* (Turner and Rees, 1998; Levy et al., 2001). Plasmapheresis consists of removal of 50mL/kg (for a maximum of 4L) of plasma with replacement with a 5% albumin solution, performed daily for at least 14d or until circulating antibody levels become undetectable (Levy et al., 2001). In those patients with pulmonary hemorrhage, clotting factors should be replaced by administering fresh-frozen plasma at the end of each treatment. Similarly to the regimen described for ANCA-associated vasculitis, prednisone is started at 1mg/kg/d (for a maximum dose of 60mg daily) and tapered after the first month over a period of 4–5 months. The role of high-dose intravenous methylprednisolone pulses (7mg/kg/d ×3d for a maximum dose of 500mg daily) remains unproven in the treatment of anti-GBM disease. Nonetheless, the urgent nature of the clinical process prompts some nephrologists to administer methylprednisolone as part of induction therapy. No data is available as to the optimal modality or duration of cyclophosphamide therapy. At Hammersmith Hospital (London, UK), cyclophosphamide was given orally (2–3mg/kg/d) for up to 3 months. In patients who are dialysis-dependent, and in the absence of pulmonary hemorrhage, treatment should be discontinued after 8–12 weeks if there is no recovery of renal function (Levy et al., 2001).

Using this regimen, patient survival is approximately 85% with 40% progression to ESRD (Lockwood et al., 1976; Madore et al., 1996; Pusey et al., 1983; Pusey, 1990). These results are better than those before the introduction of plasmapheresis, when patient survival was <50% with a near 90% rate of ESRD. In a retrospective analysis of 71 patients treated with plasmapheresis, prednisolone, and cyclophosphamide, patient and renal survival were excellent among patients presenting with a serum creatinine <500µmol/L (5.7mg/dL) (100% and 95% respectively at 1 year and 94% at a median follow up of 90 months). Among patients presenting with a serum creatinine >500µmol/L but not needing dialysis, patient and renal survival were 83% and 82% respectively at 1 year and 80% and 50% respectively long term. In contrast, the outcome at 1 year of patients on dialysis was significantly worse with 65% patient survival and only 8% renal survival (Levy et al., 2001). Although no absolute degree of crescent formation alone predicted irreversible renal failure, no patient who required immediate dialysis and had 100% crescents on renal biopsy recovered renal function (Levy et al., 2001). These findings underscore the importance of early recognition of the anti-GBM positive forms of CrGN.

Once remission of anti-GBM disease is achieved with immunosuppressive therapy, recurrent disease occurs only rarely (<3%) (Levy et al., 2001). Similarly, the recurrence of anti-GBM disease after renal transplantation is also rare, especially when transplantation is delayed until after disappearance of anti-GBM antibody in the circulation (Almkuist et al., 1981). Because of the rarity of relapses, the course of immunosuppression can be brief (3–6 months) and maintenance immunosuppression is not required. Following titers of anti-GBM antibody may be of value to assess the success of treatment but this is not well established.

ANCA positive, anti-GBM positive disease (dual antibody disease)

The treatment of patients with both anti-GBM autoantibodies and ANCA follows the same treatment regimen as described for ANCA vasculitis and anti-GBM disease. If recognized early, plasmapheresis in addition to immuno-modulating therapy is indicated. In a retrospective analysis comparing patients with anti-GBM (n = 13), MPO-ANCA (n = 46) and both (n = 10), 'double positive' patients and those with anti-GBM autoantibodies presented with significantly higher serum creatinine (10.3 ± 5.6 and 9.6 ± 8.1 respectively) than patients with MPO-ANCA alone (5.0 ± 2.9). Thus, 1-year renal survival was best among patients with MPO-ANCA alone (63%) as compared to the double positive group (10.0% p = 0.01) and the anti-GBM group (15.4%; p = 0.17) (Rutgers et al., 2005). Patient survival at 1 year was best among patients with anti-GBM alone, although the differences did not reach statistical significance.

In patients who have both circulating anti-GBM and ANCA, the chance of recovery of renal function may be better than that of patients with anti-GBM alone. In these patients, immunosuppressive therapy should not be withheld, even in those presenting with advanced renal failure requiring dialysis (Jayne et al., 1990; Levy et al., 2004; Rutgers et al., 2005).

Practical recommendations

The general principles that should guide therapy of CrGN are given in Table 10.4. Treatment recommendations for the specific pathogenetic sub-varieties of CrGN are given below.

Pauci-immune necrotizing and crescentic glomerulonephritis ANCA positive

Patients with ANCA-positive P-INCGN should receive induction therapy with pulse methylprednisolone for 3d, followed by prednisone (1mg/kg/d, not to exceed 60mg daily) for the first 4 weeks followed by a taper over the subsequent 4 months. Considering the data regarding the adverse effects of pulse intravenous cyclophosphamide vs. the daily oral regime, it is reasonable to start induction therapy with pulse intravenous cyclophosphamide (0.5–0.75g/m^2 body surface area every 4 weeks). Patients who do not respond to this form of therapy within about 3 months, or those with a rapid relapse after discontinuing a course of IV cyclophosphamide can be switched to a regimen of daily oral cyclophosphamide (2mg/kg/d titrated to keep the WBC count >3000 cells/mL).

Patients who are in complete clinical remission can be switched after 3–4 months to a maintenance regimen with azathioprine (2mg/kg/d titrated to keep the WBC count >3000 cells/mL). Patients who are intolerant of azathioprine can be switched to a maintenance regimen with MMF with a target dose of 1g bid. The optimal duration of therapy is unclear. Patient who are at high risk of relapse with a history of at least one risk factor (PR3-ANCA, or lung or upper respiratory tract involvement), and patients who are persistently PR3-ANCA positive, should receive maintenance therapy for a total of 12–18 months. On the other hand, immunosuppressive therapy can probably be discontinued after a 6-month course of cyclophosphamide in patients with no risk factors for relapse (MPO-ANCA and no history of lung or upper respiratory tract involvement) who are in complete remission.

Patients with advanced renal failure requiring or nearing the need for dialysis, and those with pulmonary hemorrhage should receive a course of plasmapheresis in addition to glucocorticoids and cyclophosphamide. Patients with persistent or progressive disease despite glucocorticoids, and cyclophosphamide can benefit from the addition of intravenous gammaglobulin (IVIg) *or* plasmapheresis, *or* rituximab *or* infliximab.

The treatment of disease relapse should be tailored to the severity of the disease. Patients with recurrent glomerulonephritis and loss of GFR, and those with pulmonary hemorrhage or severe subglottic stenosis, life- or organ-threatening disease should receive therapy with glucocorticoids and cyclophosphamide as described above. Patients with mild-to-moderate relapse (with mild upper respiratory tract disease) may receive therapy with daily glucocorticoids and azathioprine or MMF. Patients who suffer a relapse while on maintenance therapy with azathioprine or MMF can be treated with the addition of rituximab, *or* IVIg, *or* infliximab.

Treatment of patients with P-INCGN who are persistently ANCA negative and anti-GBM antibody negative follows the same recommendations as for those with a positive ANCA test. Cyclosporin has been used successfully to treat ANCA-positive CrGN, but a high relapse rate is to be expected (Allen et al., 1993). Cyclosporin has been used successfully to prevent reactivation of disease, but this has not been subjected to a randomized trial (especially in comparison to MMF or azathioprine maintenance regimens) (Haubitz et al., 1998) and this approach is not widely used.

Immune complex crescentic glomerulonephritis (ANCA negative and anti-GBM antibody negative)

In the absence of evidence for underlying systemic autoimmune disease, infection, or occult malignancy, the treatment of idiopathic immune complex glomerulonephritis consists of daily glucocorticoids, with consideration for induction therapy with pulse methylprednisolone and cyclophosphamide or MMF for patients with more advanced renal impairment or extensive crescent formation seen on biopsy.

Anti-GBM disease

These patients should receive induction with oral glucocorticoids, cyclophosphamide, and plasmapheresis as described above. Patients with severe renal disease should probably also receive pulse methylprednisolone for induction

(7mg/kg/d ×3 [≤ 500mg/d]). The risk-benefit ratio of such therapy should be carefully assessed for an individual patient presenting at or near dialysis, and the likelihood of dialysis-free survival at 12 months is only in the order of 10%. Long-term maintenance immunosuppression is usually not needed due to the rarity of relapses.

Anti-GBM and ANCA dual positive disease

These patients should receive induction therapy with pulse glucocorticoids, cyclophosphamide, *and* plasmapheresis as described for ANCA-positive patients and anti-GBM antibody positive patients. Such patients with severe renal impairment may have a better prognosis than those with anti-GBM alone, but this is not consistently found, and in general the outcome of the disease in these patients with therapy is similar to those with anti-GBM disease only, at comparable degrees of renal function at presentation.

Transplantation

Pauci-immune necrotizing and crescentic glomerulonephritis ANCA positive

Renal transplantation is well-recognized as an option of renal replacement therapy in patients with ANCA-associated P-INCGN with or without systemic small vessel vasculitis (Wegener's granulomatosis or MPA). Successful renal transplantation in patients with ANCA-associated SVV has been reported in patients who were in full remission and with negative ANCA titers, in patients with positive ANCA titers (Morin et al., 1993; Frasca et al., 1996; Rostaing et al., 1997), and even in patients with evidence of active vasculitis at the time of transplantation (Schmitt et al., 1993). Recurrent systemic vasculitis after transplantation has been described as occurring from a few days (Reaich et al., 1994) to several years post-transplantation (Fogazzi et al., 1993). Reported recurrences after transplantation involve a spectrum of various organs and are not limited to the transplanted kidney.

Based on a pooled analysis (Nachman et al., 1999), ANCA-associated SVV recurs in about 19% of all patients, with an average time from transplantation to relapse of disease in the graft of 31 months. The presence of ANCA at transplantation does not appear to increase the rate of relapse post-transplantation. Patients with Wegener's granulomatosis had a relative risk of relapse of 2.75 when compared with patients with MPA or P-INCGN alone. Conversely, ANCA pattern (c-ANCA or p-ANCA) or antigen specificity (PR3 or MPO) was not associated with differences in recurrence rate post-transplantation. A recent report describes the outcome of 35 patients who received a kidney transplant between 1996–2005 (Gera et al., 2007). The most common post-transplant immunosuppressive therapies were antibody induction, glucocorticoids, MMF, and tacrolimus. The overall and death censored graft survivals were 94% and 100%, respectively, at 5 years post-transplantation. Non-renal recurrence occurred in only three patients, at 20, 24, and 68 months post-transplantation. The rate of recurrence was significantly different between patients who were ANCA-positive at the time of transplant and those who were ANCA-negative. There is no indication that a negative ANCA test is necessary prior to transplantation in order to avoid recurrence of disease in the graft. The prognosis for ANCA-positive renal transplant recipients is good also in the long-term. In a retrospective study the 10-year patient survival was 87% in vasculitic patients vs. 90% well matched controls and the 10-year death-censored graft survivals were respectively 84 and 100% (Moroni et al., 2007).

A review of the reports of recurrent ANCA-associated SVV post-transplantation reveal a good response to cyclophosphamide in the treatment of relapsing disease, although recurrent disease can lead to graft loss and even patient death.

In summary, renal transplantation is a beneficial option in the management of patients with ANCA-associated SVV and ESRD. Although the presence of circulating ANCA is not a sufficient contraindication to transplantation, it is current practice not to perform transplantation in patients with clinically active vasculitis, but to delay surgery until the disease is in remission. No data are currently available about the need to wait a certain period of time after remission is attained before proceeding to transplantation.

Anti-GBM disease

The risk of recurrent disease in renal allografts is low for patients with anti-GBM disease. Although recurrence of anti-GBM disease after transplantation has been reported (Khandelwal et al., 2004), its frequency is very low, especially in patients who have negative anti-GBM titers at the time of transplantation. Traditionally, transplant has been delayed for 12 months after the anti-GBM titers become negative, although there is no direct evidence to substantiate this recommendation. Nevertheless it seems reasonable to delay transplantation until negative (or very low and stable) anti-GBM titers are attained. In cases of recurrent disease post-transplantation, patients should be treated with pulse methylprednisolone, oral cyclophosphamide and plasmapheresis (Khandelwal et al., 2004).

References

Allen N., Caldwell D., Rice J., et al. (1993). Cyclosporin A therapy for Wegener's granulomatosis. In W. L. Gross (ed), *ANCA associated vasculitides: immunological and clinical aspects*, pp.473–6. Plenum Press, New York, NY.

Almkuist RD, Buckalew VM, Jr., Hirszel P, et al. (1981). Recurrence of anti-glomerular basement membrane antibody mediated glomerulonephritis in an isograft. *Clinical Immunology Immunopathology* **18**:54–60.

Aries PM, Hellmich B, Both M, et al. (2005). Lack of efficacy of rituximab in Wegener's granulomatosis with refractory granulomatous manifestations. *Annals of Rheumatic Diseases* **65**:853–8.

Bariety J, et al. (2003). Glomerular epithelial-mesenchymal transdifferetiation in pauci-immune crescentic glomerulonephritis. *Nephrology Dialysis Transplantation* **18**:1777–84.

Bariety J, et al. (2005). Podocyte involvement in human crescentic glomerulonephritis. *Kidney International* **68**:1109–19.

Bautz DJ, et al. (in press). Antibodies with dual reactivity to plasminogen and complementary PR3 in Pr3-ANCA vasculitis. *Journal of the American Society of Nephrology.*

Behmoaras J, Bhangal G, Smith J, et al. (2008). Jund is a determinant of macrophage activation and is associated with glomerulonephritis susceptibility. *Nature Genetics* **40**:553–9.

Billheden J, et al.(1997). Glomerular basement membrane antibodies in hantavirus disease (hemorrhagic fever with renal syndrome). *Clinical Nephrology* **48**:137–40.

Bonsib SM (1985). Glomerular basement membrane discontinuities: Scanning electron microcopic study of acellular glomeruli. *American Journal of Pathology* **19**:357–60.

Bonsib SM, Goeken JA, Kemp JD, Chandran P, Shadur C, and Wilson L (1993). Coexistent anti-neutrophil cytoplasmic antibody and antiglomerular basement membrane antibody associated disease = report of six cases. *Modern Pathology* **6**:526–30.

Border WA, et al. (1979). IgA antibasement membrane nephritis with pulmonary hemorrhage. *Annals of Internal Medicine* **91**:21–5.

Borgmann S, Haubnitz M (2004). Genetic impact of pathogenesis and prognosis of ANCA-associated vasculitides. *Clinical and Experimental Rheumatology* **6**(Suppl. 36) s79–s86.

Borza DB, et al. (2005). Recurrent Goodpasturess disease in a monoclonal IgA1-kappa antibody autoreactive with the alpha1/alpha2 chains of Type IV collagen. *American Journal of Kidney Diseases* **45**:397–406.

Borza DB, et al. (2003). Pathogenesis of Goodpasture's syndrome– a molecular perspective. *Seminars in Nephrology* **23**:522–31.

Booth A, Harper L, Hammad T, et al. (2004). Prospective study of TNFalpha blockade with infliximab in anti-neutrophil cytoplasmic antibody-associated systemic vasculitis. *Journal of the American Society of Nephrology* **15**:717–21.

Cameron JS (1977). The long-term outcome of glomerular disease. In RW Schrier, Gottschalk AR (eds). *Diseases of the Kidney,* pp.1929–35. Little Brown, Boston, MA.

Cameron JS (1998) Crescentic nephritis secondary to infection, systemic disease and other glomerulopathies. In C Pusey, A. Rees (eds), *Rapidly Progressive Glomerulonephritis,* pp.207–35. Oxford University Press, Oxford.

Clatworthy MR, Wallin EF, Jayne DR (2008). Anti-glomerular basement membrane disease after alemtuzumab. *New England Journal of Medicine* **359**:768–9.

Cohen Tervaert JW, Huitema MG, Hene RJ, et al. (1990). Prevention of relapses in Wegener's granulomatosis by treatment based on antineutrophil cytoplasmic antibody titre. *Lancet* **336**:709–11.

Couser WG (1988). Rapidly progressive glomerulonephritis: classification, pathogenetic mechanisms, and therapy. *American Journal Kidney Diseases* **11**:449–64.

Davenport A, Lock RJ, and Wallington T (1995). Clinical significance of the serial measurement of autoantibodies to neutrophil cytoplasm using a standard indirect immunofluorescence test. *American Journal Nephrology* **15**:201–7.

de Groot K, Adu D, and Savage CO (2001). The value of pulse cyclophosphamide in ANCA-associated vasculitis: meta-analysis and critical review. *Nephrology Dialysis Transplantation* **16**:2018–27.

de Lind van Wijngaarden RA, et al. (2006). Clinical and histologic determinants of renal outcome in ANCA-associated vasculitis. A prospective analysis of 100 patients with severe renal involvement. *Journal of the American Society of Nephrology* **17**:2264–74

de Lind van Wijngaarden RA, Hauer HA, et al. (2007). Chances of renal recovery for dialysis-dependent ANCA-associated glomerulonephritis. *Journal of the American Society of Nephrology* **18**:2189–97.

de Lind van Wijngaarden RA (2008). Hypotheses on the etiology of antineutrophil cytoplasmic autoantibody associated vasculitis. The cause is hidden, but the result is known. *Clinical Journal of the American Society of Nephrology* **3**:237–52.

De GK, Rasmussen N, Bacon PA, Tervaert JW, et al. (2005). Randomized trial of cyclophosphamide versus methotrexate for induction of remission in early systemic antineutrophil cytoplasmic antibody-associated vasculitis. *Arthritis Rheumatism* **52**:2461–69.

De'Oliviera J, Gaskin G, Dash A, Rees AJ, and Pusey CD (1995). Relationship between disease activity and anti-neutrophil cytoplasmic antibody concentration in long-term management of systemic vasculitis. *American Journal of Kidney Diseases* **25**:380–9.

Dewan D, Gulati S, Sharma RK, Prasad N, Jain M, Gupta A, Kumar A (2008). Clinical spectrum and outcome of crescentic glomerulonephritis in children in developing countries. *Pediatric Nephrology* **23**:389–94.

Dickenmann M, Oettl T, Mihatsch MJ (2008). Osmotic nephrosis: acute kidney injury with accumulation of proximal tubular lysosomes due to administration of exogenous solutes. *American Journal of Kidney Diseases* **51**:491–503.

Eriksson P (2005). Nine patients with anti-neutrophil cytoplasmic antibody-positive vasculitis successfully treated with rituximab. *Journal of Internal Medicine* **257**:540–8.

Falk RJ, et al. (1990) Clinical course of anti-neutrophil; cytoplasmic auto-antibody associated glomerulonephritis and systemic vasculitis. The Glomerular Disease Collaborative Network. *Annals of Internal Medicine* **113**:656–63.

Ferrario F, Tadros MT, Napodano P, Sinico RA, Fellin G, and D'Amico G (1994). Critical re-evaluation of 41 cases of "idiopathic" crescentic glomerulonephritis. *Clinical Nephrology* **41**:1–9.

Ferrario F and Rastaldi MP (1998). Pathology of rapidly progressive glomerulonephritis. In C Pusey, A. Rees (eds), *Rapidly Progressive Glomerulonephritis*, pp.207–35. Oxford University Press, Oxford.

Finkelman JD, Lee AS, Hummel AM, et al. (2007). ANCA are detectable in nearly all patients with active severe Wegener's granulomatosis. *American Journal of Medicine* **120**:643–14.

Fischer EG, Lager DJ (2007) Anti-glomerular basement membrane glomerulonephritis: a morphologic study of 80 cases. *American Journal of Clinical Pathology* **125**:445–50.

Fisher M, et al. (1997). Susceptibility to anti-glomerular basement membrane disease is strongly associated with HLA-DRB1 genes. *Kidney International* **51**:222–9.

Fogazzi GB, et al. (1993). Late recurrence of systemic vasculitis after kidney transplantation involving the kidney allograft. *Advances in Experimental Medicine and Biology* **336**:503–6.

Frasca GM, et al. (1996). Renal transplantation in patients with microscopic polyarteritis and anti-myeloperoxidase antibodies: report of three cases. *Nephron* **72**:82–5.

Gaskin G and Pusey (1998). Clinical aspects of systemic vasculitis. In C Pusey, A Rees (eds), *Rapidly Progressive Glomerulonephritis*, pp.207–35. Oxford University Press, Oxford.

Gera M, Griffin MD, Specks U, Leung N, Stegall MD, and Fervenza FC (2007). Recurrence of ANCA-associated vasculitis following renal transplantation in the modern era of immunosupression. *Kidney International* **71**:1296–1301.

Glassock R, Cohen A, and Adler S (1995). Primary glomerular disease. In BM Brenner (ed), *The Kidney*, pp.1402–10. Saunders, Philadelphia, PA.

Guillevin L, Cohen P, Gayraud M, Lhote F, Jarrousse B, and Casassus P (1999). Churg–Strauss syndrome. Clinical study and long-term follow-up of 96 patients. *Medicine* (Baltimore) **78**:26–37.

Guillevin L, Cordier JF, Lhote F, et al. (1997). A prospective, multicenter, randomized trial comparing steroids and pulse cyclophosphamide versus steroids and oral cyclophosphamide in the treatment of generalized Wegener's granulomatosis. *Arthritis Rheumatism* **40**:2187–98.

Hagen EC, et al. (1998). Diagnostic value of standardized assays for anti-neutrophil cytoplasmic antibodies in idiopathic systemic vasculitis: EC/BCR project for ANCA Assay Standardization. *Kidney International* **53**:743–53.

Han WK, et al. (2003). Serial ANCA titers: useful tool for prevention of relapses in ANCA-associated vasculitis. *Kidney International* **63**:1079–85.

Haubitz M, et al (1998). Cyclosporin for the prevention of disease re-activation in relapsing ANCA-associated vasculitis. *Nephrology Dialysis Transplantation* **13**:2074–6.

Hauer HA, et al. (2002). Determinants of outcome in ANCA-associated glomerulonephritis: a prospective clinico-histopatholgical analysis of 96 patients. *Kidney International* **62**:1732–43.

Heckmann M, et al. (2008). The Wegener's granulomatosis trait lcous on Chromosome 6p21.3 as characterized by taqSNP genotyping. *Annals of Rheumatic Disease* **67**:972–9.

Heeringa P, Brouwer E, Klok PA et al. (1996). Autoantibodies to myeloperoxidase aggravate mild anti-glomerular-basement-membrane-mediated glomerular injury in the rat. *American Journal of Pathology* **149**:1695–706.

Hellmark T, Niles JL, Collins AB, McCluskey RT, and Brunmark C (1997). Comparison of anti-GBM antibodies in sera with or without ANCA. *Journal of the American Society of Nephrology* **8**:376–85.

Hellmich B, Csernok E, Fredenhagen G, and Gross WL (2007). A novel high sensitivity ELISA for detection of antineutrophil cytoplasm antibodies against proteinase-3. *Clinical Experimental Rheumatology* **25**:S1–S5.

Herody M, Bobrie G, Gouarin C, Grunfeld JP, and Noel LH (1993). Anti-GBM disease: predictive value of clinical, histological and serological data. *Clinical Nephrology* **40**:249–55.

Hogan SL, Falk RJ, Chin H, et al. (2005). Predictors of relapse and treatment resistance in antineutrophil cytoplasmic antibody-associated small-vessel vasculitis. *Annals of Internal Medicine* **143**:621–31.

Hogan SL, et al. (2007). Association of silica exposure with anti-neutrophil cytoplasmic autoantibody small-vessel vasculitis: a population-based, case-control study. *Clinical Journal of the American Society of Nephrology* **2**:290–9.

Holdsworth SR, et al. (1998). Immunopathogenesis of crescentic glomeruloephritis. In C Pusey, A Rees (eds), *Rapidly Progressive Glomerulonephritis*, pp.12–42. Oxford University Press, Oxford.

Hu W, Liu C, Xie H, Chen H, Liu Z, and Li L (2008). Mycophenolate mofetil versus cyclophosphamide for inducing remission of ANCA vasculitis with moderate renal involvement. *Nephrology Dialysis Transplantation* **23**:1307–12.

Huang XR, et al. (1994). Evidence for delayed type hypersensitivity mechanisms in glomerular crescent formation. *Kidney International* **46**:69–78.

Isaacs JD, Manna VK, Rapson N, Bulpitt KJ, Hazleman BL, Matteson EL, St Clair EW, Schnitzer TJ, and Johnston JM. (1996). CAMPATH-1H in rheumatoid arthritis--an intravenous dose-ranging study. *British Journal of Rheumatology* **35**:231–40.

Jayne D, Rasmussen N, Andrassy K, et al. (2003). A randomized trial of maintenance therapy for vasculitis associated with antineutrophil cytoplasmic autoantibodies. *New England Journal of Medicine* **349**:36–44.

Jayne DR (2002). Campath-1H (anti-CD52) for refractory vasculitis: retrospective Cambridge experience 1989-1999. *Cleveland Clinical Journal Medicine* **69**:SII–129.

Jayne DR, Chapel H, Adu D, et al. (2000). Intravenous immunoglobulin for ANCA-associated systemic vasculitis with persistent disease activity. *Quarterly Journal of Medicine* **93**:433–9.

Jayne DR, Gaskin G, Rasmussen N, et al. (2007). Randomized trial of plasma exchange or high-dosage methylprednisolone as adjunctive therapy for severe renal vasculitis. *Journal of the American Society of Nephrology* **18**:2180–8.

Jayne DR, Marshall PD, Jones SJ, Lockwood CM (1990). Autoantibodies to GBM and neutrophil cytoplasm in rapidly progressive glomerulonephritis. *Kidney International* **37**:965–70.

Jennette JC, Falk RJ (1990). Antineutrophil cytoplasmic autoantibodies and associated diseases: a review. *American Journal of Kidney Diseases* **15**:517–29.

Jennette JC, Falk RJ (1991). Diagnostic classification of antineutrophil cytoplasmic autoantibody- associated vasculitides. *American Journal of Kidney Diseases* **18**:184–7.

Jennette JC, Falk RJ (2008). New insights into the pathogenesis of vasculitis-associated with anti-neutrophil cytoplasmic autoantibodies. *Current Opinion in Rheumatology* **20**:55–60.

Jennette JC, et al. (1994). Vasculitis affecting the skin. *Archives of Dermatology* **130**:899–906.

Johnson RJ, et al. (1994). Renal manifestations of hepatitis C virus infection. *Kidney International* **46**:1255–63.

Joy MS, Hogan SL, Jennette JC, Falk RJ, and Nachman PH (2005). A pilot study using mycophenolate mofetil in relapsing or resistant ANCA small vessel vasculitis. *Nephrololgy Dialysis Transplantation* **20**:2725–32.

Kalluri R, Danoff T, and Neilson EG (1995). Murine anti-alpha3(IV) collagen disease: a model of human Goodpasture syndrome and anti-GBM nephritis. *Journal of the American Society of Nephrology* **6**:833.

Kalluri R, Meyers K, Mogyorosi A, Madaio MP, and Neilson EG (1997). Goodpasture syndrome involving overlap with Wegener's granulomatosis and anti-glomerular basement membrane disease. *Journal of the American Society of Nephrology* **8**:1795–1800.

Keogh KA, Wylam ME, Stone JH, and Specks U (2005). Induction of remission by B lymphocyte depletion in eleven patients with refractory antineutrophil cytoplasmic antibody-associated vasculitis. *Arthritis Rheumatism* **52**:262–8.

Khan SB, et al. (2005) Antibody blockade of the TNF-alpha receptor reduces inflammation and scarring in experimental crescentic glomerulkonephritis. *Kidney International* **67**:1812–20.

Khandelwal M, McCormick BB, Lajoie G, Sweet J, Cole E, and Cattran DC (2004). Recurrence of anti-GBM disease 8 years after renal transplantation. *Nephrology Dialysis Transplantation* **19**:491–4.

Kirk AD, Hale DA, Mannon RB, et al (2003). Results from a human renal allograft tolerance trial evaluating the humanized CD52-specific monoclonal antibody alemtuzumab (CAMPATH-1H). *Transplantation* **76**:120–9.

Kitching AR, et al. (1999). Il-12 directs severe renal injury, crescent formation and the Th1 responses in murine glomerulonephritis. *European Journal of Immunology* **29**:1–10.

Klemmer PJ, Chalermskulrat W, Reif MS, Hogan SL, Henke DC, and Falk RJ (2003). Plasmapheresis therapy for diffuse alveolar hemorrhage in patients with small-vessel vasculitis. *American Journal of Kidney Diseases* **42**:1149–53.

Koukoulaki M and Jayne DR (2006). Mycophenolate mofetil in anti-neutrophil cytoplasm antibodies-associated systemic vasculitis. *Nephron Clinical Practice* **102**:c100–c107.

Kriz W and Le Hir M. (2005). Pathways to nephron loss starting from glomerular disease- insights form animal models. *Kidney International* **67**:404–19.

Lamprecht P, Till A, Steinmann J, Aries PM, and Gross WL (2007). Current state of biologicals in the management of systemic vasculitis. *Annals of the New York Academy of Sciences* **1110**:261–70.

Lan HY, et al. (1997). Local macrophage proliferation in the pathogenesis of glomerular crescent formation in rat glomerular basement membrane (GBM) glomerulonephritis. *Clinical and Experimental Immunology* **110**:233–40.

Le Hir M, et al. (2001). Podocyte bridges between the tuft and Bowman's capsule: an early event in experimental crescentic glomerulonephritis. *Journal of the American Society of Nephrology* **12**:2060–171.

Leaker B and Neild GH (1991). Effect of enalapril on proteinuria and renal function in patients with healed severe crescentic glomerulonephritis. *Nephrology Dialysis Transplantation* **6**:936–8.

Levy JB, Turner AN, Rees AJ, and Pusey CD (2001). Long-term outcome of anti-glomerular basement membrane antibody disease treated with plasma exchange and immunosuppression. *Annals of Internal Medicine* **134**:1033–42.

Levy JB, et al. (2004). Clinical features and outcome of patients with both ANCA and anti-GBM antibodies. *Kidney International* **66**:1535–40.

Lionaki S, Jennette JC, Falk RJ (2007) Anti-neutrophil cytoplasmic (ANCA) and anti-glomerular basement membrane (GBM) autoantibodies in necrotizing and crescentic glomerulonephritis. *Seminars in Immunopathology* **29**:459–74.

Little MA and Pusey CD. (2004). Rapidly progressive glomerulonephritis: current and evolving treatment strategies. *Journal of Nephrology* **8**(Suppl.b):510–19.

Lockwood CM, Rees AJ, Pearson TA, Evans DJ, Peters DK, and Wilson CB (1976). Immunosuppression and plasma-exchange in the treatment of Goodpasture's syndrome. *Lancet* **1**:711–15.

Ma KW, et al. (1978). Glomerulonephritis with Hodgkin's disease and herpes zoster. *Archives of Pathology & Laboratory Medicine* **102**:527–9.

Madore F, Lazarus JM, and Brady HR (1996). Therapeutic plasma exchange in renal diseases. *Journal American Society Nephrology* **7**:367–86.

Maes B, et al. (1999) IgA anti-glomerular basement membrane disease associated with bronchial carcinoma and monoclonal gammopathy. *American Journal of Kidney Diseases* **33**:E3

Martinez V, Cohen P, Pagnoux C, et al. (2008). Intravenous immunoglobulins for relapses of systemic vasculitides associated with antineutrophil cytoplasmic autoantibodies: results of a multicenter, prospective, open-label study of twenty-two patients. Arthritis Rheumatism **58**:308–17.

Metzler C, Miehle N, Manger K, et al. (2007). Elevated relapse rate under oral methotrexate versus leflunomide for maintenance of remission in Wegener's granulomatosis. *Rheumatology* (Oxford) **46**(7):1087–91.

Morgan MD, et al. (2006). Anti-neutrophil cytoplasm-associated glomerulonephritis. *Journal of the American Society of Nephrology* **17**: 1224–34.

Morin MP, Thervet E, Legendre C, Page B, Kreis H, and Noel LH (1993). Successful kidney transplantation in a patient with microscopic polyarteritis and positive ANCA [letter]. *Nephrology Dialysis Transplantation* **8**:287–88.

Moroni G, Torri A, Gallelli B, et al. (2007). The long-term prognosis of renal transplant in patients with systemic vasculitis. *American Journal of Transplantation* **7**: 2133–9.

Mukhtyar C. et al. (2008). Outcomes from studies of anti-neutrophil cytoplasmic antibody associated vasculitis: a systematic review by the European League Against Rheumatism systemic vasculitis task force. *Annals of Rheumatic Diseases* **67**:1004–10.

Nachman PH, Hogan SL, Jennette JC, Falk RJ (1996). Treatment response and relapse in antineutrophil cytoplasmic autoantibody-associated microscopic polyangiitis and glomerulonephritis. *Journal of the American Society of Nephrology* **7**:33–9.

Nachmann P, et al. (1998) Pathogenesis of systemic vasculitis. In C Pusey, A Rees (eds), *Rapidly Progressive Glomerulonephritis*, pp.148–85. Oxford University Press, Oxford.

Nachman PH, Segelmark M, Westman K, et al. (1999). Recurrent ANCA-associated small vessel vasculitis after transplantation: A pooled analysis. *Kidney International* **56**:1544–10.

Neild GH, Cameron JS, Ogg CS, et al. (1983). Rapidly progressive glomerulonephritis with extensive glomerular crescent formation. Quarterly Journal of Medicine **52**: 395–416.

Ng YY, et al. (1999) Glomerular-epithelial-myofibroblast transdifferentiation in the evolution of glomerular crescent formation. *Nephrology Dialysis Transplantation* **14**:2860–72.

Pagnoux C, et al. (2008). Predictors of treatment resistance and relapse in antineutrophil cytoplasmic antibody-associated small-vessel vasculitis: Comparison of two independent cohorts. *Arthritis and Rheumatism* **58**:2908–18.

Phoon RK, Kitching AR, Odobasic D, Jones LK, Semple TJ, Holdsworth SR (2008). T-bet deficiency attenuates renal injury in experimental crescentic glomerulonephritis. *Journal of the American Society of Nephrology* **1**:477–85.

Pusey CD (1990). Plasma exchange in immunological disease. *Progress Clinical Biological Research* **337**:419–24.

Pusey CD, Lockwood CM, and Peters DK (1983). Plasma exchange and immunosuppressive drugs in the treatment of glomerulonephritis due to antibodies to the glomerular basement membrane. *International Journal Artificial Organs* **6**(Suppl.1):15–18.

Pusey C and Rees A (eds) (1998). *Rapidly Progressive Glomerulonephritis.* Oxford University Press, Oxford .

Reaich D, Cooper N, and Main J (1994). Rapid catastrophic onset of Wegener's granulomatosis in a renal transplant. *Nephron* **67**:354–7.

Rees A, Peters DK, Amos N, et al. (1984). The influence of HLA-linked genes on the severity of anti-GBM antibody mediated nephritis. *Kidney International* **26**:445–50.

Rostaing L, Modesto A, Oksman F, Cisterne JM, Le Mao G, and Durand D (1997). Outcome of patients with antineutrophil cytoplasmic autoantibody- associated vasculitis following cadaveric kidney transplantation. *American Journal of Kidney Diseases* **29**:96–102.

Rutgers A, Slot M, van Passen P, van Breda Vriesman P, Heeringa P, and Tervaert JW (2005). Coexistence of anti-glomerular basement membrane antibodies and myeloperoxidase-ANCAs in crescentic glomerulonephritis. *American Journal of Kidney Diseases* **46**:253–62.

Salama AD, et al. (2003). Regulation by CD28+ lymphocytes of auto-antigen specific T-cell responses in Goodpasture's (anti-GBM) disease. *Kidney International* **64**: 1685–94.

Sanders JS, Huitma MG, Kallenberg CG, and Stegeman CA (2006). Prediction of relapses in PR3-ANCA-associated vasculitis by assessing responses of ANCA titres to treatment. *Rheumatology* (Oxford) **45**:724–9.

Savage CO and Lockwood CM (1990). Antineutrophil antibodies in vasculitis. *Advances Nephrology Necker Hospital* **19**:225–36.

Schmitt WH, Haubitz M, Mistry N, Brunkhorst R, Erbsloh-Moller B, and Gross WL (1993). Renal transplantation in Wegener's granulomatosis [letter]. *Lancet* **342**:860.

Sneller MC, Hoffman GS, Talar-Williams C, Kerr GS, Hallahan CW, and Fauci AS (1995). An analysis of forty-two Wegener's granulomatosis patients treated with methotrexate and prednisone. *Arthritis Rheumatism* **38**:608–13.

Stasi R, Stipa E, Poeta GD, Amadori S, Newland AC, and Provan D (2006). Long-term observation of patients with anti-neutrophil cytoplasmic antibody-associated vasculitis treated with rituximab. *Rheumatology* (Oxford) **45**:1342–6.

Stassen PM, Cohen Tervaert JW, and Stegeman CA (2007). Induction of remission in active anti-neutrophil cytoplasmic antibody-associated vasculitis with mycophenolate mofetil in patients who cannot be treated with cyclophosphamide. *Annals Rheumatic Diseases* **66**:798–802.

Stevenson A, et al. (1995) Biochemical markers of basement membrane disturbances and occupational exposure to hydrocarbons and mixed solvents. *Quarterly Journal of Medicine* **88**:23–8.

Stone JH (2003). Limited versus severe Wegener's granulomatosis: baseline data on patients in the Wegener's granulomatosis etanercept trial. *Arthritis Rheumatism* **48**:2299–2309.

Thorner PS, et al. (2008). Podocytes contribute to the formation of glomerular crescents. *Journal of the American Society of Nephrology* **19**:495–502.

Tipping PG and Holdwworth SR (2006) T-cells in crescentic glomerulonephritis. *Journal of the American Society of Nephrology* **17**:1253–63.

Tsuchiya N, et al. (2006). Association of HLA-DRB*0901-DQB1*0303 haplotype with microscopic piolyangiitis in Japanese. *Genes and Immunity* **7**:81–4.

Turner AN, Rees AJ (1998). Anti-glomerular basement membrane disease. In C Pusey, A Rees (eds), *Rapidly Progressive Glomerulonephritis*, pp.108–24. Oxford University Press, Oxford.

Weschsler E, et al. (2008). Anti-glomerular basement membrane disease in an HIV-infected patient. *Nature Clinical Practice Nephrology* **4**:167–71.

Weidanz F, Day CJ, Hewins P, Savage CO, and Harper L (2007). Recurrences and infections during continuous immunosuppressive therapy after beginning dialysis in ANCA-associated vasculitis. *American Journal Kidney Diseases* **50**:36–46.

Wiggins RC. (1998). Rapidly Progressive glomerulonephritis; resolution and scarring. In C Pusey, A Rees (eds), *Rapidly Progressive Glomerulonephritis*, pp.43–58. Oxford University Press, Oxford.

Xenocostas A, et al. (1999). Anti-glomerular basement membrane glomerulonephritis after extra-corporeal shock wave lithotripsy. *American Journal of Kidney Diseases* **13**:128–32.

Xiao H, Schreiber A, Heeringa P, et al. (2007). Alternative complement pathway in the pathogenesis of disease mediated by anti-neutrophil cytoplasmic antibodies. *Am J Pathol* **170**:52–64.

Yang J, Bautz DJ, Lionaki S, et al. (2008). ANCA patients have T cells responsive to complementary PR-3 antigen. *Kidney International* **74**:1159–69.

Chapter 11

Other primary glomerular diseases

Claudio Ponticelli and Richard Glassock

Fibrillary glomerulonephritis/immunotactoid glomerulopathy (Table 11.1)

Introduction and overview

Fibrillary glomerulonephritis (FGN) and immunotactoid glomerulopathy (ITG) are both glomerular diseases characterized histologically by a diffuse increase in mesangial matrix due to deposits having a fibrillary structure by electron microscopy, which are negative for Congo-red stains but positive for immunoglobulin deposition. Most patients present with proteinuria, often in a nephrotic range, microhematuria, and hypertension. Almost half of patients have a reduced renal function at presentation. Although FGN and ITG have quite similar light microscopical and clinical features the current opinion is that they represent two separate diseases. FGN is an idiopathic (primary) condition characterized by polyclonal immune deposits with restricted gamma isotypes. Most patients present with significant renal insufficiency and have a poor outcome despite immunosuppressive therapy. By contrast, ITG very often contains monoclonal IgG deposits and has a significant association with underlying monoclonal paraproteinemia and hypocomplementemia. ITG is more properly classified as a mono-clonal immunoglobulin deposition disease (MIDD). Differentiation of FGN from the much more rare entity ITG appears justified on immunopathologic, ultrastructural, and clinical grounds (Fogo et al., 1993; Bridoux et al., 2002; Rosenstock et al., 2003). Both will be discussed together, although only FGN should be regarded as a primary glomerular disease, as defined in this monograph.

Pathology

Light microscopy FGN may show different histological patterns. According to Rosenstock et al. (2003) the most common pattern (44% of patients) was membranoproliferative glomerulonephritis, with mesangial expansion, foci of mesangial interposition and replication of glomerular basement membrane

Table 11.1 Common and different features of fibrillary glomerulonephritis (FGN) and immunotactoid glomerulopathy (ITG)

Pathology:	Both FGN and ITG may show a pattern of membranoproliferative glomerulonephritis with deposits of IgG and C3. On electron microscopy fibrils are randomly arranged and intermingled with the mesangial matrix in FGN while in ITG there are larger microtubuli in parallel arrays, with a distinct hollow core and well defined borders of deposits
Pathogenesis:	Unidentified serum precursors could be responsible for fibril deposition in FGN, the abnormal structure and physicochemical properties of monoclonal proteins together with tissue affinity may be responsible for crystallization and microtubular formation in ITG.
Etiology:	Unknown. One-third of cases of FGN are associated with autoimmune diseases, while ITG is more frequently associated with hematological malignancy
Clinical presentation:	Both FGN and ITG usually present with proteinuria in a nephrotic range, hematuria and various degrees of renal insufficiency
Prognosis:	Usually severe
Treatment:	No specific treatment is available. Rare cases responded to glucocorticoids or cytotoxic agents

(GBM) (see Atlas plate 18). Isolated mesangial proliferation or sclerosis was seen in 21% of cases. A pattern of diffuse endocapillary proliferation was observed in 15% of cases. A membranous-like pattern with subepithelial fibrillar deposits was seen in 7% of patients. In the remaining 13% advanced glomerular sclerosis was seen. Cellular or fibrocellular crescents were seen in 31% of all biopsies. ITG had similar patterns, although in no case crescents were observed.

Immunofluorescence microscopy Both FGN and ITG display diffuse, glomerular positivity for IgG (almost 100% of cases), IgM (about 50%), C3 (86–100%), and less frequently for IgA and C1q. Although IgG4 is the most frequent IgG, all the subclasses of IgG may be found. The deposits are usually polyclonal in FGN and monoclonal in ITG. Glomerular deposits are diffuse, in some cases irregular, predominantly located in the sub-epithelium and more rarely in the mesangium. Neither FGN nor ITG deposits react with histochemical dyes Congo red and Thioflavin T, thus both are classified as Congored negative fibrillary glomerulopathies.

Electron microscopy In FGN the glomerular deposits are fibrils, which are more frequently detected in the mesangium (98%) or within the GBM (92%). Fibrils are randomly arranged and intermingled with the mesangial matrix or GBM (see Atlas plate 18). They usually have a diameter comprised between 12–24nm, larger than amyloid fibrils but smaller than the fibrils seen in ITG.

In ITG, the deposits consist of microtubular structures which often measure >30nm and are usually organized in parallel arrays.

Unfortunately size alone is not sufficient for a differential diagnosis between FGN and ITG as microtubules with a diameter between 16–22nm have been reported. Moreover the distinction between fibrils and microtubules requires meticulous morphologic analysis on high-quality ultrathin sections. According to Bridoux et al. (2002) there are three key features for recognizing microtubular deposits: i) an arrangement in parallel arrays; ii) the presence of a distinct hollow core; iii) well defined borders of deposits. Other fibrillar or microtubular deposits that may enter a differential diagnosis are amyloid deposits (the fibrils have a fiameter between 8–15nm, and react with Congo red and thioflavin T), cryoglobulinemic deposits (microtubular indistinguishable from ITG), deposits in lupus nephritis (that have a fingerprint appearance).

Pathogenesis

The pathogenesis of FGN has not been elucidated. The deposition of fibrils is, in general, limited to the kidney, although there have been occasional reports of extra-renal involvement. The predominantly renal and glomerular involvement indicates that the specific glomerular environment and the physico-chemical properties of the deposited immunoglobulins are the factors that favor fibrillogenesis. The staining for IgG and C3 and presence of polyclonal IgG suggest an autoimmune process. Rostagno et al. (1996) found that a serum fibrillar cryoprecipitate, obtained from a patient with fibrillary glomerulonephritis, consisted of immunoglobulins, heavy chains gamma and mu, light chains kappa and lambda, and fibronectin, similar to the proteins identified by immunofluorescence and immunoelectron microscopy in the glomerular fibrils. According to these findings some unidentified serum precursors may be the source of the fibrillar deposits. The hypothesis of circulating factor(s) is also supported by the high incidence of recurrence of FGN after transplantation.

The pathogenesis of formation of microtubules in ITG is not known. As in FGN, the deposition of the microtubules is generally limited to the kidney. The abnormal structure of the monoclonal protein, together with its physicochemical properties and tissue affinity, seem to be the key factors governing the crystallization and the unique microtubular appearance. ITG has been reported in association with lymphoproliferative disorders, hepatitis C virus infection, leukocytoclastic vasculitis and hypocomplementemia, conditions likewise associated with type II cryoglobulinemia. Type II cryoglobulins have also been detected occasionally in patients initially diagnosed as having ITG (Ivanyi and Degrell, 2004). The overlaps in the ultrastructural morphology of the deposits and the underlying diseases have led to the hypothesis that some cases of ITG, and possibly even FGN, may represent a *forme fruste* of type II cryoglobulinemia.

Etiology

The etiology of FGN is unknown and the disease is considered as a primary glomerular disease. In about one-third of cases FGN may be associated with diabetes mellitus, malignancy, hepatitis C, systemic lupus erythematosus, thyroiditis, rheumatoid arthritis, or vasculitis. On the other hand, ITG is frequently associated with lymphoproliferative disorders, paraproteinemia, and, more rarely, with autoimmune diseases. In some cases a latent B-cell lymphoma may be discovered years after the diagnosis of ITG.

Clinical presentation

FGN may occur at any age, but often presents at an age between 55–60 years. The disease occurs more frequently in women (Fogo et al.,1993; Rosenstock et al., 2003). Patients typically present with proteinuria, which is in a nephrotic range in about 50% of cases. Hematuria is frequent. Most patients have renal insufficiency of various degrees at presentation and about 60% are hypertensive. No clinical laboratory findings are specific for FGN (Alpers and Kowalewska, 2008).

The clinical features at presentation in ITG are similar to those observed in FGN, although in ITG the severity of renal insufficiency is usually lower. Patients with ITG have a high incidence of serum or urine monoclonal gammopathy, underlying lymphoproliferative disorders, and hypocomplementemia.

Epidemiology

Both diseases are very rare. In a retrospective French review only nine cases of FGN and fourteen cases of ITG were found by reviewing the biopsies of fifteen nephrology departments between 1980 and 1997 (Bridoux et al., 2002). At the Renal Pathology Laboratory of Columbia University in New York the diagnosis of FGN was made in 0.6% of 10,108 renal biopsies and that of ITG in 0.06% (Rosenstock et al., 2003). Ninety per cent of patients are Caucasian.

Natural history

The outcome for patients with FGN is frequently poor. Progression to endstage renal failure occurs in approximately half of the patients within 2 years from presentation (Fogo et al., 1993). Serum creatinine at presentation and severity of interstitial fibrosis at initial renal biopsy are independent predictors of progression (Rosenstock et al., 2003).

The prognosis of ITG is less severe as the disease usually shows a slower progression. When ITG is associated with malignancy or infection the prognosis is mainly related to that of the underlying monoclonal gammopathy.

Specific treatment

The apparent role of Ig in the pathogenesis of FGN has led to a variety of immunotherapies. However, only transient response to glucocorticoids and immunosuppressive drugs has been reported in some patients with FGN. Few patients responded to fludaribine or mituximal (Rosenstock et al., 2003, Collins et al., 2008). The experience with ITG is also limited and anecdotal. Therapeutic trials with steroids alone, steroids with cytotoxic agents, and steroids with plasmapheresis have been associated with clinical remission of proteinuria in <10% of the cases (Schwartz et al., 2002). Sporadic cases of long-term remission of monoclonal paraprotein-induced ITG have been reported after high-dose chemotherapy for the plasma cell neoplasia.

Practical recommendations

Although FGN and ITG are rare diseases, their prevalence is probably under-appreciated. As a matter of fact, electron microscopy is not performed routinely by many nephrologic units, and without ultramicroscopic examination the diagnosis of glomerular deposition diseases is generally overlooked. It is possible that some cases of membranoproliferative or membranous glomerulonephritis actually mask an underlying FGN. The presence of monoclonal light chains in the urine may raise the suspicion for an underlying ITG. Once a diagnosis of fibrillary deposits is made or suspected, staining with Congo red may ascertain or exclude an amyloidosis. Immunofluorescence indicates whether the disease is Ig-derived or not (diabetes mellitus). The differential diagnosis with cryoglobulinemia, monoclonal gammopathy, or lupus nephritis is usually easy on the basis of clinical and laboratory features. The differential diagnosis between FGN and ITG is based on the diameter, the morphology, and the array of fibrils evaluated with a properly calibrated electron microscope.

Whether and how to treat these patients remain unanswered questions. The diseases are rare and the reports on therapeutic attempts are scanty. Symptomatic treatment should be maximized (see Chapter 1). Treatment with glucocorticoids and cyclophosphamide may be tried if there are not clinical contraindications keeping in mind, however, that <10% of patients will respond. Theoretically agents that interfere with Ig production, i.e., fludaribine, rituximab, or alemtuzumab, might be of benefit but information about their efficacy in FGN and ITG is lacking.

Transplantation

By reviewing the literature, Samaniego et al. (2001) reported fourteen cases of FGN who received renal transplantation. Histological recurrence was diagnosed in six patients (44%); four of them lost their allograft respectively 4, 5, 11, and 13 years after transplantation. Another patient died with stable graft function 7 years after transplantation. Rosenstock et al. (2003) reported two further cases. One patient had no clinical evidence of recurrence 8 years after transplantation with normal creatinine and no proteinuria. The other patient died 4 years after transplantation due to colon cancer with a stable creatinine of 2.2mg/dL. Thus, renal transplantation may be considered as a viable option for patients with FGN or ITG, but with the expectation of a frequent recurrence of the same disease in the renal allograft, which may impair long-term graft survival. A case of *de novo* FGN has also been reported after renal transplantation (Gough et al., 2005).

Collagenofibrotic glomerulopathy (Table 11.2)

Introduction and overview

Collagenofibrotic glomerulopathy is a rare primary glomerular disease in which accumulation of collagen III fibrils progressively accumulates within the mesangial matrix and subendothelial space. The disease has been included in the classification of primary glomerular diseases by the World Health Organization (Churg et al., 1995). Pathological features include lobulation and enlargement of glomeruli due to massive accumulation of fibrillar material as

Table 11.2 Main characteristics of collagenofibrotic glomerulopathy

Pathology:	Glomeruli appear expanded with a lobular aspect caused by eosinophilic subendothelial and mesangial deposits. Immunochemistry shows abundant staining for collagen type III in mesangium and GBM. On electron microscopy there is a wide accumulation of fibrillar material in the mesangium and subendothelial space
Pathogenesis:	The disease is probably related to an increase in serum type III procollagen peptide leading to abnormal subendothelial and mesangial deposits of collagen III
Etiology:	Unknown, no good evidence for a genetic transmission
Clinical presentation:	Most patients present with proteinuria in a nephrotic range, hypertension and anemia
Prognosis:	The disease may follow an unremitting course leading about half of patients to end-stage renal disease within 10 years from presentation
Treatment:	No specific treatment is available

seen at ultramicroscopic examination. Clinically the disease is characterized by proteinuria, often in a nephrotic range, hypertension and progression to renal failure. There is a typical increase in serum type III procollagen peptide (PIIINP) levels. Most of the few reported cases have been observed in Japan, suggesting a geographic or ancestral influence.

Pathology

The main pathological features have been carefully described by Alchi et al. (2007) in their excellent review of the literature.

Light microscopy The glomeruli appear expanded by eosinophilic subendothelial and mesangial deposits giving a clear lobular aspect to glomeruli (see Atlas plate 19). Congo red and thioflavin T stains are negative. There is neither mesangial cell proliferation nor cell infiltration. Peripheral capillary walls are thick and often show double-contour appearance, similar to that in membranoproliferative glomerulonephritis. In advanced stages, tubular atrophy and interstitial fibrosis are present, capillary lumens are narrowed by the expanded mesangium, and thickened capillary walls and glomeruli show a nodular appearance suggestive of Kimmelstiel–Wilson lesions in patients with diabetic nephropathy.

Immunofluorescence microscopy Focal and segmental staining for IgM, IgG, and C3 may be found in subendothelial deposits. Immunohistochemistry shows abundant staining for collagen type III in the expanded mesangium and thickened glomerular capillary walls.

Electron microscopy The extracellular space of the mesangium and subendothelial space of the GBM are markedly expanded, giving a lucent or lytic appearance to these structures. In both spaces, there is a marked accumulation of fibrillar material. The fibers have a transverse band structure, with a distinctive periodicity of approximately 60nm, exactly the same as that of type III collagen. The fibers tend to be curved or frayed, forming irregularly arranged bundles on longitudinal section and flower-like or ragged moth-eaten appearance on cross-section (see Atlas plate 20).

Pathogenesis

This disease is clearly related to abnormal subendothelial and mesangial deposits of collagen III Type III collagen is a ubiquitous structural protein of the extracellular matrix which is particularly abundant in tissues showing elastic properties, such as skin, blood vessels, and various internal organs. In normal human kidney, type III collagen is present in only the interstitium and blood vessels, but not in glomeruli. It may be found in the glomerular mesangium in patients with various types of glomerulonephritis and in the vascular pole in patients with progressive renal disease.

It is still unkown whether in collagenofibrotic glomerulopathy abnormal collagen originates from within the glomeruli or derives from an extrarenal source (Alchi et al., 2007). Collagen fibers in glomeruli often are located near mesangial cells, which can produce type III and IV collagen fibres. Experimental studies showed that IL-4 can stimulate the production of collagen III and cause glomerulosclerosis in transgenic mice suggesting its possible role for the over-production of type III collagen fibres. Glomerular epithelial cells potentially can synthesize collagen type III. However, it is unclear whether epithelial cells or even endothelial cells are responsible for the production and/or deposition of type III collagen fibers in this disease. Alternatively, type III collagen glomer-ulopathy might be a systemic disorder with abnormal metabolism of type III collagen. The finding of abnormally high serum PIIINP levels suggests the systemic nature of this condition, a hypothesis also supported by the rising of PIIINP after transplantation (Suzuki et al., 2004).

Etiology

The causes are entirely elusive. Although the disease is mostly sporadic, a few cases occurred in siblings whose parents had no renal disease. This led to the assumption that collagenofibrotic glomerulopathy is a genetic disease trans-mitted as an autosomal recessive trait (Gubler et al., 1993), but, as pointed out by Alchi et al., (2007) numbers of patients and kindreds analyzed to date have not allowed an inheritance pattern to be definitely established.

Clinical presentation

The disease can affect all age groups without difference in gender. The most common presenting feature is proteinuria that may reach the nephrotic range in approximately 60% of patients. About two-thirds of patients have hyperten-sion at the time of presentation. Anemia is frequent even before renal failure develops. The only specific laboratory finding is represented by elevated serum PIIINP levels.

Epidemiology

Most cases reported in the literature occurred in Asian patients, particularly in Japanese population. However cases have also been observed in Caucasian patients (Imbasciati et al., 1991; Gubler et al., 1993). Most cases occurred spo-radically, but familial cases transmitted according to an apparently autosomal recessive trait have also been described (Gubler et al., 1993).

Natural history

The disease is usually progressive, although it may follow a slow renal functional deterioration. Both in children and adults the nephropathy follows an unremitting course and may eventually lead to ESRD after several years. However, it is difficult to establish the long-term prognosis as in many cases the follow-up was relatively short. In a Japanese retrospective investigation on patients followed by different hospitals a 10-year renal survival of 49% was reported (Suzuki et al., 2004).

Specific treatment

Specific treatment is not available. Theoretically, glucocorticoids might be of some help as these agents may suppress type III collagen synthesis in the dermis. Hisakawa et al. (1998) treated with prednisolone (40mg/d) a 68-year-old Japanese man and reported some improvement of renal function, anemia, and proteinuria, which paralleled decreases in serum PIIINP levels.

Symptomatic treatment should be directed to control hypertension, correct anemia, and reduce proteinuria with ACE inhibitors and angiotensin receptor blockers (see also Chapter 1).

Practical recommendations

The diagnosis of this disease is quite difficult and it is easy to miss. Histological pattern may resemble that of a membranoproliferative glomerulonephritis, but in collageno-fibrotic disease there is no glomerular hypercellularity and at immunofluorescence, IgG and C3 deposits are scanty and focal, when present. With light microscopy a differential diagnosis with thrombotic microangiopathy may be difficult, but the clinical features and ultrastructural investigation may orientate towards a correct diagnosis. Amyloidosis may be ruled out as the collagen III deposits do not stain with Congo red or thyoflavin T. Electron microscopy is needed for a correct differential diagnosis with other fibrillary diseases. In type III collagen glomerulopathy, electron-dense immune complex-type deposits usually are not present; although subendothelial dense deposits can be seen infrequently. Unique microtubular structures as seen in immunotactoid glomerulopathy, fibrin, and amyloid fibrils are not observed. In contrast to nail-patella syndrome, the lamina densa of the glomerular basement membrane in patients with collagenofibrotic glomerulopathy is of normal thickness and lacks the lucent areas or so-called 'moth-eaten appearance.' Various degrees of effacement of epithelial foot processes usually are seen.

Unfortunately, however, when the diagnosis is made there is not an available specific treatment. A trial with glucocorticoids may be attempted, following proteinuria and serum PIIINP levels to evaluate the response. Otherwise patients should be given symptomatic therapy.

Transplantation

To the best of our knowledge, only one young Japanese woman received a kidney transplantation. Her post-operative course was uneventful with good renal function 3 years after transplantation. The immunosuppression consisted of methylprednisolone, tacrolimus, and basiliximab. Although urinary protein was negative, the serum level of PIIIP gradually increased suggesting new collagen production in the graft and the presence of a systemic factor that stimulated collagen III production (Suzuki et al., 2004).

Thin basement membrane nephropathy (Table 11.3)

Introduction and overview

Thin basement membrane nephropathy (TBMN), also called benign familial hematuria or benign essential hematuria, is a primary glomerular disorder characterized clinically by isolated microscopic hematuria and pathologically by diffuse uniform thinning of the glomerular basement membrane (GBM) on

Table 11.3 Main characteristics of thin basement membrane nephropathy (TBMN)

Pathology:	At optic microscopy the glomeruli appear normal. Immunofluorescence is negative. On electron microscopy there is an uniform thinning of GBM
Pathogenesis:	In TBMN there are defects of type IV collagen, a fundamental component of GBM
Etiology:	The disease is caused by a disorder of *COL4A3/CL4A4* genes which are responsible for the synthesis of collagen IV. In about half of cases there is an autosomal dominant transmission of the disease
Clinical presentation:	The disease is usually asymptomatic. It can be diagnosed by the discovery of a persistent dysmorphic hematuria or by an occasional macroscopic hematuria. Proteinuria is mild or absent. The differential diagnosis with Alport syndrome may be difficult. Type IV collagen chains α 3 to α 5 are usually absent in Alport syndrome
Prognosis:	Most patients do not show any progression of the disease but sporadic cases may develop proteinuria and progressive renal failure
Treatment:	No treatment is required. In the rare cases with proteinuria, ACE-inhibitors or angiotensin receptor blockers may be used

electron microscopy examination. In the majority of cases, TBMN is caused by a disorder of *COL4A3/COL4A4* genes responsible for the synthesis of the alpha 3/4 chains of type IV collagen, a fundamental component of GBM. TBMN is often discovered incidentally and usually has an excellent long-term prognosis. About 50% of cases of TBMN show a familial aggregation most often in an autosomal dominant pattern. Unlike X-linked Alport syndrome, affected father to affected son transmission may be seen. Occasionally some patients develop proteinuria and impaired renal function, but it is difficult to be certain that these patients did not have autosomal recessive Alport syndrome or hemizygous (female) X-linked Alport syndrome. Together with Alport syndrome and IgA nephritis, TBMN is one of the most frequent causes of microhematuria. Thin basement membranes may be observed in 1–10% of the population as a whole.

Pathology

Light microscopy The glomeruli appear normal or show mild mesangial cellular proliferation and matrix expansion. Slight attenuation of the GBM sometimes can be observed by Jones methenamine silver or periodic acid- Schiff stains, suggesting GBM thinning.

Immunofluorescence microscopy It is usually negative but there is sometimes positivity for IgM or C3 and rarely IgG or IgA.

Electron microscopy It reveals the typical feature of TBMN, i.e., thinning of the GBM (Fig 11.1). However, the diagnosis may be difficult as the GBM thickness varies with age, sex, and the different methods of tissue preparation and measurement (Foster et al., 2005). The GBM thinning in TBMN is uniform, it appears as a trilaminar structure with a central lamina densa an inner lamina rara interna, and an outer lamina rara externa. According to Churg et al. (1995) the threshold for assessing a thin GBM is 250nm for adults and 180nm for children between 2–11 years of age. According to Vogler et al. (1987), the criteria for TBMN in children vary between <200 and <250nm, and in adults from <200nm to <264nm. This variation is due to difficulties in standardizing the technical methods. Sometimes, rare regions are observed with lamellation or regional thickening, a feature typically seen in Alport syndrome. This may pose a problem in differentiating between TBMN and Alport syndrome, as electron microscopic analysis at early stages of Alport syndrome can reveal similar uniform thinning of the GBM (Tryggvason and Patrakka, 2006).

Immunohistochemical evaluation of the type IV collagen α3 to α5 chains in renal biopsy has become of major importance as a method to use in differentiating between TBMN and early stages of Alport syndrome with thin GBM,

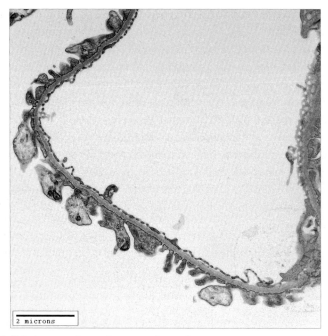

Fig. 11.1 Thin basement membrane nephropathy.

as these chains usually are either absent or abnormally distributed in Alport syndrome. Normal children and some patients with minimal change nephropathy or other glomerulonephritis may also show thin GBM but thinning is usually focal and not uniform as in TBMN.

Pathogenesis

In the majority of cases TBMN is a genetic disorder of type IV collagen mainly related to mutations in locus *COL4A3/COL4A4*. In many families the development of autosomal dominant TBMN involves heterozygous mutations in either *COL4A3 or COL4A4*, whereas homozygosity or combined heterozygosity of mutations in these genes results in autosomal recessive Alport syndrome. About 20 *COL4A3 or COL4A4* mutations have been found in TBMN. It is still unknown, however, what happens in families in whom hematuria does not segregate with the locus *COL4A3/COL4A4*. There are reports that a single heterozygous mutation in *COL4A3 or COL4A4* can cause Alport syndrome, suggesting that some mutations are particularly serious, but it cannot be excluded that in these cases, there is another unknown mutation somewhere else in the other allele or gene that could lead to absence of the chain. To date, too few mutations have been identified in TBMN and autosomal dominant Alport for making conclusions about the differences in pathogenesis (Tryggvason and Patrakka, 2006).

In summary, many different *COL4A3 and COL4A4* mutations may cause TBMN and autosomal recessive Alport syndrome. However, testing for *COL4A3 and COL4A4* mutations to diagnose TBMN is difficult because of the frequent polymorphism of these genes and the likelihood of a further gene locus. From a clinical point of view it is simpler to perform genetic testing to exclude or confirm an Alport syndrome, which is the disease that enters more frequently in the differential diagnosis with TBMN (Rana et al., 2005).

Etiology

In most cases, TBMN is an inherited disorder of type IV collagen. At least 50% of patients with TBMN have an autosomal dominant transmission. Type IV collagen is a specific triple-helical structural component of basement membranes. There are six distinct collagen IV α chains, α1 to α6 that are encoded, respectively, by the specific genes *COL4A1 to COL4A6*.The most common form of type IV collagen molecules contains α1 and α2 chains in a 2:1 ratio. In GBM, this form of collagen IV is replaced after birth by molecules with the chain composition α3:α4:α5. This isoform of collagen IV is essential for the integrity of GBM, as well as for some other specialized basement membranes in the inner ear and lens capsule. Patients with TBMN are heterozygous for mutations in either *COL4A3 or COL4A4*, and they represent a carrier status for autosomal recessive Alport syndrome, in a similar manner as female individuals with mutations in one *COL4A5* allele are carriers for X-linked Alport syndrome in male individuals.

Clinical presentation

TBMN is often diagnosed when there is persistent dysmorphic hematuria, with no or mild proteinuria, without other renal or extra-renal abnormalities. Many patients have relatives with isolated microhematuria. At least a single episode of macroscopic hematuria is observed in 5–22% of patients, typically manifesting after exercise or during infection The age at diagnosis varies considerably, from as early as age 1 year up to an elderly age. Occasionally, the hematuria has disappeared over time.

Epidemiology

TBMN is estimated to affect up to about 10% of the general population and has been reported in all geographic regions of the world and in all ancestries but most cases have been reported in developed countries. Hematuria has been diagnosed at all ages. It is still uncertain whether the disease is or is not more frequent in females. Exact prevalence of the disease is difficult to appreciate as not all the patients have persistent isolated microhematuria, many of them are not submitted to renal biopsy and electron microscopic analyses is performed only in a limited number of cases. This may explain a large disparity in the prevalence of TBMN in the general population that has been estimated to range between 1–10% (Tryggvason and Patrakka, 2006).

Natural history

TBMN is considered to be a benign disease. In the great majority of patients TBMN does not show any impairment of renal function over time. Some patients followed for up to 30 years maintained a persistent microhematuria, sometimes intervalled by episodes of macrohematuria. However, sporadic cases develop proteinuria and progressive renal failure. It is unclear whether these patients are affected by a form of TBMN caused by heterozygous *COL4A3 or COL4A4* mutations, by a disease caused by mutations of other genes, by a coexistent renal disease (particularly IgA nephritis), or by a misdiagnosed Alport syndrome (Gregory, 2005).

Specific treatment

Most patients with TBMN do not require any treatment. Patients showing signs of progressive renal disease may benefit from treatments that may reduce proteinuria, i.e., ACE-inhibitors, angiotensin-receptor blockers, and spironolactone (see Chapter 1).

Practical recommendations

The first problem for the nephrologist confronted by a patient with persistent microscopic hematuria is to accurately and fully assess the diagnosis. A careful study of the urine sediment by phase contrast microscopy showing >75–80% distorted (dysmorphic) red blood cells is very strongly suggestive of a glomerular disease. The finding of >4–5% acanthocytes (ring-formed cells with one or more protrusions of different shape and size) is essentially equivalent to a diagnosis of aglomerular disease. To ascertain the diagnosis of TBMN a renal biopsy with ultrastructural examination is absolutely necessary and indispensable. As pointed out earlier, the differential diagnosis with Alport syndrome may be difficult and the threshold for deciding whether GBM may be considered *thin* has been differently estimated and is variable with the age. Moreover, while many investigators think that in TBMN there is a uniform thinning of GBM, some investigators pointed out that a considerable number of patients with TBMN display segmental GBM attenuation (Ivanyi et al., 2006). Immunohistochemical evaluation of the type IV collagen α3 to α5 chains may help for the differential diagnosis as these chains are usually absent in Alport syndrome. Some clinical features may help in the differential diagnosis. Typical Alport syndrome findings, such as hearing loss, lenticonus, and, develop usually first during adolescence. Approximately 95% of the hemizygous female carriers of X-linked Alport syndrome have hematuria, but they cannot easily be distinguished from individuals with authentic TBMN, without a study of the presence of the alpha3-5 chains of type IV collagen in glomeruli, Bowman's capsule, tubular basement membrane, or skin basement membrane. However, knowledge about hearing loss, lenticonus, or retinopathy in other relatives can give a hint about X-linked Alport syndrome. Sequencing of the *COL4A3* and *COL4A4* genes is possible in specialized laboratories. It would be important to be able to provide DNA sequencing of the *COL4A3*, *COL4A4*, and *COL4A5* genes for making an accurate genetically-based diagnosis of TBMN and the various forms of Alport syndrome.

Despite the generally excellent outcome, very occasionally patients with apparent TBMN may develop renal function impairment, most often in association with the appearance of qualitatively abnormal proteinuria. It is therefore recommended that patients with a diagnosis of TBMN are regularly monitored, at least once a year, to check the absence of significant proteinuria, arterial hypertension and/or renal function impairment.

Transplantation

The few patients who develop end-stage renal failure and receive a renal transplant may show recurrence of TBMN on the allograft. However, the effects, if any, of the thinned membranes on allograft function remain unclear. It is possible that these 'recurrences' might be due to the inadvertent transmission of a 'latent' disease from an asymptomatic donor.

Lipoprotein glomerulopathy (Table 11.4)

Introduction and overview

Lipoprotein glomerulopathy (LPG) is a rare disorder in which lipoprotein thrombi are seen in glomerular capillaries. The disease may be familial or sporadic. It mainly affects Japanese or Chinese patients. The disease usually presents with proteinuria and hypertension, and frequently progresses to renal failure. Glomeruli on biopsy are large, and their capillaries contain pale-staining amorphous thrombi staining positive for lipid (Oil Red-O stains) in non-ethanol fixed specimens. Although total cholesterol, low-density lipoprotein (LDL), cholesterol, or triglyceride levels may be elevated, the only abnormality seen in every patient with lipoprotein glomerulopathy has been increased serum apolipoprotein E (apoE) levels.

Table 11.4 Main characteristics of lipoprotein glomerulopathy (LPG)

Pathology:	Light microscopy shows marked dilatation of the capillary lumen of glomeruli by a pale stained substance. On electron microscopy the substance appears composed by granules and vacuoles of various sizes forming concentric lamellae. Immunochemical studies show that there are deposits of apolipoproteins A, B, and E
Pathogenesis:	The disease probably results by interactions between genetic factors and kidney intrinsic factors. Abnormal apolipoprotein variants may concentrate and aggregate in the glomerular flow and may deposit in capillary walls or around the mesangium. Accumulation of abnormal lipoproteins may be facilitated by dysfunction of Fc receptors that dysregulate the uptake and clearance of lipoproteins
Etiology:	LPG is caused by mutations of apolipoproteins E that may diminish their capacity to bind to LDL receptor and may decrease their uptake from endothelial and mesangial cells
Clinical presentation:	Proteinuria and hypertriglyceridemia are constant features. Most patients present with a nephrotic syndrome
Prognosis:	About half of patients may develop end-stage renal disease but the rate of progression is extremely variable
Treatment:	Lipid-lowering agents including fibrates were able to halt the progression of the disease in a few patients

Pathology

Light microscopy the light microscopy shows marked dilatation of the capillary lumen in glomeruli filled by a pale stained substance. Foam cells rarely are seen in either glomeruli or interstitium (see Atlas plate 21).

Electron microscopy shows thrombus-like substances in glomerular capillaries, composed of granules and vacuoles of various sizes, forming concentric lamellae, like a fingerprint (see Atlas plate 22).

Immunohistochemical studies in snap-frozen renal sections, show deposition of apoB and apoE, and lipid droplets in the thrombus-like substances (Saito et al., 2006; Zhang et al., 2008).

Pathogenesis

The development of LPG is probably the result of interactions between genetic factors and kidney intrinsic factors. The trigger of the disease is an apoE variant called apoE Sendai. The substitution of proline (Arg145Pro) in apoE Sendai may produce severe structural changes in the middle of the helix in apoE and may alter the 3-dimensional conformation of the protein. These abnormal lipoproteins containing apoE Sendai may concentrate and aggregate in the glomerular flow and may deposit in capillary walls or around the mesangium. Some apoE variants of LPG, e.g., apoE Kyoto and apoE5(Gln3Lys), may produce lipid peroxidation and a direct damage to glomerulus. Moreover the negatively charged apoE variants cause hypetriglyceridemia, which in turn promotes the increase in apoE, apoC-III, and electronegative LDL. It should be also pointed out that apoE is synthesized in human kidney and regulates mesangial cell proliferation and matrix overproduction in experimental models. Therefore, apoE seems to act as an autocrine regulator of mesangial and glomerular function, and intrarenal dysfunction induced by apoE abnormality may contribute to the induction of LPG (Saito et al., 2006).

Intrinsic glomerular factors may also interact with apoE variants and lipoprotein abnormalities for induction of LPG. This hypothesis is also sustained by the association of LPG with other glomerulonephritis. A possible pathogenetic role may be played by a dysfunction of Fc receptors. A dysfunction of mesangial Fc receptors may dysregulate the uptake and clearance of LDL leading to the accumulation of lipoproteins in mesangial and endothelial cells, even in the absence of atherogenic changes (Kanamaru et al., 2002), with formation of lipoprotein thrombi, lipid granules, apoA and apoE deposits with a fingerprint pattern.

Etiology

Lipoprotein glomerulopathy is associated with novel mutations in apoE, the gene that encodes apolipoprotein E 2. This novel apoE variant (Arg145Pro) has been termed apoE Sendai, representing the name of the city where the patients lived (Oikawa et al., 1997). Subsequently, other apoE variants, apoE Kyoto, apoE Tokyo, apoE Maebashi, apoE Guangzhou, and apoE Tsukuba have been described in patients with LPG, although the majority had apoE Sendai. The discovery of novel mutants in apoE suggested that lipoproteins with these variants have an etiological role in LPG. Probably these mutations diminish the capacity of apolipoprotein E to bind to the low-density lipoprotein receptor and also decrease its uptake by endothelial and mesangial cells. The causative role of apoE mutations was confirmed by the demonstration that LPG may be induced by virus-mediated transduction of apoE Sendai in apoE-knockout mice (Saito et al., 2006).

Clinical presentation

Although the age at presentation may range from 4–69 years, most afflicted patients are in the third and fourth decades of life (Sam et al., 2006). Blood pressure in most patients is normal or moderately elevated. Protein excretion exceeds 1g/d in almost all patients, and about 60% of patients are nephritic and present with edemas. Microscopic hematuria mostly is absent. One-third of patients have impaired renal function at presentation. Most patients have hyperlipemia with predominance of triglycerides (Zhang et al., 2008). In detailed assays for plasma lipoproteins isolated by means of ultracentrifugation, high cholesterol levels in very-low-density and intermediate density lipoprotein fractions were observed. In the review of Sam et al. (2006) all except one patient had elevated plasma apoE levels (4.0 to 38mg/dL).

Epidemiology

According to Saito et al. (2006) a total of 65 cases have been reported before 2006. Of them, most were from the eastern area of Japan and some patients were Chinese. After that paper the number of reports from China and Taiwan increased. Only two French cases were patients of Caucasian origin but recently Rovin et al. (2007) described LPG in two American men of European ancestry. Among the reported cases, about one-third of patients had a positive family history.

Natural history

It is difficult to know the outcome for patients with LPG, as many of the described cases had a short-term follow-up. It is likely that most patients have a relentless course to end-stage renal failure. In the review of Saito et al. (2006) half the patients developed renal failure at 1–27 years after onset.

Specific treatment

Glucocorticoids immunosuppressants, and anticoagulants are ineffective. Intensive therapy using lipid-lowering agents, including fibrates, was reported to halt the progression of renal dysfunction in sporadic cases, although there was not any impact on proteinuria (Sam et al., 2006). In a patient, complete disappearance of lipoprotein thrombi was shown in serial renal biopsies, in addition to decreases in serum cholesterol, triglyceride, and apoE levels (Ieiri et al., 2003). These findings suggest that hyperlipidemia mediated by the environment also is an important factor in the development of LPG, although LPG essentially is based on the genetic abnormality of apoE.

Practical recommendations

LPG is an exceptionally rare disorder and its diagnosis can be easily missed. According to Saito et al. (2006) the diagnosis should be suspected in the presence of:

- Mild-to-severe proteinuria.
- Dilatation of glomerular capillary lumina with pale-stained substances on light microscopy.

◆ Stone or sand-like granules occupying the capillary lumina on electron microscopy (so-called lipoprotein thrombi).

◆ Type III HLP with high apoE concentration, usually associated with a heterozygous apoE phenotype, E2/3 or E2/4, but sometimes with an uncommon type, e.g., E1/3 or others.

Treatment of LPG should be based on symptomatic therapy (see Chapter 1), maximizing the doses of fibrates and statins, under strict surveillance of creatine-phosphokinase enzyme levels in the serum in order to detect and prevent rhabdomyolysis.

Transplantation

Recurrence has been reported in the few patients who received a kidney allograft either from living or deceased donors, suggesting a role for humoral components resulting from abnormal lipoprotein metabolism, probably linked to apolipoprotein E. Although the majority of patients lost their allograft after recurrence, a French woman with LPG has stable graft function 14 years after histological recurrence was documented (Mourad G, personal communication)

'Pure' mesangial proliferative glomerulonephritis
(Table 11.5)

Introduction and overview

'Pure' mesangial proliferative glomerulonephritis (MesPGN), as defined below, is an uncommon cause of primary glomerular disease. It is more often

Table 11.5 Main characteristics of 'pure' mesangial proliferative glomerulonephritis

Pathology:	Increased number of nucleated (presumably intrinsic mesangial) cells per glomerular lobule. Capillary walls thin and delicate. No necrosis or crescents. Ig and /or C3 in mesangium (but not IgA or IgM). Electron dense deposits in mesangium may be observed
Pathogenesis:	Unknown, but probably an 'immune-complex' mediated disease
Etiology:	Unknown, but some cases might be a resolving form of post-infectious glomerulonephritis.
Clinical presentation:	Usually glomerular hematuria with variable degrees of proteinuria, including the nephrotic syndrome.
Prognosis:	Variable. Persisting nephrotic syndrome may be a feature of an evolution to FSGS and progressive renal failure
Treatment:	Not well established. A trial of steroids, cytotoxic agents or calcineurin inhibitors may be indicated for severe nephrotic syndrome and/or a progressive course

associated with a variety of systemic illness, predominately SLE and other auto-immune diseases, and infections. 'Pure' MesPGN must also be separated from other primary glomerular diseases that can manifest pathologically as a diffuse mesangial proliferative lesion, including IgA nephropathy, IgM and C1q nephropathy (see Chapter 8 and below) that are distinguished based upon immunofluoresence microscopy patterns of Ig and complement component deposition. The group of disorders included in the rubric of 'pure' mesangial proliferative glomerulonephritis are undoubtedly very heterogeneous with respect to pathogenesis and etiology (Adler and Cohen, 2001). Considered here will be the collection of primary glomerular disorders having in common some degree of pathological mesangial cell hypercellularity unaccompanied by any disturbance in the architecture of the peripheral capillary wall, and in which IgA, IgM, and C1q nephropathy have been excluded by an appropriate immunofluorescence microscopy study of a renal biopsy. Thus, this group can also be separated from membranoproliferative glomerulonephritis (also known as mesangiocapillary glomerulonephritis) based on the absence of thickening or reduplication of the peripheral capillary walls of the glomeruli (see Chapter 9). Most of the patients falling to this category of primary glomer-ular disease will have some combination of proteinuria and hematuria, and nephrotic syndrome may also develop (Adler and Cohen, 2001). The out-come is highly variable, but a portion of the patients will progress to end-stage renal disease (ESRD), often with the development of persistent, steroid-resist-ant nephrotic syndrome and superimposed focal and segmental glomerular sclerosis (FSGS) or more rarely crescentic glomerulonephritis (see Chapters 6 and 10).

Pathology

Light microscopy Mesangial hypercellularity is usually defined by ≥ three nucleated (non-polymorphonuclear, non-monocytic) cells (presumptively mesangial cells) per mesangial zone or lobule. In MesPGN the hypercellularity is rather uniformly expressed among all of the lobules, although it varies in degree. (see Atlas plate 23). Necrosis, exudation (presence of circulating poly-morph nuclear or monocytic leukocytes) segmental sclerosis, adhesions, cres-cents, and thickening of the periphery of the capillary walls are absent. Milder degrees of mesangial hypercellularity are quite common in other primary glomerular diseases, including Minimal change lesion (Andal, et al., 1989).

Immunofluorescence microscopy According to the definition used here, deposits of IgA, IgM, or C1q should be absent or inconspicuous. However, deposits of polyclonal IgG and/or C3 may be evident, and a fraction of cases have no immune deposits (Orfila, et al, 1980; Sato et al., 1993). Those cases with C3-only deposits may represent stages of an acute, post-infectious (streptococcal) glomerulonephritis (see Chapter 4). Isolated C3 deposits may also be seen in a rare form of membranoproliferative glomerulonephritis associated with abnormalities in the complement regulatory protein H (CFH) (see Chapter 9). Monoclonality of the IgG deposits strongly suggests an underlying monoclonal immunoglobulin deposition disease.

Electron microscopy The hypercellularity of the mesangium can be easily demonstrated. Electron dense deposits are quite variable, but often present. There may be focal effacement of the podocytes, but when this is very extensive the diagnosis of minimal change lesion or FSGS (see Chapters 5 and 6) should be considered, especially when the mesangial hypercellularity is mild or moderate and when diffuse foot process effacement is observed in electron microscopy.

Pathogenesis

The pathogenesis of MesPGN is largely unknown. When polyclonal IgG deposits are present by IF microscopy and electron dense deposits found by EM, then an immune-complex mediated disorder can be suspected. Very rarely linear deposits of IgG are found by IF, possibly indicating a role for anti-GBM auto-antibodies.

Etiology

The etiology of MesPGN is unknown, but the clinical and pathological features often suggest that an infectious disease is involved in some fashion. The late discovery of MesPGN with isolated deposits of C3 and persistent hematuria may suggest a resolving form of post-streptococcal glomerulonephritis (see Chapter 4).

Clinical presentation

The typical presentation of MesPGN is a combination of glomerular hematuria and proteinuria. Nephrotic syndrome may be present (Bhasin et al, 1978). Renal function is typically normal, but progression of disease may be seen, especially if the lesion 'evolves' to one of FSGS. Complement levels are normal and serological evaluation for SLE, vasculitis, monoclonal paraprotein diseases, and infection should be negative. Many patients have isolated recurrent gross or microscopic hematuria with minimally elevated levels of urinary protein excretion. Since renal biopsies are seldom carried out in these clinical situations, the overall occurrences of MesPGN may have been underestimated.

Epidemiology

The incidence and prevalence of MesPGN is not well known. Among patients presenting with nephrotic syndrome it is quite uncommon, accounting for

<5% of cases (Adler and Cohen, 2001). Mild degrees of mesangial proliferation may accompany other lesions such as the minimal change lesion and focal and segmental glomerulosclerosis, so it is possible that some cases may mistakenly be assigned to the category of MesPGN, at least initially. As stated above, IgA nephropathy, IgM nephropathy, C1q nephropathy, SLE and resolving post-infectious glomerulonephritis need to be excluded. Ascertainment bias (indications for renal biopsy) may contribute to the relative infrequency of MesPGN in descriptions of prevalence.

Natural history

The evolution of MesPGN is not well understood. It is very clear that some patients may evolve into a picture of typical FSGS (particularly when there are diffuse mesangial deposits of IgM, see below). When the mesangial cell proliferation is mild, many cases cannot be clinically distinguished from the evolution of the minimal change lesion (Andal, et al., 1989) Spontaneous remission may develop, but more often the disease persists and if nephrotic syndrome is present, progression to focal and segmental glomerulosclerosis and renal failure is more common. Patients with isolated glomerular hematuria or those with minimal degrees of proteinuria tend to have a benign evolution.

Specific treatment

Due to the absence of randomized, prospective controlled trials of therapy for MesPGN, the efficacy and safety of various proposed treatment regimens are very uncertain (Adler and Cohen, 2001). Due to their likely benign prognosis, patients with isolated microscopic hematuria or those with minimal degrees of proteinuria (<1.0g/d) probably do not require any therapy, other than vigorous control of blood pressure. Those with nephrotic syndrome have usually been treated with oral glucocorticoids in a fashion similar to that described for FSGS (see Chapter 6). A response (partial or complete remission) is observed in about 50–70% of patients so treated. A role for cytotoxic agents, such as cyclophosphamide, azathioprine or mycophenolate mofetil (MMF) is unknown, but many patients resistant to the effects of glucocorticoids and with persistent nephrotic syndrome and worsening renal function are offered these options, with variable results. Calcineurin inhibitor therapy (cyclosporin or tacrolimus) has been anecdotally effective, particularly when there is a high suspicion of an underlying FSGS.

Practical recommendations

Patients with 'pure' MesPGN and isolated hematuria and/or minimal proteinuria do not require any specific therapy, other than control of blood pressure. Those with more severe degrees of proteinuria, including nephrotic syndrome, should be given a trial of oral glucocorticoids similar to that recommended for FSGS (see Chapter 6). If the patient proves to be 'steroid-resistant' and still has relatively well-preserved renal function (serum creatinine of <2.0mg/dL) a trial of either oral cyclophosphamide or a calcineurin inhibitor could be considered. Calcineurin inhibitors might be preferred if the biopsy showed lesions suspicious for FSGS, while cyclophosphamide might be preferred if the findings on renal biopsy were more suggestive of a minimal change lesion. A therapeutic role for MMF or azathioprine is quite uncertain.

Transplantation

The risk for a recurrence of the original disease in renal transplants is unknown. However, since many cases originally diagnosed with MesPGN may 'evolve' into a picture of focal and segmental glomerulosclerosis, it may be presumed that a risk of recurrence is quite real. Indeed, patients with FSGS who also have superimposed MesPGN may have an increased risk for recurrent disease in the renal transplant (see Chapter 6).

IgM nephropathy (Table 11.6)

Introduction and overview

The lesion of *IgM nephropathy* was first described by Cohen, Border, and Glassock in 1978 (Cohen et al, 1978). This original description incited much controversy since deposits of IgM were often found 'non-specifically' in many

Table 11.6 Main characteristics of IgM nephropathy

Pathology:	Diffuse and generalized mesangial IgM deposition, often with C3 in the same distribution accompanied by a light microscopic appearance of mesangial proliferative glomerulonephritis. Electron dense deposits present in the mesangium
Pathogenesis:	Unknown. Thought to be an immune-complex disease, but IgM deposition may be 'non-specific'
Etiology:	Unknown. No known infectious agent produces this lesion. Can be associated with focal and segmental glomerulosclerosis
Clinical presentation:	Often with glomerular hematuria and/or nephrotic syndrome
Prognosis:	Progressive if associated with persisting nephrotic syndrome. May evolve to a picture of focal and segmental glomerulosclerosis over time
Treatment:	Not well understood. Some patients (50%) may respond to steroids and /or cytotoxic agents. Treatment programs are similar to those used for primary focal and segmental glomerulosclerosis

disorders, including minimal change lesion and focal and segmental glomerulosclerosis (Pardo, et al, 1984; Andal, et al., 1989). Thus, some held that IgM nephropathy was not a 'clinico-pathologic' entity (Kasap, et al., 2008). However, the diagnosis of *IgM nephropathy* is more properly restricted to a group of patients manifesting: i) hematuria and variable degrees of proteinuria, including the nephrotic syndrome; ii) renal biopsies demonstrating variable but distinct degrees of mesangial proliferation without obvious segmental sclerosis; iii) diffuse and generalized mesangial deposits of IgM accompanied by discrete electron dense deposits in the mesangium. Many authors agree that if these criteria are fulfilled then a distinctive natural history and response to treatment can be delineated (Lawler et al, 1980; Helin et al, 1982). Widely scattered mesangial IgM deposits in a biopsy that reveals features quite compatible with the minimal change lesion are not sufficient to define *IgM nephropathy*. In addition, a renal biopsy which reveals the characteristic features of FSGS and also shows segmental deposits of IgM is not *IgM nephropathy*. Thus, in part, a diagnosis of IgM nephropathy is one of exclusion. Many, indeed most, patients with *IgM nephropathy* will also display features of MesPGN (see above) and vice versa, thus there is substantial overlap between MesPGN and IgM nephropathy in the literature. Rarely, IgM nephropathy may present as a familial disorder (Scolari, et al., 1990), including an association with familial Mediterranean fever (Said and Hamzeh, 1990).

Pathology

Light microscopy The glomeruli appear hypercellular in the mesangial zones, but the peripheral capillary walls are thin, delicate, and free of proteinacious deposits. No focal and segmental glomerulosclerosis should be observed, but there may be a variable increase in the mesangial matrix. Variable degrees of tubulo-interstitial fibrosis and/or mononuclear cell infiltration can be seen.

Immunofluorescence microscopy By definition, heavy diffuse and generalized deposits of IgM must be present in the mesangial zones (Fig 11.2). Lesser degrees of IgG and or IgA may also be seen. C3 and C1q deposition are quite common and may be intense. The C3 deposits are in the same pattern as the IgM deposits.

Electron microscopy Small discrete electron dense deposits are regularly found in the mesangium, but there are no deposits in or on the capillary walls. Variable degrees of an increase in mesangial matrix and mesangial cell proliferation are also observed. The podocytes are effaced but not uniformly, unless severe proteinuria is present. Extensive and diffuse podocyte effacement with a more focal distribution of IgM and no electron dense deposits by electron

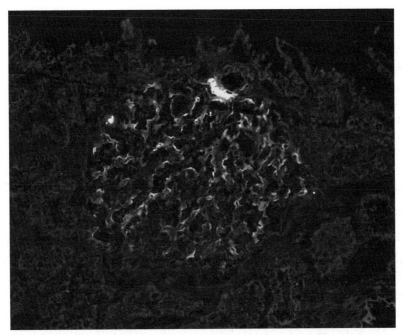

Fig. 11.2 IgM nephropathy (anti-IgM antibody fluorescent conjuguates).

microscopy should suggest a minimal change lesion with superimposed non-specific IgM deposition, instead of IgM nephropathy.

Pathogenesis

The pathogenesis of IgM nephropathy is unknown. It is possible that the deposits represent 'immune-complexes' to an undefined autogenous or exogenous antigen.

Etiology

The etiology of IgM nephropathy is unknown.

Clinical presentation

The clinical presentation of IgM nephropathy is quite varied. Some patients may present with only hematuria and variable degrees of proteinuria (Myllymäki et al., 2003). A larger number of patients present with more severe proteinuria, including the nephrotic syndrome, frequently accompanied by microscopic hematuria. Serum C3 levels are normal (or sometimes elevated) and there is no serological evidence of a systemic 'auto-immune,' neoplastic or infectious disease. IgM levels may be elevated, but IgA levels are normal. Renal function is typically normal at presentation but may progress to severe degree of renal impairment or even ESRD. Various ages may be affected and males are affected twice as commonly as females. Rarely a familial aggregation may be observed. Rare cases associated with familial Mediterranean fever have been reported.

Epidemiology

IgM nephropathy accounts for about 10% of all primary glomerular diseases in adults, however, this may be an overestimate since it includes some patients with minimal change disease or FSGS and 'non-specific' IgM deposition. It apparently has a world-wide distribution. There is no evidence that it is increasing in frequency unlike focal and segmental glomerulosclerosis.

Natural history

The natural history of the untreated disorder is not well understood since most reports included patients who were actively treated. It does seem clear that many patients evolve over time into a picture more compatible with focal and segmental glomerulosclerosis (Zeis, et al., 2001). Some patients may remain stable for many years (Vangelista, et al, 1981).Over a 15-year follow up period about 40–60% can be expected to develop some degree of renal impairment and 20–30% will reach ESRD (O'Donoghue, et al, 1991). The outcome is much poorer for those with persistent nephrotic syndrome than those presenting with hematuria and/or low-grade proteinuria. A high serum C3 level may predict a poor outcome (Myllymäki et al., 2006). Spontaneous remissions may occur, but are rather infrequent. Interstitial fibrosis and global glomerulosclerosis indicate a less favorable outcome.

Specific treatment

In the absence of controlled trials, it is difficult to determine the efficacy of treatment. In retrospective, uncontrolled observations about 60% of patients presenting with the nephrotic syndrome will be responsive to steroids, and frequent relapses and steroid dependence may commonly develop (Zeis et al., 2001; Myllymäki et al., 2003). Cytotoxic drugs may be helpful in the steroid resistant cases, but this has not been documented by randomized trials. A role for calcineurin inhibitor or MMF therapy is unknown. A complete or partial remission is associated with an improved prognosis.

Practical recommendations

Patients with isolated hematuria and/or minimal proteinuria need not be treated other than to control blood pressure, if elevated. Patients with nephrotic syndrome should receive a trial of oral glucocorticoids using the regimen described for treatment of focal and segmental glomerulosclerosis (Chapter 6). Relapsing diseases should be treated in the manner described for the minimal change lesion (Chapter 5). Steroid-resistant cases could be given a trial of oral cyclophosphamide (10–12 weeks) or a calcineurin inhibitor (6 months) but the overall effectiveness for this approach is not well understood.

Transplantation

The risk of recurrence of IgM nephropathy in the renal transplant is probably similar to that described for MesPGN (see above). Patients who 'evolve' into a picture of steroid-resistant FSGS probably have an appreciable risk of recurrence of the original disease in renal allograft (perhaps approaching 30–40%) (see also Chapter 6).

C1q nephropathy (Table 11.7)

Introduction and overview

The clinico-pathologic entity known as *C1q nephropathy* was first described by Jennette and Hipp in 1985 (Jennette and Hipp, 1985a,b; Jennette and Falk, 2001). Like IgA nephropathy and IgM nephropathy it is defined by immunofluorescence examination of renal biopsy material. Such studies reveal the characteristic presence of heavy deposits of C1q in the glomerular mesangium usually accompanied by IgG and/or IgM and by C3 in a similar distribution. The disease is uncommon and has a predilection for children and young adults (particularly African-Americans). By definition, no clinical or laboratory features indicative of a systemic 'auto-immune' disease (such as SLE) are present, and nephrotic syndrome with progressive renal failure is common. Patients with

Table 11.7 Main characteristics of C1q nephropathy

Pathology:	Marked deposition of C1q, often with immunoglobulins, resembling lupus nephritis (but without any serological features of SLE). Light microscopy findings highly variable but focal and segmental glomerulosclerosis, mesangial proliferation and membranoproliferative patterns most common
Pathogenesis:	Unknown. May be an immune complex mediated disease
Etiology:	Unknown. Lesion has features suggesting SLE but serology and clinical findings routinely negative for an auto-immune disease
Clinical presentation:	Nephrotic syndrome with hematuria and progressive renal failure are common
Prognosis:	Variable, but often poor especially in the presence of persisting nephrotic syndrome
Treatment:	Uncertain. Most patients are resistant to therapy

C1q nephropathy are not infrequently labeled as 'sero-negative' lupus nephritis (Sharman et al, 2004).

Pathology

Light microscopy The features by light microscopy are quite varied and can include minimal change lesion, MesPGN, or focal and segmental glomerulosclerosis (Jennette and Hipp, 1985b). The latter lesion is the most common in most series (Markowitz et al, 2003). Some investigators believe that C1q nephropathy should be classified as a 'variant' of 'idiopathic' FSGS (see Chapter 6). Collapsing lesions have been observed but necrosis and crescents are uncommon, seen in <5% of cases.

Immunofluorescence microscopy The characteristic feature is intense granular or amorphous deposition of C1q in the mesangial and in a few capillary loops (Jennette and Hipp, 1985b). Polyclonal IgG and IgM along with C3 deposits are also seen in 85–95% of cases. IgA deposition is much less frequent.

Electron microscopy Mesangial electron-dense deposits are found quite frequently and the peripheral capillary walls show only a few deposits. Tubuloreticular inclusions are seen rarely (in contra-distinction to lupus nephritis) (Sharman et al., 2004).

Pathogenesis

The pathogenesis of **C1q nephropathy** is unknown but all of the immunopathologic features of the disorder suggest that deposition or in-situ formation of immune complexes, involving an unknown antigen, are involved. Some suggest that C1q nephropathy is a part of the spectrum of minimal change lesion and focal and segmental glomerulosclerosis (Markowitz et al, 2003) and that the C1q and Ig deposits are a "non-specific" feature of abnormal protein traffic across the glomerular capillary bed.

Etiology

The etiology of C1q nephropathy is unknown.

Clinical presentation

The clinical features of C1q nephropathy are quite varied, but proteinuria, often in the nephrotic range is very characteristic (Jennette and Hipp, 1985b; Lau et al., 2005). Hypertension is present in about 50% of patients. Signs and laboratory features of a systemic (auto-immune) disease (such as SLE) are uniformly absent, by definition. Males outnumber females by about 1.8 to 1. African-Americans are more commonly affected. Any age may be affected, but most cases are seen in children and in young adults. A presentation with asymptomatic urinary abnormalities in children is uncommon (Nishida, 2005). Rarely, acute nephritic syndrome with hypocomplementemia may be the presenting features (Imai et al., 1996). Renal insufficiency at the time of presentation is quite frequent. The C3 levels are nearly always normal, and anti-C1q auto antibodies are absent (unlike lupus nephritis). Very rarely a vasculitis, tubulo-interstitial nephritis and hypocomplementemia may be observed (Imai et al, 1996). Familial cases have been described.

Epidemiology

C1q nephropathy is an uncommon condition. It accounts for <3% of all forms of primary nephrotic syndrome of all ages (Jennette and Hipp, 1985b; Markowitz et al., 2003). It is more common in African-Americans, in children, and young adults. It apparently has a world-wide distribution, but most cases have been reported from the USA.

Natural history

Persisting proteinuria and nephrotic syndrome is the rule. Spontaneous remissions are uncommon, but have been reported to occur (Nishida et al., 2000), perhaps more frequently in children. Renal insufficiency is eventually seen in the majority of cases, and the 3 year renal survival is about 80% (Kersnik Levart et al., 2005; Fukuma et al, 2006;) A lesion of focal segmental glomerulosclerosis portends a poor outcome.

Specific treatment

The treatment of C1q nephropathy is uncertain, but most studies have indicated that a poor response to glucocorticoid therapy (10-20% compete or partial remission) is to be expected (Jennette and Hipp, 1985b; Markowitz et al., 2003). Patients with the minimal change lesion may respond better than those with the lesion of FSGS. Glucocorticoid therapy may be associated with a somewhat higher likelihood of a partial remission, but no controlled trials are available to validate this effect. The benefits or lack thereof for cytotoxic drugs, MMF or calcineurin inhibits is not known. Impaired renal function at presentation usually will indicate unresponsiveness to therapy.

Practical recommendations

A trial of oral glucocorticoids similar to that described for treatment of FSGS (see Chapter 6) would seem to be indicated unless contraindications exist. A better response to this therapy would be expected in those with the minimal change lesion than those with an underlying lesion of FSGS. No clear rationale exists for the use of cytotoxic drugs, MMF or calcineurin inhibitors. A complete or partial remission to therapy would likely be associated with an improved long-term outcome. Patients with persistent proteinuria should be treated with ACE inhibitors and/or angiotensin receptor blockers.

Transplantation

No reports of recurrence of C1q nephropathy in a renal allograft have yet appeared. However, it is possible that some of the recurrences reported in patients with 'primary' or 'idiopathic' focal and segmental glomerulosclerosis may have been in patients with unrecognized C1q nephropathy in which immunofluorescence microscopy was not performed.

Idiopathic nodular glomerulosclerosis (Table 11.8)

Introduction and overview

This recently recognized clinico-pathologic entity is characterized by glomerular lesions virtually indistinguishable from the diabetes-related Kimmelstiel–Wilson lesions but developing in the absence of any abnormality in glucose homeostasis (Herzenberg et al., 1999; Markowitz et al., 2002; Navantheethan et al., 2005; Nasr and D'Agati, 2007). In addition, other lesions causing 'nodules' to form in the intercapillary zones of the glomeruli, such as kappa light chain glomerulopathy, other monoclonal immunoglobulin deposition diseases, idiopathic and secondary membranoproliferative glomerulonephritis type I,

Table 11.8 Main characteristics of idiopathic nodular glomerulosclerosis

Pathology:	Intercapillary nodular and diffuse mesangial sclerosis, closely resembling the diabetes-related Kimmelstiel–Wilson lesion by light, immunofluorescent and electron microscopy. Diabetes, monoclonal immunoglobulin deposition diseases (kappa light chain nephropathy), thrombotic microangiopathy and membranoproliferative glomerulonephritis must be excluded. A diagnosis of exclusion only.
Pathogenesis:	Unknown, but believed to be due to chronic or intermittent endothelial cell injury
Etiology:	Unknown. Thought to be due to glomerular endothelial cell injury from cigarette smoking and/or intermittent hypoxia
Clinical presentation:	Proteinuria, nephrotic syndrome, and progressive renal failure are observed. Hypertension is common but glucose intolerance and proliferative retinopathy are absent (by definition)
Prognosis:	Generally poor. Progression to ESRD is common. No spontaneous remissions.
Treatment:	None available other than control of blood pressure and proteinuria with agents affecting the rennin–angiotensin–aldosterone system

chronic thrombotic microangiopathy (including atypical hemolytic uremia syndrome), and fibrillary glomerulonephritis must be excluded. It is a quite rare disorder, occurring in <0.5% of native renal biopsy specimens.

Pathology

Light microscopy The glomeruli reveal diffuse and nodular mesangial sclerosis, and thickening of the glomerular basement membrane (Markowitz et al., 2002) (see Atlas plate 24). Severe, arteriolo- and arterial-nephrosclerosis is also present. Abnormalities of the endothelial cells and 'neo-vascularization' is common in the glomeruli, but lacking in the retina. Congo red stains for amyloid are negative.

Immunofluorescence microscopy Glomerular deposits of immunoglobulin or complement are lacking but linear albumin deposits may be present.

Electron microscopy Electron dense deposits are absent. No fibrillary deposits are seen. The mesangium is greatly expanded and the glomerular basement membrane is thickened.

Pathogenesis

The pathogenesis of idiopathic nodular glomerulosclerosis is unknown. Certain features suggest prominent injury to endothelial cells with attempts at repair (neovascularization) (Markowitz et al., 2002; Nasr and D'Agati, 2007). Exactly why the lesion is confined to the kidney is a mystery.

Etiology

The etiology of idiopathic nodular glomerulosclerosis is unknown. The strong association to excessive and prolonged cigarette smoking has suggested that a primary chronic or recurring injury to the endothelium induced by components of cigarette smoke combined with transient hypoxia, even in the absence of an abnormality in glucose homeostasis, can give rise to lesions resembling diabetic nodular glomerulosclerosis (Nasr and D'Agati, 2007).

Clinical presentation

The patients are typically over age 65 years, male or female and have had long-standing hypertension (Markowitz et al., 2002). A history of diabetes is typically absent. A history of heavy smoking can almost invariably also be obtained. Renal insufficiency, heavy proteinuria (including the nephrotic syndrome) and hypertension are very common. Blood sugar and hemoglobin A1c are normal. Complement levels are normal. No monoclonal immunoglobulin paraproteins are present in serum or urine. Hypercholesterolemia and extra-renal vascular disease is also very common (most probably secondary to hypertension and smoking).

Epidemiology

The disorder is rather uncommon having been seen in <0.5% of a large renal biopsy series from Columbia University, New York (Markowitz et al, 2002). Males and females appear to be about equally affected, but most are older adults. The lesion has not yet been observed in children. Its geographic distribution is unknown.

Natural history

A progressive course to ESRD is seen in >50% of patients. The median time from biopsy to ESRD was only about 2 years in the Columbia University series of 23 patients. Elevated serum creatinine at discovery and persistent nephrotic range proteinuria are indicators of an adverse prognosis. Spontaneous remissions are very infrequent if they occur at all.

Specific treatment

There is no known treatment for this condition other than stopping smoking and treatment of the hyperlipidemia and hypertension. Inhibition of the angiotensin II system is indicated in all cases.

Practical recommendations

There is no proven effective therapy for this condition. All patients should be strongly encouraged to stop smoking and should have their blood pressure brought under strict control, (<130/80mmHg) preferably with inhibitors of angiotensin II or renin. There are no indications for the use of glucocorticoids or cytotoxic agents.

Transplantation

No information is yet available regarding the recurrence of this disorder in the renal allograft. Kappa light chain disease, which may mimic this disorder, is well known to recur in the renal allograft (Ots et al., 2001, and may easily be mistaken for the *idiopathic* form of nodular glomerulosclerosis if the abnormal monoclonal light chains (usually kappa) are not sought for in serum and urine.

References

Adler SG and Cohen AH. (2001). Mesangial Proliferative glomerulonephritis. In S Massry and R Glassock (eds), *Textbook of Nephrology*, 4th edn, pp.717–19., Lippincott, Williams and Wilkins, Philadelphia, PA.

Alchi B, Nishi S, Narita I, Gejyyo F (2007). Collagenofibrotic Glomerulopathy: Clinicopathologic overview of a rare glomerular disease. *American Journal of Kidney Diseases* **49**:499–506.

Alpers CE, Kowalewska J (2008). Fibrillary Glomerulonephritis and Immunotactoid Glomerulopathy. *Journal of the American Society of Nephrology* **19**:34–7.

Andal A, Saxena S, Chellani HK, et al. (1989). Pure mesangial proliferative glomerulonephritis: A clinicopathologic analysis and its possible role in morphologic transition of minimal change lesions. *Nephron* **51**:314–19.

Bhasin HK, Abuelo JG, Nayak R, et al. (1978). Mesangial proliferative glomerulonephritis. *Laboratory Investigation* **39**:21–9.

Bridoux F, Hugue V, Coldefy O et al. (2002). Fibrillary glomerulonephritis and immunotactoid (microtubular) glomerulopathy are associated with distinct immunologic features. *Kidney International* **62**:1764–75.

Churg J, Bernstein J, Glassock R (1995). *Renal Disease: Classification and Atlas of Glomerular Diseases* 2nd edn., Igaku- Shoin, New York.

Cohen AH, Border WA, Glassock RJ (1978). Nephrotic syndrome with glomerular mesangial IgM deposits. *Laboratory Investigation* **38**:610–19.

Collins M, Navaneethan SD, Chung M et al. (2008). Rituximab treatment of fibrillary glomerulonephritis. *American Journal of Kidney Diseases* **52**:9958–62.

Fogo A, Qureshi N, Horn RG (1993). Morphologic and clinical features of fibrillary glomerulonephritis versus immunotactoid glomerulopathy. *American Journal of Kidney Diseases* **22**:367–77.

Foster K, Markowitz GS, D'Agati VD (2005). Pathology of thin basement membrane nephropathy. *Seminars in Nephrology* **25**:149-58.

Fukuma Y, Hisano S, Segawa Y, et al. (2006). Clinicopathologic correlations of C1q nephropathy in children. *American Journal of Kidney Diseases* **47**:412–18.

Gough J, Yilmaz A, Yilmaz S, et al. (2005).Recurrent and de novo glomerular immune-complex deposits in renal transplant biopsies. *Archives Pathology Laboratory Medicine* **129**:231–3.

Gregory MC (2005). The clinical features of thin basement membrane nephropathy. *Seminars in Nephrology* **25**:140–5.

Gubler MC, Dommergues JP, Foulard M, et al. (1993). Collagen type III glomerulopathy: a new type of hereditary nephropathy. *Pediatric Nephrology* **7**:354–60.

Helin H, et al. (1982). IgM-associated glomerulonephritis. *Nephron* **31**:11–16.

Herzenberg AM, Holden JK, Singh S, et al. (1999). Idioapthic nodular glomerulosclerosis. *American Journal of Kidney Diseases* **34**:560-564.

Hisawaka N, Yasuoka N, Nishiya K, et al. (1998). Collagenofibrotic glomeulonephropathy associated with immune complexes. *American Journal Nephrology* **18**: 134–41.

Ieiri N, Hotta O, Taguma Y (2003). Resolution of typical lipoprotein glomerulopathy by intensive lipid-lowering therapy. *American Journal of Kidney Diseases* **41**:244–9.

Imai H, Yasuda T, Satoh K, et al. (1996). Pan-nephritis (glomerulonephritis, arteriolitis and tubulo-interstitial nephritis) associated wtih predominant mesangial C1q deposition and hypocomplementemai: a variant type of C1q nephropathy. *American Journal of Kidney Diseases* **27**:583–7.

Imbasciati E, Gherardi G, Morozumi K, et al. (1991).Collagen type III glomerulopathy: a new idiopathic glomerular disease. *American Journal Nephrology* **11**:422–9.

Ivanyi B, Degrell P (2004). Fibrillary glomerulonephritis and immunotactoid glomerulopathy. *Nephrology Dialysis Transplantation* **19**:2166–70.

Ivanyi B, Pap R, Ondrik Z (2006). Thin basement membrane nephropathy: diffuse and segmental types. *Archives of Pathology & Laboratory Medicine* **130**:1533–7.

Jennette JC, Hipp CG (1985a). Immunohistological evaluation of C1q in 800 renal biopsy specimens. *American Journal of Clinical Pathology* **83**:415–20.

Jennette JC, Hipp CG (1985b). C1q nephropathy: a distinct pathologic entity usually causing nephrotic syndrome. *American Journal of Kidney Diseases* **6**:103–10.

Jennette JC, Falk RJ (2001). C1q Nephropathy. In S Massry and R Glassock (eds), *Textbook of Nephrology*, 4th edn, pp.730–133, Lippincott, Williams and Wilkins, Philadelphia, PA.

Kanamaru Y, Nakao A, Shirato I, et al. (2002). Chronic graft-versus host autoimmune disease in Fc receptor γ chain-deficient mice results in lipoprotein glomerulopathy. Journal of the American Society of Nephrology 13:1527–33.

Kasap B, Türkmen M, Sarioğlu S, et al. (2008). The relation of IgM deposition to clinical parameters and histomorphometry in childhood mesangial proliferative glomerulonephritis. Pathology, Research and Practice 204:149–53.

Kersnik Levart T, Kenda RB, Avgustin Cavić M, et al. (2005). C1q nephropathy in children. *Pediatric Nephrology* **20**:1756–61.

Lau KK, Gaber LW, Delos Santos NM, et al. (2005). C1q nephropathy: features at presentation and outcome. *Pediatric Nephrology* **20**:744–9.

Lawler W, Williams G, Tarpey P, et al. (1980). IgM associated primary diffuse mesangial proliferative glomerulonephritis. *Journal of Clinical Pathology* **33**:1029–38.

Markowitz GS, Lin J, Valeri AM, et al. (2002). Idiopathic nodular glomerulosclerosis is a distinct clinico-pathologic entity linked to hypertension and smoking. *Human Pathology* **33**:826–35.

Markowitz GS, Schwimmer JA, Stokes MB, et al. (2003). C1q nephropathy: a variant of focal segmental glomerulosclerosis. *Kidney International* **64**:1232–40.

Myllymäki J, Saha H, Mustonen J et al. (2003). IgM nephropathy: clinical picture and long-term prognosis. *American Journal of Kidney Diseases* **41**:343–50.

Myllymäki J, Saha H, Pasternack A, et al. (2006). High serum C3 predicts poor outcome in IgM nephropathy. *Nephron. Clinical Practice* **102**:c122–7.

Navantheethan SD, Singh S, Choudry W. (2005). Nodular glomerulosclerosis in a non-diabetic patient: case report and review of the literature. *Journal of Nephrology* **18**:613–15.

Nasr SH and D'Agati VD (2007). Nodular glomerulosclerosis in the non-diabetic smoker. *Journal of the American Society of Nephrology* **18**:2032–6.

Nishida M, Kawakatsu H, Komatsu H, et al. (2000). Spontaneous improvement in a case of C1q nephropathy. *American Journal of Kidney Diseases* **35**:E22.

Nishida M, Kawakatsu H, Okumura Y, et al. (2005). C1q nephropathy with asymptomatic urine abnormalities. *Pediatric Nephrology* **20**:1669–70.

O'Donoghue DJ, et al. (1991). IgM-associated primary diffuse mesangial proliferative glomerulonephritis: natural history and prognostic indicators. *Quarterly Journal of Medicine* **79**:333–50.

Oikawa S, Matsunaga A, Saito T, et al. (1997). Apolipoprotein E Sendai (arginine 145!proline): A new variant associated with lipoprotein glomerulopathy. Journal American Society Nephrology 8:820–3.

Orfila C, Pieraggi MT, Suc JM. (1980). Mesangial isolated C3 deposition in patients with recurrent or persistent hematuria. Laboratory Investigations **43**:1–8.

Ots, M, Kulla A, Luman M, et al. (2000) Non-diabetic nodular glomerulosclerosis recurring in a renal graft. Nephrology Dialysis Transplantation **15**:2053–6.

Pardo V, Riesgo I, Zilleruelo G, et al. (1984). The clinical significance of mesangial IgM deposits and mesangial hypercellularity in minimal change nephrotic syndrome. *American Journal of Kidney Diseases* **3**:264–269.

Rana K, Wang YY, Buzza M, et al. (2005). The genetics of thin basement membrane nephropathy *Seminars in Nephrology* **25**:163–70.

Rosenstock JL, Markowitz GS, Valeri AM, et al. (2003). Fibrillary and immunotactoid glomerulonephritis: Distinct entities with different clinical and pathologic features. *Kidney International* **63**:1450–61.

Rostagno A, Vidal R, Kumar A, et al. (1996). Fibrillary glomerulonephritis related to serum fibrillary immunoglobulin-fibronectin complexes. *American Journal of Kidney Diseases* **28**:676–84.

Rovin BH, Roncone D, McKinley A, et al. (2007). APOE Kyoto mutations in European Americans with lipoprotein glomerulopathy. *New Engl J Med* **357**:2522–

Said R and Hamzeh Y (1990). IgM nephropathy associated with familial Mediterranean fever. Clin Nephrol **33**:227–31.

Saito T, Matsunaga A, Oikawa S (2006). Impact of lipoprotein glomerulopathy on the relationship between lipids and renal diseases. *American Journal of Kidney Diseases* **47**:199–211.

Sam R, Wu H, Yue L et al. (2006). Lipoprotein glomerulopathy: A new lipoprotein E mutation with enhanced glomerular binding. *American Journal of Kidney Diseases* **47**:539–48.

Samaniego M, Nadasdy GM, Laszik Z, et al. (2001). Outcome of renal transplantation in fibrillary glomerulonephritis. *Clinical Nephrology* **55**:159–66.

Sato M, Kojima H, Nabeshima K, et al. (1993). Primary glomerulonephritis with predominant mesangial immunoglobulin G deposits—a distinct entity? *Nephron* **64**:122–8.

Schwartz MM, Korbet SM, Lewis EJ (2002). Immunotactoid glomerulopathy *Journal American Society Nephrology* **13**:1390–7.

Scolari F, Scaini P, Savoldi S, et al. (1990). Familal IgM mesangial nephropathy: a morphological and immunogenetic study of three pedigrees. *American Journal of Nephrology* **10**:261–8.

Sharman A, Furness P, Feehally J (2004). Distinguishing C1q nephropathy from lupus nephritis. *Nephrology Dialysis Transplantation* **19**:1420–6.

Suzuki T, Okubo S, Ikezumi Y, et al. (2004). Favorable course of collagenofibrotic glomerulopathy after kidney transplantation and questionnaire survey about the prognosis of collagenofibrotic glomerulopathy. *Nippon Jinzo Gakkai Shi Japanese Journal Nephrology* **46**:360–4.

Tryggvason K, Patrakka J (2006). Thin basement nephropathy. *Journal of the American Society of Nephrology* **17**:813–22.

Vangelista A, Frascá G, Biagini G, et al. (1981). Long-term study of mesangial proliferative glomerulonephritis with IgM deposits. *Proceedings of the European Dialysis and Transplant Association* **18**:503–7.

Vogler C, McAdams AJ, Homan SM (1987). Glomerular basement membrane and lamina densa in infants and children: an ultrastructural evaluation. *Pediatric Pathology* 7:527–34.

Zeis PM, Kavazarakis E, Nakopoulou L, et al. (2001). Glomerulopathy with mesangial IgM deposits: long-term follow-up of 64 children. *Pediatric International* 43:287–92.

Zhang B, Liu ZH, Zeng CH, et al. (2008). Clinicopathological and genetic characteristics in Chinese patients with lipoprotein glomerulopathy. *Journal of Nephrology* 21:110–7.

Index